comprehensive family and community health nursing

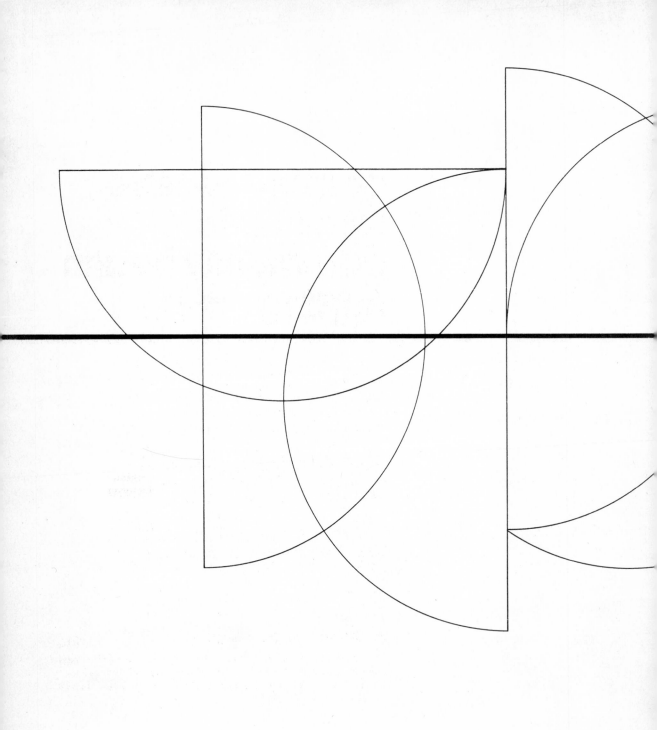

comprehensive family and community health nursing

Susan Ann Clemen, R.N., M.P.H.
Associate Professor and Clinical Director
Community Health Nursing Graduate Program
School of Nursing, University of Michigan

Diane Gerber Eigsti, R.N., M.S.
Assistant Professor, Community Health Nursing
School of Nursing, University of Rochester

Sandra L. McGuire, R.N., M.P.H.
Assistant Professor, Community Health Nursing
School of Nursing, University of Michigan

McGraw-Hill Book Company

New York   St. Louis   San Francisco   Auckland   Bogotá   Guatemala   Hamburg
Johannesburg   Lisbon   London   Madrid   Mexico   Montreal   New Delhi
Panama   Paris   San Juan   São Paulo   Singapore   Sydney   Tokyo   Toronto

NOTICE

Medicine is an ever-changing science. As new research and clinical experience broaden our knowledge, changes in treatment and drug therapy are required. The editors and the publisher of this work have made every effort to ensure that the drug dosage schedules herein are accurate and in accord with the standards accepted at the time of publication. Readers are advised, however, to check the product information sheet included in the package of each drug they plan to administer to be certain that changes have not been made in the recommended dose or in the contraindications for administration. This recommendation is of particular importance in regard to new or infrequently used drugs.

Library of Congress Cataloging in Publication Data

Clemen, Susan Ann.
    Comprehensive family and community health nursing.

    Bibliography: p.
    Includes index.
    1. Community health nursing. 2. Family— Health and hygiene.
3. Community health nursing—United States.
I. Eigsti, Diane Gerber, joint author. II. McGuire, Sandra L., joint author. III. Title.
RT98.C56   610.73′43   80-23913
ISBN 0-07-011324-6

Comprehensive Family and Community Health Nursing

1 2 3 4 5 6 7 8 9 0   DODO   8 9 8 7 6 5 4 3 2 1 0

This book was set in Baskerville by Waldman Graphics, Inc. The editors were David P. Carroll and Moira Lerner; the production supervisor was Jenet C. McIver. The designer was Elliot Epstein. The drawings were done by ECL Art Associates, Inc.
R. R. Donnelley & Sons Company was printer and binder.

Part 2 opening photo by Abigail Hyman, © Magnum Photos, Inc.
Part 3 opening photo © Hanna Schreiber, Rapho/Photo Researchers, Inc.

To Our Significant Others:

Verna Gearhart Clemen, a fifty-year nursing graduate, for encouraging and supporting independent thinking even when this was not the norm.

Al J. Clemen, who we wish was here to see this publication in print.

John and Sharon Clemen and Sara and Henry Parks, for their caring and interest.

Ike, Heiki-Lara, and Inge-Marie Eigsti, for their patience and loving.

Joseph, Matthew, and Kelly McGuire, for being there and being themselves.

Donald and Mary Lue Johnson, for their support and encouragement, which will never be forgotten.

Arthur and Sally Johnson, for the belief they instilled in the value of education and their faith in others.

All of our friends who "understood."

contents

Community health nursing is an exciting, challenging, and changing field which integrates all areas of nursing practice. The dimensions of community health nursing practice are expanding in many directions. Nurses in the community work daily with individuals, families, and populations at risk across the lifespan in a variety of health care settings. Community health nurses provide direct services to families, participate in health planning, and utilize the principles of management to manage health care resources effectively and to evaluate the quality of health care provided. They recognize the need for comprehensive, continuing health services and focus their attention on the population as a whole. The community is the client for the community health nurse, and the family is the basic unit of service.

The unique perspective that the community health nurse brings to any health care team is a holistic philosophy derived from a synthesis of nursing and public health knowledge. Preventive activities at all three levels—primary, secondary, and tertiary—are implemented by the community health nurse to enhance the state of wellness in a community. The community health nurse respects cultural differences and varying life-styles and analyzes sociocultural, political, economic, and environmental forces that influence consumer interests, needs, beliefs, and values. This text has addressed the unique role of the community health nurse by

· Analyzing the scope of community health nursing practice

· Integrating nursing and public health knowledge throughout the text

· Presenting the family-centered approach to nursing care, with emphasis on examining significant structural and process parameters of family functioning

· Utilizing a developmental model to address the health needs of populations across the life-span and to plan appropriate health services for populations at risk

· Discussing in depth the health and welfare

systems and how the community health nurse can facilitate client utilization of health and welfare resources

· Presenting specific federal legislation that provides funding for health care services and that affects the delivery of nursing services

· Including the principles of management and quality assurance utilized by community health nurses to manage and evaluate the multiple responsibilities assigned to them

· Integrating theoretical concepts and clinical data in case situations to illustrate the application of nursing and public health theory in the practice setting

· Presenting tools currently being used by practitioners which assist them in delivering quality nursing services to clients

· Including selected bibliographies which expand on the theoretical concepts presented in the text and which describe the multiple situations encountered by the community health nurse

The organization of this text stems from the philosophy of community health nursing practice delineated in the American Nurses' Association's definition of this specialty area. The three major parts of this book explore how community health nurses utilize concepts from nursing and public health to provide comprehensive, continuous, preventive health services for groups (families, populations at risk, and communities). Part 1 presents a philosophical framework for nursing practice in the community. It analyzes the origin and scope of current community health nursing practice and examines community dynamics and social, cultural, political, and economic factors that influence the delivery of health and welfare services. Part 2 focuses on the direct service functions of the staff community health nurse.

It discusses why the family is viewed as the unit of service in community health and outlines relevant theoretical concepts essential for understanding family dynamics. Special emphasis is placed on analyzing how the community health nurse utilizes the nursing process to implement and evaluate intervention strategies with families. Part 3 stresses the value of working with populations at risk in the community. Population groups, delineated by age, are examined in terms of developmental characteristics, health needs, health and welfare services, barriers to the utilization of health and welfare services, and the role of the community health nurse in meeting the needs of high-risk groups. The epidemiological process and the principles of health planning are presented as the tools for studying the determinants of health and disease frequencies in populations and for planning health promotion and disease control programs. Management concepts are included because they help community health nurses to integrate and handle their multiple professional commitments in a meaningful way.

The logo for the book, interconnecting systems and subsystems on a continuum, emphasizes a major focus in community health nursing practice—helping clients to fit together effectively community systems and subsystems in their environment—and is stressed throughout all six units. One will frequently find, when working in the community setting, that clients (individuals, families, populations at risk, and communities) have not reached their maximum potential because the environment they are functioning in does not enhance the growth process. Community health nurses can and frequently do alter this occurrence. They have unique skills which assist them to bring together in a meaningful way all the systems encountered by their clients.

ACKNOWLEDGMENTS

The authors are greatly indebted to family, friends, colleagues, students, former faculty advisors, and associates for their support, guidance, and assistance. Special appreciation is extended to the following:

Beverly Smith, our administrative secretary, whose painstaking efforts, patience, and dedication to our project made it a reality. This book could never have been published without her help.

Bill Smith, whose "it only takes a little more to do it right" encouragement provided the impetus to move forward. His gracious hospitality and willingness to share his wife's time will never be forgotten.

Mona Tremblay Kaser and Myrna Kay Schuiling, two community health nursing graduate students who constructively criticized our entire manuscript. Their theoretical knowledge of community health concepts and their clinical expertise helped us to provide a balance between the ideal and the reality.

Carol Loveland-Cherry, who assisted us in conceptualizing the organization of this text and who reviewed selected chapters for content accuracy.

Kathryn Robeson, colleague and friend, who constructively reviewed the organization of this text and selected chapters. Her ideas and thoughts guided our focus and stimulated an interest in the historical as well as the current aspects of community health nursing practice.

Lorraine Black, Joan Ceglarek, Dorothy Donabedian, Joan Goldstein, Dorothy Quigley, and Sandy Walls, colleagues from service and academia, who criticized selected chapters and provided a stimulus for learning.

Ann Welber, friend and colleague, whose encouragement and assistance facilitated an understanding of family dynamics and the completion of this text.

Colleagues from the University of Michigan School of Nursing for their encouragement and aid.

Leslie Davis and Ike Eigsti for helping us with our artwork and photography.

Former faculty at Goshen College, Michigan State University, St. Vincent's School of Nursing, Tulane University, and the University of Michigan, who encouraged critical thinking. Many of their ideas and thoughts are reflected in the philosophy of community health nursing practice promoted in this text.

Moira Lerner, editing supervisor, who patiently and supportively spent considerable time and effort in refining our manuscript.

David Carroll, Elliot Epstein, Dorothy Hoffman, Dave Horvath, Margaret Jack, Bob McGraw, Nancy Parisotti, Mary Ann Richter, and Gary Snyder, McGraw-Hill staff members, who were never too busy to listen and who facilitated the production process.

Publishers and authors who graciously granted us permission to use information from their writings.

Susan Ann Clemen
Diane Gerber Eigsti
Sandra L. McGuire

comprehensive family and community health nursing

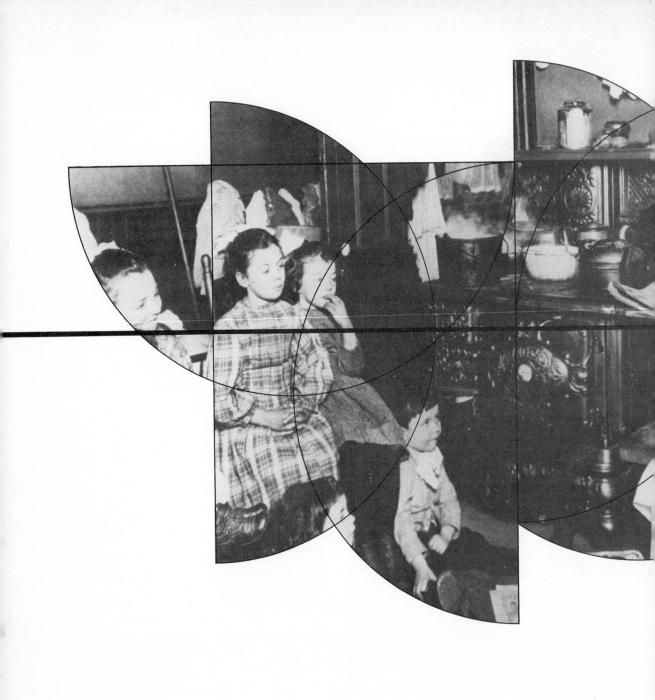

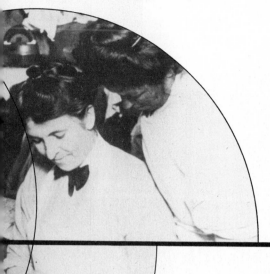

part one

a framework for community health nursing practice

Public health nurses have been leaders in improving the quality of health care for people since the late 1800s. They have been the vanguard of change for both the nursing profession and society as a whole. They stressed the importance of establishing standards for nursing practice, nursing education at the university level, and social reform to improve the quality of life for all individuals. They quickly recognized the need to deal with community dynamics and to influence legislative processes and the direction of our health and welfare systems at the local, state, and national level.

In order for community health nurses to continue the progress made by their early leaders, they must understand where and how they began, the nature of current community health nursing practice, and how community forces contribute to, or distract from, the health of families and populations at risk. Part 1 examines these aspects of community health nursing practice.

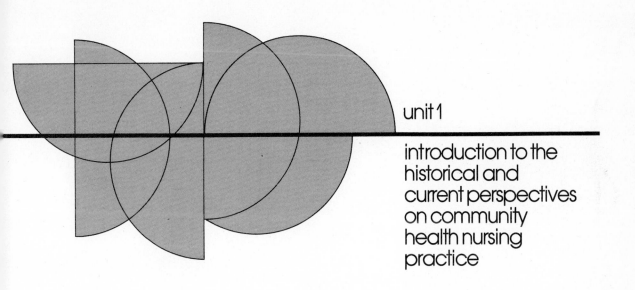

unit 1

introduction to the
historical and
current perspectives
on community
health nursing
practice

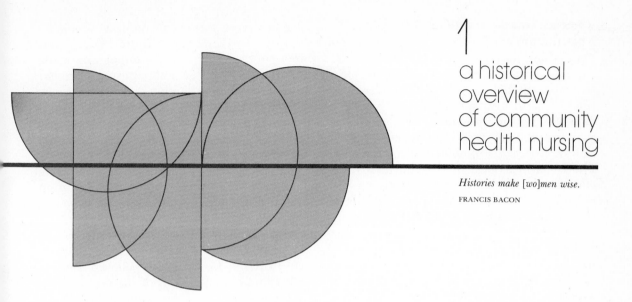

Histories make [wo]men wise.
FRANCIS BACON

Today's nurse should be proud of the founders of public health nursing! They are heroines who are role models for persons committed to nursing and to working for the improvement of health care services. Lavinia Lloyd Dock, one early public health nurse pioneer, was picketing, parading, and protesting 60 years ago. Dock, a feminist, scholar, and accomplished musician, devoted 20 years of her life to helping women gain the right to vote (Christy, 1969).

To understand the role the legendary Lavinia Dock and her peers played in establishing public health nursing, we must go farther back into the history of nursing. Looking at significant public health nursing pioneers and events helps us to understand how public health nursing was shaped and how areas of concern within public health nursing developed.

IN THE BEGINNING

Nursing began when humanity began.

The word nurse is a reduced form of the Middle English *nurice,* which was derived, through the old French *norrice,* from the Latin *nutricius* (nourishing). In Roman mythology, the Goddess Fortuna, in addition to her usual function as Goddess of Fate, was also worshipped as Jupiter's nurse (Fortuna Praeneste) and prayed to for hygiene in the public baths (Fortuna Balnearis). From the dawn of civilization, mankind has sought to acquire a knowledge of pain-relieving remedies and to discover ad-

ditional means of preventing disease. To alleviate human suffering, man has also developed nursing roles. (Kalisch and Kalisch, 1978, p. 1)

In 1916, Mary Sewall Gardner, another public health nurse pioneer, published the "first really comprehensive and authoritative presentation on the subject of public health nursing" (Nelson, 1954, p. 38). Gardner wrote that "the true ancestors of the modern nurse are the noble abbesses and early Christian women who were trying to do for their day what the nurse of today is trying to do for her's" (Gardner, 1919, p. 3).

Visiting nursing, or the care of ill people at home by a specialized group, has probably existed down through the ages. The New Testament is replete with stories of how the sick were visited. The Apostle Paul wrote of Phoebe in Rom. 16:1–2, "I commend to you our sister Phoebe, a deaconess of the church at Cenchreae, . . . help her in whatever she may require from you, for she has been a helper of many and of myself as well." Phoebe is probably the first visiting nurse we know by name.

The Middle Ages, with the subsequent rise of monasteries and convents, contributed to nursing a specialized effort to care for the ill. Specific convents had as their stated reason for existing the nursing care of sick people. To perform acts of mercy for the well-being of one's eternal soul was, during this time, a common and accepted reason for entering nursing convents. These early nurses included among their numbers males who were drawn into military nursing orders as a result of the Crusades (1091–1291). The Crusades were religious wars between the Turks and the Christians which encouraged both the spread of disease and the exchange of ideas between East and West. It has been well documented that nurses of high intellectual capacity responded to the needs of society in times of war and persecution (Dolan, 1978).

The Renaissance (about 1500 to 1700) brought about great political, social, and economic expansion. Two names of this period that are important to public health nursing are St. Vincent de Paul and Mademoiselle Le Gras. Gardner says of de Paul that "there is no more prominent figure in the history of nursing and social welfare" (Gardner, 1919, p. 9).

In 1617, de Paul organized the Sisterhood of the Dames de Charité. The ladies went from home to home, visiting the sick. As the movement spread and its numbers increased, dif-

ficulties arose because of the lack of supervision of work done by them. St. Vincent reorganized this group by appointing Mademoiselle Le Gras as a supervisor. Together, their greatest contribution to the development of public health nursing was the idea of providing education for those persons helping the poor and the sick, as well as recognizing the need for professional supervision of care givers. Taking care of ill people at home could not be accomplished simply with intuition; nursing practice must be based on principles somewhat akin to social work as we know it today. They felt that people could best be helped by "helping them to help themselves." De Paul and Le Gras also believed that one must find out the needs of the poor, investigate the causes, and then help supply possible solutions. Taken for granted by people today, these were entirely new concepts of charity for this time (Maynard, 1939).

The Era of Sairy Gamp

It is difficult to imagine how nursing could sink to the low levels it did during the time from the end of the seventeenth century to the middle of the nineteenth century. The change from nursing care given by devoted deaconesses to nursing care given by drunks and prostitutes is a change that is baffling. In *Martin Chuzzlewit* (1844), Charles Dickens immortalized the prototype of the nurse of this era by describing a drunk, untrained servant, Sairy Gamp, as a nurse. In order to understand what persons such as Florence Nightingale and her peers accomplished, the reader must know the nursing conditions that were in existence when they began their efforts to professionalize nursing.

The basis for the nursing care given by Phoebe and her contemporaries was charity. Thus the care was only as good as the church organization that supported it. During the time of the Reformation (the 1500s), nursing care degenerated to the greatest extent in countries where Catholic organizations were overthrown. In England, for instance, 100 hospitals were closed, and for a period of time there was no provision for the institutional care of ill people who were poor (Deloughery, 1977, p. 23). When nursing lost the importance once lent it by the church, it also lost its social standing. Thus, it was necessary to recruit nurses from distinctly lower classes, because "respectable" people would no longer do the work.

The status of women also greatly affected the change in the status of nursing. The church had given women an opportunity for a career in nursing. Love for others was the basis of the Gospel, and women were considered to be persons of worth. The Reformation and subsequent Protestant church movement changed this attitude. The general social position of women reached its lowest level in the eighteenth century.

The accompanying conditions in society during the 1600s were also dismal. The slums of European cities were huge and bred disease. Life expectancy was short and mortality rates were high. Before the Industrial Revolution (about 1750–1850) the social and economic structure of the Western world was quite simple: there were only a few large cities and work was largely agrarian. Social classes were rigidly stratified. During this time medicine was at a low level, largely because the scientific basis for it was unknown. Thus, health care was based on folklore and superstition.

Nursing existed in a low and dismal state indeed. It existed without organization and without social standing. No one who could possibly earn a living in some other way performed this service. Those who did so lost caste thereby, for as one is judged partly by the company one keeps, a woman who began to practice nursing was almost certain to become corrupted if she were not so already.[1]

[1]G. L. Deloughery. *History and trends of professional nursing* (8th ed.). St. Louis: Mosby, 1977, p. 24.

With this background, the contributions of Florence Nightingale to nursing, to public health, and to women are inestimable.

Florence Nightingale's Legacy

The family of this pioneer nurse leader was a wealthy one, and the environment into which she was born in 1820 became instrumental in her life's work. Nightingale was well educated by her father and, to her family's chagrin, longed to be a nurse. After a delay of many years, in deference to her family's wishes, she entered nurses' training with Pastor Fliedner, at Kaiserswerth on the Rhine, Germany. Her subsequent work in the Crimean War at Scutari has been chronicled by many, among them Longfellow, in his "Santa Filomena." It was there that she demonstrated that thousands of lives could be saved by intelligent nursing care and that capable nurses were needed in military hospitals. This was accomplished in the face of overwhelming obstacles. The hospital at Scutari was built for 1700 patients. When Nightingale arrived, there were 3000 to 4000 wounded men in it, lying naked with no beds, no blankets, and no eating or laundry facilities. Within days of her appearance at Scutari, she had a food kitchen operating as well as a laundry.

When Florence Nightingale began her career, it was a very dreadful thing to be a nurse. By helping establish the first modernly planned training school for nurses at St. Thomas Hospital in 1850, Nightingale set the example for Bellevue Hospital in New York City to follow in 1873. She also began the movement which led to the University Schools of Nursing at Western Reserve and Yale (Winslow, 1946, p. 331). Nightingale was the originator of the concept of the nursing process. She insisted that educated nurses were essential to perform the nurse's role. In this role she included assessment and intervention, followed by evaluation. In her famous *Notes on Nursing,* she defined nursing as that care that puts a person in the best possible condition for nature to either restore or preserve health, to prevent or cure disease or injury (Nightingale, 1859). Furthermore, from the very beginning of her career, she visualized the nurse as not merely an attendant for the sick but also a teacher of hygiene. She described the nurse as a "health missioner," a guide and teacher of health to the individual in the home. She recognized that "from the very nature of the case, compulsion can under no conditions work the changes we want to see wrought by the obedience of consent" (Winslow, p. 331). This was a very early affirmation of the principle that individuals are responsible for their own health.

THE ESTABLISHMENT OF VISITING NURSING

Visiting nursing, or district nursing, was the forerunner of public health nursing. The modern concept of a nurse who provides care to families in the home was visualized and established in 1859 by William Rathbone of Liverpool, England. "It is to Mr. Rathbone that we owe the first definitely formulated district nursing association and in that sense he may be called the father of the present movement" (Gardner, 1919, p. 14). Rathbone was a wealthy businessman and philanthropist. His wife died after a long illness, and he had been impressed and comforted by the skilled nursing care that was given her in the months before she died. Rathbone had long been interested in helping the many poor people of Liverpool. If nursing care could help his wife who had everything that money could buy, how much more might it do for poor people whose physical illnesses were made increasingly burdensome by their poverty. To test his idea, he employed Mrs. Mary Robinson, the nurse who had cared for his wife, to visit the "sick poor" in their homes. She was to give care, instruct both the patient and the family in the care of the sick, and teach hygienic practices to prevent illnesses. The experiment was so successful that Rathbone decided to establish a permanent system of district or visiting nursing in Liverpool (McNeil, 1967, p. 1).

Rathbone's first problem was that there were no nurses in Liverpool to do this difficult work. So, with the help and advice of Florence Nightingale, he founded a school in 1859 for the training of visiting nurses on the grounds of the Liverpool Infirmary. Within 4 years, 18 nurses were working in this same city, demonstrating dramatically the organization and success of the venture. Even at this early date, these visiting nurses were visualized not only as people who cared for the sick but also as social reformers.

Visiting Nurses in the United States

As is already evident from this historical overview, trends within nursing are directly influenced by trends in society. The development of visiting nursing in the United States was no exception.

By the late 1800s, organized nursing care in hospitals had been demonstrated to be effective. Germ theory was used as the basis for communicable disease control. Poverty was beginning to be seen as the result and cause of multiple social problems.

Florence Nightingale's work and the establishment of her school of nursing in England were well known. Her concept that better nursing care could be given if nurses were educated for the position became more clearly understood.

The growth of our nation's cities as well as the waves of immigrants to America, the "land of opportunity," were two underlying reasons for the development of visiting nursing. Although every city had its rich people, the poor greatly outnumbered them (Kalisch and Kalisch, 1978, p. 225).

New York had the largest settlement of immigrants and thus faced the most problems concerning them. Dismal tenement houses were built for this huge influx of people, and living conditions were horrible. Very young children were expected to work 12 to 14 hours a day in dark, airless factories.

Visiting nursing in the United States, just as in England, was begun by groups of people who were greatly distressed by the conditions in which many poor people lived. Then, as now, the most serious public health problems were in slum areas, and visiting nurse agencies were often located in buildings in low-income areas. Nurses from these organizations provided care to the sick in their homes and gave instruction to families as well. Buffalo, Boston, and Philadelphia developed such services during 1885 and 1886, about 25 years after Rathbone's experiment. The Philadelphia Visiting Nurse Society cared for the sick as well as for the poor and, at a very early date, established a fee for services given.

Visiting nursing in this country did not follow the English system established by Rathbone (Gardner, 1919, p. 29). In England, Queen Victoria's Jubilee Institute for Nurses was founded in 1889, and it set standards for the preparation of visiting nurses as well as for the care given by them. In 1890 in the United States, there were 21 separate organizations engaged in visiting nursing. These organizations had no connection with each other and also had no common standards of educational preparation for the care givers. Each city and town established its own visiting nurse service so that there was great diversity in the quality of organization and care given.

In 1896, the Nurses' Associated Alumni (now the American Nurses' Association) was formed and helped to organize the nurses of the country into a professional group. This was the beginning of "group consciousness" among the visiting nurses of the United States.

Enter Lillian Wald

The person who coined the expression *public health nursing* was Lillian Wald. Nightingale had originated the idea of "health nursing"; it was Wald who placed the word *public* in front of it so that all people would know that this type of service was available to them (Haupt, 1953, p. 81). Wald was the "predecessor of the modern public health nurse in the United States" (Christy, 1970, p. 50). *The House on Henry Street* is her story of the work she did as director of the Henry Street Settlement House. Her accomplishments are legendary. She originated the idea and then helped to establish the U.S. Children's Bureau, as well as school and rural nursing in the Red Cross Town and Country Nursing Service. Wald was also instrumental in securing changes in child labor laws, better housing conditions in tenement districts, city recreation centers, more and better parks, pure food laws, graded classes for mentally handicapped children, and humanistic provisions for immigrants to the United States. What a role model for public health nurses today! And how appropriate the title, "predecessor of modern public health nursing"!

Lillian Wald was born in 1867 and spent her growing years in Rochester, New York. Though her family was not wealthy, her father, an optical goods dealer, provided a comfortable living for them. She studied at a private school and was an excellent student. Wald chanced to meet a graduate of the Bellevue Hospital Training School for Nurses who had assisted her sister during pregnancy. In this manner, Wald became interested in nursing and entered training at New York Hospital in 1891, where she spent 2 years.

After graduating, she supplemented her nursing instruction with a period of study at a medical college. During this time of study, she was asked to give classes in home nursing and bedside care to a group of women in the Lower East Side tenement district. This was a turning point of Wald's career:

From the schoolroom where I had been giving a lesson in bed-making, a little girl led me one driz-zling March morning. She had told me of her sick mother, and gathering from her incoherent ac-count that a child had been born, I caught up the paraphernalia of the bed-making lesson and carried it with me.

The child led me over broken roadways,—there was no asphalt, although its use was well established in other parts of the city,—over dirty mattresses and heaps of refuse,—it was before Colonel Waring had shown the possibility of clean streets even in that quarter,—between tall, reeking houses whose laden fire escapes, useless for their appointed purpose, bulged with household goods of every description. The rain added to the dismal appearance of the streets and to the discomfort of the crowds which thronged them, intensifying the odors which as-sailed me from every side. Through Hester and Division Streets we went to the end of Ludlow; past odorus fish-stands, for the streets were a market-place, unregulated, unsupervised, unclean; past evil-smelling, uncovered garbage-cans; and—per-haps worst of all, where so many little children played—past the trucks brought down from more fastidious quarters and stalled on these already over-crowded streets, lending themselves inevitably to many forms of indecency.

The child led me on through a tenement hallway, across a court where open and unscreened closets were promiscuously used by men and women, up into a rear tenement, by slimy steps whose accu-mulated dirt was augmented that day by the mud of the streets, and finally into the sickroom.

All of the maladjustments of our social and eco-nomic relations seemed epitomized in this brief journey and what was found at the end of it. The family to which the child led me was neither crim-inal nor vicious. Although the husband was a crip-ple, one of those who stand on street corners ex-hibiting deformities to enlist compassion, and masking the begging of alms by a pretense at sell-

ing; although the family of seven shared their two rooms with boarders,—who were literally boarders, since a piece of timber was placed over the floor for them to sleep on,—and although the sick woman lay on a wretched, unclean bed, soiled with a hem-orrhage two days old, they were not degraded hu-man beings, judged by any measure of moral val-ues.

In fact, it was very plain that they were sensitive to their condition, and when, at the end of my min-istrations, they kissed my hands (those who have undergone similar experiences will, I am sure, un-derstand), it would have been some solace if by any conviction of the moral unworthiness of the family I could have defended myself as a part of a society which permitted such conditions to exist. Indeed, my subsequent acquaintance with them revealed the fact that, miserable as their state was, they were not without ideals for the family life, and for society, of which they were so unloved and unlovely a part.

That morning's experience was a baptism of fire. Deserted were the laboratory and the academic work of the college—I never returned to them. On my way from the sickroom to my comfortable stu-dent quarters my mind was intent on my own re-sponsibility. To my inexperience, it seemed certain that conditions such as these were allowed because people did not know, and for me there was a chal-lenge to know and to tell. When early morning found me still awake, my naive conviction remained that, if people knew things,—and "things" meant everything implied in the condition of this family,— such horrors would cease to exist, and I rejoiced that I had had a training in the care of the sick that in itself would give me an organic relationship to the neighborhood in which this awakening had come. (Wald, 1915, pp. 4–8)

This experience was the cause for the cre-ation of the Henry Street Settlement House in 1893. Along with Mary Brewster, another New York Hospital graduate, Wald elicited funds from wealthy people and founded a place where care was offered to needy people.

Wald's settlement house changed the focus of nursing service: the only other visiting nurses during this period were those associ-ated with sectarian organizations or free dispensaries. Wald felt that a nurse could be most effective if she were independent of any religious agency and not associated exclusively with one doctor. She insisted that nurses should be available to anyone who needed them, without the intervention of a doctor, establishing early in the history of nursing that the profession should be an independent one. She also believed that nurses should live in the neighborhood where they practiced so that they could identify with the needs of the family served, as Wald herself did.

School Nursing Develops

The nursing care of children in public schools began with an idea by Lillian Wald. In 1902 health conditions of school children in New York City were appalling. Thousands of students were sent home from school with diseases such as trachoma (an infectious eye disease), pediculosis, ringworm, scabies, and impetigo. They then played outside with the children from whom they had previously been excluded in the classroom (Wald, 1915, p. 51). Wald offered to show school officials in New York that with the assistance of a well-prepared nurse fewer children would lose valuable school time. It would also be possible to bring under treatment those who needed it. The experiment was to be paid for with public funds. One month's trial with Lina Rogers, a nurse from Henry Street, proved to be immensely successful. Thirty thousand dollars was approved by the Board of Estimate and Apportionment for the employment of trained nurses, the first municipalized school nurses in the world (Wald, p. 53).

Maternal-Infant Care Becomes a Concern

An appreciation of the needs of children, demonstrated in part by the rise of settlement houses like Henry Street, was a part of the social consciousness of the early 1900s. There

were spasmodic efforts to help children to better health, and in 1909 these were united into action at a Conference on Infant Mortality called by the American Academy of Medicine. Finally in 1912, the Children's Bureau was created by Congress to draw the attention of the highest levels of government to the needs of children. Though many nurses and lay associations contributed to its formation, Lillian Wald's activities, initiative, and remarkable skill in securing support for new ideas was fundamental to the establishment of the Children's Bureau (Stewart and Austin, 1938, p. 197).

The passage of the Shepherd-Towner Act of 1921 was a historic milestone in the evolution of public health and public health nursing. Studies by the Children's Bureau at the federal level showed that the United States had a higher maternal death rate than most other developed countries. This act, administered by the Children's Bureau, gave grants to states to develop programs that provided care to that population group.

Marie Phelan was appointed in 1923 as the first nurse consultant to the federal government in peacetime. At the request of state health departments, she helped to develop programs that promoted the health of mothers and children. Her work had the effect of creating a demand for nurses to work with established county or official agencies to begin demonstration programs with mothers and infants (Figure 1-1). The results of these nurses' work is difficult to measure, but the maternal death rate was reduced from 7.1 per 1000 live births in 1915 to 6.7 for the years between 1925 and 1929. In a final report on the program, the chief of the Children's Bureau noted that "a nurse working alone had frequently afforded a starting point for the development of full-time health departments" (Roberts, 1954, p. 196). As a result of strong political conservatism, the Shepherd-Towner Act was permitted to lapse in 1929 and was not renewed.

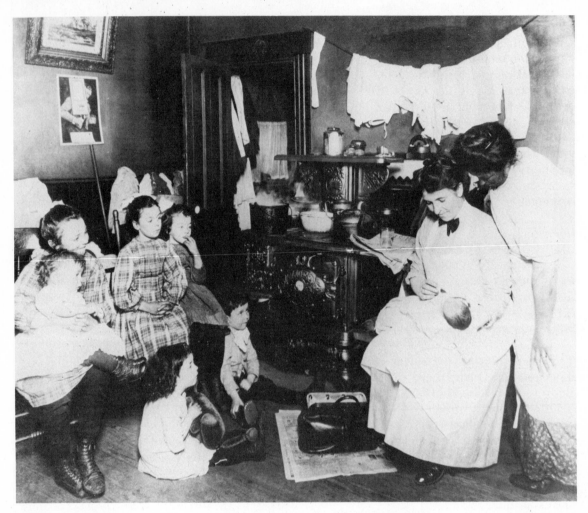

FIGURE 1-1 Involving the family in baby care, Boston, 1912. (*The Metropolitan Life Insurance Company of New York. Used with their permission.*)

Today the original Shepherd-Towner Act has been amended and broadened to include under its auspices a network of maternity and infant care programs, as well as children and youth programs, throughout the United States. Nurse-midwives, pediatric nurse practitioners, and family planning nurse practitioners are responsible for providing primary health care in many of these programs.

Metropolitan Employs PHN

In 1909 the first public health nursing program for policyholders of an insurance company was initiated (Haupt, 1953, p. 8). Lillian Wald and Lee Frankel, founder of the Metropolitan Life Insurance Company Welfare Division, convinced the board of directors at Metropolitan that healthier workers live longer and thus profit the company by purchasing insurance longer. Wald felt that nurses supplied by agencies such as Henry Street could provide skilled service needed to produce healthy workers. Increased efficiency on the workers' part could favorably influence the output of industry, which, in turn, would pay for the health services in cash and better morale.

The two principles underlying this concept were that the company should utilize existing public health nursing services rather than employing their own nurses and that services should be available to anyone, with fees based on the ability to pay. Both of these ideas are utilized today in health agencies.

The Metropolitan project was terminated in 1953 after 44 successful years. The shifting of the voluntary responsibility for health care to professional community organizations was the basis for the change.

There were numerous contributions to public health nursing as a result of this project (Haupt, 1953). Among them, the following:

1. The extension of bedside nursing care on a fee-for-service basis.
2. The establishment of a cost-accounting system for visiting nurses, which is used to this day.
3. The recruitment of nurses, aides, and home nursing programs under the Red Cross by the use of advertisements in paper and radio. This was a new concept of recruitment.
4. The reduction of mortality rates from infectious diseases. Mortality rates were reduced by half in the 44 years of the program among the Metropolitan Life Insurance policyholders.

5. The demonstration of how nursing and a business organization can work together, despite each having an interest in the promotion of its *own* goals.

Public Health Nursing in Rural Areas

While public health nursing in cities and towns was developing at a rapid rate, work in rural areas was progressing slowly. In 1912, the same year the Children's Bureau was formed, Lillian Wald asked her wealthy friend, Jacob Shiff, to donate money to the Red Cross so that a system of rural nursing could be developed (Gardner, 1919, p. 37).

Wald had been a Red Cross member in 1904 and 1905. She expressed strong dissatisfaction at seeing so potent an organization as the Red Cross limited to the uncertainty and irregularity of service in war or calamity; she felt it simply wasteful to have a national organization inactive. Wald believed that the Red Cross was a logical facility to employ in promoting public health nursing in rural areas and scattered towns on a regular national scale (Dock, Pickett, Noyes, Clement, Fox, and Meter, 1922, p. 1212).

And so it happened that the Red Cross began a new department, the Town and Country Nursing Service, which was later to be named the Bureau of Public Health Nursing. The purpose of the department was to supply rural areas and small towns with trained public health nurses and to supervise their work. The Red Cross, however, did not assume the local financial responsibility for this work. Voluntary and charitable organizations as well as fees for service financed nursing care given.

PUBLIC HEALTH NURSING BECOMES A GOVERNMENT CONCERN

Public health nursing grew out of the need recognized by groups of citizens to help poor people who suffered not only physically but in

all other areas of life as well. Thus, public health nurses were financed by voluntary agencies, depending upon contributions and

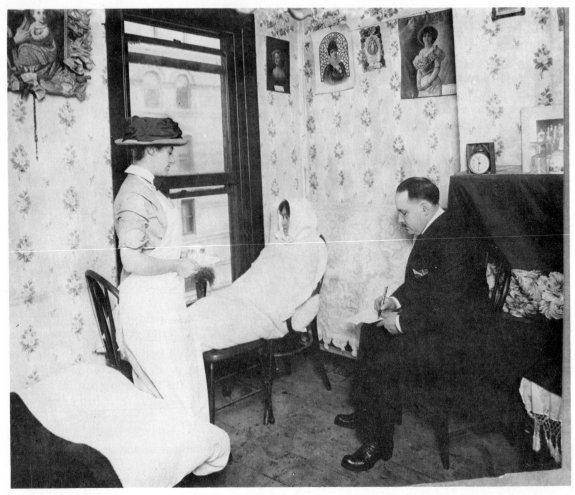

FIGURE 1-2 Convalescing from typhoid fever, New York City, 1912. (*The Metropolitan Life Insurance Company of New York. Used with their permission.*)

small service charges for financial support. The state of our nation's health forced a change.

In the nineteenth century, threats to the public's health and welfare were increasing due to diseases such as smallpox, yellow fever, cholera, typhoid, tuberculosis, and malaria (Figure 1-2). In Massachusetts in 1850, for example, the tuberculosis death rate was 300 per 100,000 population. The infant mortality rate was 200 per 1000 live births, and smallpox, scarlet fever, and typhoid were the leading causes of death (Hanlon, 1974, p. 21).

In response to these problems, some larger cities such as Philadelphia and New York established city health departments. In 1855 Louisiana set up what is called by some historians the first state health department. Its function was to deal with repeated outbreaks of yellow fever and other epidemic diseases.

In terms of the more usual concept of the general functions of a state health department, Massachusetts is usually credited with the first state health department, founded in 1869 (Hanlon, 1974, p. 23).

An early public health pioneer of this period was Lemuel Shattuck. In 1842, he helped to achieve passage of a law in Massachusetts which resulted in the statewide registration of health-related statistics. In the next few years, Shattuck compiled shocking statistics about unbelievably high infant and maternal mortality rates. The Shattuck Report, one of the first public health documents in the United States, was published in 1850. It recommended the establishment of state and local health departments as well as pointing out the need for sanitary surveys. It unfortunately lay unnoticed for 25 years, although much of it is relevant for today (Hanlon, 1974, pp. 22–23).

Thus the concept of the public's health developed near the turn of the century. Personal health services played an increasingly important role in community health programs. A new era was reached when, in Los Angeles in 1889, a nurse was employed by the city's health department to provide home nursing care to the sick poor (Rosen, 1958, p. 380). At this point, public health nursing began to be officially recognized and tax-supported. However, it was not until 1913 that the Los Angeles Health Department established a bureau of nursing.

In 1902 Lillian Wald had loaned a nurse to the New York City Health Department to ascertain whether or not pupil absence from the schools could be reduced with nursing care. The reader may recall that this experiment was extremely successful and that a group of nurses was then employed to work in the schools. This was the first use of trained nurses in any large number in health departments. In 1903, this same health department appointed three nurses (annual salary $900) to visit tuberculosis patients at home. The nurses were to teach the patients about sputum disposal and other aspects of care. In 1905 the number of nurses serving tuberculosis patients was increased to 14. Alabama, in 1907, was the first state to legally approve the employment of public health nurses by local boards of health (Rosen, 1958, p. 380).

By 1912 public health nurses were supported by both private and public funds. The need for the skills and knowledge of this kind of professional was generally well recognized. They could be found in many kinds of agencies as well as in both rural and urban settings. Table 1-1, compiled by public health nurse pioneer Mary Gardner, illustrates this distribution well.

ORGANIZING PUBLIC HEALTH NURSES

Leaders among public health nurses, including Lillian Wald, Mary Beard, Ellen Phillips Crandall, Jane Delano, and Mary Gardner, soon realized the need to develop professional standards for this expanding professional group. Although most agencies employing nurses were attempting to do conscientious work, there were no overall professional and ethical guidelines. These same leaders felt clearly that only a new organization "whose sole object should be public health nursing would adequately meet the need" (Gardner, 1919, p. 41).

June 7, 1912, was a momentous day in the history of American public health nursing: at the annual meeting of the American Nurses' Association and the Society of Superintendents of Training Schools, the National Organization for Public Health Nursing (now the National League for Nursing) was voted into

TABLE 1-1   Distribution of Public Health Nurses in 1912

Visiting nurse associations	205
City and state boards of health and education	156
Private clubs and societies	108
Tuberculosis leagues	107
Hospitals and dispensaries	87
Business concerns	38
Settlements and day nurses	35
Churches	28
Charity organizations	27
Other organizations	19

SOURCE: From Mary S. Gardner. *Public health nursing* (3d ed.). New York: Macmillan, 1936, p. 40.

NOTE: This list, used by the author in 1912, as secretary of a joint committee of the American Nurses' Association and the Society of Superintendents of Training Schools, to circulate names of the agencies then known to be engaged in public health nursing, probably gives a reasonably true picture of the general distribution of nursing work among the different type of agencies. There were 78 letters sent to nurses working in that number of counties in Pennsylvania and 204 to nurses independently employed by the Metropolitan Life Insurance Company.

existence with Lillian Wald as president. The two purposes of the National Organization for Public Health Nursing (NOPHN) were the stimulation and standardization of public health nursing and the furthering of relationships among all people interested in the public's health. It was the first national nursing organization to have a headquarters and paid staff. For a long period in the development of nursing, it grew in power, set standards for practice, and influenced education by requiring certain curriculum content as a basis for employment (Fagin, 1978, p. 752). One of the unique features of the NOPHN was that membership was open to public health nursing agencies and other interested people, as well as to nurses. Collaborative relationships among health and social agencies has always been a strength among those who work in public health nursing.

Public Health Nursing Magazine

On the very day that the NOPHN was formed, the Cleveland Visiting Nurses Association presented its magazine, *The Quarterly,* to the group as a gift. *The Quarterly* later became *Public Health Nursing* and, still later, *Nursing Outlook.* It was an essential element to the development and dissemination of the public health nursing movement in the United States.

Education for Public Health Nurses

The education of public health nurses presented special problems because, traditionally, all nurses were prepared in apprentice-type programs in hospitals. Their curriculum was determined by the needs of the hospital and was controlled by physicians whose primary responsibility was service to patients rather than the education of nurses. The education was illness- and individual-oriented and did not adequately prepare (or even claim to prepare) a person to work in the community setting, where the care delivered differed from hospital care. In the community setting, nurses had a greater degree of independence; they did health teaching, carried out case finding, and made referrals; and their responsibility was to population groups.

The first course in public health nursing was offered by the Boston Instructive Nursing Association in 1906 (McNeil, 1967, p. 4). However, considering the broad scope of a public health nurse's work, it soon became apparent that education for this group was a function of the university. Because of the nurse's concern with social and educational problems, most of the early university public health nursing programs were in teacher's colleges or university departments of sociology or social work. By 1921, courses in public health nursing, which met standards developed by the NOPHN were offered by 15 colleges and universities. These courses taught "preventive medicine," covering topics such as how to examine a class of children, how to find those who were developing measles, and how to visit in a home and evaluate tuberculosis contacts (Jensen, 1959, p. 236).

The Goldmark Report

In 1919, under the auspices of the Rockefeller Foundation and at the urging of concerned nursing leaders, the Committee for the Study of Public Health Nursing Education, with C.-E. A. Winslow as chairman, began a 2-year investigation. Josephine Goldmark was secretary of the committee and the study was later to bear her name.

The purpose of the committee was to look at typical examples of public health nursing education and service and to study the education of these workers afforded by hospital training schools, graduate courses for public health nurses, and special schools of a non-nursing type (Committee for the Study of Nursing Education, 1923, p. 2). The study was expanded the following year to look at the entire field of nursing education.

Ten conclusions were reached that have profoundly affected the course of public health nursing, as well as of all nursing (Committee for the Study of Nursing Education, 1923):

Conclusion 1. That, since constructive health work and health teaching in families is best done by persons:

(a) capable of giving general health instruction, as distinguished from instruction in any one specialty; and

(b) capable of rendering bedside care at need; the agent responsible for such constructive health work and health teaching in families should have completed the nurses' training. There will, of course, be need for the employment, in addition to the public health nurse, of other types of experts such as nutrition workers, social workers, occupational therapists, and the like.

That as soon as may be practicable all agencies, public or private, employing public health nurses, should require as a prerequisite for employment the basic hospital training, followed by a postgraduate course, including both class work and field work, in public health nursing.

Conclusion 2. That the career open to young women of high capacity, in public health nursing or in hospital supervision and nursing education, is one of the most attractive fields now open, in its promise of professional success and of rewarding public service; and that every effort should be made to attract such women into this field.

Conclusion 3. That for the care of persons suffering from serious and acute disease, the safety of the patient, and the responsibility of the medical and nursing professions, demand the maintenance of the standards of educational attainment now generally accepted by the best sentiment of both professions and embodied in the legislation of the more progressive states; and that any attempt to lower these standards would be fraught with real danger to the public.

Conclusion 4. That steps should be taken through state legislation for the definition and licensure of a subsidiary grade of nursing service, the subsidiary type of worker to serve under practicing physicians in the care of mild and chronic illness, and convalescence, and possibly to assist under the direction of the trained nurse in certain phases of hospital and visiting nursing.

Conclusion 5. That, while training schools for nurses have made remarkable progress, and while the best schools of today in many respects reach a high level of educational attainment, the average hospital training school is not organized on such a basis as to conform to the standards accepted in other educational fields; that the instruction in such schools is frequently casual and uncorrelated; that the educational needs and the health and strength of students are frequently sacrificed to practical hospital exigencies; that such shortcomings are primarily due to the lack of independent endowments for nursing education; that existing educational facilities are on the whole, in the majority of schools, inadequate for the preparation of the high-grade of nurses required for the care of serious illness, and for service in the fields of public health nursing and nursing education; and that one of the chief reasons for the lack of sufficient recruits, of a high type, to meet such needs lies precisely in the fact that the average hospital training school does not offer a sufficiently attractive avenue of entrance to this field.

Conclusion 6. That, with the necessary financial support and under a separate board or training school committee, organized primarily for educational purposes, it is possible, with completion of a high school course or its equivalent as a prerequisite, to reduce the fundamental period of hospital training to 28 months, and at the same time, by eliminating unessential, non-educational routine, and adopting the principles laid down in Miss Goldmark's report, to organize the course along intensive and coordinated lines with such modifications as may be necessary for practical application; and that courses of this standard would be reasonably certain to attract students of high quality in increasing numbers.

Conclusion 7. Superintendents, supervisors, instructors, and public health nurses should in all cases receive special additional training beyond the basic nursing course.

Conclusion 8. That the development and strengthening of University Schools of Nursing of a high grade for the training of leaders is of fundamental importance in the furtherance of nursing education.

Conclusion 9. That when the licensure of a subsidiary grade of nursing service is provided for, the establishment of training courses in preparation for such service is highly desirable; that such courses should be conducted in special hospitals, in small unaffiliated general hospitals, or in separate sections of hospitals where nurses are also trained; and that the course should be of 8 or 9 months' duration; provided the standards of such schools be approved by the same educational board which governs nursing training schools.

Conclusion 10. That the development of nursing service adequate for the care of the sick and for the conduct of the modern public health campaign demands as an absolute prerequisite the securing of funds for the endowment of nursing education of all types; and that it is of primary importance, in this connection, to provide reasonably generous endowment for university schools of nursing.

The significance of this very early study is, even today, not fully understood and implemented. However, some positive changes were slowly made: poor schools were closed, qualified faculty members were hired, and the money allotted to education programs was increased.

Changes in Nursing Education

Until World War II it was believed that nurses could be prepared for public health only after they graduated from a hospital (diploma) school of nursing. It became evident, however, that graduates of collegiate schools of nursing did not need the same additional content in public health nursing as did graduates of diploma schools, because the broader background of a liberal arts education helped prepare one for this area of nursing. Content in public health became increasingly evident in collegiate schools of nursing. Finally, in 1944 the first basic collegiate program in nursing was accredited as including adequate preparation for public health nursing, so that graduates did not need additional study to practice public health nursing after graduation from the basic nursing program (National Organization for Public Health Nursing, 1944, p. 371).

During the next 30 years there were drastic changes in nursing education. Like most major changes, they were met with resistance from many sources and caused severe distress for some individuals. These changes included the following:

1. One-year practical nursing programs were established and the numbers of schools and graduates increased rapidly. More than half of these programs were offered under vocational education.

2. Two-year programs in nursing were established (1952), most of them in junior colleges. These graduates were qualified to take the examination to become registered nurses.

3. After 1963 no specialized baccalaureate program was accredited unless it prepared its graduates for public health nursing. Emphasis on comprehensive nursing care in both public health and hospital nursing revealed that all baccalaureate graduates should be prepared for staff-level positions in both hospitals and public health nursing agencies. Only three graduate schools of public health had undergraduate programs in public health nursing, and these were discontinued when the content was included in baccalaureate nursing curriculums.

4. Universities assumed more responsibility for clinical field instruction, which enriched both field and classroom teaching.

5. Members of the American Nurses' Association, in 1965, approved a position paper on the educational preparation for nurse practitioners, which stated that education for all those licensed to practice nursing should take place in institutions of higher education.

6. In 1978, the American Nurses' Association, after years of debate, resolved again that the baccalaureate degree should be the minimum preparation for entry into professional nursing practice.

The Effects of World War I on Public Health Nursing

By 1915 the role of the public health nurse was well established and the pioneer stage of this specialized area was drawing to a close. However, with the advent of World War I in 1917 and the involvement of thousands of nurses in military service, public health nurs-

ing services were threatened. The American Red Cross (which had been founded in 1882 by Clara Barton to supply nurses for war service) along with a committee chaired by Adelaide Nutting, the "far-seeing dean of American nurses," investigated methods to deal with the situation (Roberts, 1954, p. 131).

The efficient use of the limited supply of public health nurses was ensured by the Red Cross, which set up a roster of nurses who could be called upon to coordinate and supplement health resources. Emphasis was placed upon educational programs for the community as well as the control of communicable diseases.

During World War I, a nurse was loaned to the U.S. Public Health Service from the National Organization of Public Health Nursing, to develop a public health nursing program for the military outposts. This was the first public health nursing service to be established within the federal government (Gardner, 1919, p. 44).

The committee was convinced that the standards for preparing nurses must be maintained and that quick "short courses" to prepare nurses would have a disastrous effect on war and postwar health programs. To alleviate the nursing shortage and to ensure standards of care, they encouraged the development of a quality shortened program.

The Vassar Training Camp for Nurses

A unique experience in the annals of nursing education was the Vassar Camp School of Nursing. Begun in 1918 and supported by the American Red Cross and the Council of National Defense, the program was based on the principle that the 3-year nursing course could be shortened to 2 years for students who had graduated from college majoring in other subjects. It was modeled on the Plattsburg Military Camp at Plattsburg, New York, where college men were given intensive training to become

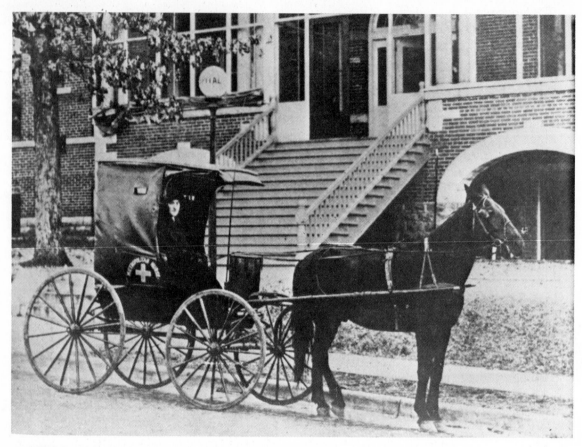

FIGURE 1-3 Public health nurse utilizing horse and buggy before the advent of the automobile. (*The Metropolitan Life Insurance Company of New York. Used with their permission.*)

army reserve officers. The purpose was to more rapidly fill the desperate need for women in nursing in wartime. Applicants to the program chose a college and were admitted into selected nursing schools across the country. Graduates of this program numbered 435; the program ended with the armistice.

This patriotic opportunity attracted both high-level faculty and students. The program produced distinguished nursing leaders of the next several decades, including people such as Katherine Densford Dreves, who became dean of the University of Minnesota School of Nursing, president of the American Nurses' Association, and second vice-president of the International Council of Nurses.

After World War I

Rapid changes came with peace. Economic prosperity, reaction to prohibition, and the increasing use of the automobile created radical changes in the way people lived. These changes brought subsequent changes in public health nursing. The use of the automobile, for instance, permitted nurses to have easy access to rural areas and made once-closed areas accessible (Figures 1-3 and 1-4).

The poor physical condition of the nation's males, made evident in wartime, shocked the nation. About 29 percent of those called for service were unfit for military duty because of problems that in many cases were preventable (Roberts, 1954, p. 164). Health programs of both official and nonofficial agencies grew as a result.

Smillie says that "beginning in 1925 and extending through the present time (1952) is the extraordinary phenomenon of the nationalization of the public health. The public health was, for generations, a community affair administered under local self-government with some slight degree of state government supervision. Public health has now become a subject of nation-wide interest and importance" (Smillie, 1952, p. 10).

By 1920 there were 28 states that had a statewide public health nursing program. However, only 5 had divisions of public health nursing within state health departments (Roberts, 1954, p. 168).

Two voluntary (non-tax-supported) agencies were very active during this time: the National Tuberculosis Association and the American Red Cross. The Red Cross supplemented but did not supplant the work of legitimate health agencies. Its goal was that public health nursing would be conducted as a public service by municipalities, counties, or states. In some states the public health nursing supervisors in state health departments also functioned as Red Cross supervisors. In 1921, state tuberculosis associations had supervising nurses in 28 states, the Red Cross in 31. In 29 states, the state board of health had a director of public health nursing or a division of child hygiene (Fox, 1920, p. 180).

The Effects of World War II on Public Health Nursing

The Depression of 1929, which preceded World War II, forced many hospitals and schools of nursing to close. The supply of nurses far exceeded the demand. In the health field as a whole, the financial crisis resulted in the wider use of national, state, and local tax funds for health and welfare services. An important aspect of this program on the national level was the passage of the Social Security Act in 1935, which introduced governmental involvement in health care on a large scale. This meant that the federal government was taking on a new role in assuming responsibility for the health of people. The individualism that was important to the founding of this country was no longer sufficient to solve all problems. The Depression also led to the rapid growth of voluntary insurance plans for financing hospital and medical care (Stewart and Austin, 1938, p. 219).

In 1933 Pearl McIver, a well-qualified pub-

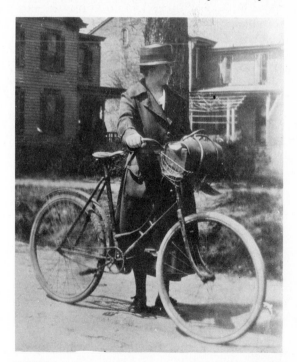

FIGURE 1-4 Public health nurses utilized bicycles before the advent of the automobile. (*The Metropolitan Life Insurance Company of New York. Used with their permission.*)

lic health nurse in the U.S. Public Health Service, was assigned as a consultant for the placement of nurses on federal relief projects. Many of these nurses were formerly hospital nurses now assigned to public health agencies and clinics, and they became interested in this new field. Thus, when the Social Security Act of 1935 made money available for the education and employment of public health nurses, many of those working on relief projects seized the opportunity to study. Other educational funds followed which made it possible for nurses to complete their education in a shorter time. These included Training for Nurses for National Defense, the GI bill, the Nurse Training Act of 1943, and Public Health and Professional Nurse traineeships. Funds were also available to help prepare nurses at the graduate level for specialties such as tuberculosis, cancer, mental health, maternal and child health, and research (McNeil, 1967, p. 6).

After the war began in 1941, the nurse shortage became acute. The problem was more serious than in World War I because of the duration and scope of the war effort. The National Nursing Council, composed of six national nursing organizations, along with the aid of the U.S. Department of Education, requested $1 million to enlarge facilities for nursing education. The administration of this money was assigned to the U.S. Public Health Service.

In 1943, the Cadet Nurse Corps was authorized by the Bolton Act. Sixty million dollars was appropriated to recruit and educate 70,000 cadets in 1125 schools between 1944 and 1946. These nurses comprised 90 percent of the total enrollment of basic nursing programs for this time. Lucille Petry, chief nurse officer, directed this remarkable program at a difficult time in our nation's history.

World War II, like World War I and the Depression, had a major impact on public health nursing:

1. The importance of public health nursing service was recognized when public health nurses were declared essential for civilian work, although many of them entered military service.

2. Maximum utilization of personnel was essential and official tax-supported public health nursing agencies combined with voluntary non-tax-supported agencies, to avoid duplication.

3. Practical nurses were accepted as an important resource for nursing service.

4. The establishment of priorities for health care became more than a topic for discussion.

5. Additional funds for nursing education became available and the fear of governmental control of education decreased. After the war, the enrollment of nurses who were veterans or widows of veterans strained the resources of universities and agencies providing field experience.

FROM WORLD WAR II TO THE PRESENT

The depressions before and after World War II, as well as the war itself, provided the milieu for the development of numerous programs designed to help the country renew itself. Chronic disease and accidents replaced infectious disease as the leading causes of death, a result of the effectiveness of new drugs and vaccines. Consequently, life expectancy increased.

The years between 1935 and 1965 produced much legislation that was aimed at improving the health, education, and housing of people, ending discrimination against minorities, and providing proper working conditions for wage earners. This legislation began with the Social Security Act of 1935; it provided monies for old-age benefits, state grants for aid to the blind and disabled, aid for dependent and crippled children, vocational rehabilitation programs, and unemployment compensation programs.

Title VI of the act focused on public health programs, and its overall purpose was to elicit a public health program that would protect and promote the nation's health. One part of title VI provided money to states and counties to establish and maintain health services. Allocations in this part of the act provided money for nurses to study public health nursing. Prior to 1935, only one-third of the states had a public health nursing section within the state health department, and only 7 percent of the public health nurses employed had taken an accredited course in public health nursing. During 1936, the first year that money became available through the Social Security Act, over 1000 nurses received money to study in a program accredited by the National Organization for Public Health Nursing.

Another part of title VI provided money for research and the investigation of diseases and problems with environmental health. Title VI was directly responsible for expanding public health nursing programs and developing new ones. As a result of this legislation, the public health nurse became an integral part of local health departments: the maternal and child health programs of the Social Security Act made the nurse's work with families essential. By 1940, 3000 nurses had received public health training in accredited schools, 970 counties had developed full-time public health services, and 1150 clinics had been added to those already working on the problems of venereal diseases (Williams, 1951, p. 156).

Later, President Kennedy's New Frontier and President Johnson's Great Society epito-

mized the era in our nation's history when the government took on even more aggressively the role of guardian of the nation's health. The rugged individualism of the early 1900s had disappeared. John Kennedy's inaugural address in 1961 is remembered for the words, "Ask not what your country can do for you— ask what you can do for your country." A new social consciousness swept the country, and the differences between black and white, poor and rich became topics for scrutiny, worth dying for.

Citizens began to see health as a right rather than a privilege, a significant change from the beginning of the century when families with large numbers of children were the norm so that at least some could be expected to live to adulthood. Parents realized that health should be the birthright of every child, not the privilege of a few.

The constitution of the World Health Organization defined health as "complete physical, mental and social well-being and not just the absence of disease." This definition reflected inclusion of the mental and social aspects of health as well as its physical aspects.

The demand for health care services on the part of an increasingly sophisticated and informed public came about in part as the result of ideas generated through television, magazines, newspapers, and radio. The ability to pay for these services led to the quest for a national compulsory health insurance.

When the war was over in 1945, President Harry Truman presented to Congress a health message with the following proposals for a health care system (Kalisch and Kalisch, 1977, p. 8):

1. Prepayment of medical costs with compulsory insurance and general revenues.

2. Protection from loss of wages as a result of sickness.

3. Expansion of services related to the public's

health and including maternal and child health services.

4. Governmental aid to medical schools for research.

5. Increased construction of hospitals, clinics, and medical institutions.

Charges of socialism from the American Medical Association ended the quest for national health insurance in 1949 and 1950 (Kalisch and Kalisch, 1978, p. 618). Much later, in 1965, a health insurance program for people 65 and older, Medicare, financed under the Social Security Act, was enacted by President Johnson.

Hospital Survey and Construction Act, 1946

Only the last of Truman's proposals was enacted. The Hospital Survey and Construction Act, also called the Hill-Burton bill, provided a 5-year program to states for the purpose of assessing needs, and then planning and constructing needed hospitals and public health centers.

The federal government provided one-third of the funds needed for the program, and each state provided the remaining two-thirds of the money. This act gave some nurses an opportunity to help plan the areas where they worked.

Organizing Public Health Nursing Services

It was at this point in our nation's history, after the war, when public health nursing seemed to become more concerned with how services were organized than with responding to health needs. The leadership among public health nurses, demonstrated by Wald and Gardner, appeared to diminish, and this specialty area entered a period in which it took a defensive stance regarding its contributions to health care and to nursing (Tinkham and Voorhies, 1977, p. 88).

In 1946, a committee of representatives from numerous agencies interested in public health nursing published guidelines upon which this area of nursing should be organized (Public Health Nursing, 1946, p. 387). The reason for the publication of these guidelines lies in the history of public health nursing. Public health nursing began with visits to the sick poor by voluntary agencies. Usually this was the only kind of care given by an agency and was the only organized program of home nursing. As the concept of public health grew, both voluntary and governmental services developed to provide public health nursing for special programs such as tuberculosis or child health. This resulted in duplication of services and unnecessary costs. Although the principal purpose of home nursing agencies was to give home care to the sick, nurses very quickly assumed the role of teaching a family to take responsibility for its own health. Thus, visiting nurses played a big part in helping to prevent and control sickness and epidemics. Gradually, city health departments became aware of the value of nursing and added nurses to their staffs to give health protection to the community as mandated by law. Nursing care of the sick was not accepted by health departments as a public health problem, so this activity remained the focus of voluntary agencies. This meant that in many communities public health nurses from two agencies (as well as an additional nurse from the school setting) might visit the same home, a problem that can still exist today in some communities.

The guidelines adopted by the committee addressed this history and resulting problems. It was agreed that a population of 50,000 was needed to support an adequate health program and that there should be one public health nurse for every 2000 people. Other principles included:

1. That each public health nurse should combine the functions of health teaching, control of disease, and care of the sick

2. That the community should adopt one of three patterns of organization that would best serve that community:

   a. All public health nursing service, including care of the sick at home, administered by the local health department

   b. Preventive services carried on by the health department with one voluntary agency, in close coordination with the health department, carrying responsibility for bedside nursing care

   c. A combination service jointly administered and financed by official and voluntary agencies with all service given by a single group of public health nurses

The Nurse Shortage

Right after World War II a serious undersupply of nurses created critical situations in hospitals and health centers. This was a result of factors including the increase in the population, the increase in insurance plans such as Blue Cross, an increase in the sophistication of surgery and medicine, which kept people alive longer, and the different situations in which nurses were increasingly employed, such as industry and schools.

Also, during the 1940s and the 1950s the place for women to be was in the home with husband and children. Married nurses were affected by this philosophy, and careers came second. It was not until the late 1960s that nurses began to develop a consciousness about their possible role in shaping the health care policies of the country, as well as their role in the political arena. Nurses were finally beginning to see themselves as the very obvious answer to the health care problems in the United States (Grissum and Spengler, 1976). This rise in activism among nurses paralleled the feminist movement among women in general.

In 1972, Nurses for Political Action was organized with headquarters in Washington, D.C. It became affiliated with the American Nurses' Association and later changed its name to N-CAP, Nurses Coalition for Action in Politics. Its purpose as a nonpartisan, nonprofit association was to obtain support for nursing from legislators, governmental officials, and the general public. At a time when a new national health care system was being developed and the present health care system was fragmented and dominated by the medical profession, nurses sought a place where they could make known their thoughts and ideas and help plan a system that comprehensively met people's health care needs.

The Federal Government Prepares Nurses

The government became involved in preparing new nurses with the passage of the Health Amendments Act of 1956. Title II authorized monies to aid registered nurses in the full-time study of either administration, supervision, or teaching.

However, in 1963 the Surgeon General's Consultant Group on Nursing reported that there were still too few nursing schools and not enough capable people being recruited into nursing. Additional problems were that nursing personnel were not well utilized and that only limited research was being done in nursing (U.S. Public Health Service, 1963).

Based upon these conclusions, the Nurse Training Act of 1964 was passed. This act provided money for loans and scholarships as well as for nursing school construction. With this act the federal government greatly helped to improve the quality of nursing in America.

The Expanding Role of the Nurse

By the 1960s the nursing profession began to look at new methods of meeting the health care needs of people, utilizing advanced nursing practice and extending the nursing role to take over some medical functions. The term *nurse practitioner* was first used at the University of Colorado in 1965 in a program that prepared nurses to provide comprehensive well-child care in ambulatory settings.

The concept of primary care nursing also became an important one. Primary care involves three important elements: first contact with the patient, continuity of care, and coordination of care. It is ambulatory care that views a person in relation to family and environment and emphasizes cure as well as prevention. Primary care can prevent both gaps and overlapping in health care services.

Public health nursing evolved from concern for the individual, the family, and the community. In fact, the early public health movement was the historical forerunner of today's primary care movement (Fagin, 1978, p. 752). Though presently other nursing specialties besides public health nursing work outside the hospital setting, and work with a person in terms of the family and the environment, public health nurses first used the concept that nursing could best meet the total health needs of people. The major difference between public health nursing and other areas of primary nursing is that public health nursing deals with the personal and environmental health of populations rather than only individuals and families. Public health practice must deal in concepts such as caseloads, clinics, counties, or census tracts to locate subgroups who have problems and are at risk.

In 1971, a bronze bust of Lillian Wald was placed in the Hall of Fame for Great Americans. An editorial about this event stated,

The kind of health care Lillian Wald began preaching and practicing in 1893 is the kind the people of this country are still crying for. She demonstrated with no need to rest on formal research that nursing could serve as the entry point—not only for health care, but for dealing with many other social ills of which sickness is only a part. She felt that nurses should go to the sick, instead of expecting the sick to come to them (and waiting for physicians to refer them); that care of persons in the home, especially

of children, was far more effective and much less expensive except perhaps for those needing, to use her own word, "intensive" care. (*American Journal of Nursing,* 1971, p. 53)

There is still not total agreement in nursing on the definition of and preparation for the expanded role of the nurse. However, increasing numbers of people are viewing primary care as the major focus of nursing (Fagin, 1978, p. 753). Attractive federal funding has encouraged the growth of practitioner programs.

The Decade of the Seventies

Public health nursing, as well as all of professional nursing, is in a state of transition. The contribution of this specialty area to the health needs of people is less clear than it was in Lillian Wald's time. She and her peers had no doubt about their mission and the goals of public health nursing. Through the 1920s and 1930s the public health nursing movement grew in power, set standards for practice, and influenced education by requiring certain content as a condition for employment.

In the seventies, all areas of nursing, including parent and child nursing, psychiatric nursing, and medical and surgical nursing, began discovering the community. These areas also began to emphasize the importance of the family to the patient, and the clear lines of distinction for what constituted public health nursing started to blur. Now, not even public health nurses agreed on the nature, standards, and scope of public health nursing practice (Ruth and Partridge, 1978, p. 625). However, it must be reemphasized that public health nursing was seen as a generalized area within nursing. Each of the other areas, medical-surgical nursing, psychiatric nursing, and parent and child nursing, had a specialized focus. Public health nursing has always been broad and comprehensive. Efforts are now being made to define the nature, standards, and scope of public health nursing practice.

Further, more and more professionals and semiprofessionals have begun to work in the community. Social workers, physical therapists, occupational therapists, as well as physicians' assistants and home health aides, are now seen in public health settings. To complicate the situation, there are numerous ways to become a "nurse"; associate degree programs, diploma programs, and baccalaureate programs all claim to prepare a different level of nurse. How these levels function in the community setting varies from agency to agency.

Voluntary agencies and health facilities have multiplied, and many of them have not been coordinated or designed with comprehensive health care plans in mind. Strong, effective official planning often has not been evident on the state and local level. Health maintenance organizations, neighborhood health centers, free clinics, and numerous home health care programs based in hospitals and "for-profit agencies" represent the conglomeration of facilities that can spring up in any one community.

The rapid development of health services and specialties has created even more confusion for people who find the present health care system difficult to negotiate. People desperately need someone to help them, and public health nurses can be the answer.

Up from Here

The struggles that public health nursing has experienced are maturing ones. Much rethinking of the goals and values of public health nursing has taken place. We do have a unique contribution to make, and we urgently need to act upon it. No other specialty area looks at the personal and environmental health of population groups. Health problems such as those seen with teenage pregnancies (which are now of epidemic proportions) will not be solved by taking care of several pregnant teenagers each month. Progress is made by looking at this population subgroup and devising strategies for prevention. Viewing the health of population groups can be a vital force in reducing disease and promoting health.

SUMMARY

The beginnings of nursing can be traced to the beginnings of humankind since there has always been a need for reducing pain with comfort measures. The early Christian church's contributions to nursing were significant, as were the organizational contributions of St. Vincent de Paul and Mademoiselle Le Gras to public health nursing. The influence of the status of women on nursing can be demonstrated by Sairy Gamp, a prostitute-nurse who cared for people in the 1700s when no "respectable" woman could take this position. Florence Nightingale's legacy to professional nursing and to public health, along with the

contributions of William Rathbone, the founder of public health nursing in England, provided the basis for public health nursing in the United States. Events in society at large have shaped nursing as a whole and the development of public health nursing. The life and work of Lillian Wald, predecessor of the modern public health nurse, was powerfully influenced by the waves of immigrants to New York City and the desperate conditions in which they lived. How public health nurses organized themselves along with methods of education for this area of nursing shaped not only the development of this specialty area but all of nursing. Gradually, the nation developed a consciousness about its collective health status, and this was demonstrated by the formation of health services on the national, state, and local level. Both world wars and the Depression forced negative as well as positive changes in public health nursing. Emphases in public health nursing as well as nursing in general are changing; the health scene is chaotic because there is no overall health plan. Public health nursing, with its focus on the health of groups, can involve nurses in health planning and in the necessary task of bringing order out of chaos.

The Appendix to this chapter presents some beginnings and developments of significance to public health nursing in a chronological chart form. It is especially important to note other contemporary social events when reviewing the historical transition of public health nursing. Societal changes tremendously influence changes that occur in a profession.

APPENDIX 1-1
Some Beginnings in and Developments of Significance to Public Health Nursing*

Nursing and public health nursing	Other significant events
	1765 First school of medicine (Philadelphia)
	1798 Marine Hospital Service (became USPHS 1912) Treasury Department
1813 Ladies Benevolent Society, Charleston, South Carolina	
	1839 First dental school (Baltimore)
1851 Florence Nightingale (1820–1910) went to Kaiserswerth	
1859 First District Nursing Association, Liverpool (William Rathbone and Mrs. Mary Robinson)	
1860 Nightingale Training School established, London	
	1861–1865 Civil War
	1864 International Red Cross (Henri Durant)
	1869 Massachusetts State Department of Health
1872 First schools of nursing in United States (New England Hospital for Women and Children, Boston, and Women's Hospital, Philadelphia)	1872 American Public Health Association founded
1873 Linda Richards, first nurse graduated in United States	
1877 New York City Mission sent trained nurses into homes of sick, poor	
	1880 National Death Registration established by U.S. Census
	1882 American Red Cross (Clara Barton)
	1882–1884 Discovery of bacteria causing tuberculosis, diphtheria, and typhoid
1885 Buffalo District Nursing Association	

*Some dates may be disputed.

Nursing and public health nursing	*Other significant events*
1886 Boston Instructive District Nursing Association and Philadelphia Visiting Nurse Association (VNA)	
1889 Chicago Visiting Nurse Association	
	1890–1910 "Golden Age of Bacteriology"
	1890 Pasteurization of milk
1892 School nursing, London (Amy Hughes)	
1893 Henry Street Visiting Nurse Service, New York (Lillian D. Wald and Mary Brewster); first milk station, New York City; American Society of Superintendents of Training Schools for Nurses (became National League for Nursing Education, 1912)	
	1894 School medical inspection, Boston
1895 Industrial Nursing, Vermont Marble Works (Ada Mayo and Stewart Markolf)	
1897 Nurses' Associated Alumnae of United States and Canada (became American Nurses' Association 1911)	1897 University of Michigan granted Master of Science degree in Hygiene and Public Health
1898 Los Angeles Health Department paid public health nurses; Detroit Visiting Nurse Association	1898 Course in social work, New York Charity Organization Society
1899 International Council of Nurses; University education for nurses, Teacher's College, Columbia University (course in hospital economics)	1899 Association of Hospital Superintendents (became American Hospital Association 1907)
1900 *American Journal of Nursing*	1900–1925 Expansion of voluntary agencies
1901 58 public health nursing associations; 130 public health nurses in United States	
1902 School nursing, New York City (Lina Rogers)	
1903 Tuberculosis nursing, Baltimore; First Nurse Practice Acts	
1904 Visiting nurses have program at Conference of Charities and Correction	1904 National Organization for the Study and Prevention of Tuberculosis (became National Tuberculosis Association)
1905 200 public health agencies; 440 public health nurses in United States	1905 Medical social work, Massachusetts General Hospital
1906 Course in district nursing offered by Boston Instructive District Nursing Association	
1907 Alabama law permitting employment of public health nurses	1907 Visiting teacher, Boston
1908 English health visitor; Detroit Health Department employed public health nurses	
1909 University of Minnesota School of Nursing	1909 National Committee for Mental Hygiene
1909 Metropolitan Life Insurance Company contracts for visiting nursing service; The *Visiting Nurse Quarterly* published by Cleveland Visiting Nurse	1909 First White House Conference; American Association for the Study and Prevention of Infant Mortality

Nursing and public health nursing	*Other significant events*
Association (later presented to NOPHN and became *Public Health Nursing* monthly until 1953)	
1910 Public health nursing program, Teachers' College, Columbia University	1910 *Medical Education in the United States and Canada,* Abraham Flexner
	1911 Boston Instructive Visiting Nurse Association added nutritional service
	1911 Joint Committee on Health Problems in Education, American Medical Association and National Education Association; county health departments in Gilford County, North Carolina, and Yakima County, Washington
1912 American Red Cross Rural Nursing Service (1200 services in 1922); National Organization for Public Health Nursing (NOPHN); U.S. Children's Bureau, Department of Labor	
1913 Division of Public Health Nursing, New York State Department of Health	1913 Harvard School of Public Health
1914 NOPHN suggested 4-month course in a visiting nurse association as essential preparation for public health nursing	
	1915 National Birth Registration Area established
	1915–1925 Wave of legislation of physical education and hygiene
1916 1922 public health nursing agencies; 5152 public health nurses: University of Cincinnati School of Nursing 5-year program leading to bachelor's degree	
	1917–1918 World War I
	1917 American Dietetic Association; Massachusetts and New York employed public health nutritionists
1918 USPHS organized a division of public health nursing to work in extracantonment zones	1918 Community chests and councils
1918–1923 Increased interest in combining local public health nursing agencies	1918 Compulsory education in all states; American Association of Medical Social Workers
1918 Maternity Center Association, New York	
1919 *Public Health Nursing,* Mary S. Gardner; increase in public health nurses and public health nursing education; public health nursing program, University of Michigan	1919–1929 Demonstrations of child health and public health services
1920 NOPHN-approved university programs in public health nursing	
1921 Industrial and school nursing sections of NOPHN; NOPHN set 1 academic year as minimum for public health nursing certificate	1921 First university program in public health education, Massachusetts Institute of Technology, Harvard; National Health Council; American Association of Social Workers
	1921–1929 Sheppard-Towner Act—federal aid for maternal and child health

Nursing and public health nursing	*Other significant events*
1922 4040 public health agencies; 11,548 nurses	1922–1935 American Child Health Association
1923 Public health nursing section, APHA; Nursing and Nursing Education in the United States ("The Winslow-Goldmark Report"); Yale and Western Reserve Universities established collegiate schools of nursing	
1924 U.S. Indian Bureau Nursing Service (Eleanor Gregg)	
1925 Frontier Nursing Service—nurse-midwives (Mary Breckenridge); first NOPHN statement of qualifications for public health nurses; John Hancock Mutual Life Insurance Company Visiting Nurse Service	
1925–1926 Chicago Infant Welfare Society and Boston and East Harlem public health nursing agencies employ psychiatric social workers	
1926 Committee on Grading of Nursing Schools began studies	
	1927–1931 Research by Committee on the Cost of Medical Care
	1929 Beginning of the Depression
1930 Unemployment of nurses	1930 Study of maternal mortality in New York City
1931 4355 public health agencies; 15,865 nurses	
1932 Final report of Commission on Medical Education; Association of Collegiate Schools of Nursing; Lobenstine Midwifery Clinic and School (Maternity Center responsible for school 1934); 7% of nurses employed in public health nursing had completed a 1-year program	
1933 Pearl McIver appointed to USPHS as a public health nursing analyst	1933 U.S. Birth and Death Registration Areas complete
1934 *Survey of Public Health Nursing,* NOPHN, published	
1935 *Facts about Nursing,* American Nursing Association (ANA)	1935 Social Security Act
	1935–1936 National Health Survey
	1937–1947 Beginning of federal appropriations for cancer, venereal diseases, tuberculosis, mental health, heart disease, etc.
	1939 Reorganization of federal agencies; USPHS transferred from Treasury Department to Federal Security Agency
	1939–1945 World War II
1940 20,434 nurses employed for public health nursing; 22% had completed 1 or more years in an approved public health nursing program	
1942 American Association of Industrial Nurses	

Nursing and public health nursing	Other significant events
1943 Bolton-Bailey Act for nursing education and Cadet Nurse Program; Division of Nursing Education, USPHS [Lucile Petry (Leone)]	1943–1947 Emergency Maternity and Infant Care Program
1944 Division of Nursing, USPHS [Lucile Petry (Leone)]; commissioned rank for nurses; NOPHN accredits only public health nursing programs with professional content of at least 1 year, which is part of program leading to a degree; Skidmore College basic nursing program approved for preparation of public health nurses	
	1945 End World War II; educational privileges provided for nurse veterans by GI Bill of Rights; publication of *Local Health Units for the Nation;* APHA accreditation of schools of public health
1946 Nurses classified as professional by U.S. Civil Service Commission	1946 Hospital Survey and Construction Act (Hill Burton)
1948 Publication of *Nurses for the Future* (Esther Lucile Brown)	1948 World Health Organization permanently established and meeting of World Health Assembly
1949 National Federation of Licensed Practical Nurses; national nursing organizations support legislation for federal financial aid for practical nursing education	
1950 25,081 nurses employed for public health work in the United States and territories; 34% had completed 1 or more years in an approved public health nursing program	
1951 National League for Nursing recommendation that collegiate basic nursing education programs include preparation for public health nursing; National Association of Colored Graduate Nurses integrated with ANA	
1952 Reorganization of national nursing organizations, major functions transferred to American Nurses' Association and National League for Nursing	
1952 Boston University program with a major in general nursing approved for preparation of public health nurses	
1952–1953 American Red Cross, Metropolitan Life Insurance Company, and John Hancock Mutual Life Insurance Company discontinue public health nursing services; *Public Health Nursing,* December 1952, last issue	
1953 *Nursing Outlook* published in January; U.S. Department of Health, Education, and Welfare including USPHS and United States Children's Bureau established with cabinet status	1953 Department of Health, Education, and Welfare established with cabinet status
1955 27,112 nurses employed in public health work in the United States and territories; 37% had completed at least 1 year of approved public health nursing program; nursing programs preparing for public health nursing:	1955 National Association of Social Workers (seven associations combined)

Nursing and public health nursing	*Other significant events*

Major in public health nursing 33
Baccalaureate basic 25
Major in general nursing 9

1959 NLN voted that no new specialized baccalaureate program be accredited and that after 1963 only baccalaureate programs that include public health nursing be accredited

1960 *NLN Criteria for the Evaluation of Educational Programs in Nursing that Lead to Baccalaureate and Master's Degrees*

1961 First White House Conference on Aging

1962 11 accredited schools of public health in United States, 2 in Canada

1963 Report of Surgeon General's Consultant Group on Nursing

1964 *NLN Statement of Beliefs and Recommendations Regarding Baccalaureate Programs Admitting Registered Nurse Students*; Nurse Training Act of 1964

1964 Economic Opportunity Act of 1964

1964 Agencies and nurses employed for public health nursing:

	Agencies	*Nurses*
Local	9,094	35,209
Board of Education	5,412	13,257
Official	2,712	14,738
VNA	682	3,826
Combination	51	1,478

Population per public health nurse in United States 5586, 43.4% of full-time nurses had completed 30 or more hours in an approved public health nursing program; 39.7% had college degrees

1965 Social Security Amendment—Medicare legislation

1966 NLN programs accredited for public health nursing—June 1966:

Masters	42
Baccalaureate basic (students with no previous nursing preparation and registered nurses)	151
Baccalaureate basic (students with no previous nursing preparation)	91
Baccalaureate basic (registered nurses only)	6

1968 Health Manpower Act (Extended Nurse Training Act of 1964)

1970 National Commission on Nursing and Nursing Education—Abstract for Action; Family Planning Services and Population Research Act;

Nursing and public health nursing		*Other significant events*
		Occupational Safety and Health Act; Comprehensive Alcohol Abuse and Alcoholism Prevention, Treatment, and Rehabilitation; the National Environmental Policy Act (established Council on Environmental Quality)
	1971	Nurse Training Act (expanded and continued nurse training provisions of the 1964 and 1968 acts); Comprehensive Health Manpower Training Act; Sickle Cell Anemia Act; National Cancer Act
	1972	Communicable Disease Control Amendments Act; Social Security Amendments regarding Medicare and Medicaid; National Heart, Blood Vessel, Lung, and Blood Act
	1973	The Health Maintenance Organization (HMO) Act
1974 Formation of Nurses Coalition for Action in Politics; first certification examinations by the ANA for excellence in practice	1974	The Health Planning and Resources Development Act
	1975	Health Services, Health Revenue Sharing, and Nurse Training Act (NTA)
	1976	Costs for health care in the United States rose 14% over 1975
1977–1978 Designated the "Year of the Nurse" by ANA to help the public better understand nursing	1977	Passage of the Rural Health Clinic Services bill— Public Law 95-210
1978 Massachusetts becomes the seventh state to mandate continuing education as a requirement for relicensure of both registered and practical nurses	1978	President Carter vetoes the Nursing Training Act
1978 Robert Wood Johnson Foundation finances $5 million program to train nurses as school nurse practitioners and place them in areas where children now receive inadequate care		
1979 ANA board determined that future ANA conventions and conferences will be held only in states that have ratified the Equal Rights Amendment; Maryland passes law which requires insurance companies to provide reimbursement "for any service which is within the lawful scope of a duly licensed health care provider"; ANA sponsors a Study of Credentialing in Nursing, which spurs nationwide discussion and debate; N-CAP survey shows that nurses act on their political convictions and back candidates on the basis of issues, not party philosophy (they also vote and let officials know what they think)	1979	Due to antirecession lobbying by nurses and others, NTA funds were cut $15.75 million rather than Carter's $84 million; President Carter's fiscal 1980 budget cut nursing education funds to $15 million in contrast to current levels of $122 million (only nurse practitioner programs fared well); President Carter sent to Congress a national health insurance bill which would require minimum benefits for employed people and upgrade coverage for the poor, aged, and disabled; he became the first president to formally back a plan with the underlying concept that health care is a basic human right
	1979	President Carter's cost containment bill designed to limit annual revenue for the nation's hospitals ran into many snags and has slim chance of passing.

SOURCE: Used by permission of Ella McNeil, Professor Emeritus of Public Health Nursing, School of Public Health, University of Michigan, Ann Arbor, Michigan. Original compilation of important beginnings was updated to reflect significant changes in the late seventies.

REFERENCES

Christy, T. E. Portrait of a leader: Lavinia Lloyd Dock. *Nursing Outlook,* June 1969, *17,* 72–75.

———. Portrait of a leader: Lillian Wald. *Nursing Outlook,* March 1970, *18,* 50–54.

Committee for the Study of Nursing Education. *Nursing and nursing education in the United States.* New York: Macmillan, 1923.

Deloughery, G. L. *History and trends of professional nursing* (8th ed.). St. Louis: Mosby, 1977.

Desirable organization of public health nursing for family service. *Public Health Nursing,* August 1946, *38,* 387–389.

Dock, L., Pickett, S. E., Noyes, C. D., Clement, F. E., Fox, E. E., & VanMeter, A. R. *History of American Red Cross nursing.* New York: Macmillan, 1922.

Dolan, J. A. *Nursing in society. A historical perspective.* Philadelphia: Saunders, 1978.

Fagin, C. M. Primary care as an academic discipline. *Nursing Outlook,* December 1978, *26,* 750–753.

Fox, E. G. (Ed.). Red Cross public health nursing. *Public Health Nursing,* February 1920, *12,* 175–181.

Gardner, M. S. *Public Health Nursing* (3d ed.). New York: Macmillan, 1919.

Grissum, M., & Spangler, C. *Woman power and health care.* Boston: Little, Brown, 1976.

Hanlon, J. J. *Public health administration and practice* (6th ed.). St. Louis: Mosby, 1974.

Haupt, A. C. Forty years of teamwork in public health nursing. *American Journal of Nursing,* January 1953, *53,* 81–84.

Jensen, D. M. *History and trends of professional nursing* (4th ed.). St. Louis: Mosby, 1959.

Kalisch, P., & Kalisch, B. J. *Nursing involvement in the health planning process.* (DHEW Publication No. HRA 78-25). Hyattsville, Md.: Department of Health, Education, and Welfare, 1977.

———&———. *The advancement of American nursing.* Boston: Little, Brown, 1978.

Maynard, T. *The apostle of charity: The life of St. Vincent de Paul.* New York: Dial Press, 1939.

McNeil, E. E. Transition in public health nursing. John Sundwall Lecture, University of Michigan, Feb. 27, 1967.

National Organization for Public Health Nursing. Approval of Skidmore College of Nursing as preparing students for public health nursing. *Public Health Nursing,* July 1944, *36,* 371.

Nelson, S. C. Mary Sewall Gardner. *Nursing Outlook.* January 1954, *2,* 37–39.

Nightingale, F. *Notes on nursing.* London: Harris and Sons, 1859 (Philadelphia: Lippincott, 1946).

A prophet honored (Editorial). *American Journal of Nursing,* January 1971, *71,* 53.

Roberts, M. M. *American nursing, history and interpretation.* New York: Macmillan, 1954.

Rosen, G. *A history of public health.* New York: MD Publications, 1958.

Ruth, M. V., & Partridge, K. B. Differences in perception of education and practice. *Nursing Outlook,* October 1978, *26,* 622–628.

Smillie, W. G. *Preventive medicine and public health* (2d ed.). New York: Macmillan, 1952.

Stewart, I. M., & Austin, A. L. *A history of nursing* (5th ed.). New York: Putnam, 1938.

Tinkham, C. W., & Voorhies, E. F. *Community health nursing. Evolution and process* (2d ed.). New York: Appleton-Century-Crofts, 1977.

U.S. Public Health Service. *Toward quality in nursing: Needs and goals. Report of the surgeon general's consultant group on nursing.* Washington, D.C.: Government Printing Office, 1963.

Wald, L. *The House on Henry Street.* New York: Holt, 1915.

Williams, R. *The United States public health service.* Bethesda, Md.: Commissioned Officers Association of the U.S. Public Health Service, 1951.

Winslow, C.-E. A. Florence Nightingale and public health nursing. *Public Health Nursing,* July 1946, *38,* 330–332.

SELECTED BIBLIOGRAPHY

Bishop, W. J. Florence Nightingale's message for today. *Nursing Outlook,* May 1960, *8,* 246–249.

Boardman, M. T. Rural nursing service of the Red Cross. *American Journal of Nursing,* September 1913, *13,* 937–939.

Brainard, A. M. *The evolution of public health nursing.* Philadelphia: Saunders, 1922.

Dock, L. L., & Stewart, I. M. *A short history of nursing.* New York: Putnam, 1931.

Ehrenreich, B., & English, D. *Witches, midwives, and nurses. A history of women healers.* Old Westbury, N.Y.: Feminist Press, 1973.

Fitzpatrick, M. L. Nursing and the Great Depression. *American Journal of Nursing,* December 1975, *75,* 2188–2190.

Foley, E. L. Standing orders. *American Journal of Nursing,* March 1919, *13,* 451.

Gardner, M. S. The national organization for public health nursing. *Visiting Nurse Quarterly,* July 1912, *4,* 13–18.

Heide, W. S. Nursing and woman's liberation: a parallel. *American Journal of Nursing,* May 1973, *73,* 824–827.

Kark, S. *Epidemiology and community medicine.* New York: Appleton-Century-Crofts, 1974.

Lewis, R. A. *Edwin Chadwick and the public health movement, 1832–1854.* New York: Longmans, 1952.

Nelson, S. C. Mary Sewall Gardner. *Nursing Outlook,* January 1954, *2,* 37–39.

Rathbone, W. *History and progress of district nursing.* New York: Macmillan, 1890.

Terris, M. Evolution of public health and preventive medicine in the United States. *American Journal of Public Health,* February 1975, *65,* 161–169.

Tucker, K., & Hilbert, H. *Survey of public health nursing, administration and practice.* New York: Commonwealth Fund, 1934.

U.S. Department of Health, Education, and Welfare, Secretary's Committee to Study Extended Roles for Nurses. *Extending the scope of nursing practice: A report of the secretary's committee.* Washington, D.C.: Government Printing Office, 1972.

Wald, L. *Windows on Henry Street.* Boston: Little, Brown, 1934.

Watson, J. The evolution of nursing education in the United States: One hundred years of a profession for women. *Journal of Nursing Education,* September 1977, *16,* 31–37.

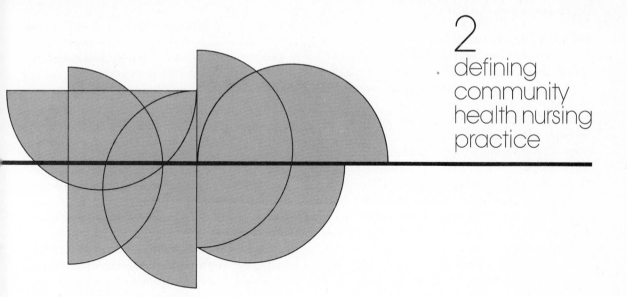

When public health nursing began in the early 1900s, it was a simple matter to define it as a specialty area within nursing. Public health nursing took place outside the hospital setting; it was "nursing without walls," nursing that was independent and practiced primarily with families. As the focus of health care moves outside the hospital setting and as more and more nurses assume expanded, independent roles in primary care, defining community health nursing as a specialty area is less easily done.

The definition becomes sharp and clear, however, when it is understood that it is the nature of the practice and not the setting that defines community health nursing as a specialty area. Nursing outside hospital walls is not necessarily community health nursing: pediatric nurse practitioners who do assessments of newborns in physician's offices and nurses who counsel clients in mental health centers may not be practicing community health nursing. These nurses are probably practicing primary care nursing, which is not synonymous with community health nursing. Primary care

is a coordinated system of health care that emphasizes first-contact care as well as continuity. It is ambulatory care that is coordinated and holistic (Parker, 1976).

As was discussed in Chapter 1, the expanded role of the nurse is not new to community health nursing. In many areas, nurses historically functioned in independent positions in collaboration with physicians. Today, nurses in numerous settings are routinely assessing the health of individuals and families, providing care during normal pregnancies and deliveries, providing family planning services, and managing care for specific clients which includes prescribing as well as providing the treatment. This is done in consultation with physicians and members of other disciplines.

Community health nurses deal with both the personal and the environmental health of people. Personal health involves the physical, biological, social, and psychological aspects of health, whereas environmental health deals with people's surroundings, settings such as homes, schools, work places, or recreational facilities. In community health nursing, nurses enter the environment in which people live, and they practice within this environment. This is the opposite of many nursing situations in which the client enters the nurse's environment in a hospital or clinic. In addition to the one-to-one or single-family approach to health care, the community health nurse thinks in terms of populations such as caseloads, clinics, districts, census tracts, and cities. Groups at risk within these populations, including families at risk, are identified so that preventive measures can be targeted for them. In this manner, available resources can be wisely utilized (Ruth and Partridge, 1978, p. 625). Resource distribution is discussed in Chapters 9 through 18.

An example illustrates the difference between community health nursing practice and primary care. One community health nurse was assigned a census tract as her population to be served. This census tract was located in a decaying area of town with substandard housing and no transportation, playgrounds, or parks. A large industrial complex lay in the census tract, and consequently large numbers of young laborers and their families lived there. There was no hospital located in the area and only one physician. The community health nurse received numerous referrals from the physician and outlying hospitals to visit young mothers with newborns who needed support with parenting their children. The nurse assessed the need for a parenting group by talking with the families whom she served, as well as with her supervisors. She and the families she visited planned a weekly sharing and support group that met in a neighborhood church. The group was well attended and continued to function after the nurse left. The nurse demonstrated the focus in community health on planning preventive health measures for groups at risk, which is a step beyond giving primary health care to families who need it.

One-to-one clinical practice, illustrated by pediatric nurse practitioners and family nurse practitioners, certainly has a place in community health nursing when it is performed for the explicit purpose of improving the level of health in a community. Nurses in these roles can have the expertise to plan for populations at risk and also act as consultants to other community health nurses. One official health department has a pediatric nurse practitioner who holds well-child conferences weekly in impoverished rural areas where there is almost no other health care available. This nurse is serving the high-risk population of children, from birth through 5 years of age, in that county. Other staff nurses in the agency use her as a resource person when they have questions about the children they serve.

The World Health Organization has defined three necessary components of community health nursing practice that further delineate the uniqueness of this specialty area (WHO, 1974):

1. A sense of responsibility for coverage of needed health services in a community. It is not necessary that community health nursing provide these services. The sense of responsibility for their provision, however, must be present.

2. The care of vulnerable groups in a community is a priority. The basis for involvement in the health care of groups is based upon their vulnerability. The long involvement of community health nursing in maternal child health is based upon this component.

3. The client (family, group, community) must be a partner in planning and evaluating health care.

THE ANA DEFINES COMMUNITY HEALTH NURSING

The American Nurses' Association (ANA) Division on Community Health Nursing Practice defines community health nursing as

a synthesis of nursing practice and public health practice applied to promoting and preserving the health of populations. The nature of this practice is general and comprehensive. It is not limited to a particular age or diagnostic group. It is continuing, not episodic. The dominant responsibility is to the population as a whole. Therefore, nursing directed

to individuals, families or groups contributes to the health of the total population. Health promotion, health maintenance, health education, coordination and continuity of care are utilized in a holistic approach to the family, group and community. The nurse's actions acknowledge the need for comprehensive health planning, recognize the influences of social and ecological issues, give attention to populations at risk and utilize the dynamic forces which influence change. (ANA, 1973)

ANALYZING COMPONENTS OF THE ANA DEFINITION

Community health nursing is a synthesis of nursing practice and public health practice. Community health nurses use the same knowledge and skills that nurses use in other settings. In addition, community health nurses must use the knowledge and skills of the public health sciences. In 1952, Winslow described public health as the science and art of preventing disease, prolonging life, and promoting health and efficiency through organized community effort for:

a. sanitation of the environment

b. control of communicable diseases

c. education regarding personal hygiene

d. organization of medical and nursing services for early diagnosis and preventive treatment of disease

e. development of social machinery to insure everyone a standard of living adequate for health maintenance, so organizing these benefits as to enable every citizen to realize his birthright of health and longevity. (Winslow, 1952, p. 30)

The county which has environmental engineers who test well water for purity and inspect restaurants for cleanliness illustrates how the concepts in this definition are applied, as does the nurse who works with parents and newborns, teaching parenting skills.

In order to assess needs and plan health services for families, groups, and communities, a public health knowledge base is mandatory. This basic knowledge, which includes epidemiology, biostatistics, social policy, and the principles of health planning, is unique to community health nursing and will be more fully explored in this text.

THREE MAJOR CONCEPTS OF THE ANA DEFINITION: GOALS, TARGETS, AND SERVICES

The ANA definition is prefaced with the statement that "nursing practice is a direct service, goal directed, and adaptable to the needs of the individual, family and community during health and illness" (ANA, 1973). This definition combines three major concepts which reflect the goals of community health nursing services, the types of services, and the targets of those goals and services, the client population. The goal is health, the services involved

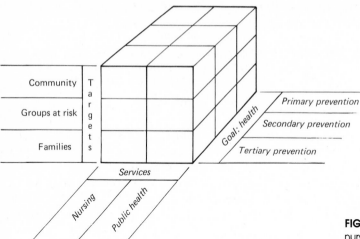

FIGURE 2-1 The process of community health nursing practice.

are nursing and public health, and the targets are families, groups at risk, and the community. Figure 2-1 depicts the process of community health nursing. It was designed to illustrate the relationships between the three major concepts in the ANA's definition of community health nursing. It shows that the community health nurse provides nursing and public health services to populations (community, groups at risk, and families) in order to promote optimal health. Prevention is essential for health maintenance and promotion.

Goals in Community Health Nursing

The goal of community health nursing practice is health—that is, helping clients to obtain their maximum level of physical, mental, and social functioning. The term *health* reflects the wellness orientation of the practice, in contrast to the illness orientation seen in other areas of nursing. All individuals, families, groups, and communities need to have their healthy as well as their problematic characteristics identified. Focusing on health broadens the community health nurse's practice. Emphasis is placed on

health-promotion activities as well as on curative services.

A health orientation reflects an assumption that people always have the potential for higher levels of functioning and that people in all stages of living, including those who are dying, are growing and developing. Community health nurses, utilizing concepts from nursing and public health, seek to intervene actively at any level to promote the health of identified clients.

The community health nurse works with all three levels of prevention: primary, secondary, and tertiary (Leavell and Clark, 1965, p. 21). Primary prevention deals with health promotion and specific protection from health problems. Immunizations, family planning services, antepartal care, classes for retirement preparation, dental prophylaxis, poison-control teaching, anticipatory guidance in family health and child care, and counseling on accident prevention are all examples of primary prevention activities.

Secondary prevention or health maintenance focuses on early diagnosis and prompt intervention to limit disabilities. The community health nurse, observing poor maternal-infant bonding and providing a role model for new interaction techniques, illustrates this concept. Also, assessing for developmental delays in the young child, teaching and reinforcing the need to do self-examination of the breasts, and encouraging regular medical, dental, and ophthalmologic examinations can be part of the effort toward secondary prevention.

Tertiary prevention refers to activities that help rehabilitate clients and restore them to maximum levels of functioning. The nurse who teaches a client with arthritis how to rest at intervals throughout the day provides an example of tertiary prevention. Assisting the post–cerebrovascular accident client to continue with a physical and speech therapy regimen is also carrying out aspects of tertiary prevention. Chapter 17 discusses in depth the role of the community health nurse in rehabilitation.

To achieve the goal of community health nursing, optimal health, all three levels of prevention—primary (promotion), secondary (maintenance), and tertiary (rehabilitation)—must be implemented. Populations must develop behaviors that promote health as well as prevent disease in order to achieve an optimal level of functioning.

The Targets of Community Health Nursing

The target of community health nursing practice is defined in the statement, "The dominant responsibility is to the population as a whole." A subconcept related to this statement is that of the client of the community health nurse, i.e., the individuals, families, groups, communities, and populations at risk. The ANA definition specifies that the nurses' major responsibility is to the population as a whole as opposed to individuals or groups of specific people. "Nursing directed to individuals, families, or groups contributes to the health of the total population." This emphasizes a holistic approach to the family, group, and community, and especially to "populations at risk." Though it is difficult to care for entire populations, care given to at-risk groups contributes to the overall health of populations. Care given to infants at risk is a good example, because healthy infants ensure healthy succeeding generations of citizens. However, community health nursing must continually reflect a primary concern for the health of the total population. Providing immunization clinics at "preschool roundups" is a way in which nurses affect the health of a population group.

The word *client* rather than *patient* is used for a purpose in community health nursing. It reflects a wellness orientation in addition to an active, independent relationship, the opposite of the passivity denoted in the word *patient*. The client asks questions and is a participant in assessing needs and in planning and implementing the plan of care. Care is not given *to* clients; rather, they have a full part *in* their care. Remember, the client may be an individual, a family, a group, or a community.

Two other subconcepts related to the targets of practice are reflected in the terms *generalized and comprehensive* and *continuing*. The targets of service are not restricted to a particular age or diagnostic category or to an event or time frame. Services to an individual extend to his or her family. In fact, community health nursing is defined by a lack of boundaries. Thus the community health nurse's concern encompasses all of the human population over time, reflecting a concern for the future as well as the present. This is the opposite of the focus on disease in acute care. For this reason, persons involved in community health nursing must be concerned with "comprehensive health planning, recognize the influences of social and ecological issues, give attention to populations at risk and utilize dynamic forces which influence change." It is impossible to be comprehensive in care and not plan for the future.

The Services Involved in Community Health Nursing

The services of community health nursing are defined as a "synthesis of nursing and public health." Both nursing and public health are concerned with the health of people. Nursing traditionally focuses on individuals and views them from the illness perspective; public health views groups from the preventive perspective. Community health nursing embodies the entire health-illness continuum and practices with families, small groups, and large populations.

The nature of community health nursing services is, again, like the target, general, comprehensive, and continuing. It reflects a holistic approach to practice in which all needs, physical, mental, and social, are assessed and provided for by the nurse-client relationship.

The community health nurse implements such activities as health promotion, health maintenance, and health education, and makes provision for the coordination and continuity of care in order to provide holistic care to the target of the interventions. In addition, the community health nurse is involved in comprehensive health planning (general and comprehensive care over time), recognizes the influence of social and ecological issues, and utilizes dynamic forces that influence change. Such forces include research, leadership, political strategies, and change-agent skills directed toward the improvement of the health of populations.

Nurses are becoming increasingly involved in the political process at the local, state, and even national levels because they understand that, ultimately, problems such as equal distribution of health professionals, transportation, and the availability of health care for everyone must be solved outside the nurse-family relationship. One nurse, a state senator, has been called one of the most influential people in her state in health care matters. She has helped to sponsor much valuable health care legislation for her state that directly affects the health of many people (*American Journal of Nursing*, 1979, p. 146).

Maintaining the health of people is a complex task. In order to accomplish this task, community health nurses must analyze carefully and apply the concepts delineated in the ANA definition of community health nursing practice. In summary, this definition specifies the health of the total population as the goal; identifies the targets as families, groups at risk, and the community; and describes community health nursing services as comprehensive, general, and continuing. In addition, it stresses that community health nurses provide both nursing and public health services to the targets they serve. Through the provision of these services, they promote health and prevent disease.

SETTINGS, ROLES, AND WORK FORCE IN COMMUNITY HEALTH NURSING

How do community health nurses carry out the practice of community health nursing? What are some of the roles in which they participate so that quality service is provided to families, groups, and communities? In what settings do they practice?

Settings in Which Community Health Nurses Function

Community health nurses have traditionally been employed by health departments or other tax-supported agencies, visiting nurse associations or other non-tax-supported agencies, and schools and occupational health programs.

Such nurses have always functioned rather independently in a way that corresponds to the current definition of the expanded or extended role of the nurse. In addition to the above settings, health maintenance organizations, neighborhood health centers, and home health care services have also used community health nurses in an expanded role as the source of primary health care.

Roles of the Community Health Nurses

There are numerous roles used by nurses to deliver community health nursing services. Other chapters in this text discuss these roles in depth. Below is a listing of the types of roles community health nurses assume:

1. *Case finder.* The community health nurse looks for clients at risk among the population being served. Chapters 12 through 19 discuss ways nurses serve as case finders.

2. *School nurse.* Chapter 14 presents the role of the nurse with this vital population group.

3. *Home visitor.* Perhaps the most unusual aspect of this specialty area is that the community health nurse enters the client's setting. The nurse not only assesses the environment but also works within it. Home visitors are able to gather environmental data as well as data about how a family system functions within that environment.

4. *Clinic nurse.* Chapter 19 expands on the role of the nurse in the ambulatory care setting.

5. *Group leader.* Chapter 19 also discusses the role of the nurse who works with groups in practice.

6. *Teacher.* Utilization of teaching-learning principles in facilitating behavioral change among clients is a basic intervention strat-

egy in community health. Chapter 7 presents the role of the nurse when she or he utilizes the educative intervention strategy with families.

7. *Epidemiologist.* The community health nurse uses the epidemiological method to study disease and health among population groups. Chapter 10 explains this role.

8. *Occupational health nurse.* Chapter 16 presents this expanding and changing area of community health nursing.

9. *Health planner.* Providing health programs for populations at risk is described in Chapters 11 through 18.

There are many other roles assumed by the community health nurse; those described above are not all-inclusive. The excitement of this specialty area lies in its diversity.

After surveying a large number of community health nurses who identified themselves as community nurse practitioners, Archer (1976, p. 500) systematically classified community health nursing practice according to functions, primary activity, clientele, focus of practice, kinds of decision making involved, and site of practice (Table 2-1). She also classified their work as either direct, semidirect, or indirect client services (Figure 2-2).

Direct client services usually involve a personal relationship between the nurse and client (which can be a person, a family, a group, or the community). Direct service includes teaching, assessing needs and strengths, providing care, and providing for continuity of care for clients.

Well-functioning semidirect and indirect client services offer to the community health nurse the support that is needed to continually plan and give quality care.

Figure 2-2 demonstrates the relationship of the indirect, semidirect, and direct services to the client and to each other. "The funnel anal-

TABLE 2-1. Typology of Community Health Nursing Practice by Characteristics and Client Subsystems

| Characteristics | Subsystems by nature of client services | | |
	Direct client services	Semidirect client services	Indirect client services
Functional category	Community nursing plus diagnostic-disease-medical specialty Community nursing plus primary care Community nursing plus population group Community nursing plus place or spatial unit	Community nursing plus middle management and teaching	Administration and system maintenance
Primary activity	In-depth services to diagnostic category, usually but not always tied to illnesses Physical and psychosocial assessment; follow-up on deviations from norm and health promotion Wide-range service to designated group: positive health, overt illness, preventive actions Concern with widely defined health issues: delivery of comprehensive care to all in geographic area	Management of personnel and material resources to facilitate delivery of direct client services	Administration, research planning, system development, maintenance and repair, public relations, lobbying
Clientele	Individuals or group members who fit disease category; their family members Individual-centered. Occasionally mother-child; some total family Group and members identified by shared characteristics All those within the spatial unit; communities, especially geographic; institutions	Health workers on all levels; students on all levels	System: Institution, agency, professional organization, funding agency
Focus	Problem-centered on and related to organizing and delivering care to those in disease category Treatment and continuity of care for deviations from norm; health promotion and maintenance Range of problems in client group, especially those particularly related to group membership Part of health care team serving geographic group; widest range of practice: primary, secondary, and tertiary preventive services	Teaching, facilitating, and supervising others who deliver direct client services	Administering, planning, and evaluating direct and semidirect client services, resource development and allocation, research
Decision making	Problem-solving processes, client management, and teaching Sorting at entry point into care system: treat, consult, refer, follow Problem identification; matching resources to needs; transmission of information; advocacy	Teaching, consulting, allocating resources, evaluating those who give direct client services	Planning, evaluating, controlling, allocating, forming policy for direct and semidirect client services.

Characteristics	Subsystems by nature of client services		
	Direct client services	Semidirect client services	Indirect client services
	Assessment, client finding, counseling, teaching, referral; epidemiological investigations and data gathering		
Sites	Health agencies, inpatient and outpatient specialty clinics, occasionally specialist M.D. offices	Health service agencies, educational institutions in middle management, faculty, and discharge planner positions	Top management positions in service and educational institutions, professional organizations, research groups, management consultant firms
	HMOs, OPDs, clinics, M.D. offices, health centers, health departments, independent practice		
	Nonhealth and multipurpose agencies geared to serve client group; urban health centers, senior centers, churches, schools, social service agencies, outreach programs, OPDs		
	Local comprehensive health care centers, health departments, legislative and executive offices in branches of government		

SOURCE: From S. E. Archer. Community nurse practitioners. Another assessment. *Nursing Outlook*, August 1976, *24*, p. 500.

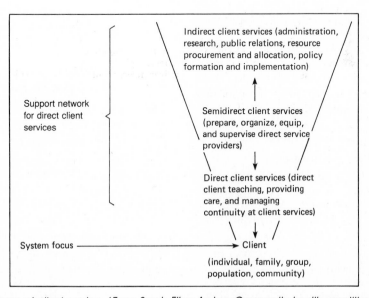

FIGURE 2-2 Subsystems of client service. (*From Sarah Ellen Archer. Community health practitioners: Another assessment. Copyright 1976, American Journal of Nursing Company. Reproduced with permission from Nursing Outlook, August 1976, 24, p. 501.*)

ogy is used to emphasize the system's focus on the client, and the two-way arrows illustrate the interdependence among the subsystems" (Archer, 1976, p. 499).

It is clear from Table 2-1 and Figure 2-2 that there are diverse settings, as well as many roles, in which community health nurses function, all using the philosophy and knowledge of community health nursing practice. Some nurses work in groups and others work alone. The goal of all those working in community health nursing should be to help clients (families, groups at risk, and the community) to attain and maintain their optimum level of functioning.

Public Health Nursing and Community Health Nursing

In Chapter 1, the term *public health nurse* was used. As was evident in that chapter, the term has its historical roots in Florence Nightingale's *health nurse* and Lillian Wald's *public health nurse*. Wald thought that the word *public* denoted a service that was available to all people; however, the public health nurse also came to be associated with the setting of a tax-supported, public agency as the service moved into official (tax-supported) health departments, as well as voluntary visiting nurse associations that are not tax-supported.

The phrase *community health nurse* has become widely used because it denotes a nurse who focuses on the community. The community health nurse deals with people from many backgrounds and cultures and with varying values and attitudes. The nurse considers individuals, families, and groups in the context of the health of the larger community. The health of any one of these affects the health of the other.

Some people use the terms *community health nurse* and *public health nurse* interchangeably. However, not every nurse who works in the community is a community health nurse. Public health or community health nurses have a definitive philosophy of practice as delineated in the ANA definition of community health nursing practice. In this text, the authors have chosen to use the terms *community health nurse* and *community health nursing* because they help to emphasize the focus of the nurse's work—the community—as well as the services given and the underlying philosophy.

Community health nursing involves a high level of independence. There are often no physician's orders to follow, and the result is that the nurse carries out nursing interventions based upon nursing theory, with the guidance of administrative nursing personnel. The community health nurse also deals with numerous other health professionals, such as sanitarians, physicians, and physical and occupational therapists, as well as community agencies. The nurse's independence ranges from developing nursing care plans to deciding what activities to schedule in any given day.

The range of services provided by community health nurses includes communicable disease control, maternal-child health care, health supervision of well families, care of chronic conditions, and concern for the environmental health of people. These services are discussed in depth in the rest of the text.

Size of the Work Force and Work Settings in Community Health Nursing

The number of nurses working in community health has increased dramatically. Some of these changes have been brought about by legislation such as the Social Security amendments of 1965, Medicare and Medicaid.

The earliest known count of public health nurses in the United States was reported by Harriett Fulmer at the International Congress of Nurses in Buffalo, New York, in 1901. At that time, there were 58 public health nursing organizations, employing about 130 nurses. In

1912 Mary Gardner found that approximately 3000 nurses were engaged in community health nursing services. From 1916 to 1931, periodic enumerations of public health nursing agencies and the nurses they employed were recorded by the Statistical Department of the National Organization for Public Health Nursing. Since 1937, the state directors of Public Health Nursing and the Division of Nursing, U.S. Public Health Service, have systematically collected and compiled data about numbers and educational preparation of nurses employed for public health work in the United States. State and local official and nonofficial (voluntary) public health agencies, boards of education, national agencies, universities, and, in some years, industries, have supplied the information. The counts were reported annually from 1937 through 1953, and then in 1955 and 1957, and biennially since 1960 (*Source Book,* 1975, p. 187). Table 2-2 shows the distribution for 1972.

In 1972, there were 11,455 national, state, and local health agencies in the United States, Puerto Rico, Guam, and the Virgin Islands, employing 58,241 registered nurses for public health work. Of all agencies reporting, local official health agencies ranked as the largest employers of nursing staff; they employed nearly 24,000 registered nurses (RNs) and licensed practical nurses (LPNs), or 39 percent of all those in public health. Local boards of education employed the second largest number, accounting for 35 percent of nurses in public health community nursing services.

TABLE 2-2   Nurses in Public Health, 1972

Type of agency	Number of agencies	Number of nurses		
		Total	RNs	LPNs
National agency	8	886	885	1
University	270	916	916	
State agency	151	2,194	2,140	54
Local agency:	11,026	57,550	54,300	3,250
Official agency	2,950	23,854	22,436	1,418
Visiting nurse association and other nonofficial	648	6,118	5,511	607
Combination agency	70	2,341	2,177	164
Organized home health and categorical program	657	3,812	3,061	751
Board of education	6,701	21,425	21,115	310
Total	11,455	61,546	58,241	3,305

SOURCE: From *Source Book, Nursing Personnel, December 1974.* Bethesda, Md.: Government Printing Office, DHEW Publication No. HRA 75-43, 1975, p. 188.

The total numbers of registered nurses employed by health agencies and boards of education for public health-community health services in the United States and territories tripled in the 35 years from 1936 to 1972; the increase from 1962 and 1972 was 60 percent. Figure 2-3 graphically shows the change from 1962 to 1972 (*Source Book,* 1975, p. 188).

SUMMARY

The following typical day in the life of a community health nurse, described in a local newspaper story, illustrates several important concepts (Haradine, 1978): the community health nurse is a generalist and serves all population groups. She or he works in the setting where the client is at home, utilizing principles of primary, secondary, and tertiary intervention. The community health nurse also serves population groups in clinics and schools; concepts from the public health sciences of biostatistics, epidemiology, and administration help the

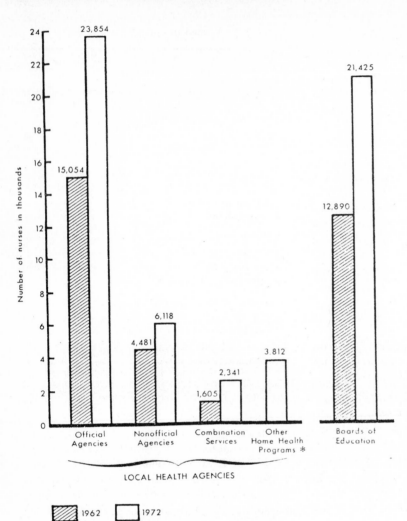

FIGURE 2-3 Registered nurses employed for public health work in local agencies and boards of education, 1962 and 1972. (*Note:* Organized services not included in 1962.) [*From Source Book, Nursing Personnel, December, 1974. (DHEW Publication No. HRA 75-43). Bethesda, Md.: Government Printing Office, 1975, p. 188.*]

community health nurse to identify needs of these populations.

Her first stop by 8 A.M. each day is at her desk in the health department to pick up messages from the day before, make phone calls and plan her day's schedule.

After morning coffee with the other nurses, which offers time for comparisons, she starts her calls.

"Sometimes you've had a dark day and you need input, you need to talk to someone," she explains.

"I could get depressed if I allowed myself, but I realize whose problem it is. It's not my problem. It's only my place to help when I'm accepted."

Many calls start with a request from a school or another public health nurse, or Charlene's own case finding.

Her first stop on a gray, cheerless day recently was a happy one, to visit a new baby. Paul Daniel Conner had spent two months in a hospital nursery after being born prematurely, weighing only 3 pounds, 7 ounces.

Now 2½ months old, he has adjusted easily to his mother's style in the two weeks he has been home.

"He's a perfect baby," says his mother, Julie. "He doesn't ever cry." But she does have a few questions, written on a scrap of paper.

"I was surprised how easy it has been. I've been just really relaxed with him," she tells Charlene.

The routine on a visit to a new baby includes leaving a sheaf of pamphlets for the mother's spare-time reading. Topics include first aid, exercises for the mother, feeding, birth control and descriptions of the free services offered by the health department.

Charlene advises Mrs. Conner not to put Paul Daniel to bed with a bottle.

"A baby will get a pool of milk, juice or Kool-Aid in its mouth that causes tooth decay. I see children with nothing but little brown stubs left of their teeth," she explains.

"You can use your blender to make baby food from table food, then freeze it in an ice cube tray and put it in a bag. But be sure to freeze it."

The telephone number for the Western Michigan Poison Center and instructions on taking a baby's temperature are all part of the routine which ends with a full examination of the baby and measuring its height and weight.

Charlene tells Mrs. Conner she can take her baby to the health department's well-baby clinic in the Belmont area, for children from birth to school age.

"It's one of your benefits as a taxpayer. You can take the baby in for his shots, but continue to see the doctor."

The idea appeals to Mrs. Conner. She takes the information, the telephone number she would use for an appointment.

"You can call me anytime," Charlene says as she leaves. "I'm usually in early in the morning."

Few newborns in Kent County are seen by a public health nurse. Many don't need it; more probably do. All it would take is a call—from the hospital, from the mother, or even from a relative.

"There are many out there I'm not getting, mothers who are having problems adjusting to a new baby, who didn't like children or babies before and now overcompensate," Charlene explains.

A stop at West Oakview School is squeezed in before the students' lunch break to check a girl with bites on her arms and legs (probably flea bites from a cat, Charlene thinks) and a progress report from a class for emotionally impaired youngsters.

At North Oakview School, after lunch, Charlene calls in to her office for messages. Then she visits a "readiness room" for 5-to-7-year-olds taught by Ann Westerhof.

"If Charlene didn't come in once a week, I don't know what I'd do," Mrs. Westerhof exclaims. "She's the go-between for me and the families. She helps me know what I can and can't do."

The "star" of this visit is Jim Fragale, 6, who is sporting a new brace, an unusual contraption with a tripod base and straps that keep his legs bent to aid healing of the hip joints.

The cause of Jim's hip problem is unknown, Charlene explains. "The ball joint of the hip softens, then starts coming back. But the regeneration is dependent on rest and nutrition."

Jim had a little trouble balancing when he was first fitted with the brace, and even fell backwards, Mrs. Westerhof explains. "And he was a little embarrassed by it at first. But now he can show the other students tricks they can't do."

Charlene's link was knowing what agency to contact to make the brace a reality. "So many times, parents can't afford the treatment needed, and Char knows how to get it," Mrs. Westerhof adds.

From the young to the old—that switch in thinking is typical for public health nurses.

Twice a month, Charlene is in charge of the well-baby clinic in Belmont. She sees humanity at its beginnings there, in the tots brought in for free care—routine physical examinations by a doctor, immunizations and advice for parents.

Although the wait can be long, the time can be used to ask a public health nurse about the little doubts, those questions that seem too insignificant for the doctor.

"I thought he'd outgrow it by this time. I guess he won't," one mother was overheard commenting to one of the three nurses staffing the clinic.

These chats, informal and friendly, offer help on parenting to start the young out right.

When the young, at 14 or 15, stumble along the way, Charlene and the other public health nurses are there, just a telephone call away.

Sometimes it's the child's problem, and sometimes it's the parent's, spreading over to the child. "Rare is the teen-ager who will say, 'Hey, I've got a problem,' " Charlene notes. "Some social workers do refer kids to me.

"We see some child abuse cases and we see neglect, which is so hard to prove. It's insidious and camouflaged. Sometimes the parents are too wrapped up in themselves, or it might be a lack of resources, of money.

"We have to know what help is available from the different agencies."

The old pose a different problem, when loneliness and loss have taken their toll. Charlene pulls into a driveway along the Grand River, next to a small house with a tidy yard at 4566 Abrigador Trail NE. It's a call to the other end of life.

"They say I'll live to be 90, but I don't care to," says Josephine Robbins as Charlene takes her blood pressure.

"I know that," Charlene replies, acceptingly, as she removes the blood pressure cuff from the arm of the woman, who is 80.

The youngest of seven, Josephine says, "The others, they're all gone. My sister was 92."

Her husband, Lloyd, died in March. "What do I have to live for?" she asks.

In answer to Charlene's questions on her health, she reports only "a catch in my side" now and then. But she takes "just a little Lydia Pinkham's and it goes away."

An active woman now very lonely and anxious, Josephine looks forward to the weekly nurse visit. "You're not taking any of those pills are you?" Charlene asks in a warning tone.

"No, I threw them out." A neighbor had given Josephine two drugs, Librium (a tranquilizer) and nitroglycerine (a heart drug), saying, "They always helped me. Maybe they'll help you."

Charlene had become aware of them on her last visit when she had asked what medications Josephine was taking.

Josephine worries about getting her things in order, her will, her records and being able to pledge her eyes and kidneys before she dies. "They said I had to come down and sign in front of two witnesses, but I can't get down there," she tells the nurse. Not necessary; just witnesses, there in her home.

Besides the decisions for her will, on the who and what of all she owns, Josephine must finish the mural she is painting on one wall, then paint a scene in a window and refinish some furniture. And then . . .

"There's just an awful lot of red tape," the gray-haired woman comments sadly. "I'm never going to be through."

The public health nurse visits often when the need is great, then as the crisis eases, the visits taper off, to make time and room for someone else with other pressing needs.

Days are filled with joy and sadness. Charlene believes she gets as much as she gives in her 8–5 job. "I need people. I see myself as a helping person and they are fulfilling to me."

But in public health the rewards are seldom quick in coming. "You see something grow. You see a person who has never had any self-confidence make strides.

"I'm really in preventive medicine," Charlene says. "By educating others and by my intervention, I believe I'll make a difference."

REFERENCES

American Nurses' Association. Profile. Health care is a political issue for this nurse. *American Journal of Nursing,* January 1979, *79,* 146.

Archer, S. E. Community nurse practitioners: Another assessment. *Nursing Outlook,* August 1976, *24,* 499–503.

Community health nursing, 1974. WHO Expert Committee Report No. 558. Geneva: World Health Organization, 1974.

Haradine, J. Public health nurse makes a difference. *Grand Rapids Press,* Dec. 3, 1978, 29–33.

Leavell, H. R., & Clark, E. G. *Preventive medicine for the doctor in his community. An epidemiological approach* (3d ed.). New York: McGraw-Hill, 1965.

Parker, E. W. Normative approach to the definition of primary health care. *Milbank Memorial Fund Quarterly,* Fall 1976, *54,* 415–438.

Ruth, M. V., & Partridge, K. B. Differences in perception of education and practice. *Nursing Outlook,* October 1978, *26,* 622–628.

Source Book, Nursing Personnel, December 1974. Bethesda, Md.: Government Printing Office, DHEW Publication No. HRA 75–43, 1975.

Standards, community health nursing practice. Kansas City, Mo.: American Nurses' Association, 1973 (unnumbered pages).

Winslow, C.-E. A. *Man and epidemics.* Princeton, N.J.: Princeton University Press, 1952. Reprinted by permission of Princeton University Press.

SELECTED BIBLIOGRAPHY

Ackerman, N., & Baisel, S. An internship in community health nursing. *Nursing Outlook,* June 1975, *23,* 374–377.

Bernal, B. Levels of practice in a community health agency. *Nursing Outlook,* June 1978, *26,* 364–369.

Davis, A. J., & Underwood, P. Role, function, and decision making in community health nursing. *Nursing Research,* July–August 1976, *25,* 255–258.

Davis, M. Z., Kromer, M., & Strauss, A. L. *Nurses in practice. A perspective on work environments.* St. Louis: Mosby, 1975.

Fagin, C. M. Primary care as an academic discipline. *Nursing Outlook,* December 1978, *26,* 750–753.

Freeman, R. The nurse practitioner in the community health agency. *Journal of Nursing Administration,* November–December 1974, *4,* 21–24.

Heagarty, M. C., Grossi, M. I., & O'Brien, M. Pediatric associates in a large official agency: Their education, productivity, and cost. *American Journal of Public Health,* September 1977, *67,* 855–858.

Highriter, M. E. The status of community health nursing research. *Nursing Research,* May–June 1977, *26,* 183–192.

Igoe, J. B. The school nurse practitioner. *Nursing Outlook,* June 1975, *23,* 381–384.

Levin, L. S. Patient education and self-care: How do they differ? *Nursing Outlook,* March 1978, *26,* 170–175.

O'Brien, M., Manley, M., & Heagarty, M. C. Expanding the public health nurse's role in child care. *Nursing Outlook,* June 1975, *23,* 369–373.

Skrovan, C., Anderson, E. T., & Gottschalk, J. Community nurse practitioner: An emerging role. *American Journal of Public Health,* September 1974, *64,* 847–853.

Werner, J. R. Effective community health nursing: A framework for actualizing standards of practice. *Nursing Forum,* 1976, *15* (3), 265–276.

Williams, C. A. Community health nursing—What is it? *Nursing Outlook,* April 1977, *25,* 250–254.

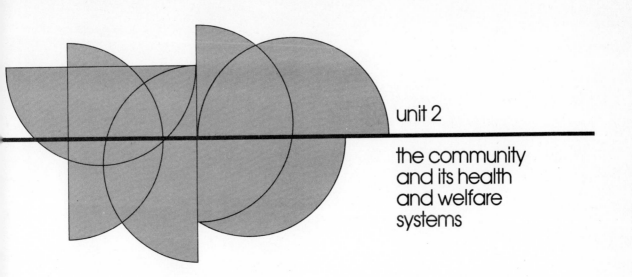

unit 2

the community
and its health
and welfare
systems

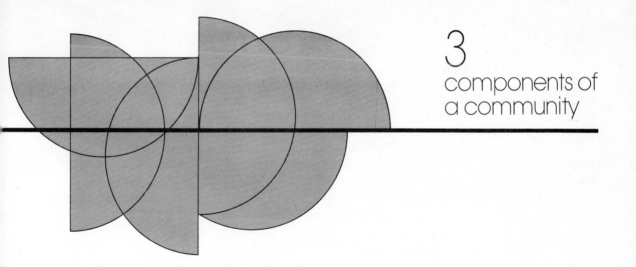

The health problems, solutions, and planning with which the community health nurse is concerned are deeply embedded in the structure of the community. Families, as part of the community, contribute to the health of the community, just as the health of the community contributes to the health of the family. As is stated in the American Nurses' Association definition of community health nursing, "The dominant responsibility is to the population as a whole." Therefore, nursing activities directed to individuals, families, or groups contribute to the health of the total population. The purpose of this chapter is to provide a conceptual framework for the word *community*, which is the "population as a whole," for the community health nurse.

DEFINING COMMUNITY

Physical, social, and political scientists have developed many definitions for the word *community*. Some of these definitions are concrete and relate mainly to legal jurisdictions such as cities, towns, or municipalities, whereas others are more abstract and examine how a group of people is organized to achieve common goals. In this text, the term *community* will be used in its broadest sense: a community is a group of people, in an environment that has the ability to meet their life goals and needs. A community is part of a larger society and has patterns of communication, leadership, and decision making which either facilitate or inhibit interactions within the community and between the community and the larger society.

In order for a community to achieve its goals, it must be organized. It must contain a set of institutions—industry, stores, churches, organizations, schools, and government—so its residents can carry out life within its bounds (Warren, 1972, p. 6). A community encompasses a variety of health care resources which provide both inpatient and outpatient health care services. Often, anything outside the inpatient settings (hospitals, nursing homes, and extended care facilities) is labeled "the community." However, these health care resources are as much a part of the community as are other resources such as the health department, social service agencies, and private practitioners. A community must have inpatient care settings in order to provide comprehensive health care services for members of the community. Without these resources, it would be impossible for a community to meet the emergency, long-term, and acute care needs of its citizenry. It is important for a community health nurse to recognize this fact so that health-planning efforts (see Chapter 12) will be directed toward improving the health services for individuals who have emergency, acute, and long-term needs as well as for individuals who have preventive, diagnostic, and rehabilitative needs.

COMPONENTS OF A COMMUNITY

Communities have the common components of people, goals, needs, environment, service systems, and boundaries. The people of a community have demographic, biologic, social, and cultural characteristics that influence their actions and interactions. They have shared goals and needs related to survival and self-fulfillment that become the essence of community functioning. The community's environment includes (1) *physical characteristics* such as geography, climate, terrain, natural resources, and structural entities (buildings such as schools, workplaces, and homes); (2) *biological and chemical characteristics* such as flora, animal reservoirs, vectors, bacteria, agents, toxic substances, and food supplies; (3) *social characteristics* such as economics, education, health and welfare services, leadership, recreation, and religion. These characteristics combine to make each community unique and will have a major impact on the health and welfare resources a community can provide for its population.

The service systems of a community assist in meeting the goals and needs of the community. Sanders (1966) views the major systems of the community as (1) health, (2) social welfare, (3) education, (4) economic, (5) government, (6) recreation, and (7) religious. These systems have a network of resources that have a philosophy, that deliver services to community members, and that maintain linkages with other systems. A primary function of a community is to mobilize services so that the needs of its population are met (Bevis, 1973).

Community systems are extremely important to the community health nurse because it is through them that many services are provided for individuals, families, and populations at risk. The nurse should take the time to assess all community systems and identify the services they provide, the linkages (communication patterns) between them, how to utilize them effectively, and how each fits into the overall structure and function of the community. All of these systems are essential for maintaining and promoting wellness in a community; their relative importance is influenced by both community needs and community interests. The health system is the central focus for the community health nurse. However, the economic system (economic sufficiency) is the usual focus for the citizenry and leadership of the community (National Commission on Community Health Services, 1966, p. 7). Until a community's basic economic needs are met, it is not likely that people will work diligently on other needs, such as health.

The community components of people,

shared goals and needs, environment, and service systems have boundaries; these boundaries serve to regulate the exchange of energies between a community and its external environment. In general, boundaries may be concrete (definite, spatial) or conceptual (elusive, nonspatial). Concrete boundaries are more absolute and easier to see and to define. They include geographic boundaries (mountains, valleys, and deserts), political boundaries (cities, towns, counties, states, and nations), and situational boundaries (home, school, and work). Conceptual boundaries are less definite and do not necessarily fit into a defined space. They can be such things as interest-area, problem solving, or service-area boundaries.

A community's boundaries are often not concrete. Instead, they conform to the service areas of the community, are flexible, dynamic, and ever changing. Communities may overlap and intermingle and will not always conform to the boundaries of a local political jurisdiction, such as a town or city.

Population Groups in the Community

A community is made up of various population groups. Population groups are clusters of two or more persons with a common characteristic. Population groups can be based on an infinite number of characteristics, including age, sex, race, marital status, religion, occupation, education, income, health conditions, recreational and social activities, neighborhoods, and ethnic origin. Individuals are members of a number of population groups. The community health nurse's role in providing services to population groups based on age-related developmental tasks and populations at risk is discussed throughout this text. A population group that has special significance to this chapter is that cluster of people who make up a neighborhood. The community health nurse works extensively with clients in the neighborhoods in which they live.

Neighborhoods

Neighborhoods have a specific population and boundaries and may provide resources to meet the needs of residents, such as recreational facilities, schools, and shops. A neighborhood is usually unable to meet all the health and welfare needs of its population and must have ties with the larger community. People may identify more closely with their neighborhood than with the community as a whole. Neighborhoods can be looked at in terms of *interaction* in the neighborhood, *identification* with the neighborhood, and *connections* outside the neighborhood (Warren and Warren, 1975, pp. 72–76). Neighborhoods vary greatly in leadership, cohesiveness, self-sufficiency, and ties with the larger community. These neighborhood variances play a significant role in relation to the health services the community health nurse is able to provide residents. Warren (1977, pp. 224–229) has elaborated on this variance in neighborhoods by using the following classifications to identify differences between neighborhoods:

INTEGRAL: The individuals in this setting have frequent face-to-face contacts. The norms, values, and attitudes of the neighborhood support those of the larger community. People are cohesive within the neighborhood but belong to other groups outside their area of residence. There is a form of power, authority, and leadership within this type of neighborhood which aids its members to reach out to the larger society for assistance when a problem arises that cannot be handled internally.

PAROCHIAL: People in this setting also have face-to-face contacts, but there is an absence of ties to the larger community. These neighborhoods tend to be protective of their status, screen out values that do not conform to their own, and enforce their own beliefs within the neighborhood. The power, authority, and leadership structure within this type of neigborhood encourages isolation from the larger community.

DIFFUSE: Neighbors within this type of environment interact infrequently with each other and have few ties with the larger community. There is often a lack of shared norms, values, and attitudes. A primary tie between these neighbors is geographic proximity to one another. There may be little or no leadership in these areas. When leadership exists, it is often not representative of the entire neighborhood, but is composed of an "elitist" leadership that ignores or subverts the values of most residents. Groups of residents, such as those living in a public housing unit, may be categorized and separated from the mainstream of the neighborhood.

STEPPING-STONE: This type of neighborhood is characterized by a rapid membership turnover and families who have a weak sense of identity with the neighborhood. Members are willing to give up the ties established in the neighborhood if other commitments arise; they strive to attain a higher social status. Residents of these areas do, however, have close ties to the larger community and do interact regularly with neighbors. Leadership is usually not effective because of the high rate of mobility; conflicts arise between the needs of the local neighborhood and the values of social mobility.

TRANSITORY: Members of this kind of neighborhood fail to participate in or identify with the local community. There is an emphasis on people keeping to themselves, because links with others may interfere with the goals of the individual and the family. There may be a widespread feeling of mistrust in this type of neighborhood.

ANOMIC: Such a neighborhood is completely disorganized; its residents lack participation in and a common identification with the neighborhood or the larger community. This neighborhood reflects mass apathy and is not likely to influence or alter the values of its residents through any form of socialization. There is little interaction between people within the neighborhood or between the neighborhood and the larger community, and leadership activity is largely lacking.

Identifying the type of neighborhood in which one is working helps the community health nurse to assess and plan for meeting health needs. For example, if a community health nurse is working in a parochial neighborhood, it would be imperative for her or him to work closely with neighborhood leaders in the delivery of health care services. The nurse may find that the parochial neighborhood readily becomes involved in providing services for its residents. However, there also may be more resistance in this neighborhood to health services proposed by the larger community which do not coincide with neighborhood values and beliefs. In an anomic neighborhood, on the other hand, the community health nurse may find little neighborhood leadership and may want to invest effort in developing this leadership to facilitate implementation of health care services. In addition, the nurse may find that the anomic neighborhood offers few services to its residents and that services need to be sought extensively from outside the neighborhood.

Whatever the type of neighborhood, its structure has implications for the activities of the community health nurse. Neighborhoods, as part of the community, play an important role in providing for the needs of the population. Communities meet these population needs by carrying out specific functions.

COMMUNITY FUNCTIONS

In order to provide for the life goals and needs of its population, the community carries out a number of functions. Warren (1972, p. 167) lists the following functions of a community:

1. *Production-distribution-consumption.* The community produces, distributes, and utilizes goods and services that are essential for meeting the health and welfare needs of its residents. This triad of activities provides opportunities which help community residents to carry out activities of daily living, and it involves extensive resource coordination. Establishing and supporting local companies and businesses are an integral part of this function, because community residents need employment to meet their basic needs (food, clothing, and shelter) and the community needs funds from taxes to maintain its systems. Tax funds from industry and business significantly contribute to the economic stability of a community.

2. *Socialization.* This is the process by which prevailing knowledge, values, beliefs, customs, and behavior are transmitted to a community's members. It is a lifelong process which helps persons to learn how to effectively relate in a social environment and to develop a philosophy of life.

3. *Social control.* The community influences the behavior of its members through norms and rules of social control. Social control has a legal component that is often enforced through law agencies, courts, and the government. It also has a "social sanction" component that is enforced by the family, neighborhood residents, friends, and the educational, religious, and recreational systems. Social control helps to safeguard and protect the community.

4. *Social participation.* People have basic needs for self-expression and self-fulfillment. These needs are largely met through interaction with others. Social participation is primarily carried out through the community's private sector. This function provides opportunity for members of the community to achieve psychosocial wellness.

5. *Mutual support.* This involves people lending help and assistance to one another. It is frequently offered through family, friends, neighbors, and religious groups, as well as official health departments and departments of social service within the community.

The ability to carry out these functions is a major determinant of whether or not a community really exists. These functions provide for the services and activities necessary for community life. The community health nurse must be aware of these functions and how a community implements them in order to effectively assess and plan for essential nursing services in the community.

The way in which a community carries out all of its functions makes an impact on how well the community health nurse will be able to meet the needs of the population being served. For example, if there is a gap in production-distribution-consumption, the community may not have the health resources to meet the health needs of its population. If people have not been socialized to value preventive health care, or if they have customs (such as religious fasting) that affect the delivery of health care services, the nurse's ability to effectively implement preventive health care services can be hindered. If there is no adequate community health policy and enforcement of social control, the biopsychosocial health of the community may be in jeopardy. If the members of the community do not value social interaction and participation, the community's response to clinics, classes, and other group activities may not be maximized. If a community does not lend mutual support to its residents, there may be few health and welfare assistance programs that provide community services.

COMMUNITY DYNAMICS

Community dynamics occur as a result of interactions within the community and between the community and the larger society. Critical to the dynamics of the community are its patterns of communication, leadership, and decision making.

Communities have both horizontal and vertical patterns of communication (Warren, 1972, p. 237). *Vertical patterns* of communication link the community to the larger society (state, national, and international); *horizontal patterns* of communication link the community to itself, its people, environment, and systems. The strength, cohesiveness, and ease with which these patterns operate will largely determine the extent to which the community is able to be self-sufficient and provide for the needs of its membership. The horizontal patterns of communication are especially important, because they influence the internal dynamics of the community.

The *leadership* and *decision-making* processes within a community critically influence how well a community will function. The community usually has elected, appointed, and legal (official, manifest) leadership, such as a mayor or city council. However, much of a community's leadership is less obvious and takes more effort to decipher and detect. A community may have the obvious political leadership of a mayor but also many other leaders that are unofficial. This nonofficial leadership includes the "heroes" of the community, those whom the people in the community revere and respect, plus people of power and authority. The local community religious leader whom people often go to for advice and guidance and the wealthy philanthropist that heavily subsidizes community activities are examples of nonofficial leaders. These people may have more influence, power, and control over community decision making and action than the elected government leaders. They are also more diverse and numerous.

The leadership in the community needs to be assessed by the community health nurse, because community leaders greatly influence what type of services will be available for community residents. The nurse should be aware of official leaders and their health and welfare responsibilities within a community, as well as the nonofficial leaders. Knowing these leaders

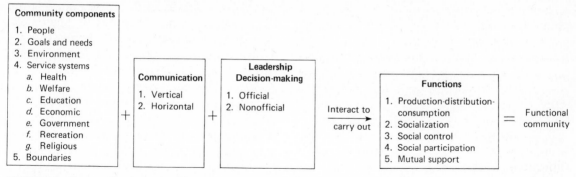

FIGURE 3-1 Community dynamics. [*Service systems data from I. T. Sanders. The community: An introduction to a social system (2d ed.). New York: Ronald, 1966. Communication and function data from R. I. Warren. The community in America (2d ed.). Chicago: Rand-McNally, 1972, pp. 167 and 237.*]

and their patterns of functioning can facilitate the implementation of health care services in the community.

One major community system may have a form of leadership or authority over another. The religious system is a good example, because it influences the health practices of its members. The religious practices of fasting, eating or not eating certain foods, and prohibiting the use of certain health care services, such as general medical care, blood transfusions, and family planning methods, are examples of how religious beliefs make an impact on the health care delivery system.

The dynamics of a community result in community action, change, and development. They will determine the community's ability to be self-sufficient and affect community health and well-being. Figure 3-1 summarizes these dynamics.

THE HEALTH SYSTEM AND THE COMMUNITY

The health system is a major community system. It consists of facilities, organizations, a work force, and funding to implement health care services. The health of a community will depend upon its ability to work toward common health goals and upon adequate distribution of health resources to all members (Hanchett, 1979, p. 46). The priority a community places on health varies and will affect health care resources and their distribution. Health care resources include individuals and groups or agencies, such as private health practitioners, volunteers, hospitals, clinics, pharmacies, nursing homes, health departments, and departments of social services. These resources are both governmental and private (Chapters 4 and 5). Utilization of these resources is presented in Chapter 9.

Private-sector provision of health care services in the community is based on supply and demand and fee-for-service. The government (official) sector provides traditional public health services, such as communicable disease control, through official health departments at no or little cost to the consumer.

The health service area for a community is the area within which a problem can be defined, dealt with, and solved (Ruybal, Bauwens, and Fasla, 1975, p. 365). Within this health service area, the nurse must be familiar with the health needs of the people and available health resources and services. In order to meet client needs, the community health nurse often utilizes health resources outside the confines of a political jurisdiction. For instance, she or he may refer families to a medical center in another area, because the medical care needs of these persons cannot be met by local community resources.

Difficulties in the Community Health System

When the nurse analyzes the community's health system, there are several concerns that may become apparent. Communication between the health care system and the other community systems has historically been weak (see Chapter 5). In many communities, official local health departments have little contact with private health care resources and other official health and welfare resources. The health system of the community also may have little direct communication with the people of the community.

No one agency has statutory (legal) responsibility for coordinating the health resources and services in the community, and the responsibility for management of these resources is often vague. Having one agency whose major role is to coordinate health services and to function as a health information center for the community would facilitate more effective delivery and utilization of community health resources.

Not only is the overall management of the health system weak, but the management skills of individual health practitioners are also weak. Health practitioners frequently do not have educational experiences which prepare them to manage health care resources (see Chapter 20). Health care professionals must understand the principles of management if the health care system is to exist effectively and carry out its functions (National Commission on Community Health Services, 1966, p. 134).

Another problem community health nurses frequently experience is the community's adherence to traditional stands on health. American communities have historically reacted better to disaster and catastrophic health events than to providing ongoing, preventive community health services. There is usually general indifference to a health problem as long as no serious or long-term effects are apparent (Smolensky, 1977, p. 52). The feeling within the community that the responsibility for health concerns rests with official health departments, private health care practitioners, and health care facilities deters community involvement in health. This is unfortunate, because "health is a community affair" (National Commission on Community Health Services, 1966).

The community may not actively support health activities (Smolensky, 1977, p. 52). This occurs for a variety of reasons, including other community priorities, a lack of information on health issues and resources, and a lack of understanding about the role the community can play in establishing and promoting positive health practices for its membership. The health system often does not include the community in health planning, implementation, and evaluation. There is a need for increased cooperation and collaboration between the community and the health care delivery system; an appreciation of all aspects of health, as well as a plan to meet future health needs, could evolve from such efforts.

The National Commission on Community Health Services issued the following futuristic goals for community health systems:

All communities of this nation must take the action necessary to provide comprehensive personal health services of high quality to all people in the community. These services should embrace those directed toward promotion of positive good health, application of established preventive measures, early detection of disease, prompt and effective treatment, and physical, social, and vocational rehabilitation of those with residual disabilities. This broad range of personal health services must be patterned so as to assure full and intelligent use by all groups in the community.

Success in this endeavor will mean change. It will require removal of racial, economic, organizational, residential, and geographic barriers to the use of health services. It will require strengthened and expanded licensure and accreditation of services, manpower, and facilities. It will require maximum coverage through health insurance and other prepayment plans, and extension of such insurance to cover the broad range of services both in and out of hospitals. Finally, success will require citizenry that is sufficiently well informed and motivated to follow established principles conducive to good health services in all phases of prevention and treatment of illness and disability.

IMPLICATIONS OF COMMUNITY DYNAMICS FOR THE COMMUNITY HEALTH NURSE

The community health nurse is in the unique position of being able to see the community carry out its functions and activities on a day-to-day basis. Unlike many other health practitioners, the community health nurse is out in the community on a regular basis, working with its people and systems. She or he provides services in homes, schools, clinics, industry, and other settings and thus has multiple opportunities to collect data about community dynamics and to comprehensively assess the community. Through the knowledge gained from these opportunities, the community health nurse has a base for analyzing strengths and deficiencies in the health care delivery system. Community data need to be gathered systematicallly and community diagnoses must be made (Chapter 11). There is an abundance of instruments for collecting and systematizing community data (Christianson, 1977, p. 9). One such tool is provided in the Appendix to this chapter.

When there are service gaps in the community, many options are open to the nurse through the health planning process (Chapter 12). The nurse knows that without adequate resources and services within the various community systems, community functions will not be carried out.

The community health nurse is often an employee of an official health department. These health departments generally operate at the state, county, and city levels of government and limit service provision to the specific political jurisdiction that they represent. The community health nurse hired by a health department provides services for clients in a specified political jurisdiction. However, the community health nurse must realize that political jurisdictions do not always reflect a community, or correspond to a community's health needs or service area.

Working with clients (individuals, families, populations at risk, and communities) becomes far more exciting when the community health nurse understands the dynamics of the community. Having this knowledge, coupled with flexibility in meeting the changing health needs of the community, facilitates high-level wellness.

SUMMARY

The community is not an easily or consistently defined entity. It is a nebulous, complex concept. However, it is within the confines of the community that nurses discover and then help to solve health problems. Community health nurses focus attention on the population as a whole, groups at risk, and health-planning activities that meet the needs of all community members. Developing a conceptual understanding of the word *community* and how health problems are generated and solved within the community setting is the first step in carrying out the unique responsibilities of the community health nurse.

APPENDIX 3-1
Community Assessment Tool: Overview of Its People, Environment, and Systems

Community_____ Date_____

Check (✔) appropriate column	Strengths	Potential need	Problems
I. PEOPLE			
A. Vital and demographic statistics			
1. Population density			
2. Population composition			
a. Sex ratio			
b. Age distribution			
c. Race distribution			
3. Population characteristics			
a. Mobility			
b. Socioeconomic status			
c. Employment status			
d. Years of school completed			
e. Marriage rate			
f. Divorce rate			
g. Dependency ratio			
h. Fertility rate			
4. Mortality characteristics			
a. Crude death rate			
b. Infant mortality rate			
c. Maternal mortality rate			
d. Age-specific death rate			
e. Leading causes of death			
5. Morbidity characteristics			
a. Incidence rate (specific diseases)			
b. Prevalence rate (specific diseases)			
B. History of community (i.e., founding, growth)			

Check (✔) appropriate column	Strengths	Potential need	Problems
C. Ethnic origin			
D. Values, attitudes, and norms			
E. Family systems 1. Types of families (i.e., head of household)			
2. Number of children per family			
F. Housing (types available by percent, condition, percent rented, percent owned)			
II. ENVIRONMENTAL *A*. Physical 1. Natural resources			
2. Geography			
3. Climate			
4. Terrain			
B. Biological and chemical 1. Animal reservoirs or vectors			
2. Toxic substances			
3. Food supply			
4. Pollutants			

Check (✔) appropriate column	Strengths	Potential need	Problems
5. Flora and fauna			
C. Is this a predominately urban, suburban, or rural community?			
III. SYSTEMS A. Health 1. Preventive health care practices and facilities (list)			
2. Treatment health care facilities (i.e., acute care, medical and surgical hospitals) (list)			
3. Rehabilitation health care facilities (i.e., alcoholism) (list)			
4. Long-term health care facilities (list)			
5. Respite care services for special population groups (list)			
6. Hospice care services			
7. Catastrophic health care facilities and services			
8. School health services (what and how provided)			

Check (✔) appropriate column	Strengths	Potential need	Problems
9. Occupational health services			
10. Sanitation services			
11. Health work force (population ratios)			
12. Health education activities			
13. Methods of health care financing (approximate percent) *a.* Private pay			
b. Health insurance			
c. HMO			
d. Medicaid/Medicare			
14. Prevalent diseases and conditions (list)			
15. Linkages with other systems			
16. Health care resource overall availability			
17. Health care resource overall utilization			

Check (✔) appropriate column	Strengths	Potential need	Problems

B. Welfare
   1. Official (public) welfare resources (list)
     a. General (i.e., Department of Social Services)			

b. Safety and protection (i.e., fire department)			
2. Transportation resources (public and private)			
3. Facilities to meet needs (i.e., shopping areas, public housing)			
4. Resource accessibility			
5. Resource utilization			
C. Education 1. Public educational facilities (i.e., schools, colleges)			
2. Private educational facilities (list)			
3. Libraries (list)			
4. Educational services for special populations a. Pregnant teens			
b. Adults			
c. Developmentally disabled children			

Check (✔) appropriate column	Strengths	Potential need	Problems
d. Other			
5. Resource accessibility			
6. Resource utilization			
D. Economic 1. Major industry and businesses (list)			
2. Banks, savings and loan, credit unions (list)			
3. Major occupations (list)			
4. General socioeconomic status of population			
5. Median income			
6. Percent of population below poverty level			
E. Government and leadership 1. Elected (official) leadership (list with title)			
2. Nonofficial leadership (list with title affiliations)			
3. City offices (location, hours, services)			
4. Accessibility to constituents			

Check (✔) appropriate column	Strengths	Potential need	Problems
5. Support of community resources			
F. Recreation 　　1. Public facilities (list)			
2. Private facilities			
3. Recreational activities frequently utilized (list)			
4. Leisure activities frequently utilized (list)			
5. Coordination with educational recreation facilities and programs			
6. Programs for special population groups 　　　　*a.* Elderly			
b. People who are handicapped			
c. Other			
7. Resource accessibility			
8. Resource utilization			
G. Religion 　　1. Facilities by denomination (list)			
2. Religious leaders (list)			

Check (✔) appropriate column	Strengths	Potential need	Problems
3. Community programs and services			
4. Resource accessibility			
5. Resource utilization			
IV. COMMUNITY DYNAMICS (describe) A. Communication (diagram and describe) 1. Vertical (community to larger society)			
2. Horizontal (community to itself)			
3. Specific resources (i.e., TV, radio, newspapers)			
V. MAJOR SOURCES OF COMMUNITY DATA A. Government (i.e., local health department, city office)			
B. Private (i.e., chamber of commerce)			

QUESTIONS FOR THE COMMUNITY HEALTH NURSE

1. In general, are resources readily available and accessible?

2. How does the community view and utilize the health care system?

3. What does the community see as its major strengths and needs?

4. How self-sufficient is the community in meeting its perceived needs?

5. What does the community health nurse see as the community's major strengths and needs?

6. What goals does the community have and how does it plan to meet them?

Goals	Activities to implement

Assessor_____ Date_____
Assessor_____ Date_____
Assessor_____ Date_____

NOTE: The material presented in Chapters 3, 4, 5, 11, and 12 is especially helpful to the nurse when utilizing this tool. The nurse would initially collect the data in this tool and then add to it on an ongoing basis.

REFERENCES

Bevis, E. M. *Curriculum building in nursing: A process.* St. Louis: Mosby, 1973.

Christianson, J. Z. A community data base record. Houston: University of Texas Health Science Center, unpublished Master of Public Health thesis. March 1977.

Hanchett, E. S. *Community health assessment.* New York: Wiley, 1979.

National Commission on Community Health Services. *Health is a community affair.* Cambridge, Mass.: Harvard University Press, 1966.

Ruybal, S. E., Bauwens, E., & Fasla, M. J. Community assessment: An epidemiological approach. *Nursing Outlook,* June 1975, *23,* 365–368.

Sanders, I. T. *The community: An introduction to a social system* (2d ed.). New York: Ronald, 1966.

Smolensky, J. *Principles of community health* (4th ed.). Philadelphia: Saunders, 1977.

Warren, R. I. *The community in America* (2d ed.). Chicago: Rand McNally, 1972.

———(Ed.). *New perspectives on the American community* (3d ed.). Chicago: Rand McNally, 1977.

Warren, R. L., & Warren, R. B. Six kinds of neighborhoods. *Psychology Today,* June 1975, 72–76.

SELECTED BIBLIOGRAPHY

ANA divisions report on practice . . . . Community health. *American Nurse,* Oct. 15, 1978, *10,* 7.

Bertrand, A. L. *Social organization: A general systems and role theory perspective.* Philadelphia: Davis, 1972.

Flynn, B. C. One master's curriculum in community health nursing. *Nursing Outlook,* October 1978, *26,* 633–637.

Greenburg, M. A concept of community. *Social Work,* January 1974, *19,* 64–72.

Hawley, A. H. *Human ecology: A theory of community structure.* New York: Ronald, 1950.

Kaplan, B. H. (Ed.). *Further explorations in social psychology.* New York: Basic Books, 1974, pp. 195–209.

Klein, D. C. *Community dynamics and mental health.* New York: Wiley, 1968.

Mercer B. E. *The American community.* New York: Random House, 1956.

Ostrand, L., & Willis, W. Faculty preparation: An MPH or MSN degree? *Nursing Outlook,* October 1978, *26,* 637–740.

Ruybal, S. E. Community health planning. *Family and Community Health,* April 1978, *1,* 81–90.

Sanders, I. T. The community: Structure and function. *Nursing Outlook,* September 1963, *11,* 642–645.

———. *Rural society.* Englewood Cliffs, N.J.: Prentice-Hall, 1977.

Warren, R. L. (ed.). *Perspectives of the American community.* Chicago: Rand McNally, 1966.

Williams, C. A. Community health nursing . . . . What is it? *Nursing Outlook,* April 1977, *25,* 250–254.

Wilson, P. Linkages among organizations: Considerations and consequences. *Health and Social Work,* May 1978, *3,* 13–33.

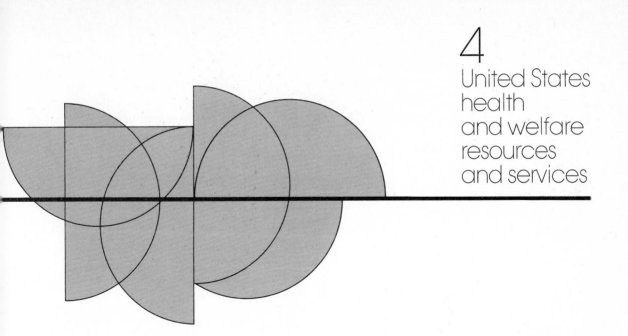

Health and welfare practices have evolved over the ages. It is known that as early as 1500 B.C. the Hebrews had a written hygienic code in Leviticus that dealt with personal and community hygiene (Hanlon, 1974, p. 14). The Egyptians and Romans of 1000 B.C. had elaborate sewage, drainage, and water supply systems, provisions for keeping public streets clean, pharmaceutical preparations, surgical treatments, and rigorous personal hygiene measures. However, during the Middle Ages (A.D. 500 to 1350) many of these past practices were ignored. Humankind has continually changed health and welfare policies to meet the demands and societal attitudes of the time. Examining the reasons for these changes helps one to understand the origins of many contemporary health and welfare practices and how they are changing.

This chapter was designed to create an awareness of the historical evolution of the health and welfare systems in the United States, as well as an understanding of current legislative trends and existing health and welfare services and resources. It is an overview and does not examine structural-functional relationships or apply the concepts presented. Application of this information to community health nursing practice is discussed throughout the text; the organization of these resources is discussed in Chapter 5.

EUROPEAN INFLUENCE ON UNITED STATES HEALTH AND WELFARE POLICY

European influence has been singled out because of the significant impact it had on the development of United States health and welfare policy. Health and welfare policies in the United States reflect a background that is European, primarily English.

Europe was not always a pacesetter in health practices. Europeans of the Middle Ages chose to ignore many of the health practices of previous times and cultures. They allowed refuse

The authors are indebted to Professor Dorothy Donabedian, colleague and friend, whose efforts have stimulated both student and faculty awareness of the health and welfare systems, as they apply to community health nursing practice. Her enthusiasm, encouragement, and suggestions in this work have been greatly appreciated.

to accumulate in streets and dwellings, dumped human waste into public water supplies, improperly stored and prepared foods, and often ignored personal hygiene. These practices did little to promote health, but did much to establish European trade routes as the demand for perfumes and spices rose.

During this time, epidemics of cholera, smallpox, typhoid, plague, and diphtheria raged. In the 1300s, bubonic plague came close to exterminating the human race, killing nearly one-half of the world's population. Epidemics have never been seen since at such magnitude. There was little government intervention in matters of public health, and the major impetus to the development of public health practices was the control of communicable disease.

During the Middle Ages in Europe, the sick, disabled, and poor were largely ignored as a public responsibility. Self-help, the responsibility of individuals to care for themselves, was the prevailing policy, and poverty was often equated with crime. Beggars and vagrants could be physically punished or imprisoned. The belief in divine causation, that conditions reflect the will and judgment of God, flourished and greatly influenced the direction of health and welfare policies. Conditions such as poverty, illness, and disability were viewed as originating in divine causation rather than societal causation. Any welfare assistance that existed was usually church-sponsored and -administered, rather than government-controlled. A step toward government involvement in welfare programs occurred in 1601 with the enactment of the Elizabethan Poor Law.

The Elizabethan Poor Law of 1601

A severe economic depression spurred the enactment of the Elizabethan Poor Law of 1601. Large-scale, involuntary unemployment and the fear of insurrection stimulated the govern-ment to provide welfare aid for select persons (Coll, 1971, p. 5). This law granted the right to assistance through taxation, and established three major categories of dependent people: the vagrant, the involuntarily unemployed, and the helpless (Coll, 1971, p. 5). The helpless included widows, the disabled, and dependent children. The last two categories were deemed as the "worthy" poor. Poor law concepts included:

1. *Local administration.* Administration was at the local level, usually through the church parish. The locality decided on the amount and type of aid to be given and who would receive it.

2. *General aid.* Aid was usually available to the worthy poor, and others could be jailed or physically punished.

3. *Responsible relative.* Relatives could be held responsible for the financial support of each other.

4. *Restrictive residence.* The locality of the individual's origin was responsible for the financial support of the individual. An indigent who migrated from his or her locality of origin could be returned to it.

5. *Individual means test.* Aid was administered on an individual basis through determination of means and needs. Local jurisdictions exercised the right to use moral qualifications to determine who was worthy of assistance.

6. *Minimal subsistence.* A recipient was to receive no more assistance than what was necessary to exist.

7. *Compulsory work or service.* Work or service by the recipient was often compulsory to obtain assistance, and refusal to work could be a punishable crime. Workhouses for the indigent were commonplace.

8. *Funding through taxation.* Funds to administer the poor law were raised through local taxes.

The Elizabethan Poor Law was a forerunner of United States welfare policy, and all of the original 13 colonies adopted it in some form. Following poor law tradition, the United States left administration of assistance programs largely under a local control, implemented responsible relative clauses, administered means tests, provided only minimal subsistence, encouraged or mandated work or service, imposed restrictive residency, and derived revenues through taxation. Restrictive residency laws have since been found to be unconstitutional in the United States. However, most original poor law concepts are still evident in our health and welfare policy.

In 1832, the English Parliament appointed a royal commission to revise the poor law, and in 1834 the revisions were implemented. Edwin Chadwick was a member of this commission and later, in 1842, he published the *Report of the Labouring Population and on the Means of Its Improvement.* It detailed the unsanitary conditions under which the laborers lived, the lack of proper refuse disposal, contaminated water supplies, and generally poor living conditions. He cited these conditions as the primary reasons for public health problems, such as high morbidity and mortality rates, rather than divine causation. Chadwick's report helped to bring about the passage of the English Public Health Act of 1848. The health practices of the time still dealt largely with the control of communicable disease, rather than with the preventive aspects of health. Government intervention in matters of health was minimal.

The following years saw significant strides worldwide in health theory and practice. Advances were made in health as disease conditions were recognized and differentiated; the sciences of bacteriology, virology, immunology, and pharmacology emerged; antibiotics and sterile techniques were developed; the importance of vectors in disease transmission and control became known; and advanced training for health professionals was enlarged.

UNITED STATES SOCIETAL INFLUENCE ON HEALTH AND WELFARE POLICY

The concepts of divine causation, self-help, minimal government intervention, and control of communicable disease prevailed in the United States. The word *health* was left out of the United States constitution, and each state was made responsible for legislating its own health law. Federal intervention in public health and welfare assistance programs was almost nonexistent in our early history. When government health and welfare programs existed, they were largely administered by the individual states.

The Shattuck Report

A major impetus to developing United States public health policy was the Shattuck Report, written in 1850 by Lemuel Shattuck, a teacher, statistician, and legislator. This report recommended such measures as the creation of state and local boards of health; collection of vital statistics; supervision of housing, factories, sanitation, and foods; procurement of immunizations; community health control measures; and school health and health education (Georke and Stebbins, 1968, p. 27). The majority of Shattuck's recommendations are accepted today as sound public health practice.

At the time of Shattuck's report, institutions and almshouses (poorhouses) were the major form of welfare assistance in this country. These were residential placements that separated the poor, disabled, and ill from the mainstream of the general population. With the advent of the Social Security Act of 1935, and the availability of financial assistance for the elderly, many almshouse placements were no longer necessary. However, institutions are still a part of our country's health and welfare tradition. The constitutionality of institutional placements for individuals, such as people who are mentally retarded, is currently being challenged in the United States court system.

Development of Voluntary Agencies

By the 1870s voluntary agencies were beginning to emerge and to work with America's health and welfare problems. In 1872, the American Public Health Association (APHA) was founded by Dr. Stephen Smith. This voluntary health association was concerned with protecting and promoting the health of the nation.

In 1877, the first charity organization society was founded in Buffalo, New York, to coordinate private, voluntary (nonprofit) welfare assistance activities. Many similar organizations developed in other cities. By the early twentieth century, groups such as the American Red Cross, the Rockefeller Foundation, the Commonwealth Foundation, and the Kellogg Foundation were established as private, voluntary health and welfare organizations. At this time, private profit-making health insurance programs were emerging as well. Voluntary organizations and individuals are an integral part of our health and welfare services. This voluntary tradition is to be applauded and is discussed in depth in Chapter 5.

Establishing Government Involvement in Health and Welfare

The U.S. Public Health Service was established in 1798. In 1879, the National Board of Health, forerunner of the Department of Health, Education, and Welfare, was established. In 1912, the United States enacted a Public Health Act. Involvement by the federal government in public health and welfare was minimal, and health and welfare services were largely left to the states. The system of federal grant-in-aid to states originated in 1919 and supplied revenue to states for health and welfare programs.

By 1919, all states had a government branch dealing with health, often known as the state department of public health (Smolensky, 1977, p. 168). State public health programs focused on the control of communicable disease and maternal-child health problems. Also by this time, many states had a government branch dealing with welfare, often a state department of social services. State welfare assistance programs largely focused on providing services to widows, dependent children, and the indigent elderly. State welfare insurance programs, in the form of workers' compensation, began to evolve in 1911. State and local taxes comprised the major source of revenue for health and welfare assistance programs.

The Great Depression

The Great Depression started with the stock market crash of 1929 and reached a peak in 1933 when 13 million persons, 25 percent of the work force, were unemployed. Neither privately nor government-funded health and welfare programs could handle the health and welfare demands created by this event, and possibly no other single event has had such an impact on United States health and welfare policy. The Depression showed the general public that anyone could become poor. It dealt a mortal blow to the belief of divine causation, because many people that the general public believed were not deserving of poverty became impoverished. There was considerable public pressure for the federal government to assist those in need.

A major concern that developed as a result of the Depression was the large, young, unemployed labor force. New jobs were hard to generate, and many jobs were held by older workers with seniority. There was no mandatory retirement age, and few retirement pension plans. The idea of mandatory retirement of workers with the retiree being eligible for a government pension emerged. This concept became a major part of the Social Security Act of 1935.

The Social Security Act of 1935

Out of the Depression came the federal Social Security Act of 1935. It has since undergone major amendment on some 15 occasions to incorporate other programs (Cohen, 1979, p.

1420). The passage of the Social Security Act gave the United States the dubious distinction of being the last of the major industrial nations to develop a federal welfare program (Institute of Gerontology, 1970, p. 2). For the first time, major health and welfare programs were consolidated under one law (Donabedian, 1980). The act established insurance programs (contributory) and assistance programs (noncontributory). Contributory programs are financed through both taxation and individual contributions, whereas assistance programs are financed only through taxation. It is a landmark piece of legislation, possibly the major one of our time.

UNITED STATES HEALTH AND WELFARE LEGISLATION

Each year many laws with health and welfare implications are enacted, and many existing laws are amended. This section is presented to give the nurse an awareness of significant health and welfare legislation, because community health nurses work daily with programs made possible by local, state, and federal legislation. An in-depth perspective on these laws can be obtained by reading materials specific to each piece of legislation in the *United States Code—Congressional and Administrative News* and the *United States Statutes at Law.*

Health and welfare legislation should be examined and understood in terms of its administration, funding, services offered, clients served, service delivery, and quality control. This type of information is needed in order for the community health nurse to effectively help clients to obtain services available to them, as well as to identify gaps in the delivery of health and welfare services. When gaps or deficiencies are identified, the community health nurse utilizes the principles of health planning to correct these problems (see Chapter 12).

Administration of Health and Welfare Legislation

Health and welfare legislation is administered through many offices, staffs, agencies, and departments of government. The responsibility to carry out this legislation is often as much a matter of historical development and organizational relationships as it is of rational decision making (Wilner, Walkley, and O'Neill, 1978, p. 34). Most federal health and welfare legislation is administered by the Department of Health and Human Services, formerly the Department of Health, Education, and Welfare.

Health and welfare administration varies in each state; it is not always identical to the federal system of administration. Some states have "super agencies," much like the Department of Health and Human Services, that incorporate a variety of health and welfare programs. Other states separate health and welfare components and administer them by separate agencies. State welfare services are often administered by a department of social services;

health services are often administered by a department of public health. State governments must adhere to federal health and welfare law, and are only allowed to exercise the powers delegated to them by the federal government.

Local health and welfare administration also varies. Each locality has its own agencies, ordinances, rules, and codes. Local governments must adhere to state and federal laws. If a locality is unable or refuses to enforce health and welfare law, the state can assist it or assume control.

The specific organization of health and welfare resources and services will be discussed in Chapter 5. It is a complicated system, but one with which the community health nurse should be familiar in order to facilitate the utilization of services by clients.

Major United States Health and Welfare Legislation

There were several acts of legislation that had a major impact on the development of health and welfare policy and practices in the United States. Of these, the Social Security Act of 1935 and the Public Health Service Act of 1944 are probably the most significant. Many new laws are amendments to these two acts; a large number of the health and welfare resources that the community health nurse will utilize on behalf of clients relate to these pieces of legislation. When examining the legislation presented, please note that federal laws are designated as Public Law and are followed by the number of the congressional session and the sequential number of the law.

Social Security Act of 1935 (Public Law 74-721) as Amended

The Social Security Act was a giant step toward safeguarding the health and welfare of Americans. When the act was passed in 1935, it included both welfare insurance and welfare assistance programs. Originally its *welfare insurance*

programs included the federal program of Old Age Insurance (OAI) and the federal-state program of Unemployment Insurance. Its categorical *welfare assistance* programs were originally the federal-state programs of Aid to the Blind (AB), Old Age Assistance (OAA), and Aid to Dependent Children (ADC). It also provided funds for services to crippled children and high-risk mothers and children. Shortly after it was passed, it was amended to include welfare insurance for qualifying survivors of workers, and the program under the act became Old Age and Survivors Insurance (OASI).

Over the years, the Social Security Act has been amended to include other benefits. In 1950, amendments of the act established the federal-state welfare assistance program of Aid to the Permanently and Totally Disabled (APTD), and expanded the ADC program to include the relative with whom the child was living. The ADC program then became Aid to Families of Dependent Children (AFDC), the program we know today. These changes significantly broadened the number of people who could receive benefits under the act.

In 1956, amendments to establish disability insurance were enacted. The federal insurance program under the act became Old Age, Survivors, and Disability Insurance (OASDI). The act did not include any major health assistance or insurance programs until 1965. In 1965, amendments provided for the establishment of the health insurance program of Medicare (title XVIII) and the health assistance program of Medicaid (title XIX). The federal insurance program under the act became Old Age, Survivors, Disability, and Health Insurance (OASDHI), the program now in existence. In 1972, a major reorganization of the welfare assistance programs occurred. Amendments established the welfare assistance program of Supplemental Security Income (SSI) to replace the categorical assistance programs of OAA, AB, and APTD, as of January 1, 1974. The welfare assistance programs under the act became SSI and AFDC. The 1972 amendments also mandated the establishment of Professional Standards Review Organizations (PSROs) in the health care field, as a means of evaluation and quality control (see Chapter 21).

Over the years there have been many other amendments to the Social Security Act. These amendments are discussed in appropriate chapters throughout this book. They provide funding for services such as maternal-child health programs, mental retardation programs and facilities, and crippled children's services. In the 1960s and 1970s, amendments to the act took significant strides to overcome sex discrimination and other biases under the act. The age at which men and women could receive benefits under the act became standardized, and benefits for widowed fathers with dependent children were established; it was also stipulated that benefits could not be barred or terminated because of marriage or remarriage; the duration of marriage requirement for divorced spouses' benefits was reduced from 20 years to 10. The elimination of sex bias was an important step in providing equal benefits to all under the act. In addition to sex bias changes, amendments have been made in the last two decades to strengthen the financing of the social security system through increased contributions and other means and to provide more comprehensive benefits. Very likely the act will continue to be amended significantly to provide funds for needed health and welfare services. Table 4-1 illustrates some of the major Social Security Act programs with which the community health nurse will have contact and their sources of administration.

Today, nearly every American family is involved with the Social Security Act in some form. Employers, employees, and the self-employed pay into the insurance programs of the act, and almost 90 percent of all United States workers contribute to these programs. The so-

cial security insurance protection (OASDHI) earned by a worker stays with the worker and his or her family even in a new job or residence. The contributions made by a worker will determine eligibility and the amount of benefits. When the contributing worker's earnings stop or are substantially reduced because of retirement, disability, or death, insurance benefits can be paid to the worker or qualifying survivors. The worker or survivors must apply for these benefits in order to obtain them.

Determining social security insurance eligibility is handled through local Social Security Administration offices. Determination of eligibility for Social Security Act assistance programs is handled through a number of federal, state, and local agencies. Welfare assistance funds are not based on the amount of contributions made into the social security program. Rather, they are allocated according to a means test.

There are federal Social Security Administration offices throughout the country and representatives are sent to communities that do not have offices. Applications for Old Age, Survivors, Disability, and Health Insurance (OASDHI) and Supplemental Security Income (SSI), which can be made in person, over the phone, or on behalf of someone else, are made at these offices. One should contact the office in advance to determine what information is necessary to complete the application.

Public Health Service Act of 1944 (Public Law 78-410) as Amended

The Public Health Service Act of 1944 consolidated and revised the laws relating to the Public Health Service and has since served to coordinate national public health legislation. It is the major piece of health legislation in the country, but does *not* have administration over the health programs, Medicaid and Medicare, of the Social Security Act. Over the years, this

TABLE 4-1 Some Major Social Security Act Programs and Their Source of Administration

Type of benefits	Type of programs		
	Federal programs*	State-federal programs†	Federal-state programs‡
Welfare insurance (cash benefit)	Old Age, Survivors, Disability, and Health Insurance (OASDHI)	Unemployment Insurance (Department of Labor)	None
Welfare assistance (cash benefit)	None	Aid to Families of Dependent Children (AFDC) (Social Security Administration)	Supplemental Security Income (SSI)
Health insurance	1. Medicare A—hospital insurance, prepaid through social security contributions 2. Medicare B—medical insurance, individual premium required Health components of (OASDHI)	None	None
Health assistance	None	1. Medicaid (Social Security Administration) 2. Miscellaneous maternal and child health programs (i.e., services to crippled children, PRESCAD) (Public Health Service)	None

*Administered *federally* through the Social Security Administration and/or the Public Health Service.
†Administered through the *state* government. Federal sharing agency is indicated by program.
‡Administered federally through the Social Security Administration. State sharing agency will vary in each state.
NOTE: Programs such as workers' compensation, general assistance, and food stamps are not provided for under the Social Security Act of 1935 and will be discussed later in this chapter.

law has been frequently amended and its programs now provide financing for the building and modernization of health care facilities; traineeships for health care professionals (nurse training acts and traineeships for graduate students in public health); grants-in-aid to schools of public health; construction of mental retardation, developmental disability, and community mental health centers and facilities; national comprehensive health planning and resource development; the development of health maintenance organizations (HMOs); health services for migratory workers; family planning services and communicable disease control; emergency medical services; and research and facilities for the prevention and control of conditions such as heart disease, cancer, stroke, kidney disease, sudden infant death syndrome, arthritis, Cooley's anemia, sickle-cell anemia, and diabetes mellitus. The 1975 amendments to this act provided a bill of rights for the developmentally disabled and established protection and advocacy services for them. Amendments such as the Heart Disease, Cancer, and Stroke Amendments of 1965 (Public Law 89-239) and 1970 (Public Law 91-515) gave research and service priority to some of the leading causes of death in this country. In Chapter 12, the Comprehensive Health Planning and Public Health Service Amendments of 1966 (Public Law 89-749) and the National Health Planning and Resources

Development Act of 1974 (Public Law 93-641) of the Public Health Service Act are discussed.

The areas covered under the Public Health Services Act are broad and comprehensive. Many of them, including chronic disease, communicable disease, and family planning, should be known to community health nurses because they work with them extensively.

Occupational Safety and Health Act of 1970 (Public Law 91-956)

Two major pieces of legislation have been enacted in the last decade to protect the rights of workers. In 1969, the Federal Coal Mine and Safety Act (Public Law 91-173) was passed to deal with problems in the mining industry. The Occupational Safety and Health Act of 1970 that followed is the most comprehensive piece of legislation on occupational health and safety in the United States. Championed by organized labor, its intent is to protect the health of the worker, and it also made worker health a public concern. The United States was the last major industrial nation to enact such a law; it will be discussed in depth in Chapter 16.

Vocational Rehabilitation Act of 1920 (Public Law 66-236) and the Rehabilitation Act of 1973 (Public Law 93-112)

The Vocational Rehabilitation Act of 1920 was an outgrowth of the health care needs evidenced by veterans after World War I. It provided training for the physically handicapped and was one of the first federal-state grant-in-aid programs to be established. The Rehabilitation Act of 1973 replaced the 1920 act but kept its major components. This new act extended and revised the authorization of grants to states for vocational rehabilitation services, emphasized services to those with severe handicaps, expanded federal responsibilities and training programs, defined services necessary for rehabilitation programs, established the National Architectural and Transportation Barriers Board to enforce legislation designed to remove architectural barriers for the handicapped, and began affirmative action programs to facilitate employment of the handicapped. Its ultimate goal is to help persons to become productive members of society. This act is further elaborated on in Chapter 17.

Economic Opportunity Act of 1964 (Public Law 88-452)

The Economic Opportunity Act of 1964 was designed to mobilize the human and financial resources of the nation to combat poverty. It included work-training and study programs, established the Office of Economic Opportunity, authorized Volunteers in Service to America (VISTA), the Job Corps, Upward Bound, Neighborhood Youth Corps, Head Start, neighborhood health centers, and community action programs. An impetus to antipoverty programs, it also incorporated establishment of urban and rural community action programs and assistance to small businesses and work experience programs. The future of Public Law 88-452 is now questionable.

Civil Rights Act of 1964 (Public Law 88-352)

The Civil Rights Act of 1964 forbade discrimination on the basis of race or sex in public accommodations, public facilities, and public education. It also enforced the constitutional right to vote. In addition, it established a Commission on Equal Employment Opportunity and attempted to ensure fair employment practices. Since 1972, if a state or local government is found to be practicing discrimination, the federal attorney general can sue to have that state's revenue-sharing funds cut off. This act and its subsequent amendments were designed to ensure fair and equal treatment for all.

State Workers' Compensation Acts

The state workers' compensation acts are the oldest form of government health and welfare insurance in this country. The first act was legislated in 1911, and by 1948 all states had such acts. Approximately 88 percent of the United States work force is covered by workers' compensation legislation (Price, 1979, p. 7). There are no mandatory federal standards for state workers' compensation legislation, and programs vary greatly from one state to another.

The stated purpose of workers' compensation is to provide income replacement and health care to workers who suffer work-related injury, disability (permanent or temporary), or death. Compensation is awarded regardless of who is at fault for the occurrence; this no-fault principle precludes legal suits against employers when the acquired disability is covered under the workers' compensation program.

Each state regulates its own program, but few states assume administrative responsibility for the program. Employers are allowed to self-insure, contract with commercial insurance providers, or purchase a policy with the state-operated insurance fund (Price, 1979, p. 4, 8). The employer is liable for the cost of the program. Many states provide limited or no workers' compensation coverage to farm and domestic workers.

The amount of the compensation awarded to the worker is related to the degree and permanence of the injury as well as the number of the worker's dependents (Wilner, Walkley, and O'Neill, 1978, p. 152). In some cases, if the worker is injured but suffers no loss of ability to work, such as in the case of certain types of hearing loss, the injury may not be compensated. Loss of ability to work is generally a criterion for awarding a workers' compensation claim. If a worker is able to return to work, his or her compensation award is usually discontinued or substantially reduced. Workers may receive benefits only for a specified period of time, even if the disability is permanent. Workers are often subject to waiting periods before the compensation award can begin.

The amount a worker receives under workers' compensation is considerably less than the wage received prior to work disability. In 1976 the average weekly wage replacement under workers' compensation programs was 64 percent of the worker's pay; the average amount of money received in 1976 was approximately $133 per week (Price, 1979, p. 13). This reduction in pay can cause financial hardship for a family in addition to all the other adjustments the family is making in relation to the disability. The nurse should be aware that some disabled workers and their families may also be eligible for benefits under other programs, including Old Age, Survivors, Disability, and Health Insurance (OASDHI), and Supplemental Security Income (SSI).

THE UNITED STATES HEALTH CARE SYSTEM

Silver (1974) provides what is possibly the best description of health care in America by utilizing the following passage from the *Book of Common Prayer*:

We have left undone those things which we ought to have done and we have done those things which we ought not to have done, and there is no health in us.

In the United States, comprehensive health services exist, but they are unequally distributed, fragmented, expensive, and often of questionable quality. Almost any type of health care service is available in the United States, but often these services are neither accessible nor affordable. Health care resources and services are found in both government (official) and private sectors.

There is often little coordination between health care resources—the hospital with the local health department or the local health department with private health care resources. There is no central system or group responsible for health resource coordination. An overview of some health resources and services in the United States follows in Table 4-2. This table vividly demonstrates the great complexity and diversity in the United States health care delivery system. Although diversity can be advantageous, it also presents major problems when one is attempting to coordinate available services and resources.

For a variety of reasons (discussed in Chapter 9 under barriers to utilization of resources), many people are not making use of available health resources. Free or low-cost immunization clinics are numerous in this country, yet many children and adults are not immunized or are inadequately immunized. Preventive health care is available, but many people do not utilize it. In 1976, it was estimated that almost 13 percent of the deaths from heart disease and cancer could have been prevented with early medical intervention (USDHEW, 1978, pp. ii, iii). It is also known that many Americans do not follow the preventive dental health practice of seeing a dentist annually.

Health care is sought and offered in this country largely on a diagnosis and treatment basis rather than on a preventive one. Despite these and other discrepancies in health care theory and practice, Americans are among the healthiest people in the world. The average life expectancy of Americans continues to increase, the death rate is historically low, and the infant mortality rate continues to decline.

We appear to make these advances in spite of ourselves.

Health Care Facilities and the Work Force

Health care resources exist autonomously, are fragmented, unequally distributed, and increasingly expensive. Accessibility to these resources is affected by individual and resource variables, such as cost, geographic location, and time factors. Because there is little coordination between health care resources, it is difficult to ensure continuity and quality of care. It is no wonder that the American public is becoming increasingly dissatisfied with the system.

There are more than 6500 acute care hospitals, 600 long-term hospitals, and 20,000 nursing homes in the United States (USDHEW, 1978, pp. 349–350). There are also more than 140,000 private physician's offices, 85,000 dentist's offices, and 52,000 drugstores according to the Committee on Economic Development (CED) (1973, p. 31). There are thousands of state and local health departments and departments of social services, as well as many private agencies and individuals who provide health care services.

Hospitals and physician's offices provide the majority of health care services in this country. Physician's offices are part of the private sector; however, hospitals have mixed government and private ownership. Government ownership of hospitals amounts to approximately 36 percent of all hospitals and includes armed forces, Public Health Service, and prison hospitals; state long-term psychiatric care facilities, mental retardation facilities, and state university medical school hospitals; and city and county hospitals for the medically indigent. Private hospitals are primarily private, nonprofit facilities.

Nursing homes are increasing in number in

TABLE 4-2 An Overview of Some United States Health Resources and Services

Government (official) resources			Private resources	
Federal	*State*	*Local*	*Profit*	*Nonprofit (voluntary)*
DIRECT SERVICES				
Department of Health and Human Services	State Department of Health	Local health department	Facilities (i.e., hospitals, nursing homes, extended care facilities, home care facilities)	Facilities (i.e., nursing homes, extended care facilities, home care facilities)
Communicable disease control (i.e., biologics, standards)	Communicable disease control (i.e., biologics immunization programs)	Communicable disease control (i.e., immunization clinics, individual CD follow-up)	Private practitioners	Professional grops (American Nurses' Association, National League for Nurses, American Medical Association)

Enforcing standards:
  Occupational health
  Environmental health
  Food and drug
  Interstate commerce
	Enforcing standards:
	  Occupational health
	  Environmental health
	  Food and drug
	  State public health Code
		Enforcing state and local health standards (i.e., environmental health)		

Maternal-child health programs	Maternal-child health programs	Maternal-child health programs	Commercial health industry (i.e., drugstores, medical supply)	Volunteerism—individuals, agencies, and groups
Adult health programs	Adult health programs	Adult health programs		
Consultation	Consultation	Consultation	Commercial health insurance	Health insurance
Laboratory services	Laboratory services	Laboratory services	Consultation	Consultation
Medicare	Workers' compensation	Clinic services (i.e., family planning, VD, antepartal)	"Fee-for-service" services	Health assistance programs
Medicaid	Medicaid	Home visits to clients		Accreditation of professional schools (i.e., NLN for schools of nursing)
Vocational rehabilitation	Vocational rehabilitation	Health classes (i.e., diabetes, hypertension)		
Hospitals (i.e., armed forces, veteran's hospitals)	Long-term care facilities (i.e., institutions for people who are mentally ill and mentally retarded)	Health care facilities (i.e., county hospital)		
Indian health service programs				
INDIRECT SERVICES				
Health planning and evaluation	Health planning and evaluation	Health planning and evaluation	Research	Research

Setting national standards:
  Occupational health
  Environmental health
  Food and drug
	Setting state standards:
	  Occupational health
	  Environmental health
	  Food and drug
		Setting local standards:
		  Environmental health
		  Health department services
			Collection and dissemination of health statistics	Collection and dissemination of health statistics
				
				Setting professional standards

TABLE 4-2 An Overview of Some United States Health Resources and Services (*Continued*)

Government (official) resources			Private resources	
Federal	*State*	*Local*	*Profit*	*Nonprofit (voluntary)*
Interstate commerce	State public health code			
Collection and dissemination of national health statistics	Collection and dissemination of state health statistics	Collection and dissemination of local statistics		
Funding for national health activities including building and modernizing of health care facilities	Funding for state and local health activities	Funding for local health activities		
Health care professional training, traineeships, and continuing education	Subsidy of state universities and health care training	Inservice for local health department staff		
International health activities	Licensing of state health professionals and facilities	Recruitment of local health department staff		
Research	Research	Research		

the United States, and their ownership is largely in the private profit-making sector. Today, 1 in 20 Americans aged 65 and over occupy a bed in a nursing or related home, and 90 percent of nursing home clients are over 65 years of age (Wilson and Neuhauser, 1976, p. 36). Nursing homes are licensed by the state and are usually certified for Medicaid and Medicare funding.

There are more than 6 million people employed in health care occupations in the United States (DHEW, 1978, p. 333). Health care is the nation's third largest employer (CED, 1973, p. 31). Education, certification, and licensing help to identify and distinguish various health care workers. There has been an increase in federal funding since World War II to train various health professionals, especially in schools of public health. Today we have 18.4 physicians, 45.1 registered nurses, 5.2 dentists, and 5.7 pharmacists per 10,000

population in the United States (Health Insurance Institute, 1978, p. 78).

There is a great disparity between the number of health care providers in urban, rural, and inner-city areas. Time after time, studies have shown rural and inner-city areas to have a significantly smaller health work force than more suburban areas. Resource distribution is also often related to the affluence of the area. The more affluent the area, the more available the health work force. The federal government is attempting to use financial incentives, to alter the training and distribution of health care personnel by offering fellowships and grants to students who commit themselves to serving in shortage areas. The government also offers financial incentives to universities and colleges that make a commitment to increase their output of health practitioners to areas where there is a shortage of health care personnel.

Cost

In general, health care in the United States is uneconomical and disproportionately inflationary. The health care financing system is diverse, is dominated by cost-increasing incentives such as fee-for-service, and is almost void of economic competition or regulations. Hospitals are reimbursed for costs and therefore are rewarded with more revenues for generating costs. Furthermore, health insurees have little incentive to question escalating costs. Health care spending accounts for approximately 8 percent of our gross national product. The following are some health care spending statistics for the United States in 1977 (USDHEW, 1978, pp. 377, 387–388):

- The total amount spent for health care was $162.6 billion, an average of $736.92 per person, and an average expenditure of $445 million a day.

- Spending for health care was 42.1 percent funded by federal, state, and local governments and 57.9 percent private (of private expenditures, approximately 26 percent was paid by insurance and 32 percent was paid out-of-pocket).

- Forty percent of all health care spending was for hospital services.

- Twenty percent of all health care spending was for physicians' services.

- Six percent of all health care spending was for dentists' services.

- Eight percent of all health care spending was for nursing home care.

- Of the $5.5 billion spent on health research, $3.7 billion was government spending, amounting to 2.3 percent of total government health care spending.

- Medicare and Medicaid accounted for 62 percent of total government health care expenditures.

Health care expenditures rise each year, and the cost of health care makes it inaccessible to many people. Some cost controls implemented in recent years have been certificate of need before a health facility can be constructed, deductibles and coinsurance as financial deterrents to a client's using unnecessary services, utilization reviews, and rate-setting commissions. The federal government has influenced the financing of health care through tax subsidies and incentives, including provisions for deductions of medical expenses with personal income tax, allowing employer's contributions to health insurance plans to be nontaxable, allowing income tax deductions for contributions made to charitable organizations engaged in health care, and extending tax exempt status to nonprofit health care resources.

Health care is financed through individual payment, insurance, and assistance programs. These methods of payment are discussed in this chapter because the health resources and services that an individual will use are largely dependent on the method of payment available.

RESOURCES FOR HEALTH CARE FINANCING IN THE UNITED STATES

The methods for health care financing in the United States are diverse, complicated, and confusing. Health care services often are not utilized because the individual is unable to afford them. Both the government and private sectors are active in health care financing, and both methods of financing are discussed here. To help make this varied system of financing clearer, the following outline will be used:

1. Individual payment (direct, out-of-pocket)
2. Health insurance
    a. Government
        (1) Medicare
        (2) Workers' compensation
    b. Private
        (1) Blue Cross-Blue Shield
        (2) Commercial insurance
        (3) Self-insurance
        (4) Health maintenance organizations (HMOs)
    c. National Health Insurance
3. Health assistance
    a. Government
        (1) Medicaid
        (2) Maternal-child health (MCH)
    b. Private
4. Health service programs
    a. Government
    b. Private

Individual Payment (Direct, Out-of-Pocket)

Individual payment for health care services is exactly what it says—the individual pays for the health care directly out of his or her own pocket. For people who are not covered under health insurance and assistance programs, individual payment becomes more of a reality.

Even with health insurance, many persons are involved in some form of individual payment due to insurance deductibles, coinsurance, fixed payment amounts, and uncovered services. A *deductible* is a set expense that must be paid by the insuree before the insurer will reimburse for services (e.g., $100 deductible). With *coinsurance,* the insuree pays a percentage of the covered health care expenses, which is often in addition to a deductible (e.g., 20 percent coinsurance rate). *Fixed payments* are arrangements whereby only a specified amount for a health service is paid by the insurer, regardless of the cost to the client (e.g., $300 for antepartal care). *Uncovered services* are easily understood: they are services that the insurer does not pay for, and payment is left to the insuree (e.g., prescriptions are not covered).

For whatever reason, many people are involved in direct payment for health care costs; in 1976, it accounted for 32.5 percent of personal health care expenditures in the United States (Wilner, Walkley, and O'Neill, 1978, p. 138). If individual payment for health care becomes excessive, it can place the individual at great financial risk. A form of health care financing that helps to protect the individual from the financial risk of health care is health insurance.

Health Insurance

Health insurance is a contractual agreement between an insurer and an insuree for the payment of costs of health care. The insuree pays a prepaid premium for specified benefits; the benefits under the insurance program are variable. Health insurance is administered by both government and private agencies. Private health insurance programs serve the majority of the American people, whereas government programs are limited largely to serving the aged and disabled.

Most health insurance programs cover hospital and surgical costs for the insuree because these costs are the most predictable and insurable of health care costs. Many insurance plans do not include regular medical, major medical, disability, or dental insurance. Some insurance plans do not cover the cost of prescription medications or health care equipment. Approximately 15 percent of the American population is not covered by any form of health insurance program. The following are some forms of health insurance coverages:

HOSPITAL: Insurance covering the cost of inpatient hospital expenses.

SURGICAL: Insurance that covers physicians' fees for surgical care.

REGULAR MEDICAL: Insurance that pays for physicians' fees for non-surgical care. There are usually maximum benefit amounts for specified services.

MAJOR MEDICAL: Insurance that helps protect against large, unpredictable medical costs usually supplements an existing insurance program, frequently has maximum benefit limits, and is subject to deductibles and coinsurance.

DENTAL: Insurance providing payment for the cost of specified dental care.

DISABILITY: Insurance that protects against wages lost from disability. This insurance may provide long-term or short-term benefits.

According to the Health Insurance Institute (1978, p. 9), the following numbers of persons had private health insurance protection of various types in the United States in 1977:

Insurance type	Number of persons covered
Hospital	178,968,000
Surgical	167,220,000
Regular medical	160,429,000
Major medical	139,362,000
Dental	53,510,000
Short-term disability	64,627,000
Long-term disability	19,364,000

These insurance statistics demonstrate that many people are not covered by comprehensive health insurance, are vulnerable to the cost of health care services, and could meet with disastrous financial consequences in the event of long-term disability.

Government

Federal government health insurance did not exist in any significant form until 1965, with the passage of Medicare under the Social Security Act. Government health insurance incorporates many of the same types of coverage as private health insurance. There are two major forms of government health insurance: Medicare and workers' compensation programs. Medicare is a federal program, and workers' compensation is a state program.

Medicare is a federally administered health insurance program created by the 1965 amendments to the Social Security Act. It provides health insurance for eligible persons age 65 and over and for qualifying people who are disabled, with no age restrictions. In 1977, it covered 26.5 million people at a cost of $20.5 billion (Health Insurance Institute, 1978, pp. 35–37).

Medicare is a contributory program, paid into during the insuree's working years. The program is administered through the Social Security Administration, Bureau of Health Insurance. Clients apply for it at local Social Security Administration offices. Reimbursement for Medicare services is provided through private insurance companies, "intermediaries," under contract with the federal government. These intermediaries are often Blue Cross-Blue Shield organizations.

There are two parts to Medicare: Medicare A and Medicare B. Medicare A is a hospital insurance program, financed through individual social security contributions; it had a deductible of $160 in 1979. In addition to inpatient hospital care, Medicare A covers selected posthospitalization home health care services, such as skilled nursing care, and physical or speech therapy on a qualifying basis. It has limits on the number of hospital and extended care facility days that will be covered and is subject to yearly changes in services and deductibles.

Medicare B is a voluntary, supplementary medical insurance program. In 1979, the monthly premium paid by the insuree electing this program was $8.70, with a deductible of $60 and a coinsurance rate of 80 percent. A qualifying individual may enroll in this program during the first 3 months of any year at a Social Security Administration office.

Medicare B covers physicians' services; limited services by dentists, podiatrists, optometrists, and chiropractors; hospital outpatient services; 100 home health service visits each year; outpatient physical therapy and speech therapy; specified equipment; radiation therapy; and other services on a qualifying basis. It excludes coverage for prescription drugs, glasses, dentures, hearing aids, yearly physical examinations, dental care, and routine foot care. Because of many of these exclusions, approximately 60 percent of persons 65 and older in this country have obtained supplemental private health insurance policies to augment their Medicare benefits (Health Insurance Institute, 1978, p. 20).

Workers' compensation has been discussed under the legislative section in this chapter.

These state programs include health and disability insurance from occupational illness or injury. Workers' compensation health care benefits cost the individual states more than $2.4 billion in 1976 (Price, 1979, p. 3).

Private

A forerunner of private health insurance in the United States was the Baylor University Plan of 1929. It had a monthly premium of 50 cents and offered 21 days of semiprivate care at Baylor Hospital, Dallas, Texas (Wilner, Walkley, and O'Neill, 1978, pp. 138–139). Out of this plan came the Blue Cross-Blue Shield concept of 1939. In 1939 less than 9 percent of the civilian, noninstitutionalized population was covered by any kind of private health insurance (Stevens and Stevens, 1974, p. 20).

In the 1950s health insurance became a major point in employees' collective bargaining, and United States industry became increasingly involved in prepayment of health care services. Today, health insurance plans are often a part of employee work benefits, and private health insurance is predominantly paid for by industry. It covers more than 150 million Americans (CED, 1973, p. 14).

Americans are protected by private health insurance offered through more than 700 private profit-oriented (commercial) insurance companies, and private nonprofit companies consisting of 69 Blue Cross and 69 Blue Shield organizations (Health Insurance Institute, 1978, p. 20). The most common forms of health insurance in this country are Blue Cross-Blue Shield, commercial insurance, self-insurance, and health maintenance organizations (HMOs). Each of these forms will be discussed here.

Blue Cross and Blue Shield are nonprofit (voluntary) organizations. Blue Cross provides protection against the cost of hospital care, and Blue Shield provides protection against the cost of medical and surgical care. They are tax-exempt organizations and exist through state legislation enabling them to provide health insurance. The state insurance commissioner usually has powers of regulation over these programs, with rate increases being approved by the commissioner and subject to public hearings. These organizations are the only organizations allowed to contract with providers of service for agreed-upon fees (Wilner, Walkley, and O'Neill, 1978, pp. 85–86).

Blue Cross and Blue Shield are legally independent of each other but usually work in close cooperation. They have boards of directors with evenly distributed representation from the public, the contracting providers, and their own organization. Many of these Blue Cross-Blue Shield plans do not cover dental, disability, or major medical health care expenses. Major medical, as well as preventive aspects of health care, may be made available at an additional cost to the insuree. Payment for service is made directly to the provider of service. These organizations provide services to 84 million persons under Blue Cross and 70 million persons under Blue Shield (Health Insurance Institute, 1978, p. 20).

Commercial insurance companies are profit-making organizations. They provide health insurance for more than 100 million Americans and cover services similar to those offered under Blue Cross-Blue Shield plans. Commercial insurers provide competition to Blue Cross-Blue Shield and have pioneered several types of health insurance coverage now common to other carriers, including major medical care, prescription drugs, and posthospitalization home care services (Wilner, Walkley, and O'Neill, 1978, p. 143). These plans usually do not cover dental services, and many do not offer disability coverage. Commercial insurers contract with clients for prepaid premiums and benefits. Clients are expected to pay the service provider and are then reimbursed by the insurer for the agreed-upon cost.

Self-insurance was stimulated by the passage of the Employee Retirement Income Security Act of 1974 (Health Insurance Institute, 1978, p. 20). Under this act, corporations and organizations can establish self-funded, non-profit health plans and escape the taxes and regulations of state insurance laws. Self-insurance plans are relatively new and statistics are not readily available on them.

Health maintenance organizations (HMOs) provide a wide range of comprehensive health care services for a specified group at a fixed, prepaid cost to the insuree (Health Insurance Institute, 1978, p. 72). Health maintenance organizations combine the principles of health insurance and group health practice and stress the preventive aspects of health care. The Health Maintenance Organization Act of 1973 (Public Law 93-222), an amendment to the Public Health Service Act of 1944, provided financial and other assistance to aid in HMO development. There are over 100 operational HMOs in this country, serving more than 6 million Americans (Wilner, Walkley, and O'Neill, 1978, p. 144). These organizations are characterized by:

· Direct service provision to enrollees on a prepayment basis, with each enrollee paying a fixed amount regardless of the volume or expense of the services utilized.

· Service provision through physicians, nurses, and other health care providers, who are under contractual agreement with the HMO. Their practice is limited to the HMO, and subscribers to the HMO are limited to usage of the health workers employed by the plan.

· Comprehensive services that include both inpatient and outpatient care and emphasize preventive health practices.

· Internal, self-regulatory mechanisms to ensure quality of care and cost control.

National Health Insurance

There is *no* form of national health insurance in this country. Each year, national health insurance legislation is introduced in Congress, but to date no plan has been passed. Different plans are supported by various individuals and groups. Most of the proposed plans involve employer and employee contributions, tax credits, or payroll taxes. Generally, they include provisions that would provide basic health care for the entire population and that would eliminate financial hardship as a result of catastrophic illness. Proposed programs generally vary as to whether they will be federally or privately administered, who will be covered, what will be covered, how they will be funded, and what quality control measures will be taken. Table 4-3 is a summation of some of the major proposals pending for national health insurance. Possibly the biggest barrier

to passage of a national health insurance plan is the proposed cost to the taxpayer.

Somers (1971, pp. 136–141) believes that a comprehensive national health insurance program should include coverage for the entire civilian population, comprehensive benefits, adequate income for care providers, incentives for efficiency and economy, equitable financing, administrative feasibility and acceptance to consumers, and flexibility. Health care professionals must monitor carefully all proposed legislation to ensure that the proposed program actually provides the services needed by the population as a whole.

Health Assistance

Health assistance resources provide health services for a qualifying individual without the prepayment of premiums by the individual,

TABLE 4-3 Proposals for National Health Insurance

Proposal	Funding	Coverage Catastrophic only	Coverage Comprehensive	Private carrier involvement	Federal contract with providers
Catastrophic Health Insurance Act and Medical Assistance Reform Act	1% payroll tax	Covers expense over $2000	No	No	No
Comprehensive Health Insurance Plan	Employer-employee tax	—	Yes	Share	No
Comprehensive Health Insurance Act	Employer tax; employee voluntary; federal subsidy for poor	—	Yes	Yes; with federal certification of provisions	No
National Health Care Services Reorganization and Reform Act	Same as above	—	Yes	Same as above	No
National Health Care Act	Same as above	—	Yes	Same as above	No
Health Security Act	3.5% payroll tax	—	Yes	None	Yes; amounts appropriated annually

SOURCE: From R. M. French. *Dynamics of health care* (3d ed.). New York: McGraw-Hill, 1979, p. 190.

and generally without the individual participating in cost-sharing for the services rendered. These programs are largely noncontributory ones.

Government

The major government health assistance programs are the federal-state, state-administered program of Medicaid and a number of maternal-child health programs. The private-sector health assistance programs are diverse and belong largely to the private nonprofit (voluntary) sector.

Medicaid was created by the 1965 Social Security Act amendments that created Medicare. It is a noncontributory health assistance program that provides both medical and hospital services for the qualifying medically indigent; however, its services are provided as health insurance to the client. The client does not pay for medical and hospital services. The federal government contracts with intermediaries, usually Blue Cross-Blue Shield organizations, to insure the client against health costs. It is a health assistance program, operating on a health insurance principle.

Both federal and state funds pay for Medicaid services, with the ratio of federal funding varying from 50 to 83 percent, depending on the state's economic status (French, 1979, p. 188). This program is administered through the Medical Services Administration of the Social and Rehabilitation Service under the Social Security Administration on a federal level. Each state administers its own Medicaid program through varying offices of state government.

Medicaid benefits vary from one state to another. Federal law does not mandate that a state operate a Medicaid program. If the state does operate the program, it must include in-hospital services, outpatient hospital services, laboratory and x-ray services, skilled nursing home services, physician's services, a screening program for children under 21 years of age for defects and chronic conditions (Early, Periodic Screening, Diagnosis, and Treatment—EPSDT), and family planning services. Medicaid does not pay for the services of podiatrists or chiropractors.

All states have established Medicaid programs. There is no residency or age requirement for the program. Anyone is eligible to receive Medicaid if he or she is receiving welfare assistance (e.g., Aid for Families of Dependent Children, Supplemental Security Income, or General Assistance) or qualify as medically needy. A person receiving Medicare may also be eligible for Medicaid.

Maternal-child health programs (MCH) have traditionally been a major source of funding for activities carried out by local health departments to meet the needs of high-risk mothers and children. These activities include nutrition programs such as Women, Infants, and Children (WIC), medical or dental care, and comprehensive preventive medical care services through centers such as PRESCAD (Preschool, Schoolage, and Adolescent). These services are discussed more extensively in Chapter 13.

Private

Volunteerism is evidenced in this country to a greater degree than in other nations of the world. In the health field, volunteerism is prevalent, with many people donating time, money, and effort to help procure health services for others. The candy stripers in the local hospital, as well as the readers for the blind, are examples of volunteers who are helping clients to obtain health care services.

Service groups such as the American Cancer Society, American Diabetes Association, American Heart Association, Associations for Retarded Citizens, Lion's Clubs, Rotarians, Goodfellows, Knights of Columbus, church groups, and Visiting Nurse Associations provide cash and service benefits in the health field. A majority of United States hospitals operate on a voluntary, nonprofit basis. The dedicated leadership, financial support, and personal service of volunteers and voluntary agencies (non-tax-supported) has greatly aided the health care delivery system in this country, and an extension of this voluntary tradition is essential to continuing health services (National Commission on Community Health Services, 1966, p. 160).

Health Service Programs

There are some government and private health service programs that are administered through an organization for the benefit of specified employees or service groups. These programs often encompass a combination of insurance and assistance benefits.

Government

Government programs have been generally established to meet the health care needs of specific population groups. Health service programs for veterans, military personnel, merchant marines, American Indians on reservations, and federal employees are available in the United States. These programs vary in relation to the type of services and benefits offered, and one should check with the resource provider to determine what benefits are available to the client.

Private

Private service programs are usually part of a benefit package for employees in the work setting. In addition to payment of employee health insurance premiums, many industries provide on-grounds employee health services. These services are usually preventive and treatment-oriented for work-related disease and disability. In addition, there are some industry-sponsored group health maintenance organization plans such as Kaiser-Permanente (French, 1979, pp. 187–188).

THE UNITED STATES WELFARE SYSTEM

The primary task of the welfare system is to alleviate the hardships of the most disadvantaged. Welfare programs reflect an effort to ensure a basic standard of living and to promote social well-being. Like the health care financing system, the welfare system is complex. In this text, programs are arbitrarily divided into welfare insurance and assistance programs. The following outline is used to familiarize the reader with these programs:

1. Welfare insurance

   a. Government

      (1) Old Age, Survivors, Disability, and Health Insurance (OASDHI)

      (2) Unemployment insurance

      (3) Workers' compensation

      (4) Retirement programs for railroad and federal employees

   b. Private

2. Welfare assistance

   a. Government

      (1) Aid to Families of Dependent Children (AFDC)

      (2) Supplemental Security Income (SSI)

      (3) Food Stamps

      (4) General assistance

   b. Private

Welfare Insurance

Welfare insurance programs are contributory. The individual or someone on behalf of the individual, such as the employer or the government, pays a premium, and benefits are awarded by virtue of these past premium contributions. Welfare insurance programs are found in both the government and private sectors.

Government

The federal government became extensively involved in welfare insurance programs with the passage of the Social Security Act in 1935. This act and its amendments are the basis for existing federal government welfare insurance programs today. State governments are also involved in the provision of welfare insurance. A discussion of the major government welfare insurance programs follows.

Old Age, Survivors, Disability, and Health Insurance (OASDHI) is the federal welfare insurance component of the Social Security Act of 1935. It should be noted that health insurance is a major component of this program. The health insurance component, Medicare, has been discussed previously. The welfare component is Old Age, Survivors, and Disability Insurance (OASDI).

Old Age, Survivors, and Disability Insurance is the largest social insurance program in the United States and is commonly called *social security*. Cash benefits for the program are awarded on the basis of money paid in, as well as time spent in the program. Benefits are paid on a monthly basis or in lump sums. The old age component of the program is often called retirement insurance. A worker often begins to receive retirement benefits at age 65. If a worker retires before the age of 65, the amount of his or her check is reduced permanently. If a worker returns to work after beginning retirement benefits, there is a ceiling limit on the amount that the worker can earn and still collect retirement benefits.

The survivors component provides benefits to survivors in the family of a deceased, qualifying worker. Monthly cash payments or a lump sum payment can be made. An application for lump sum benefits must usually be made within 2 years after the worker's death.

Disability benefits are payable to qualifying persons under 65 years of age on the basis of medical evaluations and the person's continued inability to work. After age 65, the disabled worker can apply for the old age component of the insurance program.

Unemployment insurance provides protection against earnings lost as a result of unemployment. It is a federal-state cost-sharing program provided by the Social Security Act of 1935 and is *state* administered. A worker who becomes unemployed on a job covered by unemployment insurance and who has worked a specified amount of time can apply for these benefits. The worker must remain registered to work and must actively seek employment while collecting benefits. There is a potential for coverage of up to 65 weeks after employment has been terminated, but there is no long-term coverage under the program.

Employers pay into the program on behalf of the employee while the employee is working for them. There is no commercial insurance and no self-insurance by employers. Benefits and contributions are determined primarily by state law, but federal law sets minimum standards. The federal government pays the costs of administration and makes loans to states when their unemployment insurance accounts run low. There is great variation in this program from state to state. In 1977, unemployment insurance serviced 2,647,364 workers with an average weekly benefit amount of only $78.77 (Simanis, 1979, p. 63). A separate federal unemployment system exists for railroad workers.

Workers' compensation is discussed under the legislative section on state workers' compensation laws in this chapter. Please refer to that section for information.

Retirement programs for railroad and federal employees are other welfare insurance programs which exist in the United States. The Railroad Retirement Acts of 1937 and 1974 provided for the Railroad Retirement Insurance program and gave welfare insurance protection to railroad workers. This welfare insurance program is financed by compulsory employer and employee contributions. Employees of the federal government also have their own retirement insurance program, and similar programs are administered by the states and localities for their employees. In addition, these government employees usually qualify for OASDHI.

Private

Private welfare insurance is available through a number of agencies. A major form of private welfare insurance in this country is employer-employee–funded retirement insurance; another form is disability insurance. Many persons are covered by private retirement insurance as well as the government program of OASDHI. Retirement and disability insurance can be purchased by individuals who desire to have additional financial protection when they are no longer working. Millions of American workers are covered by private retirement insurance through their place of work. The Retirement Income Security Act of 1974 helped to safeguard the financial integrity of these private retirement programs. Disability insurance was discussed under health insurance in this chapter.

Welfare Assistance Programs

Welfare assistance programs are noncontributory or minimally contributory programs for qualifying indigent individuals, and they provide cash and service benefits (e.g., food, shelter, clothing). They exist largely as a result of state and federal legislation and are locally administered. Once a person's eligibility for a categorical government welfare assistance program has been determined, he or she receives cash benefits, social service benefits, and medical benefits through Medicare or Medicaid (Donabedian, 1980). The individual is generally eligible for food stamps also. Welfare assistance programs include both government and private programs.

Government

Government welfare assistance programs provide subsistence benefits for those without other resources. Applicants often apply for these programs through local departments of social service or through the Social Security Office, depending on the program. An applicant is generally asked to provide the following information when applying for government assistance programs:

· Proof of residence

· Proof of gross income from all sources, for all household members

· Record of all property, including savings accounts, checking accounts, bonds, and land owned

· Record of house payments or rent and also insurance and taxes

· Record of utility bills

· Record of current medical and dental expenses

· Birth dates and social security numbers of household members

· Records of child support and alimony

· Proof of tuition and other required educational expenses

· Records of child care payment for employment or training purposes

Some major categorical government welfare assistance programs include the AFDC and SSI. Other government assistance programs include general or direct assistance and food stamps. These programs are discussed below.

Aid to Families of Dependent Children (AFDC) is the federal-state program provided for under the Social Security Act of 1935 that helps needy families with children. In 1977, over 3.5 million families received $10.6 billion in AFDC benefits, amounting to approximately $3030 per family per year or $254 per family per month (USDHEW, 1979). This amount of financial assistance puts AFDC families below the poverty level of income.

AFDC furnishes financial and other assistance to encourage the care of dependent children in their own homes, to help parents become capable of self-support, and to maintain family life. In order for a family to qualify for AFDC, there must be children who are deprived of the financial support of one parent because of death, disability, absence from the home, or, in some states, unemployment. The family's income must fall below a "needs standard" set by each state. The actual amount of the AFDC payment will depend on the number of persons in the family and the amount of other income. The following are selected characteristics of families who are receiving AFDC, according to the Department of Health, Education, and Welfare (1979, p. 1):

· Almost all AFDC families had one adult recipient

· AFDC families had an average of 2.2 children in 1977

· Ninety-three percent of the children who received AFDC lived with their mothers

· Almost all AFDC families received food stamps

· Almost all AFDC families (80 percent) lived in metropolitan areas

Any United States citizen or legal alien can apply for AFDC; there is no age requirement. Federal AFDC funds are available to pregnant women, and in most states, a woman can apply for AFDC or for an increase in her present allotment once a physician has verified in writing that she is pregnant.

In 1967, the Work Incentive Program (WIN) was added to AFDC to encourage employment in AFDC families. The WIN program requires adult recipients of AFDC without preschool children to register for employment. The working mother is allowed work expenses, including necessary day care for children, plus a certain amount of her earnings, before calculation of her eligibility for AFDC. In 1975, the Child Support Enforcement Division of the Department of Health, Education, and Welfare was formed to help obtain support from parents who had deserted their families, for the purpose of decreasing the amount of money spent on welfare assistance. This legislation required states to establish an office to enforce regulations in relation to paternity, locating absent parents, and obtaining child support.

Supplemental Security Income (SSI) is a federal-state assistance program that is *federally* administered through the Social Security Administration. It provides aid to qualifying aged, blind, and disabled people who have limited financial resources. The objective for establishing this program was to develop a uniform national minimum cash income for the indigent aged, blind, and disabled. In 1979, this federal standard before state supplementation was approximately $208 per month for an individual and $312 per month for a couple (Donabedian, 1979, p. 94). Federal monetary benefits under the program remain constant throughout the nation, but many states supplement the program with additional cash benefits. State supplementary benefits vary and may be made directly to the beneficiary or paid through the federal Social Security Administration. Adults are usually the beneficiaries of SSI, but a child may be eligible if he or she suffers from an impairment expected to last a year or longer, such as mental retardation, terminal illness, or blindness. Applications for SSI are made at local Social Security offices. Qualifying United States citizens and legally admitted aliens are eligible.

The food stamp program was established to improve the nutritional adequacy of low-income individuals and families. It is a federal-state program with *state* administration, general federal funding, and federal-state sharing on administrative costs. The federal sharing agency is the Department of Agriculture, and the state agency usually in charge is the Department of Social Services. Persons must qualify on the basis of financial need. With only a few exceptions, all those qualifying between the ages of 18 and 65 must register to work; refusal to register can terminate eligibility. A household on food stamps that is intending to move to another area may apply for transfer of certification before moving and then request re-certification with the administering agency within 60 days after its move. Federal law states that the food stamp office must determine eligibility within 30 days after a signed application is submitted.

Food stamps are mandated in all counties in the nation. Coupons purchased are used like money and are worth more than their purchased price. An eligible household with an extremely low income may be eligible for food stamps at no cost. Food stamps can only be used to purchase edible items; no imported foodstuffs can be bought with them. They are not transferrable to another person but must be used by the person who purchased them. Food stamp regulations apply nationwide and most grocery stores are authorized to accept

food stamps. This is the most rapidly growing form of public assistance in the country.

General assistance is a state- and locally-funded and -administered program which is not offered by all states. The program is often administered through the state's department of social services or a comparable department and is frequently referred to as direct assistance.

General assistance is usually made available to indigent persons who do not meet the criteria for other forms of welfare insurance or assistance but are unable to meet their basic survival needs of food, shelter, and clothing. This may be the only form of government assistance available for individuals who are poor but who do not qualify for AFDC or SSI monies. In many states, general assistance is limited to emergency relief (i.e., for a catastrophic event such as a flood), short-term relief, and burial benefits. Any citizen or legally admitted alien may apply. In some states, people receiving general assistance do not receive cash benefits but instead receive vouchers for food, rent, or clothing. In 1978, there were 773,000 recipients of general assistance with an average monthly payment of $116.54 (Social Security Bulletin, 1979, *42*, p. 54).

In addition to the cash benefit programs discussed, many state and local governments offer a number of other welfare services. The following list itemizes some of these services (Michigan Department of Social Services, 1977):

- Adoption services: accepting and placing children for adoption, recruiting adoptive families, and supporting the adoption placement

- Foster care: funding, licensing, and monitoring

- Day care: locating suitable day-care placements for children during part of the day, licensing and monitoring such placements, and funding services provided by them

· Counseling: counseling individuals, parents, and children with personal or family problems to strengthen family functioning and to prevent family breakdown

· Chore services: paying part or all of the cost for unskilled help with household tasks, personal care, home maintenance, or other activities for qualifying aged and disabled

· Education or training: providing funds and counseling services so that persons can improve their job skills through education and training programs

· Employment: helping people find jobs

· Family planning: providing information and referral to appropriate agencies

· Homemaking: teaching people about home management

· Housing: helping people to find or improve housing and landlord-tenant relations

· Information and referral: helping people to learn about community services

· Mental health treatment and rehabilitation: providing services to persons with mental health problems through community mental health agencies

· Money management: helping people to learn to budget and to use credit

· Placement: helping to place youth and adults in appropriate living facilities with follow-up

· Problem services: investigating reports of abuse and neglect and providing counseling

services to prevent recurrence of such problems, counseling services for runaway youth, foster care or housing in emergency situations, and protection of aging clients and children from abuse and neglect (protective services)

Private

The United States is one of the few countries in the world to offer so many and so comprehensive an array of private welfare assistance programs. Most offer short-term, acute relief, but do not provide long-term assistance for chronic problems. These programs offer services to meet homemaker, health care, counseling, and adoption needs; residential services for the handicapped; day care; recreational activities; Meals-on-Wheels; etc. The indigent may be helped with temporary food, shelter, clothing, emotional support, or other services through a variety of community groups such as Goodfellows, Lions, Rotarians, Community Self-Help, and the Salvation Army.

Knowledge of private as well as of all other health and welfare resources is essential when one is nursing a community. Though these systems are complex, time and effort spent learning them will equip the community health nurse to more effectively deal with the situations encountered daily in the practice setting. Chapter 12 discusses ways the community health nurse can become involved in making these health and welfare systems more efficient and effective.

SUMMARY

Community health nurses must be aware of the major legislation affecting health and welfare policy and practices in the United States, as well as the services provided by this legislation, in order to fulfill their responsibilities

to clients in the community. Programs enacted through the Social Security Act of 1935 and the Public Health Service Act of 1944 are extensively used by community health nurses functioning in the clinical setting. The Social

Security Act provides for the major government health and welfare insurance and assistance programs in the United States today. Although the nurse is becoming increasingly involved, through occupational health nursing, with the Occupational Safety and Health Act of 1970, the full impact of this act has yet to be seen in nursing.

The health and welfare systems in the United States are complex, diverse, and poorly coordinated. The community health nurse is in a favorable position for explaining the relationship between these system resources and services in a way that few other professionals can. The community health nurse is integrally linked with the health care system, and through community affiliations she or he is in continual contact with the welfare system as well. For many clients, basic welfare needs are a higher priority than health needs; health needs may not be viewed as a priority until the nurse can help the client meet his or her welfare needs.

The nurse should be aware of resources and services in the private sector as well as the government sector. Keeping up with private-sector resources requires diligent effort on the part of the nurse because these resources will vary greatly from locality to locality and are frequently not as obvious as government resources. Contact with local leadership, clients, other nurses, service groups, and professional organizations is helpful to the nurse who desires to remain informed.

REFERENCES

Cohen, W. J. Social security: Current myths and reality—The need for its preservation and reform. *Wayne Law Review*, September 1979, *25*, 1419–1445.

Coll, B. D. *Perspectives in public welfare*. Washington, D.C.: Government Printing Office, 1969.

Committee for Economic Development. *Building a national health-care system*. New York: Committee on Economic Development, 1973.

Donabedian, D. Conversation with author on health and welfare systems as they apply to nursing. Ann Arbor, Mich.: January 25, 1980.

———. *Health and welfare systems*. Ann Arbor, Mich.: University of Michigan School of Nursing, 1979.

French, R. M. *Dynamics of health care (3d ed)*. New York: McGraw-Hill, 1979.

Georke, L. S., & Stebbins, E. L. *Mustard's introduction to public health (5th ed.)*. New York: Macmillan, 1968.

Hanlon, J. J. *Public health administration and practice (6th ed.)*. St. Louis: Mosby, 1974.

Health Insurance Institute. *Source book of health insurance data: 1977–78*. New York: Health Insurance Institute, 1978.

Institute of Gerontology. *Social security the first thirty-five years*. Ann Arbor, Mich.: University of Michigan Press, 1970.

National Committee on Community Health Services. *Health is a community affair*. Cambridge, Mass.: Harvard University Press, 1966.

Price, D. N. Workers' compensation program in the 1970's. *Social Security Bulletin*, May 1979, *42*, 3–24.

Public assistance recipients and average monthly payments per recipient, by program, 1940–78. *Social Security Bulletin*, February 1979, *42*, 54.

Services for individuals and families. Lansing, Mich.: Michigan Department of Social Services, 1977.

Silver, G. A. *Family medical care: A design for health maintenance*. Cambridge, Mass.: Ballinger, 1974.

Simanis, J. G. Unemployment insurance: Selected data on state programs, 1940–1978. *Social Security Bulletin*, February 1979, *42*, 63.

Smolensky, J. *Principles of community health*. Philadelphia: Saunders, 1977.

Somers, A. R. *Health care in transition*. Chicago: Hospital Research and Educational Trust, 1971.

Stevens, R. B., & Stevens, R. *Welfare medicine in America: A case study of Medicaid*. New York: Free Press, 1974.

U.S. Department of Health, Education, and Welfare. *Aid to families with dependent children: A chartbook.* Washington, D.C.: Government Printing Office, 1979.

————. *Health and United States 1978.* Washington, D.C.: Government Printing Office, 1978.

————. *Social Security information for young families.*

Washington, D.C.: Government Printing Office, 1977.

Wilner, D. M., Walkley, R. P., & O'Neill, E. J. *Introduction to public health* (7th ed.). Macmillan, New York: 1978.

Wilson, F. A., & Neuhauser, D. *Health services in the United States.* Cambridge, Mass.: Ballinger, 1976.

SELECTED BIBLIOGRAPHY

American Public Welfare Association. The future of food stamps: Resolving the problems of the past? *Washington Report,* September 1975, 1–5.

Average monthly amount of combined federal and state payments in states with federally administered state supplementation, by reason for eligibility and state, October 1978. *Social Security Bulletin,* February 1979, *42,* 50.

Bortz, A. *Social Security sources in federal records: 1934–50.* Washington, D.C.: Government Printing Office, 1969.

Carroll, M. S. Private health insurance plans in 1976: An evaluation. *Social Security Bulletin,* September 1978, *41,* 3–16.

Cohen, W. J. Current problems in health care. *New England Journal of Medicine,* July 1969, *281,* 193–197.

————. United States health policy. Sinai lectureship, University of Michigan School of Public Health, Ann Arbor, Oct. 6, 1968.

Compilation of selected public health laws (vol. 1). Washington, D.C.: Government Printing Office, 1971.

Copeland, L. S. Worldwide developments in social security: 1975–77. *Social Security Bulletin,* May 1978, *41,* 3–8.

Davis, K. *National health insurance: Benefits, costs and consequences.* Washington, D.C.: The Brookings Institution, 1975.

Dolfman, M. L. The concept of health: An historical and analytic examination. *The Journal of School Health,* October 1973, *43,* 491–497.

Eitzen, D. C. *Social structure and social problems in America.* Boston: Allyn & Bacon, 1974.

Enthoven, A. C. Consumer-centered vs job-centered

health insurance. *Harvard Business Review,* January–February 1979, *57,* 141–152.

Freeman, H. E., & Kurtz, N. R. *America's troubles* (2d ed.). Englewood Cliffs, N. J.: Prentice-Hall, 1973.

Gibson, R. M. & Mueller, M. S. National health and welfare expenditures: 1976. *Social Security Bulletin,* April 1977, *40,* 3–22.

Goldmeier, H. Supplemental security income for children. *Children Today,* 1978, *8,* 14–17.

Kennedy, E. M. *In critical condition: The crisis in American health care.* New York: Pocket Books, 1973.

Komaroff, A. L., & Duffel, P. J. An evaluation of selected federal categorical health programs for the poor. *American Journal of Public Health,* March 1976, *66,* 255–261.

La France, A. B. *Welfare law: structure and entitlement.* St. Paul, Minn.: West, 1977.

Law, S. *The rights of the poor.* New York: Avon Books, 1974.

Leopold, B. *Scope of major social insurance and income assistance programs of necessity.* Detroit: Michigan Legal Services, 1977.

Mauksch, I. C. On national health insurance. *American Journal of Nursing,* 1978, *78,* 1323–1327.

McMillan, A. Social welfare expenditures under public assistance programs. *Social Security Bulletin,* 1979, *42,* 3–19.

Myers, R. J. *Medicare.* Homewood, Ill.: Irwin, 1970.

Odlin, S. The workers' compensation controversy: A status report. *Job Safety and Health,* April 1977, *5,* 15–21.

Poverty and sickness the inseparable twins. *Social Security,* February 1938, 12, 1 and 6.

Public welfare: Facts, myths and prospects. New York: Public Affairs Pamphlets, 1977.

Smith, M. Health Maintenance Organization Act of 1973. *Research and Statistics Note,* Mar. 12, 1974, 1–8.

Snee, J., & Ross, M. Social Security amendments of 1977: Legislative history. *Social Security Bulletin,* March 1978, *41,* 3–20.

Social security in review: Advisory council on Social Security named. *Social Security Bulletin.* May 1978, *41,* 1–2.

Social security in review: Social security and Medicare increases for 1979. *Social Security Bulletin,* January 1979, *42,* 1–2.

Social security related legislation in 1978. *Social Security Bulletin,* March 1979, *42,* 30–31.

Spiegel, A. D., & Podair, S. *Medicaid: Lessons for national health insurance.* Rockville, Md.: Aspen Systems Corporation, 1975.

Supplemental security income: number of persons, total, and average state payment, amount to persons under state administered, state supplementation programs by reason of eligibility, 1974–78. *Social Security Bulletin,* 1979, *42,* 51.

U.S. Code—Congressional and Administrative News. St. Paul, Minn.: West, selected years 1950–1979.

U.S. Department of Health, Education, and Welfare. *The cooperative federal-state-local health statistics system.* Washington, D.C.: Government Printing Office, 1973.

———. *Public attitudes toward Social Security 1935–1965.* Washington, D.C.: Government Printing Office, 1970.

———. *Social Security programs throughout the world.* Washington, D.C.: Government Printing Office, 1977.

———. *Towards a systematic analysis of health care in the United States.* Washington, D.C.: Government Printing Office, 1972.

———. *Your Social Security.* Washington, D.C.: Government Printing Office, 1978.

U.S. Department of Health, Education, and Welfare, Administration on Aging, Office of Human Development Services. *Program development handbook for state and area agencies on homemaker and home health services for the elderly.* Washington, D.C.: Government Printing Office, 1977.

U.S. Department of Health, Education, and Welfare, Social Security Administration. *Health insurance plans other than Blue Cross or Blue Shield plans or insurance companies: 1970 survey.* Washington, D.C.: Government Printing Office, 1971.

———. *How SSI can help.* Washington, D.C.: Government Printing Office, 1978.

———. *Pocket guide to supplemental security income.* Washington, D.C.: Government Printing Office, 1973.

———. *SSI for the aged, blind and disabled.* Washington, D.C.: Government Printing Office, 1977.

———. *Your Medicare handbook.* Washington, D.C.: Government Printing Office, 1977.

United States Statutes at Law. Washington, D.C.: Government Printing Office, selected years 1935–1978.

Worthington, N. L. National health expenditures, 1929–74. *Social Security Bulletin,* February 1975, *38,* 3–20.

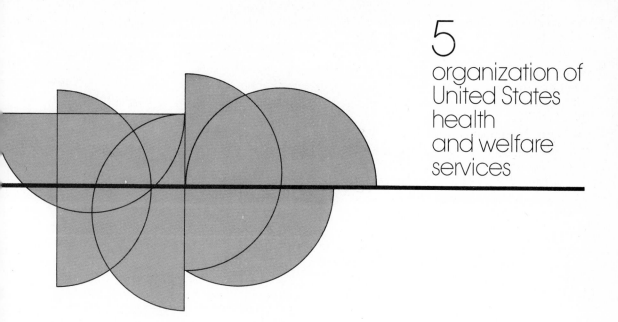

Little House on the Prairie, the best-selling children's story and popular television series, is the saga of a pioneer family living during the late nineteenth century. Health and welfare needs for these pioneers were usually met within the local community, with little government intervention. However, a rapidly growing population, increasingly complex health technology, and changing social, cultural, and economic factors have changed the organiza-tion and delivery of health and welfare services in this country. Today, health and welfare services in the United States are complex and diverse. These resources are organized in both the government and private sectors and provide many valuable services to the American public. They are too valuable to be allowed to develop and exist haphazardly. They must be organized in an effective manner.

THE HEALTH AND WELFARE LINKAGE

An individual's health and welfare needs interrelate and interact in a delicate balance. One might assume that the organization of health and welfare resources would be integrally linked to meet client needs effectively and efficiently, but this is not the case. In fact, these organizations operate autonomously and form two separate systems: a health care system and a welfare system. Lack of coordination between these two systems presents multiple problems for both providers and recipients of service. Providers of service are frustrated, because they find it difficult to know about all the resources available, to maintain effective

The authors are indebted to Loraine Black, friend and colleague, who taught both faculty and students the philosophy and practices of health care administration and who stimulated an interest in discovering how the health care system works. We appreciate her efforts in facilitating the writing of this chapter.

linkages between these two systems, and to exert influence when changes are needed to improve the quality of health care. Recipients of service are frustrated because they are not aware of resources, do not understand how to utilize them, and often receive fragmented care. A major role of the community health nurse is to explain and coordinate services provided by community resources. Lack of resource coordination adversely affects the quality of care delivered to clients. This is demonstrated in the following case situation:

John Falta, age 19, was in a motorcycle accident that necessitated an amputation below the right knee. He was hospitalized for 6 weeks and upon discharge was referred to a local visiting nurse association for skilled nursing services, the Office of Vocational Rehabilitation for rehabilitation training, and the Department of Social Services for assistance with his medical expenses. In addition, a physical therapist from the hospital saw John on a weekly basis at home, and a volunteer from a local amputee self-help group visited him regularly to help him adapt to the changes that had occurred in his life. Each of these health and welfare resources provided a valuable service, but because they were not coordinated initially, John found it difficult to understand why so many people were involved in his care. He expressed to the visiting nurse that he was confused and depressed about the onslaught of "helping agencies" and the different goals that had been set for him. The nurse suggested that a conference be arranged between John, his family, and the involved resources; John agreed that this was necessary. The conference helped to coordinate John's care as well as to stimulate John's involvement in the rehabilitation process. Because he had a clearer picture about what was happening, his depression decreased and he actively participated in establishing goals for his future.

It is not uncommon to encounter clients like John Falta in community health nursing practice. Health and welfare resources meet infrequently to plan for coordinated service delivery. When such meetings do occur, they are often arranged to deal with individual client problems rather than to *plan* for coordinated preventive health and welfare services.

Lack of coordination occurs between the health and welfare systems (intersystem) as well as within systems (intrasystem). A classic example of intersystem lack of coordination in this country is the administration of the government health insurance program of Medicare and the health assistance program of Medicaid. These programs are administered by official agencies that are traditionally considered to be welfare agencies: the Social Security Administration and state departments of social service. Official and private health agencies have little input into, control over, or administration of these two major government health programs. The case situation of John Falta evidenced both intersystem and intrasystem lack of coordination; health care and welfare professionals were not communicating with each other or with professionals from other systems.

Lack of coordination of services is evident in all sectors of our health and welfare systems. The National Commission on Community Health Services (1966, p. 132) identified that there is minimal coordination between official (goverment) and private health care agencies. The National Health Planning and Resource Development Act of 1974 (Public Law 93-64) was passed to improve the delivery and coordination of government health care services to all segments of the population. It is hoped that this legislation will improve coordination activities between local, state, and federal government agencies as well as between government and private resources.

Presently, health and welfare resources are mainly organized on a federal level through one agency, the Department of Health and Human Services, formerly the Department of Health, Education, and Welfare. State and local governments traditionally have decentralized organization of health and welfare services, with one agency administering health programs and another agency administering welfare programs. Private health and welfare service administration is diverse.

THE FEDERAL GOVERNMENT: HEALTH AND WELFARE ORGANIZATION

The word health was left out of the United States Constitution, and thus the federal government bases its health and welfare activities on the Preamble to the Constitution, which charges it with providing for the general welfare of the people. Public health is the responsibility of the individual states and is provided for through their constitutions, legislation, and public health codes.

The Surgeon General of the United States has recently issued a document which describes the potential for better health among Americans (*Public Health Reports,* 1979, p. 483). This document, "Healthy People: The Surgeon General's Report on Health Promotion and Disease Prevention," sets forth specific goals to be attained over the next 10 years. These are the following:

· A 35 percent reduction in infant mortality

· A 20 percent reduction in deaths of children age 1 to 14

· A 20 percent reduction in deaths among adolescents and adults

· A 25 percent reduction in deaths among adults age 25 to 46

· A major improvement in health, mobility, and independence among older people, measured by a 20 percent reduction in the average number of days of illness among this age group

The health problems implicit in these goals cannot be solved by individuals alone. Organized health and welfare efforts at all levels of the government are essential in order to achieve these goals. The health and welfare activities of the federal government are described below.

Functions

The federal government establishes health goals and then attempts to implement them through its various agencies and offices. In order to implement established goals, the federal government is involved in carrying out certain health functions. The functions of the federal government in relation to health and welfare issues fall into three major categories (Wilner, Walkley, and O'Neill, 1978, pp. 33–34):

1. Functions dealing with the general population

    a. Protection from hazards affecting the entire population that cannot be provided by the states

    b. Collection and dissemination of national health and welfare statistics and related data

    c. Advancement of the biologic, medical, and environmental sciences

    d. Augmentation of health facilities and certain categories of health personnel

    e. Support of state and local governments in the maintenance of public health services.

    f. Organization and support of disaster relief and civil defense

2. Functions dealing with special population groups

   a. Protection of workers from hazardous occupations and adverse conditions of work

   b. Provision of categorical and special services by state and local governments for children, the aged, the mentally ill and retarded, vocationally handicapped adults, and blind persons

   c. Purchase of medical care by state and local governments for certain dependent population groups

   d. Provision of special services for farm families and migrant workers

   e. Provision of hospital and medical services to veterans, merchant seamen, American Indians, Alaskan natives, federal prisoners, persons with leprosy, members of the armed services and their dependents, and civil service employees of the federal government who are injured as a result of their employment

   f. Hospital and medical insurance for civil service employees of the federal government

3. Functions dealing with international health and welfare

   a. Participation in international health activities

   b. Sharing of health knowledge with other nations

   c. Maintenance of membership in the World Health Organization and other international health and welfare agencies

The federal government provides funding for programs through general tax revenues and social security health insurance contributions. In 1976, the federal government spent $42.5 billion on health (Turner, 1977, p. 1443). Most of the health and welfare functions of the federal government are coordinated through the Department of Health and Human Services.

Department of Health and Human Services/Department of Health, Education, and Welfare (DHEW)

This department assumed a cabinet-level position in 1953, with a charge to safeguard the health and welfare of the nation. It has regional offices across the nation to help carry out this task. In 1980, the Department of Health, Education, and Welfare became the Department of Health and Human Services and the Department of Education. The Department of Health and Human Services is expected to carry out the health and welfare activities that have previously been the responsibility of the DHEW. The organizational structure of the Department of Health and Human Services has not yet been determined. It is assumed that this department will incorporate major DHEW branches, such as the Social Security Administration, Public Health Service, Office of Human Development, Health Care Financing Administration, and Office of Child Support Enforcement. These agencies are discussed below (Federal Information Center, 1980). Other DHEW components, especially those which have both health and educational aspects, are less definite as to their eventual place of administration. Their eventual placement is of significance to the community health nurse, because it involves legislation, including the Nurse Training Acts, which provides funding for the preparation of qualified community health nurses. Nurses should watch these developments with awareness and work with their professional organizations to monitor the distribution of funds for professional education.

Social Security Administration

This administration was established on July 16, 1946, when its predecessor, the Social Security Board, was abolished. It administers many of the assistance and insurance programs established by the Social Security Act of 1935. Other functions of this agency include research and program development to reduce poverty, and health programs, as well as statistical evaluation of social security programs and government and public education services funded by the Social Security Act. This administration is serviced by local offices across the nation and is the major federal agency dealing with social welfare programs (see Chapter 4).

Public Health Service

This agency is charged with protecting the health of the nation, as well as developing international health policies and cooperation. It is the oldest of the department's component agencies, established in 1798, and is under the direction of the Surgeon General. It primarily carries out the mandates of the Public Health Act of 1944 and is the major health agency of the federal government.

The Public Health Service collects and disseminates national health statistics, coordinates national health resource planning, operates laboratory services, funds the construction and modernization of health care facilities, conducts and supports health research, provides grants-in-aid to schools of public health, provides funding for the training of health care professionals, operates the Food and Drug Administration, National Institutes of Health, Center for Disease Control, and National Institute for Occupational Safety and Health, and works to prevent and control communicable disease. Through its Center for Disease Control, rarely used therapeutic and immunoprophylactic agents may be obtained (Benenson, 1975, p. xix).

Office of Human Development

This office assists in developing to their fullest potential at-risk Americans, such as children, the aged, the physically and mentally handicapped, and those Americans living in areas that have limited health and welfare resources. Services for high-risk population groups are discussed in Chapters 13 through 19.

Health Care Financing Administration

This agency oversees the administration of Medicare, Medicaid, and related federal quality control measures designed to improve the delivery of health care services. It was created by the DHEW reorganization of March 8, 1977. Chapters 4, 12, and 21 address issues handled by this administration.

Office of Child Support Enforcement

This office was also created by the DHEW reorganization of March 8, 1977. It develops, plans, and implements child support enforcement policy, helps to establish paternity, and obtains child support for dependent children from absent parents. It was established to decrease the amount of federal spending on welfare assistance programs.

ACTION

ACTION carries out important human service functions on both a national and international level, even though it is not a cabinet-level agency. Some of its component programs are Volunteers in Service to America (VISTA), the Peace Corps, foster grandparent programs, and other national volunteer programs. The agencies that the nurse will frequently hear about are the Peace Corps and VISTA.

The Peace Corps and VISTA are federal volunteer organizations. The Peace Corps is an international program that provides health and welfare services, through American volunteers, to nations in need. The VISTA program is a national program which brings health and welfare services to disadvantaged people in America. Many VISTA and Peace Corps volunteers are health and welfare professionals, including nurses, doctors, and social workers. Peace Corps and VISTA volunteers undergo extensve training. Peace Corps volunteers must learn to speak the local language, become familiar with local customs, and adapt to the living conditions of the area. Peace Corps and VISTA volunteers live in the communities in which they serve, in the same living conditions as the people with whom they work.

Other Federal Departments and Agencies with Health and Welfare Functions

All of the federal departments in the United States have functions which relate to the improvement of health and welfare conditions in our nation or foreign countries. These departments do not have the scope of health and welfare responsibilities that DHEW has, but they provide essential services that enhance the health status of United States residents. Briefly summarized below are some of the health and welfare functions carried out by our federal departments:

· Department of Agriculture: works to eradicate animal diseases; inspects domestic and imported meat, poultry, dairy products, and fresh and processed fruit and vegetables; operates programs of loans to protect and develop natural resources; coordinates a nationwide rural development program, and administers the food stamp, child nutrition, and supplemental food (WIC) programs (Office of Federal Register, 1977, pp. 107–141).

· Department of Commerce: promotes the nation's economic development and encourages technological advancements. Its Bureau of the Census collects and disseminates data about the economy of the country and the characteristics of population groups; census information is discussed more thoroughly in Chapter 11 (Office of Federal Register, 1977, pp. 142–164).

· Department of Defense: protects the security of our nation by maintaining sufficient military forces throughout the world and by operating the National Civil Defense Program (Office of Federal Register, 1977, pp. 165–240).

· Department of Housing and Urban Development (HUD): provides assistance for low-income housing, for the development of impoverished communities, and for the establishment of new communities. It also directs the Federal Disaster Relief Program and establishes standards for mobile homes (Office of Federal Register, 1977, pp. 283–300).

· Department of the Interior: enforces health and safety standards in mines, protects natural resources, and conducts research and health educational programs to improve the ecological conditions in our country. Its Bureau of Indian Affairs actively promotes the improvement of health and welfare conditions for our Native Americans (Office of Federal Register, 1977, pp. 301–330).

· Department of Justice: protects the health of the American public in a variety of ways. By enforcing federal laws, this department is involved in reducing many of our major health problems, including such things as homicidal deaths, accidents due to violence, and drug addiction. It also maintains a health program in federal prisons which provides medical, psychiatric, dental, and health support services for prisoners, along with environmental health, safety, and rehabilitation services (Office of the Federal Register, 1977, pp. 331–357).

· Department of Labor: responsible for helping disadvantaged segments of the population (migrant workers, Native Americans, older workers, offenders, seasonal farm workers, welfare recipients, and others) to obtain employment, for increasing workforce services to underserved areas, for coordinating federal worker compensation programs, and for enforcing safety standards and fair employment practices in the work environment. This department administers the major provisions of the Occupational Safety and Health Act of 1970 (Office of Federal Register, 1977 pp. 358–378).

· Department of the State: assists the president in formulating foreign policy for the purpose of promoting long-range security and well-being in the United States. Carries out foreign assistance programs (AID) to improve the quality of life in underdeveloped countries (Office of Register, 1977, pp. 379–402).

· Department of Transportation: protects the nation's environment by implementing the National Environmental Policy Act; by enforcing air, land, and water safety standards; and by conducting programs aimed at reducing the increasingly large number of deaths or injuries due to traffic accidents (Office of Federal Register, 1977, pp. 403–429).

· Department of the Treasury: through the U.S. Customs Service and the Bureau of Alcohol, Tobacco, and Firearms, assists other government agencies in preventing illegal drug traffic; illegal possession of firearms, alcoholic beverages, and tobacco products; transportation of diseased animals and plants; and the spread of communicable diseases (Office of Federal Register, 1977, pp. 430–455).

Besides our federal departments, there are numerous other agencies on the federal level that have significant health and welfare functions. The Veterans' Administration, for instance, provides hospital, nursing home, and domiciliary care and outpatient medical and dental care to eligible veterans of military service. This agency is also responsible for coordinating compensation, pension, and assistance programs; rehabilitation training for disabled veterans; and life insurance programs and burial services for veterans. In addition, it maintains a National Cemetery System (Office of the Federal Register, 1977, pp. 657–661). The Commission on Civil Rights, the Environmental Protection Agency, the Interstate Commerce Commission, and the Tennessee Valley Authority are a few other examples of federal agencies that work to improve health and welfare conditions in our nation. The federal agencies that carry out health and welfare activities are too numerous to describe here. The *United States Government Manual* provides detailed information about the functions of most federal departments and agencies and is updated yearly.

International Involvement

Every nation has its own health and welfare policies. However, there is international cooperation and coordination on issues related to public health and welfare. The United States is involved with a number of agencies, groups, and governments on an international level, to maintain and improve health and welfare conditions throughout the world. There are several intergovernmental agreements, especially in relation to disease control, trade, immigration, world peace, and respect for basic human rights, which have been developed to enhance the well-being of all people.

The United States is extensively involved in international health and welfare issues through the United Nations. This international assembly is dedicated to promoting welfare, peace, and health. Two major United Nations–sponsored groups with which the United States works are the World Health Organization (WHO) and the United Nations' Children's Fund (UNICEF).

World Health Organization

Efforts to organize international health activities took place between 1851 and 1909, when a series of meetings known as the International Sanitary Conferences occurred. These meetings were the precursor to the creation of the International Office of Public Health in 1909 (Wilner, Walkley, and O'Neill, 1978, p. 62). The primary focus of most international health activity is the control of communicable disease.

In 1948, the World Health Organization (WHO) was created and became a part of the United Nations. The World Health Organization is concerned with standardizing international health activities and regulations, providing statistical and health educational services, promoting research, training health workers, promoting maternal-child health, and controlling communicable diseases. Any nation can belong to WHO without being a member of the United Nations. It is an influential international health organization that has done much to promote world health.

United Nations' Children's Fund

UNICEF attempts to meet the emergency and ongoing needs of children, particularly children in developing countries. It has improved maternal and child health and welfare conditions by combating malnutrition (food programs), preventing and controlling communicable diseases (immunization and treatment programs), compiling statistics, supporting research, and providing shelter and other basic welfare needs. WHO and UNICEF work closely together to promote services for at-risk mothers and children throughout the world.

International and federal health and welfare programs are designed to safeguard the health of all citizens in the United States as well as the health of persons throughout the world. These programs help state and local governments to effectively monitor communicable diseases and to provide and evaluate needed health and welfare services in the local community. Even though their services were discussed only briefly, it must be emphasized that international and federal health programs are critical to the maintenance of health in states and local communities.

STATE AND LOCAL GOVERNMENT: HEALTH SERVICES RELATIONSHIP

In the United States, each state is responsible for providing for the health of its residents. Each state has a public health code that authorizes public health activities, and an agency, usually a state health department, to deal with health. It has been traditional for state and local governments to place health and welfare functions with separate agencies. This separation often results in lack of service coordination. When the terms *state health department* and *local health department* are used in this text, it will be in reference to official government health departments. These agencies are supported by general tax revenues and provide services at little or no cost to the general public. The services they offer are discussed later in this chapter; they will vary greatly from state to state and locality to locality.

Each state health department has local affiliates. State public health codes establish what type of relationship will evolve between state and local health departments. Miller, Brooks, DeFriese, Gilbert, Jain, and Kavaler (1977, p. 932) found that there are definite patterns of organization that exist between state and local health departments.

Patterns of Organizational Structure between State and Local Health Departments

There are three organizational patterns that characterize the administrative relationships between state and local health departments (Miller, Brooks, DeFriese, Gilbert, Jain, and Kavaler, 1977, p. 932):

1. Centralized organization: a state department of public health or a state board of health operates local health units that function directly under the state's authority, sometimes through regional administration and sometimes with the help of a local board that maintains advisory functions to the local unit.

2. Decentralized organization: local government (city, township, county, or some combination) operates a health department either directly or with the authority of a local board of health intervening. The state health department offers consultation and advice either to the local board, to the local department, or to both.

3. Shared organizational control: local government may operate a health department either directly or through a local board of health. Under circumstances that are more or less well defined, these same departments fall under the authority of state health departments. The state department sometimes retains appointive and line authority over local health officers who are also responsible to local boards or commissions. Sometimes the local departments must submit programs, plans, and budgets to the state health department in order to qualify for federal or state funds.

The relationships between state and local health departments are seldom explicit in legislation and public health codes. Authority for the promulgation of health rules and regulations is shared by state and local health departments in 68 percent of the states and held exclusively by state health departments in 30 percent (Miller, Gilbert, Warren, Brooks, DeFriese, Jain, and Kavaler, 1977, p. 935). State health departments are frequently responsible for setting statewide standards and for assisting local health departments in providing direct health care services (Black, 1977, p. 72). State health departments usually share in the cost of local health department services, but the cost-sharing ratio varies greatly. The total cost for state and local governments to provide health department services was $2.2 billion in 1976 (Turner, 1977, p. 472). Services provided by state and local health departments vary; some common service areas are discussed here.

State and Local Health Departments: Service Functions

An overall goal of state and local health departments is to enhance personal and community health. This is done through provision of public health services such as:

1. Administrative
2. Communicable disease control
3. Personal health (maternal-child health and adult health)
4. Environmental health and safety
5. Occupational health
6. Vital statistics
7. Laboratory

8. Health education, training, and research

9. Emergency and special medical

Each state determines what health services it will offer. These services are established in the state's public health code, which many states are in the process of revising. Some states are proposing certain basic health serv-ices which every citizen has a right to receive and which must be provided by state and local health departments. Only seven states have made revisions in their codes since 1965, and over half have not revised them in the last quarter century (Miller, Gilbert, Warren, Brooks, DeFriese, Jain, and Kavaler, 1977, p. 935). Many codes still deal primarily with com-municable disease control.

STATE HEALTH DEPARTMENTS

As stated previously, in most states responsi-bility for public health is lodged in a state de-partment of public health. The chief executive of the department, often called the health of-ficer or the director, is frequently appointed by the governor or legislature and is directly responsible to them. Many state health direc-tors are physicians with public health training. State health departments are charged with providing the leadership, policies, and fund-ing necessary to develop local public health programs; their services are more *indirect* then direct.

Each state authorizes specific public health services through its public health code: all state public health codes include communicable dis-ease control and collection of vital statistics; 92 percent of them include venereal disease (VD) control and quarantine; 82 percent include re-fuse disposal; and only 26 percent include family planning services (Miller, Gilbert, War-ren, Brooks, DeFriese, Jain, and Kavaler, 1977, p. 943). The state health department can del-egate authority and responsibility for certain health activities to local health departments, but ultimate responsibility rests with the state. State health departments are funded through state tax dollars and federal grant-in-aid pro-grams. The budgets of state health depart-ments will vary.

The structure of state health departments differs from state to state. Figure 5-1 is an or-ganizational chart depicting how a state health department may be organized.

Service Functions

The state health department is charged with furnishing the leadership and funding to meet state public health needs. It carries out this charge through the service functions de-scribed below.

Administrative

Promulgation and enforcement of health standards, regulations, and policies are primary functions of state health departments. They set legally enforceable health standards, regulations, and policies, based on authority from state public health codes and other legislation. These fre-quently include establishing and enforcing public health codes; determining state public health policy; providing a state public health program with clear goals and objectives; estab-lishing communicable disease regulations and programs; licensing of state health profession-als; licensing of health facilities; and monitor-ing state health insurance laws. States may del-egate enforcement of public health law and regulations to local health agencies, but this function is overwhelmingly assigned to states

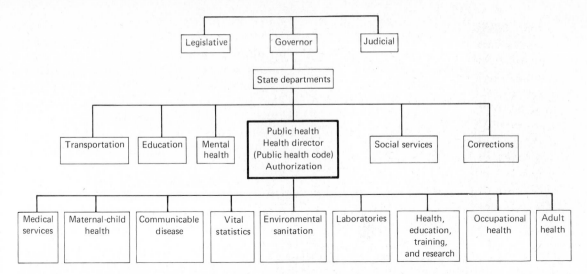

FIGURE 5-1 Organizational chart of a state public health department. *Note:* Other state-level agencies will also have health functions (Department of Social Service administering Medicaid), but the Department of Public Health is the agency traditionally in charge of public health matters. Also, the title of the health agency may vary from state to state. Some states are developing "super agencies" combining such activities as mental health, education, public health, and social services into one department.

in the public health codes. The state health department may take action against a local health department that is not adhering to state health policies. State health departments also develop standardized forms for statewide use in obtaining statistical information on births, marriages, and morbidity and mortality events. The licensing of health professionals is an important state function.

Working with local health departments to promote comprehensive, coordinated services in accordance with state health policy is extremely important. The state health department advises local health departments on health planning, programming, and enforcement, budget review, and personnel policies. It can assist them in obtaining staff members and may approve their plan of organization and function. In some states, the state health department establishes the qualifications for local health officers. It also shares the cost of service provision with local health depart-

ments, often on a per capita or straight percentage basis (e.g., 20 percent of cost).

Consultation services are provided to local health departments and other health agencies. Consultants are available in such fields as maternal-child health, nutrition, epidemiology, community health nursing, mental health, occupational health, and environmental health. These consultant activities are usually well utilized and are a major state health department service.

Administration of federally aided programs, such as maternal-child health and communicable disease control, is lodged with the state health department. The state is accountable to the federal government when federal funds are used to support such programs.

Health planning activities are carried out by the state health department. These include identification of state health needs, program development, and ongoing program evaluation. The state participates in comprehensive health planning through state and local planning agencies.

Coordination of federal, state, and local health programs and services is assumed by the state health department. It compiles data on available health resources and services offered throughout the state.

Legislation is guided and influenced by the department at both the state and federal levels. Health legislation that represents and meets the needs of the people is promoted and developed. The department may meet regularly with state legislators and congressmen.

Personnel policies, including hiring and promotional guides, grievance procedures, position descriptions, and manuals are developed by the state health department. A roster of available health personnel may be kept to help local health departments and other agencies recruit new staff.

Control of Communicable Disease

Communicable disease control is a major service function of state health departments. The state establishes immunization schedules, quarantine measures, and reportable communicable diseases, provides policies for epidemics and laboratory diagnostic services, and may supply local health departments with biologics. Local health departments must adhere to state communicable disease policies and report cases of communicable disease as determined by the state. Control of communicable disease is an extremely important function, even though the extent of communicable diseases in our country has significantly decreased in the last century.

Personal Health Services

Personal health services are all services delivered to individuals, except those related to environmental health. Both maternal-child health and adult health services are often coordi-

nated by the state health department, especially if federal or state funds or both are used to finance these programs. Maternal-child health services include administering federal programs, such as family planning, the Medicaid program of Early, Periodic Screening, Diagnosis, and Treatment (EPSDT), and services to crippled children and children with mental retardation and other developmental disabilities. The state provides program planning and evaluation consultation for many maternal-child health programs that are offered at the local level.

Adult health activities include administering federal programs for heart disease, cancer, stroke, kidney disease, arthritis, and mental health. Again, these programs are brought to a direct service level through the local health department.

Environmental Health

Environmental health activities include setting and enforcing environmental health standards for food, water, air, land usage, and sanitation. The state offers consultant services in this area. Increasingly it is being recognized that there are major environmental health problems in our country. Environmental health hazards are discussed in Chapters 13 through 18, where the major health problems of the developmental age groups are identified.

Occupational Health

Occupational health activities are frequently carried out through a state occupational safety and health administration (OSHA), which is often under the direction of the state health department. Some states may not have their own OSHA, in which case this function is largely carried out through the federal Occupational Safety and Health Administration. State occupational health and safety standards must be equal to or exceed federal standards.

Vital Statistics

Vital statistics are collected and disseminated by the state health department. To aid in this, the state develops standardized forms, including certificates of birth, death, fetal death, marriage, and divorce; licenses for marriage; and epidemiologic reporting forms. The state also disseminates statistical information to individuals and agencies, including the National Center for Health Statistics. The state health department has an abundance of statistical information about the health status of its population and the health work force and resources within the state. This information is available to the general public on request.

Laboratory Services

Laboratory Services are operated by the state health department. Specimens are sent there for analysis; the diagnostic services rendered are primarily in relation to communicable disease control and environmental sanitation. Local health departments and private physicians often utilize these services on behalf of clients. There is usually no fee, or a minimal fee, to the public for laboratory analysis of reportable communicable diseases (e.g., *Shigella* and typhoid). The laboratory also certifies vaccines and other biologics.

Health Education, Training, and Research

Education, training, and research are carried out by the state health department. The state promotes the development of new health knowledge through the support of state colleges and universities and research agencies; the dissemination of health information to the general public (printed materials, classes, and media programs); the development of training and inservice programs for state and local health department personnel; and involvement in research activities. Local health departments find state health departments to be valuable resources when health information and communications media are needed.

Emergency and Special Medical Services

Special medical services include the provision of hospital and institutional services for chronic or long-term conditions, such as mental retardation, mental illness, and tuberculosis. In the event of emergencies such as epidemics and natural disasters, emergency services ensure that the necessary public health care is made available to the community in need.

Staff

The state health department is headed by a chief executive (health officer or other title) who is usually appointed by the governor; this person is traditionally a physician. Other staff members include administrators, clerical workers, and consultants in fields such as community health nursing, occupational health, mental health, epidemiology, statistics, maternal-child health, health education, and nutrition. State health departments have legal counsel available to them, often through the state attorney general's office. States may have regional directors who serve as intermediaries between their regions and the state department. Most state health department personnel, except for the chief executive, are civil service employees.

Community health nurses are a valuable part of state health department staffs. They are hired on a consultant basis and help to establish state health policies, particularly in relation to maternal-child health and adult health services. They work closely with local health departments to improve the quality of care delivered to individuals, families, and populations at risk. Generally, community health nurses who work for state health departments are prepared at the master's or doctoral level and have past community health nursing experience.

LOCAL HEALTH DEPARTMENT

The local health department is the basic unit for delivery of direct public health services to clients. It has responsibility for a specific jurisdiction, often the political jurisdiction of a city or county. Chapter 3 discusses the framework of a community and how community health service areas may conform to a political jurisdiction. Local health departments by type of jurisdiction are seen in Table 5-1. One out of every four U.S. citizens is served by these departments each year (Miller, Gilbert, Warren, Brooks, DeFriese, Jain, and Kavaler, 1977, p. 941).

Local health departments usually have a board of health and a physician as a chief executive. An example of how an organizational structure for a local health department might look is given in Figure 5-2. Each local health department establishes its own specific organizational pattern.

Local health departments receive their funding from a number of sources, primarily state and local tax dollars. These tax dollars come from tax levies assessed on the valuation of residents' taxable property, personal in-

come, and business and industry taxes (Smolensky, 1977, p. 170). Table 5-2 presents a breakdown by funding source of the mean percentages of local health department budgets in the United States. The column does not total 100 percent because of missing data and the rounding off of percentages. This funding enables the local health department to provide a number of services at no cost, or at a low cost, to the community, many of which are carried out by the community health nursing staff.

Rural areas may have a difficult time obtaining enough tax funds, population, and health professionals to support a health department. It is recommended that an area contain at least 50,000 people before it considers establishing an independent health department (Hanlon and McHose, 1971, p. 52). Increasingly it is being found that the health needs of rural citizens are not being met.

Service Functions

Local health departments have functions similar to those carried out by the state health department, but the services they provide are more direct. Direct services offered by local health departments are extensive, but many people are often not aware of the extent of these services or that they are generally offered at little or no cost.

Administrative

The administrative functions of the local health department are identical in coverage to those implemented by the state health department, but the specific services vary.

Promulgation and enforcement of health standards, regulations, and policies are responsibilities carried out by the local health department for the jurisdiction it serves. The standards estab-

TABLE 5-1. Percent Local Health Departments in United States by Type of Jurisdiction, 1974

City	14.1
County	47.4
2 or more counties	8.4
Town	8.9
City + 1 county	15.2
City + counties	4.9
Other	1.1
Total percent	100.0
Total number	1337

SOURCE: From C. A. Miller, B. Gilbert, D. C. Warren, E. F. Brooks, G. H. DeFriese, S. C. Jain, & F. Kavaler. A survey of local public health departments and their directors. *American Journal of Public Health*, October 1977, *67*, 933.

lished by a local health department usually relate to public food handling, storage, preparation, and disposal and to public water supplies, including wells, septic systems, and pools or lakes at recreational facilities. Local health departments also supervise and license local health facilities such as hospitals and nursing homes.

Working cooperatively with local health agencies is a function of the health department. Coordinating private and official health care resources and providing advice on health matters are functions that the local health department does not always maximize to fullest potential.

Consultation services are offered by the local health department to agencies and individuals. These activities usually involve consulting services from community health nurses, environmental engineers, nutritionists, and epidemiologists. Consultation in relation to health policy, environmental safety, and personal health services is often offered to schools, industry, hospitals, and nursing homes within the health department's jurisdiction.

Health planning activities within the local health department include analyzing and determining the public health needs of the people within its jurisdiction and planning health action strategies to meet these needs. The health department also carries out an ongoing evaluation of its programs and participates in statewide health planning activities (see Chapters 12 and 21).

Coordination of health services with other community agencies is an important function of the local health department. Often the health department provides leadership for resource coordination and development within the local community.

Legislation is guided and influenced by this department, primarily on a state level. The local health department makes its legislative needs known to the state legislators and members of congress. It is imperative that local

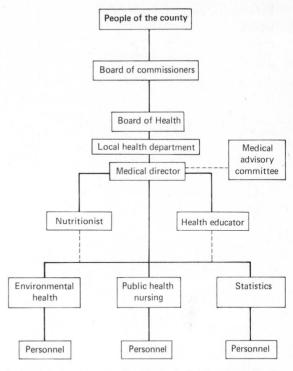

FIGURE 5-2 Organizational chart of a local health department. (*From L. Black, Community health administration. Ann Arbor: University of Michigan Press, 1977, p. 52*)

health departments assume leadership in the formulation of health policy, because they are knowledgeable about preventive health needs as well as curative needs. If local health departments do not become involved in policy making, important preventive health care services may be lacking in a community.

Personnel policies, promotion guides, position descriptions, grievance policies, and manuals are developed by local health departments to facilitate effective and efficient management of the organization. Staff turnover and job satisfaction are often directly related to how well an organization is managed (see Chapter 20). Some position descriptions and qualifications, such as health officer, may be determined by the state health department and followed by the local health departments.

TABLE 5-2 Mean Percent of Local Health Department Budget Funding by Source, United States, 1974

Budget source	Percent
Federal	8.6
State	21.6
Local	59.8
Fees (direct services, inspection, licensing)	5.3
Other (contracts, grants)	1.9
Total	97.2

NOTE: Mean total U.S. local health department budget: $759,864 per year (1974).

SOURCE: From C. A. Miller, B. Gilbert, D. C. Warren, E. F. Brooks, G. H. DeFriese, S. C. Jain, & F. Kavaler. A survey of local health departments and their directors. *American Journal of Public Health*, 1977, *67*, 933.

Some health departments use state services to recruit qualified personnel. Many local health departments are involved in working with staff unions and other collective bargaining groups. Local health department employees are frequently civil service employees.

Control of Communicable Disease

Communicable disease control is a major emphasis of the local health department. Each local health authority, in conformity with regulations of higher authority (state, national, and international), will determine what diseases are to be routinely and regularly reported, who is responsible for reporting, the nature of the reports, and the manner in which the reports are to be forwarded (Benenson, 1975, p. xxiii). Reportable communicable diseases that are required by international health regulations are cholera, plague, smallpox, and yellow fever, and those diseases under surveillance by WHO: louse-borne typhus fever and relapsing fever, paralytic poliomyelitis, influenza, and malaria (Benenson, 1975, p. xxiii). In addition, in the United States, viral hepatitis, infectious hepatitis, rubella, salmonellosis, and venereal syphilis must be reported.

Other communicable diseases reportable to

the local health authority will vary, and their selection is often dependent on the severity and frequency of the disease. Some communicable diseases will be reported on the basis of individual cases and some only if epidemics occur. Some commonly reportable individual cases of communicable diseases (in addition to those already mentioned) are diphtheria, gonorrhea, leprosy, rubeola, meningococcal meningitis, Q fever, rabies, shigellosis, tetanus, tuberculosis, typhoid, and whooping cough. Some commonly reportable disease epidemics are ringworm, conjunctivitis, staphylococcal food poisoning, viral gastroenteritis, giardiasis, bacterial pneumonia, staphylococcal disease, streptococcal disease (Group A, beta-hemolytic), and botulism.

The communicable disease services of local health departments include prevention, case finding, early diagnosis, and treatment. Many operate venereal disease, tuberculosis, and immunization clinics. These services are provided at no or little cost to the general public. Biologics for immunizations are distributed to private physicians by the health department. The department also makes epidemiological studies of suspected or reported cases of communicable disease, and the community health nurse is actively involved in this follow-up (see Chapter 10).

The health department provides other communicable disease measures, such as enforcing quarantines; conducting public food, water, and refuse disposal inspections; controlling rabies; and keeping communicable disease statistics. The environmental health division is extensively involved in these measures.

Personal Health Services

Personal health services are a major component of local health department services. They include both maternal-child health and adult health activities. To carry out these activities, the health department offers an extensive array of clinics, classes, and home visit services.

School health is a major component of maternal-child health services on the local level. Community health nurses employed by the health department often function in schools to provide health education, counseling, and direct care services to pupils. They may conduct screening programs, such as hearing, vision, and scoliosis, to identify children who have health needs. The role of the school nurse is discussed in Chapter 14.

Many other maternal-child health services are provided by the local health department. Clinic services for these two segments of the population include family planning, immunization, venereal disease, well-child, and Early, Periodic Screening, Diagnosis, and Treatment (EPSDT). Classes are offered to expectant and new parents, and home visits are made to follow up on antepartal and postpartum clients, crippled children, and high-risk infants and mothers. Counseling and health teaching in relation to immunizations, growth and development, and community resources are a few examples of the types of services provided by community health nurses when they make home visits. In addition, programs such as the nutrition program for Women, Infants, and Children (WIC), dental health, and hearing-vision conservation are often established by the local health department in order to reduce maternal and child health morbidity and mortality; consultants are often available to facilitate implementation of these services.

Adult health services also involve clinics, classes, and home visit services by the community health nurse. Community health nurses frequently visit adults to provide information about health conditions, including chronic conditions such as heart disease, diabetes, cancer, accidents, arthritis, stroke, alcoholism, and drug abuse, and to help clients experiencing these conditions to adapt to the changes occurring in their lives; the community health nurse's major goal when working with adult clients is to enhance their self-care capabilities. Classes in relation to such conditions as diabetes, hypertension, and substance abuse are also conducted by the community health nurse or other health department personnel. In addition, clinics for venereal disease, family planning, immunization, blood pressure screening, breast cancer screening, and geriatric multiphasic screening are offered to promote wellness in adults. The community health nurse works closely with community resources to assist the adult in meeting health care needs.

Environmental Health

Environmental services include but are not limited to areas concerning food, water, vectors and nuisances, land, waste disposal, air, shelters, and workplaces. These areas encompass many things. Specific environmental health services include extermination programs for nuisances and vectors (rats and mosquitoes); inspection and licensing of restaurants and other food facilities; ensuring compliance with regulations for public and private water supplies; monitoring of public recreational facilities, disposal of waste and on-site sewage, and air pollution; and controlling and giving advice on land planning, school site selection, and mobile home park and campground development. Fees may be assessed from the individual for certain permits and licenses, but most services are done at no cost.

Occupational Health

Occupational health services are usually not carried out extensively on a local level. The Occupational Safety and Health Act of 1970 allows states to establish their own occupational safety and health administrations, but occupational health activities are largely conducted on a state level. Some industries are contracting with local health departments to route workers through health department diagnostic and screening programs. Some occupational health nurses, especially those in small industries, are seeking consultation from the nursing staff in the local health department for the development of health policies and procedures and the management of clinic facilities.

Vital Statistics

Vital statistics in relation to the population that the health department serves are collected and disseminated to individuals, interested groups, and the state health department. The local health department keeps statistics on births, deaths, and reportable communicable diseases, maintains registers of individuals known to have specific communicable diseases where carrier states exist (typhoid), conducts morbidity and mortality surveys as necessary, and maintains records on jurisdictional health facilities.

Laboratory Services

Laboratory services are also provided by the local health department. However, many local health departments do not have their own laboratories and use state facilities. Laboratory services may be extended to hospitals, clinics, and private practitioners on a contractual, fee-for-service, or other basis. Laboratory services include water analysis, serology, urology, parasitology, identification of microorganisms, x-ray for tuberculosis control, sanitation laboratory services, and metabolic and genetic screening for conditions such as phenylketonuria (PKU) and sickle-cell anemia. These services are essential for communicable disease control and environmental sanitation and safety, as well as for the treatment of genetic and metabolic disorders and genetic counseling related to these conditions.

Health Education, Training, and Research

Education, training, and research are a part of local health department services. The local health department provides health education services directly to individual clients, develops and carries out community health education programs, distributes health education materials, provides classes, and serves as a health information center. Master's-prepared health educators are often hired by local health departments to coordinate health education activities.

Training activities largely involve staff in-service and continuing education programs. Some health departments offer tuition reimbursement for university course work in public health or related fields as a staff benefit.

Research activities often include morbidity, mortality, and program evaluation studies. State health departments are usually more actively involved in research, but increasingly, local health departments are recognizing the need for such activity.

Emergency and Special Medical Services

Special and emergency medical services offered by the local health department usually involve catastrophic medical care during a natural disaster or an epidemic or compulsory hospitalization through judicial admissions for acute communicable diseases such as tuberculosis. Health department personnel are also involved in health planning activities designed to meet the emergency needs of community citizens.

Overall, local health departments offer many services vital to maintaining the health of the communities they serve. Community health nurses are extensively involved in providing these services. Table 5-3 presents an overview of the types of services offered by health departments, as well as the percentage of health departments in the United States offering each specific service. These statistics were compiled by the authors of a nationwide study, who surveyed by questionnaire all the health officers in the United States. Information was received from 1345 departments, or at least 68 percent of all local health departments (Miller, Brooks, DeFriese, Gilbert, Jain, and Kavaler, 1977, p. 931).

Staff

Staff will vary from one local health department to another. The minimum staff includes (1) a health officer, (2) a community health nurse, (3) an environmental engineer (sanitarian), and (4) a clerk. Additional personnel include statistician, epidemiologist, health educator, physical therapist, occupational health specialist, nutritionist, dentist, dental hygienist, veterinarian, and social worker. To provide comprehensive community health services, a basic, multidisciplinary staff is necessary. The following staff-to-community population ratio is recommended; these numbers are not often a reality (Hanlon and McHose, 1971, p. 56):

Staff	Population
Health officer/medical personnel	1:50,000
Sanitarians (environmental engineers)	1:15,000
Community health nurses	1:5,000
Office personnel (clerk)	1:15,000

Health Officer

A health officer is usually a physician with public health training who is licensed to practice in the state. This person administers the agency; prepares and submits budgets; appoints and hires personnel; takes part in program planning, implementation, and evaluation; and serves as a consultant to health department staff and community agencies. The health officer is responsible for seeing that all divisions in the local health department

TABLE 5-3 Percent of Health Departments Providing Selected Services, United States, 1974

Services	Percent providing each service	Percent serving as sole provider of each service
Immunization programs	96.3	62.3
Environmental surveillance	96.0	70.4
Tuberculosis control	93.9	63.3
Maternal and child health	89.4	48.5
School health program	89.2	38.5
Venereal disease control	88.0	57.7
Chronic disease programs	84.3	25.7
Home care	76.7	44.8
Family planning	63.3	38.0
Ambulatory care	50.3	7.6
Mental health	47.4	5.4
Chronic institutional care	11.8	1.5
Acute institutional care	8.4	1.4

SOURCE: From C. A. Miller, B. Gilbert, D. C. Warren, E. F. Brooks, G. H. DeFriese, S. C. Jain, & F. Kavaler. A survey of local health departments and their directors. *American Journal of Public Health*, 1977, *67*, 934.

are run effectively and efficiently (Black, 1977, p. 52).

Community Health Nurse

Community health nurses carry out a variety of health activities, which are discussed throughout this text. Community health nurses utilize a synthesis of nursing and public health theory to facilitate client utilization of services in industry, schools, home, classes, clinics, and the community as a whole. They are the backbone of the personal health services of the health department and are extensively involved in most health department programs. The types of services offered by the nursing division in a local health department vary, depending on the work force available and other community resources that have been developed to meet the health care needs of community citizens. For example, if a community has a Visiting Nurse Association (VNA), community health nurses from the health department usually do not provide skilled nursing services to clients; health supervision visits would be their major focus. On the other hand, if there are no home care programs available in the community, the health department frequently provides skilled nursing services for clients in the home setting.

Environmental Engineer

The environmental engineer (sanitarian) is responsible for the elimination or reduction of hazards in the environment. He or she applies principles of education and law enforcement and uses practical and technical measures to eliminate or control environmental health problems (Smolensky, 1977, p. 154).

Clerk

The clerk is responsible for the clerical and secretarial aspects of maintaining the health department. These services are invaluable. It is extremely important to keep in mind that the clerical staff may need to be increased as new programs are developed in the health department. Without an adequate clerical staff, it is extremely difficult to effectively and efficiently manage health department services.

STATE AND LOCAL GOVERNMENT WELFARE ORGANIZATION

The provision of welfare assistance and insurance programs in every state and locality in the nation is legally mandated as a result of the Social Security Act of 1935 and other legislation. The specific services provided under the Social Security Act are discussed in Chapter 4.

The primary purpose of official welfare agencies is to assist indigent individuals in meeting their basic needs of food, shelter, and clothing. Benefits provided by these agencies are either cash or service (food and shelter). Official welfare services are organized in much the same manner as official health services. There is usually a department, such as the state department of social services, to establish rules and regulations, to set guides for service provision, and to administer services, as well as a local department of social services to provide direct services to clients. Local departments of social services administer state-subsidized programs such as Aid to Families of Dependent Children, food stamps, General Assistance, and Medicaid. Old Age, Survivors, Disability, and Health Insurance (OASDHI) and Supplemental Security Income (SSI) are administered by the federal government through Social Security Administration offices (see Chapter 4). Protective services for children and adults are often administered through departments of social service.

PRIVATE HEALTH AND WELFARE ORGANIZATION

The United States abounds in private health and welfare resources. Historically, there has been limited coordination between these and government resources. In addition, there is no central coordination of all private health and welfare resources. Both profit and nonprofit resources exist in the private health and welfare sectors.

Private profit health and welfare services include a small percentage of hospitals, a large percentage of nursing homes, health and welfare professionals in private practice, pharmacies, health business companies (medical equipment companies, hospital supplies), and proprietary social service agencies. These services are available on a fee-for-service basis and are organized primarily as companies and independent businesses.

Private nonprofit resources are known as voluntary resources. They are not mandated by any law and provide services on a nonprofit basis. They are represented by individuals, professional societies, service organizations, agencies, and facilities. Their services augment official (government) services. Voluntary resources are rather uniquely American. Individual voluntary efforts (volunteerism) have likely been with us since this country was founded. The first voluntary association, the National Tuberculosis Association, was established in 1892, and many voluntary associations have since emerged. Voluntary efforts have aided the development of American health and welfare resources, provided services that otherwise may not have been possible, and advocated health and welfare reform. Table 5-4 briefly summarizes the characteristics of voluntary resources that exist in the United States.

Today there are more than 6 million voluntary organizations in our country (Turner, 1977, p. 479). Also, millions of Americans volunteer their services to assist health and welfare programs each year. Operating funds for voluntary resources come largely from individual contributions, fees for service, membership dues, investment earnings, sales of goods and publications, bequests, grants, contracts for service, and tax funds (Turner, 1977, p. 480). Fund raising is of vital importance to these organizations, and monies are often

TABLE 5-4 Voluntary Resources: Characteristics and Classifications

CHARACTERISTICS

Voluntarily organized

Membership includes lay or professional members

Have no legal powers

Support is received primarily from voluntary contribution or fees

Activities are in research, education, and service

CLASSIFICATION

Professional societies (e.g.):

    American Medical Association (AMA)

    American Nurses' Association (ANA)

    American Public Health Association (APHA)

Service Agencies (e.g.):

    Visiting Nurse Association

    Association of Retarded Citizens

    American Cancer Society

    American Red Cross

    American Child Welfare Society

    Association of Junior Leagues of America

    Alcoholics Anonymous

    Blue Cross-Blue Shield

    Rockefeller Foundation

    Kellogg Foundation

    United Community Services

Facilities (e.g.):

    Universities

    Hospitals

    Nursing homes

    Museums

    Libraries

Individuals

SOURCE: From L. Black. *Community health and administration.* Ann Arbor: University of Michigan Press, 1977, p. 79.

raised through donation campaigns. One voluntary service agency, the United Way, represents a large number of local, voluntary resources with a central fund-raising campaign. Giving to the United Way campaign means giving to many voluntary resources with one donation. The federal government has encouraged private philanthropic giving to voluntary organizations by permitting contributions to be deducted from personal and corporate income tax.

There are usually many voluntary resources in local communities. Private profit-oriented health care agencies are emerging with increasing frequency. The Visiting Nurse Association and other home health care programs are discussed below, because home health care is becoming one of the major responsibilities of nurses in the community setting. Limiting discussion to these types of private health and welfare organizations is not meant to imply that other private agencies do not provide a valuable service to the community.

Visiting Nurse Associations (VNAs)

An especially significant voluntary organization in community health is the Visiting Nurse Association. The VNA began with the Women's Branch of the New York City Mission, which was organized in 1877 to teach hygiene in the homes of the underprivileged. In 1886, the first agency designated as a Visiting Nurse Society was established in Philadelphia (Hanlon and McHose, 1971, p. 60). Since that time, many VNAs have been established across the country. Chapter 1 discusses the historical development of these voluntary organizations.

Visiting Nurse Associations augment the services of the official health department, primarily by providing skilled nursing services (home care nursing). In recent years, there has been increased coordination between these agencies and official health departments. In some instances, combined agencies have been formed. Combination agencies are a consolidation under one centrally administered agency of official and voluntary health agency structure, function, funding, and staffing. Combined agencies have met with some success, but at times it has been found that when skilled nursing services are integrated into the health department program, health supervision and preventive activities do not receive priority. This is increasingly happening because monies for health services are less available; thus, nursing divisions are expanding their home health care programs to generate funds. Unfortunately, this expansion has resulted in less time being available for providing preventive health care services. The increasingly difficult government standards and qualifications for home care funding are also placing pressure on combined agencies to focus their attention more on home care services than on preventive health supervision activities. It will be found that standards for home care visits are better defined than standards for health supervision visits (see Chapter 21).

Visiting Nurse Associations are staffed and administered largely by nurses. They often employ master's-prepared nurses for consultant and administrative positions. The VNA is administered by a nursing director who operates under the authority of a board of directors. The board establishes policy and program emphasis and is responsible for various fund-raising activities. In contrast to the health department, the program emphasis is usually on secondary and tertiary preventive activities, rather than on primary prevention. Figure 5-3 presents a sample organizational chart for a VNA. Table 5-5 compares the administration, staffing, funding, and program emphasis of VNAs (voluntary) and official local health departments (government).

Home Health Care Programs

Home health care programs are organized in both the private profit and nonprofit sectors. Their services are delivered to individuals in

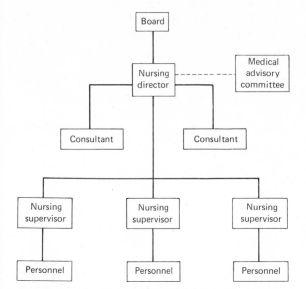

FIGURE 5-3 Organizational chart of the Visiting Nurse Association. Board = policy-making group; administrator = community health nurse; source of funds = united community services fees, contracts (schools), contributions, third-party payment (Medicaid, Medicare, Blue Cross–Blue Shield); program emphasis = primary, secondary, and tertiary prevention. (*From L. Black. Community Health Administration. Ann Arbor: University of Michigan Press, 1977, p. 81.*)

their homes and help to maintain the individual in an independent living situation. Decreasing hospital stays and reducing readmission and admission to hospitals are also goals of these programs; clients that use the services of home health care agencies are often elderly and disabled. Homemaker services are an integral part of these programs.

Home health care programs receive their funds through titles XVIII (Medicare), XIX (Medicaid), and XX (Social Services) of the Social Security Act of 1935 as amended, as well as private insurance companies. There is actually little private insurance company reimbursement for these services. Home health service programs have often been shown to be more economical than hospital care, and at least as economical as nursing home or institutional care. Keeping an individual at home has other advantages as well: families give per-

sonal, meaningful care; living in one's own home can provide a sense of security and promote feelings of self-worth (Quinn, 1975).

The American Hospital Association states that home health care programs must be able to provide the following (French, 1979, p. 53):

1. Medical care and supervision

2. Consultant services

3. Nursing care or nursing supervision

4. Hospital inpatient service

5. Social service (meal preparation, homemaker and chore services, shopping, visiting)

6. Nutritional guidance

7. Laboratory and radiology service

8. Pharmaceutical service

TABLE 5-5 Comparison of Official Local Health Department and Visiting Nurse Association

	Official local health department	*VNA*
Administration (chief executive)	Physician	Community health nurse
Personnel	Physician	Community health nurse
	Community health nurse	Clerk
	Sanitarian	
	Clerk	
Source of funds	Taxes	United community fund
	Contracts	Contracts
	Fees	Fees
	Grants	Contributions
Program emphasis	Primary prevention	Secondary, tertiary prevention

SOURCE: From L. Black. *Community health administration.* Ann Arbor: University of Michigan Press, 1977, p. 82.

Many states are including home health care agencies under their licensing laws. These agencies are growing in number. In 1975, 2254 home health service programs were certified for Medicare reimbursement; approximately 44 percent of these programs were privately organized, as illustrated in Table 5-6.

The core staff of home health agencies are community health nurses, RNs, LPNs, home health aides, and homemakers; this staff provides skilled and nonskilled nursing care and homemaker services. The staff may also include physical, speech, and occupational therapists; nutritionists; and meal and transportation aides.

Medicare has many restrictions. It limits the number of home care visits allowable each year and the services covered. In 1975, less than 15 percent of total Medicare expenditures went for home health services (Noelker and Harel, 1978, p. 40).

With the large amounts of money expended on nursing home and hospital care in this country, methods of service delivery should be

TABLE 5-6   Types and Numbers of Home Health Service Certified for Medicare Benefits, 1975

Type	Number
Government	1259
Private:	
VNA	530
Other voluntary agencies	47
Hospital-based	270
Miscellaneous	148
Total	2254

SOURCE: From R. M. French. *Dynamics of health care* (3d ed.). New York: McGraw-Hill, 1979, p. 53.

examined carefully. Home care services that maintain individual independence and preserve self-esteem should be emphasized. In 1974, the American Public Health Association Governing Council stated that up to 25 percent of the population now in institutional settings could be cared for in their own homes if organized services were available.

SUMMARY

Federal, state, and local health and welfare services are designed to safeguard the health of all citizens in our nation. Direct as well as indirect services are provided in order to meet the health needs of individuals, families, and populations at risk. International health services are also vital to the maintenance of health in the United States. The monitoring and controlling of communicable diseases, for example, require worldwide cooperation.

The community health nurse must understand how health and welfare resources are organized in this country in order to effectively enhance service coordination and to familiarize clients with the service delivery systems. Community health nurses need to be cognizant of health and welfare organization on both government and private levels. They must know what services are offered by both the state and local health departments, as well as how to help clients utilize these services. The referral process is a tool that helps community health nurses facilitate client utilization of health and welfare resources (see Chapter 9).

REFERENCES

Benenson, A. S. (Ed.). *Control of communicable diseases in man.* Washington, D.C.: American Public Health Association, 1975.

Black, L. *Community health and administration.* Ann Arbor: University of Michigan Press, 1977.

Federal Information Center. Telephone conversation. Detroit, Mich., Jan. 24, 1980.

French, R. M. *Dynamics of health care* (3d ed.). New York: McGraw-Hill, 1979.

Hanlon, J. J., & McHose, E. *Design for health* (2d ed.). Philadelphia: Lea & Febiger, 1971.

Miller, C. A., Brooks, E. F., Defriese, G. H., Gilbert, B., Jain, S. C., & Kavaler, F. A survey of local public health departments and their directors. *American Journal of Public Health,* October 1977, *67,* 931–939.

——, ——, ——, ——, ——, ——, & ——. Statutory authorizations for the work of local health departments. *American Journal of Public Health,* October 1977, *67,* 940–945.

National Commission on Community Health Services. *Health is a community affair.* Cambridge, Mass.: Harvard University Press, 1966.

Noelker, L., & Harel, Z. Aged excluded from home health care. *The Gerontologist,* January 1978, *18,* 37–41.

Office of the Federal Register. *United States Government Manual.* Washington, D.C.: Government Printing Office, 1977.

Prevention, a challenge to the nation. *Public Health Reports,* September–October 1979, *94,* 483–485.

Quinn, J. L. Triage: Coordinated home care for the elderly. *Nursing Outlook,* September 1975, *23,* 570–573.

Smolensky, J. *Principles of community health.* Philadelphia: Saunders, 1977.

Turner, J. B. (Ed.). *Encyclopedia of social work.* Washington, D.C.: National Association of Social Workers, 1977.

Wilner, D. M., Walkley, R. P., & O'Neill, E. *Introduction to public health.* New York: Macmillan, 1978.

SELECTED BIBLIOGRAPHY

Archer, S. E., & Fleshman, R. *Community health nursing.* North Scituate, Mass.: Duxbury, 1975, chap. 8.

Cohen, W. J. Current problems in health care. *New England Journal of Medicine,* July 1969, *281,* 193–197.

Committee for Economic Development. *Building a national health-care system.* New York: Committee for Economic Development, 1973.

Eitzen, D. S. *Social structure and social problems in America.* Boston: Allyn & Bacon, 1974.

Freeman, H. E., & Kurtz, N. R. *America's troubles* (2d ed.). Englewood Cliffs, N.J.: Prentice-Hall, 1973.

Gibson, R. M., & Mueller, M. S. National health and welfare expenditures: 1976. *Social Security Bulletin,* April 1977, *40,* 3–22.

Kennedy, E. M. *In critical condition: The crisis in American health care.* New York: Pocket Books, 1973.

Law, S. *The rights of the poor.* New York: Avon Books, 1974.

U.S. Department of Health, Education, and Welfare. *Towards a systematic analysis of health care in the U.S.: A report to congress.* Washington, D.C.: Government Printing Office, 1972.

——. *The cooperative federal-state-local health statistics system.* Washington, D.C.: Government Printing Office, 1973.

Wilson, F. A., & Neuhauser, D. *Health services in the United States.* Cambridge, Mass.: Ballinger, 1976.

Worthington, N. L. National health expenditures, 1929–74. *Social Security Bulletin,* February 1975, *38,* 3–20.

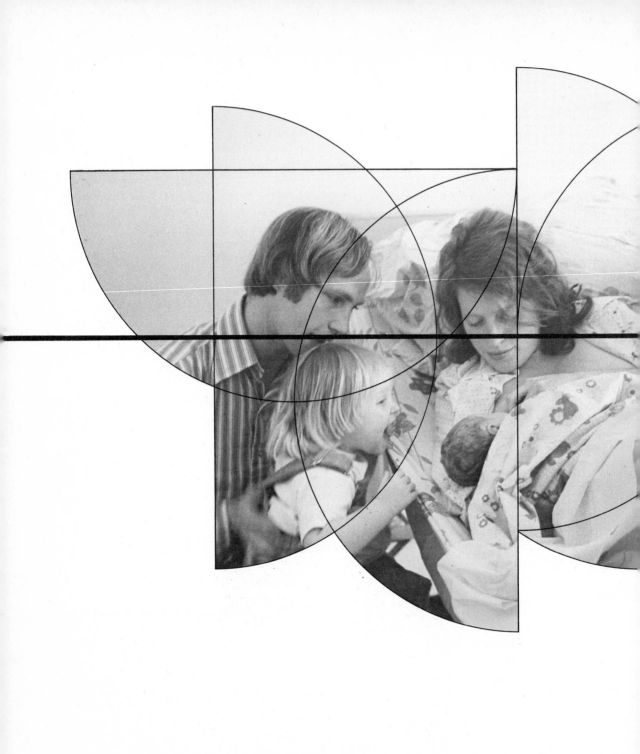

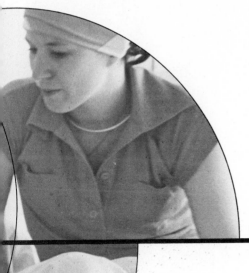

part two

working with families in the community setting

Family-centered care was historically and is still a key principle in community health nursing practice. Community health nurses believe that the health needs of individuals cannot be isolated from the interactions of the family and that stresses experienced by individual family members affect the entire family unit. They recognize that the family greatly influences the beliefs, values, attitudes, and health behaviors of its members and determines when family members will seek assistance from health care professionals.

Community health nurses use the nursing process to help families analyze the multiple forces that inhibit or facilitate their growth and to plan intervention strategies that will strengthen their self-care capabilities. Part 2 presents the theoretical concepts essential for understanding family functioning and for effectively utilizing the nursing process to provide comprehensive, continuous nursing services in the community setting.

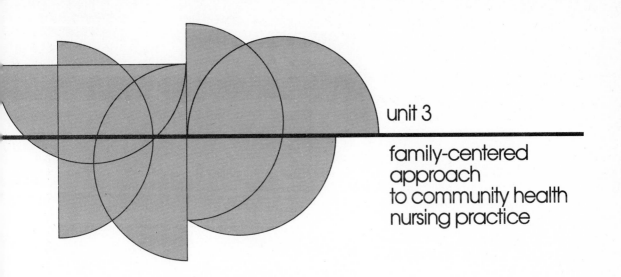

unit 3

family-centered approach to community health nursing practice

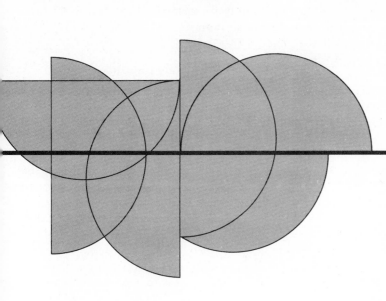

The ancient trinity of father, mother, and child has survived more vicissitudes than any other relationship. It is the bedrock underlying all other family structures. Although more elaborate family patterns can be broken from without or may even collapse of their own weight, the rock remains. In the Götterdammerung which otherwise science and overfoolish statesmanship are preparing for us, the last man will spend his last hours searching for his wife and child.

LINTON
(1959, p. 52)

Despite major societal changes in the 1960s and 1970s which have resulted in varying family forms and life-styles, the family is still the basic social unit. Although *an* American family does not exist, American families do (Howe, 1972, p. 11). Even though family structures and functions have changed, the family is still fulfilling needs in our culture. Bane (1976) and Yorburg (1973) predict that the family will continue to survive because all human beings require emotional support and nurturing over time. The bureaucratic organizations of our society cannot fulfill this need. Families must survive if individuals within our culture are to achieve emotional health and well-being. "Families are America's most precious resource and most important institution. Families have the most fundamental, powerful, and lasting influence on our lives. The strength of our families is the key determinate of the health and well-being of our nation, of our communities, and of our lives as individuals" (White House Conference on Families, 1978, p. 286).

THE AMERICAN FAMILY

Diversity is the term which best describes the American family. Cultural backgrounds, socioeconomic levels, and family structures differ throughout the country. The nuclear family unit—mother, father, and children—established through the legal sanction of marriage, is no longer the only acceptable form for family life. Alternative life-styles are becoming increasingly prevalent. Changes in societal values and attitudes are affecting both family structures and modes of living.

Scientific, technological, and sociological advances have greatly influenced societal attitudes and values about American family life.

The discovery of effective contraceptive methods, increased social mobility due to improved transportation, the women's movement, which promotes equal opportunities for women in the job market, the redefinition of sex roles, and increased health and welfare legislation have all made an impact on the American family. As a result of these events, transitions in family structure and function have occurred. Family size has decreased, with some couples voluntarily choosing not to have children. More women are becoming involved in careers outside the home. The role of the father in parenthood is examined more carefully. Families are changing their place of residence with increasing frequency. Legislation is broadening the opportunities for education, health services, and changes in marital status.

All of the above changes have provided more options in life-style for families. They have also brought new problems and stresses which require different coping mechanisms. Yorburg (1973, pp. 194–197) proposes four major problems the American family currently faces: (1) inadequate resources to meet the health, education, and welfare needs in our society of the two nonproductive generations, the young and the old; (2) lack of available support for the sharing of child-rearing responsibilities; (3) loneliness in nuclear family units who withdraw and isolate themselves; and (4) role conflicts arising from inadequate socialization for modern roles and from unrealistic expectations of family life. Yorburg believes these problems have arisen from a cultural lag between social legislation and changing societal values. An example of this is the nuclear family's difficulty in assuming all of the responsibilities once shared by the extended family. Changes in health and welfare legislation and the educational system are needed to prepare families to handle their responsibilities and to make resources available during critical transition periods. Social policy must take into consideration the needs of varying family forms and life-styles because the American family is changing.

Variations in Family Structures

Currently, several family structural forms exist in the United States. These are presented in Table 6-1. Even though all these family forms are not widely accepted, they are becoming more evident.

It is obvious from reviewing Table 6-1 that what actually constitutes a family is no longer easy to define. Varying family organizational structures have made the concept of the family an elusive one, open to numerous definitions depending on one's value system. The traditional definition of this term—a group of two or more persons related by blood, marriage, or adoption and residing together—is no longer adequate for understanding and studying the needs of the American family. It is extremely important that practitioners in the helping professions remain flexible in their interpretation of the word *family* so that social policies which enhance the growth of all types of families are developed. Families who are not legally bound together by marriage, for example, have the same needs as families who are. They need financial resources, educational opportunities, and health services to meet their basic needs. Denying them options to strengthen their family life certainly does not strengthen our nation.

In addition to reexamining the definition of the word *family*, community health nurses must also carefully identify their attitudes and values about family life, because they regularly encounter differing family forms. Although community health nurses may not choose a particular mode of living for themselves, their personal preferences should not influence their clinical judgments about the adequacy of family functioning when they work with families whose life-styles differ from theirs. Data collected from the family should be the key

TABLE 6-1 Variations in Family Life-Styles in the United States

Traditional family structures	Emerging experimental family structures

1. *Nuclear family*—husband, wife, and offspring living in a common household, established through the legal sanction of marriage
  a. Single career
    (1) Husband breadwinner, wife at home
    (2) Wife breadwinner, husband at home (usually this pattern is accepted by society only if the husband is ill, is obtaining advanced education, or is unemployed and looking for employment)
  b. Dual career
    (1) Both parents gainfully employed from the outset of the marriage
    (2) Wife's career interrupted due to child-rearing responsibilities
    (3) Wife starts career after children enter school
2. *Reconstituted nuclear family*—remarried men and women, living in a common household with children from both previous marriages, children from one previous marriage, or children from previous marriages and children from current marriage
  a. Single career
  b. Dual career
3. *Dyadic nuclear family*—childless husband and wife; one or both partners gainfully employed
4. *Single-parent family*—one parent, as a consequence of divorce, abandonment, or separation (with financial aid rarely coming from the second parent), and usually including preschool, school-age children; or both
  a. Parent working
  b. Parent not working, supported by government funds (welfare or social security), family or life insurance, and savings
5. *Single adult*—living alone, usually with a career, who may or may not desire to marry
6. *Three-generation family*—three generations or more living in a household
7. *Middle-aged or aging couple*—husband as provider, wife at home (children have been "launched" into college, career, or marriage)
8. *Kin network*—nuclear households or unmarried members living in close geographical proximity and operating within a reciprocal system of exchange of goods and services
9. *"Second-career" family*—the wife entering the work force when the children are in school or have left the parental home
10. *Institutional family*—children in orphanages, residential schools, or correctional institutions
	1. *Commune family*
	  a. Monogamous—household of more than one monogamous couple with children, sharing common facilities, resources, and appliances; socialization of the child is a group activity
	  b. Group marriage—household of adults and offspring known as one family, where all individuals are *married* to each other and all are *parents* to the children; usually develops a status system with leaders believed to have charisma
	2. *Unmarried-parent-and-child family*—usually mother and child, where marriage is not desired or possible
	3. *Unmarried-couple-and-child family*—usually a commonlaw marriage with the child their biological issue or informally adopted
	4. *Dyadic nuclear family*—husband and wife who have voluntarily chosen not to have children (national support groups are forming to help these couples maintain their position); one or both partners gainfully employed
	5. *Homosexual families*—a homosexual couple, male or female, living together with or without children; children may be informally or legally adopted
	6. *Cohabiting retired couple*—an unmarried retired couple living together, usually because financial hardship would result if they married (retirement benefits would decrease)

SOURCE: Adapted from M. B. Sussman (Chairperson). Changing families in a changing society. *1970 White House Conference on Children, Forum 14 report.* Washington, D.C.: Government Printing Office, 1971, pp. 228–229.

factor by which the community health nurse determines strengths and needs in relation to a family's functioning. A single-parent mother, for instance, may be meeting the needs of her child much more appropriately than a married couple who are having conflicts in their marriage. Assumptions about how well a family is providing for its members should not be made solely on the basis of the family's organizational structure.

THE FAMILY AS A UNIT OF SERVICE

Despite the changing nature of the American family, community health nurses still subscribe to the philosophy that the family is the basic unit of service in community health nursing practice. They recognize that the family, as the major socializing unit of society, determines how its individual members relate and act in our culture. They believe that the family greatly influences the beliefs, values, attitudes, and health behaviors of its members. They realize that the health of individual family members affects the health of the entire family unit. They see that the family provides support and encouragement at times of stress and joy. They value the role the family has in facilitating the physical and psychosocial growth of its members.

Ronald Peterson (1978) put into very simple, but impressive terms, the significance of the family in promoting the growth of its individual members when he presented the following concept of the family at a national conference on the chronic mentally ill client:

A family is a place where I think a lot of things go on. You really don't feel you're being "raised," that people are doing things to you, to raise you. Your life seems "real" and most of the time, almost everything that happens to you, you talk about it. Sometimes you have good news, sometimes you have bad news. But most of the time, it's just talking about what is going on.

It's a place you go from, to the doctor or to the hospital or the dentist, or school, or to the movies or to a job. But it's a place where you belong, where you somehow learn a lot. You change I'm sure, but usually without knowing it. And you certainly are not looked at as a patient or one who is being rehabilitated. You don't get discharged or terminated, and even when you grow up and get a job of your own and move away, it's a place you keep in touch with and visit. There's always an interest, and that's what makes the difference.[1]

Community health nurses have found, like Peterson, that families do make a difference; families provide supportive and nurturing services in a way that no other social institution provides for its members. Families influence health beliefs and attitudes, even when they are no longer physically present. They often extend themselves much further in providing assistance for their individual family members than would friends or health care professionals. It is for these reasons that community health nurses believe in the family-centered approach to nursing care.

Historically, the family-centered approach to community health nursing practice grew out of the recognition that the physical care of an individual client could not be divorced from all other aspects of a client's functioning. Innovative community health nursing leaders of the early 1900s recognized that a preventive, holistic approach to the delivery of nursing services was essential if the health of an individual, the family, and the community was to be maintained and enhanced. They saw the need to work with the family and the com-

[1]R. Peterson. What are the needs of the chronic mental patients? Presentation for the APA Conference on the Chronic Mental Patient. Washington, D.C.: Jan. 11–14, 1978.

munity in order to achieve their goals with individual clients.

The concept of family-centered care has evolved over time. Initial focus was placed on analyzing how the family could assist its individual members to achieve health and well-being. Gradually, this focus was altered, and the enhancement of the health and well-being of the entire *family unit* became the primary objective for community health nursing visits. Emphasis was placed on analyzing family dynamics which inhibited or facilitated family functioning as well as on identifying the health status of all individual family members.

Today, the family is still ideally viewed as the community health nurse's client. Historical evidence has sufficiently demonstrated the value of the family-centered approach to community health nursing practice. However, this approach to nursing care is not fully realized in the clinical setting. Lack of knowledge regarding family processes, federal legislation which financially supports services for individuals as opposed to families, insufficient criteria for judging family health, and heavy caseload demands often impede nurses' efforts to implement family care in the practice setting. Research, advocacy activities, and continuing education programs could alter this trend. Research is needed to document the value of preventive health care to families and to establish criteria for evaluating family health. Advocacy efforts which support the need for reimbursing family health care services are essential since traditionally health legislation has encouraged the delivery of curative, individual health care services. Continuing education activities aimed at increasing nurses' theoretical

base concerning family processes are necessary because many nurses have not had the opportunity to examine family theory in the educational setting.

Community health nursing leaders of the past were truly creative and innovative. They were far ahead of their time when they subscribed to the belief that family care was a key principle in community health nursing practice. It was not until the 1950s that most professional disciplines actually began to focus attention on working with families rather than with individual clients. It was only at this same time that social scientists initiated systematic theory building in relation to family processes. Thus, it is no wonder that the family-centered approach to nursing care is not completely operationalized in the practice setting. Theoretical knowledge to guide one's clinical judgments and the support for its use are needed before a particular nursing care approach can be fully implemented.

New knowledge gained about family functioning since the 1950s has made it easier for nurses to analyze family strengths and needs and to intervene appropriately with families. Selected theoretical frameworks currently being used to study the family are briefly summarized below. These frameworks help nurses to organize the family assessment process systematically and to identify the range of variables essential for understanding family relationships. They do not ensure, however, that family-centered care will be implemented. The community health nurse must internalize the belief that working with the family as a unit is important; otherwise, the goal of family-centered practice will be compromised.

THEORETICAL FRAMEWORKS FOR FAMILY STUDY

The family can be analyzed from multiple perspectives. Table 6-2, a *partial* listing of the kinds of family studies currently being conducted, illustrates the numerous disciplines involved in family research as well as the various perspectives used to gain an understanding of family dynamics. Increasingly, the importance of interdisciplinary research is being recog-

TABLE 6-2 Behavioral Sciences and Disciplines Involved in Family Study

Disciplines	*Illustrative studies*	*Representative researchers**

Anthropology:
  Cultural
    anthropology
  Social anthropology
  Ethnology
	Cultural and subcultural family forms and functions
	Ethnic, racial, and social status family differences
	Families in primitive, developing, and industrial societies
		Clyde Kluckhohn
		Oscar Lewis
		Helen and Robert Lynd
		Margaret Mead
		George Murdock

Counseling:
  Counseling theory
  Clinical practice
  Evaluation
	Dynamics of interpersonal relationships in marriage and family
	Methods and results of individual, marriage, and family
	counseling
		Rollo May
		Emily Hartshorne Mudd
		James K. Peterson
		Carl Rogers

Demography	Census and vital statistics on many facets of family life Cross-sectional, longitudinal, and record-linkage surveys Differential birth rates Family planning and population control	Hugh Carter Harold Christensen Paul Glick Philip Hauser P. K. Whelpton
Economics	Consumer behavior, marketing, and motivation research Insurance, pensions, and welfare needs Standards of living, wage scales, socioeconomic status	Howard Bigelow John Kenneth Galbraith John Morgan Margaret Reid

Education:
  Early childhood
  Early elementary
  Secondary
  College
  Parent
  Professional
	Child-rearing methods
	Developmental patterns
	Family-life education
	Motivation and learning
	Preparation for marriage
	Sex education
		Orville Brim
		Catherine Chilman
		Harold Lief
		Nevitt Sanford
		Ralph Tyler
		James Walters

History	Origins of family patterns Predictions of the future of families Social influences on the family Social trends and adaptations	Arthur Calhoun Franklin Frazier Edward Westermarck Carle Zimmerman

Home economics:
  Family relationships
  Home economics
    education
  Home management
  Nutrition
	Evaluation of family practices
	Family food habits and nutrition
	Home management practices
	Relationships between family members
		Muriel Brown
		Irma Gross
		Evelyn Spindler
		Alice Thorpe

Human development:
  Child development
  Adolescent
    development
  Middle age and aging
	Child growth and development
	Developmental norms and differences
	Nature of cognitive learning
	Cross-cultural variations
	Personality development
	Social roles of aging
		Urie Bronfenbrenner
		Erik Erikson
		Robert Havighurst
		Lois Barclay Murphy
		Bernice Neugarten
		Jean Piaget

nized. According to Duvall (1977, p. 126), this type of research adds depth to family study because concepts about several facets of family life are synthesized. Generally, scholars from the different behavioral sciences focus attention on only limited aspects of family life. Interdisciplinary research helps to bring together the various theoretical frames of reference used by different disciplines. This, in turn, gives a more comprehensive view of family functioning.

Theory building, in relation to the family,

TABLE 6-2 Behavioral Sciences and Disciplines Involved in Family Study (*Continued*)

Disciplines	Illustrative studies	Representative researchers*
Law	Adoption and child protection Child care and welfare Marriage and family law Divorce and marital dissolution Sexual controls and behavior Parental rights and responsibilities	Paul Alexander John Bradway Marie Kargman Harriet Pilpel Max Rheinstein Lenore Weitzman
Psychoanalysis	Abnormal and normal behavior Clinical diagnosis and therapy Foundations of personality Stages of development Treatment of mental illness	Nathan Ackerman Erik Erikson John Flugel Irene Josselyn Harry Stack Sullivan

Psychology:
  Clinical
  Developmental
  Social
	Aspirations and self-concepts
	Drives, needs, and hungers
	Dynamics of interpersonal interaction
	Learning theory
	Mental health
	Therapeutic intervention
		Rosalind Dymond
		Gerald Gurin
		Robert Hess
		Eleanore Luckey
		Frederick Stodtbeck
		John Whiting

Public health	Epidemiology and immunization Family health and preventive medicine Maternal and infant health Pediatric health education Venereal disease	Cecelia Deschin Nicholson Eastman Earl L. Koos Niles Newton Clark Vincent
Religion	Church policies on marriage and family Families of various religions Interfaith marriage Love, sex, marriage, divorce, and family in religious contexts	Stanley Brav Roy Fairchild Seward Hiltner John L. Thomas John C. Wynn

Social work:
  Family casework
  Group work
  Social welfare
	Appraising family need
	Devising constructive programs for family assistance
	Measuring family functioning
		Dorothy F. Beck
		L. L. Geismer
		James Hardy

Sociology	Courtship and mate selection Family formation and functioning Effects of social change on families Family crises and dissolution Prediction of family success Social class influence on families	Charlotte Towle Ernest W. Burgess Ruth S. Cayan Harold Christensen Reuben Hill Judson Landis Marvin Sussman

*Illustrative of those research workers whose published findings may be available to students of the family in various disciplines; not an all-inclusive listing.
SOURCE: E. M. Duvall. *Marriage and family development* (5th ed.). New York: Lippincott, 1977, pp. 127–129.

is a relatively new phenomenon. It was only three decades ago that family scholars developed an interest in theory construction. At that time began a much greater emphasis on *scientific* study to discover relationships between family concepts which could be generalized across cultures. In addition, for the first time, focus was placed on examining how cultural variables affected family dynamics (Christensen, 1964, p. 10).

The quantity and quality of family research has increased since the original thrust in the

1950s. Currently, substantive theory building in relation to the family has been organized by Carlfred B. Broderick (1971, p. 146) under the following six categories:

1. *The premarital dyad*

   a. Sexual behavior

   b. Dating and courtship behavior

2. *The marital dyad*

   a. Communication

   b. Role differentiation

   c. Morale and stability: role perception, expectations, and strain

   d. Decision making and power

3. *The parent-child dyad*

   a. Communication

   b. Socialization

   c. Decision making and power

4. *Whole family interaction*

   a. Family structure and function

   b. Family crisis

5. *Family location in larger social system*

   a. Cross-cultural studies

   b. Subcultural studies (especially black families

   c. Social class studies

6. *Family transactions with other elements in social systems*

   a. Informal transactions with kin, friends, etc.

   b. Formal transactions with economic policy and other institutions

Historically, five conceptual frameworks were utilized to study the family: interactional, structural-functional, situational, institutional, and developmental. These were first delineated by Hill and Hansen in their 1960 article, "The Identification of Conceptual Frameworks Utilized in Family Study." In 1964, Christensen devoted several chapters in his book *Handbook of Marriage and the Family* to the analysis of these frameworks. Both of these writings are now considered classics in the field of family study, because they have had a tremendous influence on the development of family theory in the 1960s.

Carlfred B. Broderick, after an extensive review of marriage and family living literature, concluded that three of the five original frameworks have survived: interactional, structural-functional, and developmental (Broderick, 1971, p. 141). In addition, he saw several new conceptual frameworks for family analysis emerging: balance theory, game theory, exchange theory, and general systems theory. A brief overview of each of these frameworks is presented below. Further personal investigation of the literature should be done to determine which framework fits one's clinical style when working with families.

Structural-Functional Approach

The structural-functional framework was developed by social scientists from sociology and social anthropology. It views the family as a social system which interacts with other social systems within society. It focuses on the analysis of family interplay between collateral systems, such as school, work, or health care worlds, and the transactions between the family and its subsystems (husband-wife dyad, the sibling cliques, and personality systems of individual family members). With this approach, emphasis is placed on examining the functions society performs for the family, as well as the functions the family performs for society and its individual family members. In addition, this framework looks at how the structure (organization) of systems affects their functioning (Hill and Hansen, 1960, pp. 303–304).

The family in the structural-functional approach is seen as open to outside influences and transactions, but both the family and its individual family members are considered to be reactive, passive elements of systems rather than active agents of change. This framework deals poorly with social change processes and dynamics. It handles well the relationships between the family and other social systems (Hill and Hansen, 1960, pp. 303–304).

Interactional Approach

Frequently labeled as the *symbolic* interactional frame of reference, this approach comes from sociology and social psychology. It views the family as a unity of interacting personalities, relatively closed to outside systems. Family members are seen as actors and reactors, who interact with their environment through symbolic communication. The interactional framework examines such parameters as family roles, decision-making processes, communication patterns, conflict, and reactions to stress. It identifies how relationships with others affect an individual's functioning. It emphasizes analysis of the internal aspects of family functioning, but neglects the family's relationships with other social systems (Hill and Hansen, 1960, pp. 302–303).

Developmental Approach

Concepts from various disciplines and approaches (rural sociology, child psychology, human development, sociology, and structural-functional and interactional approaches) were synthesized to create the developmental approach to family study. This approach looks at family development throughout its generational life cycle. It examines developmental tasks and role expectations for children, parents, and the family as a unit and how they

change throughout family life (Hill and Hansen, 1960, pp. 307–308).

Duvall (1977, p. 130) summarizes the key features of the developmental approach to family study as follows. The developmental approach:

1. Keeps the family in focus throughout its history

2. Sees each family member in interaction with all other members

3. Watches the ways in which individuals and the family unit influence one another

4. Recognizes what a given family is going through at any particular time

5. Highlights critical periods of personal and family growth and development

6. Views both the universals and the variations among families

7. Beams in on the ways in which the culture and families influence each other

8. Provides a basis for forecasting what a given family will be going through at any period in its life-span

Balance Theory

Balance theory originates in both the field of sociology and some branches of psychology. It examines adjustments made in situations where there is a discrepancy in the attitudes of two individuals concerning matters which are important to both. It postulates that there is a tendency toward symmetry or balance in any situation where two individuals have significant attitudes about an issue. For example, balance occurs between sentiment held for each other and attitudes maintained. If individuals like each other, they will each tend to like things liked by the other person, especially if the other person highly values a particular object (career and leisure activity) or viewpoint (religious values). They may, however, develop a dislike for each other if they cannot resolve the discrepancy in their attitudes about important issues (Broderick, 1971, p. 143). Some individuals, for instance, choose not to marry a particular person because conflicts about child-rearing practices or religious values cannot be resolved.

Balance theory has not been widely used by family scholars. It is believed, however, that there are several situations in which it could be applied to analyze family variables. Broderick (1971, p. 143) suggests it could be useful in examining dating, mate selection, and family relationship issues.

Game Theory

Game theory has its roots in mathematics. It examines decision making and communication processes during conflict situations. It provides a framework for analyzing interdependent behavior and for involving the client in the therapeutic process (Castles, 1973, pp. 110–111). Bernard (1964, pp. 695–696) identifies the following components in gaming models:

1. There are players who have conflicting goals.

2. Each player has alternative courses of action available from which to choose.

3. Each combination of alternatives for each player has an anticipated outcome.

4. Each outcome has a certain value or payoff for each player.

In addition to the above components, each player is given some degree of control in the situation, because players are allowed to make decisions for themselves. No player, however, has complete control, because each player is involved in a relationship with another player whose decisions affect how the game evolves. Players are not given absolute control in a gaming situation because there is an attempt to simulate real-life situations. In most interpersonal relationships, decision making is interdependent; decision making by one person in a relationship makes an impact on the decisions made by the other person in the relationship (Bernard, 1964, pp. 695–696).

Gaming is used to determine how individuals negotiate decisions when both parties in the situation will be affected by the decision. It assists in providing data about real-life interactions. Gaming is an especially useful tool when individuals under stress are having a difficult time describing how they go about making decisions; stress can often distort one's perceptions of what actually happens in decision-making processes. For example, a couple under stress may believe that shared decision making is occurring but can be helped through gaming to identify that this is not so. It is not unusual, for instance, for a couple to recognize that feelings are not being verbalized and, thus, decisions are being made without a shared data base.

Exchange Theory

Developed by sociologists and behavioral psychologists, exchange theory achieved a place of prominence in the field of family study in the 1960s (Broderick, 1971, p. 144). This theory examines human behavior from an exchange relationship perspective. The basic assumption in this framework is that human beings maintain involvement in relationships on the basis of rewards and costs. Rewarding situations are developed and maintained; nonrewarding situations are avoided or ended. For a relationship to last, each person must believe that he or she is receiving rewards equivalent to or greater than the costs. Implicit in this exchange is the principle of reciprocity—to receive, one must give (Eshleman and Clarke, 1978, pp. 12–13).

Rewards, according to exchange theorists, are not necessarily tangible objects like money or presents. A woman giving affection to her husband and children, a man sharing his time for a family outing, or an employer providing praise for a job well done are some examples of rewards in social interactions which are just as significant as tangible objects. Rewards, whether tangible or intangible, must be valued by the other person in order for them to be perceived as rewards.

Exchange theory is used to analyze interactions between people. It helps to determine why certain patterns of behavior have developed between individual family members. It also assists in explaining why some relationships are positive and others negative within the family unit. In addition, it offers a rationale for why interactions change over time; individuals who perceive that they are not being rewarded often end a relationship through divorce, separation, abandonment, or termination.

General Systems Theory

First introduced by biologist Ludwig von Bertalanffy (1968, p. 11), systems theory is currently being used in many disciplines. General systems theory is a "science of wholeness." "Its subject matter is the formulation of principles that are valid for 'systems' in general, whatever the nature of their component elements and the relations or 'forces' between them"(von Bertalanffy, 1968, p. 37). The goals of general systems study are to develop a theory which unites scientific thinking across disciplines and which provides a framework for analyzing the "whole" of any given system.

Von Bertalanffy (1968, p. 83) defines a system "as a complex of elements in interaction." Although the definition of systems varies slightly from author to author, several commonalities

emerge. It is generally agreed that a system consists of two or more connected elements which form an organized whole and which interact with each other.

Churchman (1968, p. 29) proposes five basic considerations that must be kept in mind when one is thinking about the meaning of a system:

1. The total system objectives and, more specifically, the performance measures of the whole system

2. The system's environment: the fixed constraints

3. The resources of the system

4. The components (elements or subsystems) of the system, their activities, goals, and measures of performance

5. The management of the system

Churchman, like many system scientists, uses an input-process-output-feedback model to depict the structural relationships of a system. An example of this type of model is shown in Figure 6-1. In very simplistic terms,

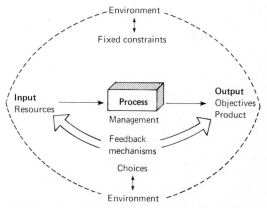

FIGURE 6-1 Structural arrangements of a system. (*Adapted from S. J. Clemen. Introduction to health care facility: Food service administration. University Park: The Pennsylvania State University Press, 1974, p. 24.*)

this model illustrates that all systems have *inputs* or resources which when *processed,* help the system to achieve its goals or *outputs.* It further shows that a system is cyclical in nature and continues to be so as long as the four parts keep interacting. If, however, there are changes in any one of the four parts, there will be changes in all of the parts. *Feedback* from within the system or the *environment* provides information which helps a system to determine whether it is meeting its goals.

When analyzing any system, it is extremely important to recognize that all systems have fixed constraints imposed on them by the environment, as well as choices that can be made about how the system will use its resources (inputs). Families, for example, must send their children to school after they reach a certain age. This is a *legal constraint,* not easily altered by a family system. To change this constraint would require consensus action by multiple systems. A family system does have some choice, however, about where the children will attend school. If a family does not like a particular public school district, this family may decide to move to another school district or to enroll the children in a private school.

No system can function in a vacuum. The environment of any system greatly affects how the system is able to function. Families' choices about educational opportunities for their children vividly illustrate this point. Some families may want to send the children to private school but are unable to do so because of *educational constraints* placed on them from the environment; in some settings private schools are unavailable. Other families may not be able to choose private school education because of *economic constraints* placed on them from the environment; their incomes may be insufficient to meet the financial requirements of a private educational system.

The processing of inputs (resources) received from the environment requires a series

of dynamic, interrelated transactions. These transactions link together the environment, the system inputs, and the system outputs.

Processes are simply "the actions needed to get the job done" (Clemen, 1974, p. 26). Different types of processes are needed to accomplish particular tasks. Those processes of special interest to community health nurses are discussed throughout this text. Presented in Chapter 8 (the nursing process) and Chapter 9 (the referral process and discharge planning) are the dynamic actions used by community health nurses to enhance client growth. Examined in Chapter 10 (epidemiological process), Chapter 11 (community diagnosis process), and Chapter 12 (planning process) are the dynamic actions integrated by community health nurses to plan and implement services for populations at risk. Covered in Chapter 20 (management process) and Chapter 21 (quality assurance process) are the dynamic actions carried out by community health nurses to ensure effective and efficient utilization of nursing time and the delivery of quality care.

The feedback mechanism is the most significant aspect of a system. It assists the system in identifying its strengths and needs and in evaluating how well it is accomplishing its goals. Feedback provides data essential for effective adaptation to internal and external system changes. It provides information which helps the system to select corrective actions when problems exist.

A system needs a mechanism that facilitates the sharing of both positive and negative feedback. A system which discourages negative input often remains static or develops dysfunctional patterns. This can lead to disorganization, confusion, or chaos. Lack of positive feedback, however, can also lead to dysfunctional behavior. Positive feedback helps to maintain healthy patterns of functioning and to stimulate creative ideas. If members of a system only receive negative feedback, they become discouraged and find it difficult to utilize their creative talents.

In addition to the input-process-output-feedback element, there are several other characteristics of all systems. The following list briefly summarizes some of the more significant ones:

1. *Boundaries.* Every system has filtering mechanisms, or boundaries, which regulate the flow of energy to and from other systems. Boundaries in a system are not physical barriers. Rather, they are *abstract* entities such as norms, values, attitudes, and rules which inhibit or facilitate human transactional processes between systems.

2. *Exchange of energy.* Energy transport is crucial to the survival of any system. Without it, dysfunctioning results. An effectively functioning system uses energy to obtain resources (inputs) from the outside, to process resources to achieve its goals, and to release outputs into the environment. Energy that promotes order in a system is labeled *negentropy.* Energy that results in chaos or disorganization, is termed *entropy* (von Bertalanffy, 1968; Wiener, 1968). All living systems contain entropy and negentropy. A system becomes distressed if extreme entropy exists for a considerable length of time. Family systems which are ineffectively dealing with crisis situations may reflect the concept of entropy. These families frequently lack energy to carry out their normal patterns of functioning and thus chaos or disorganization results.

3. *Hierarchic order.* In all systems, there is order and patterning. Von Bertalanffy (1968, p. 27) noted that fundamental to general systems theory is the concept of hierarchic order in structure (order of parts) and function (order of processes). This implies that all systems are interconnected through a complex array of processes with other systems (families), their subsystems (the family members), and suprasystems (community) and that there is a logical relationship between the parts of all systems.

4. *Open or closed systems. Open* and *closed* are terms used in general systems theory to describe how a system interfaces with its environment. A system which isolates itself from others is viewed as a closed system. A system which exchanges energy and resources with other systems is an open system. All living systems are open systems. The degree of their openness varies, however, depending on how well they transport energy to maintain themselves.

5. *Self-regulation.* An open system, through its feedback mechanism or its information processing element, obtains data needed to adjust to its environment. The circular nature of its input-process-output-feedback unit helps a system to adapt the flow of inputs and outputs so that it can achieve a balance between what is taken from the environment and what is released into the environment. It helps the system to maintain homeostasis (von Bertalanffy, 1968, pp. 160–163).

Increasingly, health care professionals and family scholars are applying the concepts, principles, and models of system theory to the study of the family. General systems theory provides a conceptual framework which is consistent with the holistic nature of humankind and professional practice. It offers a logical way to integrate all the factors that make an impact on family functioning and link the family together into a meaningful whole. It provides the basis for a humanistic philosophy of professional practice. The reason it does so is that family analysis from a systems perspective examines the family as a whole, rather than from isolated cause-and-effect relationships. Functional and dysfunctional family and individual patterns of behavior are considered to be products of system functioning vs. individual functioning. Family structure, functions, and processes are analyzed to determine why adaptive or maladaptive behavior is occurring within the family. This, in turn, negates individual blame and focuses attention on how the system must change in order to achieve productive functioning.

Use of Theoretical Frameworks in the Practice Setting

Theoretical frameworks help the practitioner to assess family structure and processes in an organized and logical fashion. They provide parameters to consider when collecting data about client situations. They facilitate the synthesis of data so that family strengths and needs can be identified. They help to explain family dynamics, which, in turn, assist the practitioner in developing appropriate intervention strategies. When a conceptual framework is lacking, it is extremely difficult to group data and to identify the relationships between the multiple variables that make an impact on the client.

Community health nurses generally utilize a combination of several theoretical frameworks to guide the family assessment process. This is appropriate because the needs of clients are varied and because there is no one framework which explains all family phenomena. Research frameworks, such as those previously discussed, tend to focus attention on some aspects of family life more than on others. In the clinical setting, it is essential for the nurse to examine the multiple aspects of internal family functioning as well as the family's relationships with other social systems. An effective management plan can only be developed after both of these areas have been assessed.

PARAMETERS TO CONSIDER DURING THE FAMILY ASSESSMENT PROCESS

In terms of the family, parameters related to both family structure and process should be considered during the family assessment process. This is true no matter what conceptual framework or combination of frameworks are selected to guide community health nursing practice. These parameters assist the nurse in obtaining a holistic view of the family. They help the nurse to identify who the family is and how family members interact to carry out their family functions.

Structural Parameters for Family Assessment

Structural components of a family are those variables which provide organization for the family system. They assist the family in coordinating their activities so that family and individual needs are met. Briar (1964, pp. 251–254) identified eight major structural characteristics of families: (1) division of labor, (2) distribution of power and authority, (3) communication, (4) boundaries of family world, (5) relations with other groups and systems, (6) ways of obtaining and giving emotional support, (7) rituals and symbols, and (8) a set of personal roles. These, as well as cultural values and attitudes and religious beliefs, are described below.

Division of Labor

Families allocate leadership responsibilities for maintaining their household in a variety of ways. Some follow traditional norms, with the man assuming major responsibility for the provider role and the woman for the homemaker role, regardless of the other role responsibilities each person has in the partnership. Some divide tasks according to their likes and dislikes or the level of competence each person has in relation to a particular task. Others share responsibilities equally, based on the demands each person has from other role positions. Nye (1976), in his text *Role Structure and Analysis of the Family,* discusses extensively the allocation of roles and the division of labor in family systems. This is a valuable reference for one who wants to review or expand knowledge in relation to role theory.

Families who rigidly define either the provider or homemaker role tend to experience more stress when family members are unable to perform their expected tasks than do families who have a flexible division of labor (Otto, 1963; Lewis, 1976; Pratt, 1976; and Beavers, 1977). It is also extremely difficult for families who have rigid patterns of functioning to mobilize new coping mechanisms when experiencing a crisis. Health care professionals, for instance, often observe confusion and disorganization when the spouse of a man or woman dies. This confusion is heightened if the man or women has not been prepared to deal with the demands of daily living. Assuming responsibilities for tasks one is not accustomed to performing is difficult at any time but especially when one is experiencing a crisis.

Identifying how the division of labor is handled by a family helps the community health nurse to understand the stresses family members are experiencing when changes have occurred in the family system. Role strain results when families do not take into consideration that role responsibilities change over time. Mothers, for example, are often confronted with excessive role demands after the birth of a child. This is especially true if husbands do not share the responsibility for housekeeping and child-care tasks. Role strain also occurs when family members are unable to perform the activities related to a given role. This is particularly noticeable when role modifications are needed because of the prolonged absence of one family member. Absences that are a result of illness, divorce, separation, or vocational responsibilities frequently require drastic modifications in a family's division of labor and result in role strain.

All family members can experience role strain. Children may be required to assume adult responsibilities which are excessive for their age and level of growth and development. This most often occurs during times of crisis or when parents have not assumed adult leadership responsibilities required to maintain their household. It has been found, for instance, that role-reversal behavior between parents and children is often present when child abuse occurs (Flanzraich and Dunsavage, 1977, p. 13). It is important for community health nurses to recognize that children do experience role strain when they assume parental functions and to avoid reinforcing role-reversal patterns. It is easy to praise a child who is functioning beyond his or her chronological age. This praise, however, may support the continuance of family patterns which are unhealthy and which adversely affect a child's emotional growth and development.

Distribution of Power and Authority

Power is conceptualized by Bredemeir and Stephenson (1965, p. 50) "as the capacity to carry out, by whatever means, a desired course of action despite the resistance of others and without having to take into consideration their needs. When power is institutionalized through respect, fear, esteem, or position, it is referred to as authority."

Several variables affect who will have power in the family system. The position of power can be *culturally* prescribed, usually with the father being in a position of authority by virtue of his role as a male. This is frequently seen in Spanish-American and Asian cultures, where male dominance is the norm. Power can also be *situationally* prescribed when family members do not necessarily follow cultural norms but develop a power structure based on their circumstances and personal interactions. The continuum of family power based on cultural and situational variables ranges from complete dominance to complete absence of power, both of which can produce dysfunctional family patterns. Complete dominance by one family member poses a threat to the self-esteem of other family members and often makes it difficult for individuals to resolve the independence-dependence conflicts which arise during adolescence and young adulthood. Complete absence of power in a family system tends to produce confusion, disorganization, and chaos. Dysfunctional families frequently exhibit power structures on either end of the continuum. Healthy families usually fall in the middle of the continuum, where power is shared by adult members, and children are involved in the decision-making process.

Exchange theory helps to explain why an equal or unequal distribution of power evolves in a family system. Sharing of power is more likely to occur when all family members perceive that they have resources to contribute which enhance the family's ability to achieve its goals and to meet the needs of individual family members. Family members who do not value their contributions or whose contributions are not valued by other family members will probably not have power within the family system.

Understanding the relationship between issues of power and decision making is essential to effect permanent changes within a family system. If the power and authority structure of a family is ignored, nursing interventions are often inappropriate and place additional stress on family members who lack the power to make decisions about needed health actions. Family members who have power must be consulted if changes in health behavior are to occur. One community health nurse, for instance, realized after several home visits to a Spanish-American family that the only way she would influence the family to obtain needed surgery for their 4-year-old preschooler was to talk with the child's father. Although the mother stated frequently that she felt it was important for her son to have surgery, no action was taken. When the mother was finally asked how her husband felt about this matter, the nurse discovered that he felt surgery was unnecessary and that he was the one who made the final decision about needed health care.

In situations where the dominant family member is temporarily immobilized, it is extremely important for the community health nurse to recognize that the family may reassign the dominant position to the nurse. Because of the nurse's professional status, families who are under stress may initially allow a nurse to assume a position of authority within the family structure. They may follow the nurse's suggestions to relieve the anxiety they are experiencing at the time. These suggestions may not necessarily be appropriate for the family, but the family may follow through on them because its anxiety level is so high. A family under stress will frequently try anything to reduce its level of discomfort. It is significant for a nurse to recognize that this does happen, because when families are experiencing pain it is easier at times to do things for them than to foster family decision making. Taking over decision making for a family is not therapeutic.

Communication Patterns

Verbal and nonverbal interactions within a family usually display significant regularities or patterns. Norms involving what is shared and not shared, as well as who shares with whom, are implicitly, if not explicitly, known by all family members. Messages are provided in a variety of ways to let family members know how to communicate within and without the family system.

The ability to communicate accurately and effectively is essential to all aspects of family functioning because communication is an integral part of daily living. It helps the family to carry out its functions, to meet the needs of individual family members, and to move toward achieving its goals.

Communication is an extremely complex process, involving not only what is said but also *how* it is said, and the *behavioral interactions* which occur during the course of a conversation. An individual can communicate even when verbal information is not shared. Watzlawick, Beavin, and Jackson (1967, pp. 48–49) noted that because all behavior in an interactional situation has message value, it is impossible for one not to communicate. They believe that "activity or inactivity, words or silence, all have message value which influence others; others, in turn, cannot avoid responding to these communications and are thus, themselves communicating." Even silence conveys a message to an individual who is sharing thoughts, ideas, or feelings.

Family communication patterns need to be analyzed along several dimensions. Verbal, nonverbal, and behavioral processes should be observed to identify the following aspects of a family's communication patterns.

1. *Content.* What actually is conveyed is known as the content of communication. Observations should be made to determine what is being shared as well as what is not being shared. It is not unusual for individuals to feel uncomfortable about sharing information concerning personal topics such as sexuality, finances, and troubled relationships

with significant others. A health care professional needs to "listen between the lines" in order to help clients verbalize areas of concern beyond those which are explicitly expressed.

2. *How content is shared.* The sharing of content does not necessarily convey to the receiver accurate knowledge, facts, or ideas, or help the receiver to understand the message one is attempting to share. Content becomes functional when there is clarity of thought, organization of ideas, and accuracy and completeness of facts. It is difficult for the receiver to understand what is being said when information is being withheld, when an overabundance of data is being shared, or when conflicting messages are being conveyed. These problems tend to distort reality and confuse the listener. They can lead to a lack of responsiveness or hostile interchange.

3. *Behavioral interactions.* How an individual responds, either verbally or nonverbally, during a conversation provides clues to others about how this individual views what is being said or how he or she regards the sender. Body mannerisms, eye contact, silence or responsiveness to content, vocal characteristics, and ways of eliciting information all provide behavioral messages which guide the course of a conversation. Behavioral messages are often *far more meaningful* in a positive or negative sense than verbal content. They may provide "double-level messages, with the voice saying one thing and the rest of the person saying something else" (Satir, 1972, p. 60). Healthy families tend to share fewer "double-level" messages than nonhealthy families.

4. *Interpretation of content and behavioral interactions.* How information and interactions are interpreted varies from one individual to another. Perceptions about messages being

conveyed are influenced by several factors, including such things as previous experiences when communicating with others, the motivations of persons involved in a conversation, feelings about oneself, and current stresses being experienced. Persons, for example, who have low self-esteem frequently find it difficult to interpret messages positively; praise is often not heard or is negated. The interpretation of messages is a key factor which determines the difference between healthy and pathological communication. When assessing family communication patterns, it is extremely important to note whether real-life events and the feelings and thoughts of others are accurately perceived. When healthy communication patterns exist, clarification is sought if individuals do not understand what is being said. Feelings such as sadness, joy, or anger are not attributed to others without validation.

5. *Ways utilized to communicate.* Satir (1975, pp. 141–149) noted that individuals use five major transactional modes to communicate when they are under stress. These are placating, blaming, superreasonable, irrelevant, and congruent modes.

    a. Placating refers to a mode of communication which entails always agreeing with what is being said, even when one does not inwardly desire to do so. The placater is trying to please others and thus does not share personal feelings and reactions. Placating may occur if an individual does not wish to engage in a conversation.

    b. Blaming patterns of behavior result when an individual has a need to prove that he or she is strong. Techniques such as fault-finding, dictatorship, or cutting remarks are used to demonstrate that one has power. Individuals who use blaming tech-

niques are usually very insecure. Often, they exert control over others, in order to achieve a sense of security through power.

    c. Superreasonable communication occurs when a person intellectualizes and avoids the sharing of feelings and emotions. Individuals who are afraid to deal with feelings and emotions frequently do not recognize the need to make constructive changes in their lives; they suppress feelings of anxiety which are needed to motivate them to examine dysfunctional patterns of behavior.

    d. Irrelevant transactions are illogical from the perspective of what is happening in an individual's environment. Irrelevant communication patterns affect the flow of a conversation as well as problem-solving and decision-making processes.

    e. Congruent interactions result when feelings and content are integrated and information sharing is logical in relation to what is happening in the environment. When using congruent communication, an individual is "real." That is, there is a consistency between what the individual outwardly shares and what is inwardly felt; this is the most functional way to interact with others. Satir (1975, p. 48) has found that when the other transactional modes of communication become patterned, psychosomatic and other illnesses often result.

6. *Linguistic characteristics.* Families have varying dialects or language differences, depending on their cultural background, their socialization process, and their geographic location. It is important for a community health nurse to note these differences, because they can interfere with communication, especially when a family's or a nurse's dialect is incongruent with the dialect of

others in their environment. Generally, clients are more than willing to help health care professionals understand language differences, if the health care professional shows an interest in learning about them.

The primary goal of observing family communication patterns is to determine if the patterns established by a particular family are functional. That is, do they help the family to carry out its functions, to relate effectively to the environment, to meet the needs of individual family members, and to achieve its goals. It is important to remember that ways of achieving functional communication between family members can vary from one family to another. In recent professional and lay literature, there has been a tendency to idealize frank, honest, self-disclosure (Briar, 1964, p. 252). Frankness may not always be functional, however; stating what one thinks without taking into consideration another person's feelings can be irresponsible. Honest interchanges in communication can occur without frank disclosure. "Being honest is saying only what you mean, not everything"(Hacker, 1979).

Hacker (1979), a health educator who specializes in sexuality counseling, has found that both clients and health care professionals are often afraid of handling sensitive topics because they are confused about the difference between honesty and self-disclosure. To her, an honest individual is one who says what he or she means and is comfortable with what is not shared. Self-disclosure is the frank sharing of one's private feelings, thoughts, and actions, often without evaluating the appropriateness of doing so in one's current situation. Hacker has found that self-disclosure is not necessarily the key to the successful handling of sexuality issues. Rather, she believes that one needs to be honest with oneself about personal sexuality concerns. Only then will one be able to deal with value issues and feelings. Shakespeare

was wise when he said in *Hamlet,* "This above all: to thine own self be true,/ And it must follow, as the night the day,/ Thou canst not then be false to any man" (*Hamlet,* act 1, sc. 3).

Boundaries of Family World

Boundary development and maintenance is essential for family survival and growth. Families must have effective filtering mechanisms so that the exchange of energies corresponds to the needs of the family. Energy exchanges which occur too rapidly or too slowly can be disruptive to the family system. Families need to bring inputs into their system and release outputs into the environment so that they can carry out their functions. However, they also need to limit the amount of input from the environment to prevent system overload and to limit the release of outputs to prevent energy depletion.

The rate of energy flow between the family and the environment must vary in order for the family to maintain the integrity of its system. Families who do not adjust their energy flow to correspond to their current circumstances have difficulty handling stress and change. In times of family stress and change, limiting the exchange of inputs and outputs conserves energy needed to carry out activities of daily living. A new mother or father, for instance, may need to reduce working hours (output) in order to conserve energy for child-care activities and to provide emotional support for others in the family system.

It is not uncommon for community health nurses to work with families who are having difficulty adjusting energy flow to and from their family system. Some of the most frequent difficulties in relation to boundary maintenance issues which will be encountered in clinical practice are summarized below:

1. *Boundaries too loose.* Disorganized, multiproblem, and crisis-prone families tend to

take little control over what comes into or leaves their environment. They have numerous outsiders, such as health care professionals or legal authorities (inputs), working with them, and often they do not set rules about how and when family members should interact outside the family system. These families usually come to the attention of health care professionals because their outputs are not acceptable to the suprasystem (community). It is not unusual, for example, for such families to be referred to the community health nurse when their children enter school, because they lacked the energy to fulfill the health requirements (immunizations and physical examinations) mandated by the educational system for school entry. Frequently in these situations, families' energies are used to deal with outsiders or crises rather than to take care of the needs of individual family members.

2. *Boundaries too rigid.* Some families allow few inputs to cross their boundaries. They isolate themselves from the larger community and thus may not obtain the resources needed for family growth. Families from differing cultural backgrounds or families who have members with a mental or physical handicap may, for instance, limit inputs from the environment because they are afraid that the larger society will not accept their differences. Conflicts between these families and their environment arise when they do not release outputs (do not send their children to school) or when their outputs are inadequate (children not prepared to handle environmental demands and pressures).

3. *Boundaries not agreed upon.* At times, community health nurses find that there is a discrepancy between the views of one family member and another regarding boundary maintenance. Families may have some boundaries which are well defined and others which are unclearly defined. They may, for example, use community resources appropriately but may not agree on how often and when they should interface with friends and the extended family. Lack of agreement on boundary maintenance issues can lead to conflict, disequilibrium, and system disintegration.

Relations with Other Groups and Systems

The development of relationships with other groups, such as extended kin or neighbors, and other systems, such as church, school, or health care agencies, is directly related to the way the family handles its boundary maintenance functions. Family boundaries can facilitate or inhibit the establishment and maintenance of interpersonal relationships with others outside the family system. Families with rigid boundaries have few contacts with persons outside their family system. Families with flexible boundaries tend to encourage close interactions with others.

When assessing family relationships outside the family system, it is important to look at the *type* of relationships they have as well as the contact allowed. Interaction with numerous people does not necessarily mean that the family is meeting their support, companionship, and growth needs. Some families develop relationships which involve more giving than receiving. In these situations, family energies are devoted to helping others, but the family receives very little support in return. In other families, individual family members are allowed to interact with anyone, even though their interactions may not be positive. Children, for example, may encounter legal difficulties because there are no controls placed on their relationships with people who are engaging in illegal activities.

Ways of Obtaining and Giving Emotional Support

Families need to achieve a balance between their relationship with others and their relationship with family members. If the family excludes itself from its external environment, there may be a lack of support from others during times of stress and crisis. If, on the other hand, the family devotes all its energy to helping others, it is highly unlikely that the family will be able to meet the emotional needs of individual family members.

Families meet their emotional needs in a variety of ways. They develop norms which regulate sources of support, provide guidelines for giving support, and define when support will be given. When assessing the ways a family obtains and gives emotional support, the following factors should be considered:

1. *Distribution of support.* All family members need support, encouragement, and praise. If support is not evenly distributed, family members who are not receiving what they need may seek support from their environment and isolate themselves from the family system. Or they may withdraw and limit contact with others outside the family as well as within the family system.

2. *When support is given.* Some families only provide support during times of stress and crisis. Others are supportive during times of stress but also during normal functioning periods. The sharing of love, attention, and affection only when family members are distressed can be dysfunctional in that it may reinforce such behaviors as illness, truancy, and other destructive activities. All human beings need emotional care and nurturing. If they are unable to obtain emotional support without manifesting symptoms of distress, they may develop physical or psychosocial difficulties in order to receive the attention needed for emo-

tional survival. Often, such individuals are unaware that they are doing this.

3. *Acceptance of family members.* How an individual family member is viewed by other family members greatly affects the amount of emotional support the individual will receive. Family goals which define desired achievements, norms which regulate acceptable and unacceptable behavior, and the emotional maturity of the family all influence how well individual family members will be accepted by other family members. Individuals within the family who do not conform to family norms and goals usually receive less support than those who do. Illustrating this is the teenager from a family with high educational aspirations who does not share these aspirations and decides not to go to college. This teenager very quickly receives a message from other family members that this is an inappropriate decision. If she or he does not alter these views, family members may withdraw support and encouragement, even if the family member succeeds outside the educational environment.

4. *How support is given.* Families use both verbal and nonverbal communication to provide support for their members. Some share support spontaneously, whereas others are more reserved and do not give support until it is elicited from them. Individuals from families who spontaneously share with each other may sense a lack of support if they marry individuals from families who were reserved in their interactions with others. This can also occur when individual family members observe how their friends' families provide support for their members. Children, for instance, may perceive that they are not loved by their parents if they observe spontaneous sharing in the homes of their friends.

Set of Personal Roles

Every family has the task of organizing its roles in a way that helps the family to achieve its goals and to carry out its functions. There is no one role-allocation pattern that works for all families. Families must allocate and differentiate roles in a manner which facilitates their functioning.

Personal roles as well as family roles evolve when families organize their role structure. Some common examples of personal roles are "the 'baby' in the family; the 'good' child; the 'bad' child; the scapegoat; the strict parent; and the 'sickest' member of the family. Such roles, even when they emerge fortuitously, can become patterned very quickly. As a result, the person may be 'locked' in the role, with important consequences for how others will treat him and what they will expect of him" (Briar, 1964, p. 254). When one is assessing family dynamics, it is extremely important to identify how personal role allocation has influenced the behavior of all family members. The "sick" member of the family, for example, is often not allowed to do things that he or she is capable of doing. Frequently, family members "take care" of this person so well that he or she never learns how to function independently.

Rituals and Symbols

Family rituals and symbols come from two major sources. First, some are adopted from the culture as a whole or a subculture within the wider culture. Second, they develop from human transactional processes which have occurred within the family system (Briar, 1964, pp. 253–254).

Family rituals and symbols develop around multiple aspects of family life. They help family members and outsiders to identify what the family views as important. They provide structure for activities of daily living and for special occasions.

Examples of the types of rituals and symbols which develop in family systems are shared below. Although some of the rituals within a family appear very similar to societal ones, family rituals usually have some very specific, unique characteristics.

1. Mealtimes: designating times for meals, seating arrangements during meals, and conversation shared

2. Family names: giving nicknames to all family members or naming children after specific family members

3. Holidays: serving specific types of food or carrying out certain kinds of activities

4. Religious observances: saying prayers at mealtime or bedtime or engaging in specific activities when a family member has died

Family rituals and symbols are extremely significant and are usually valued highly by families. They are often continued even when individual family members do not view them as important. Frequently, pressure is placed on family members to conform to family rituals and symbols until the entire family unit alters its views about them.

Cultural Values and Attitudes

There are numerous factors which influence the biological, psychosocial, and spiritual development of all human beings. Human growth and development begins with genetic characteristics inherited from parents but then branches off in different directions as one interacts with one's environment. Within this environment, the caring and nurturing by significant others greatly affects how growth progresses and what decisions are made about how to handle activities of daily living. Through environmental conditioning, people learn patterns of behavior which influence how they relate to others, how they act in social situations, and how they make decisions about significant issues. Because these patterns of behavior provide stability and security, they are not easily altered; they continuously influence the direction of one's life. They shape beliefs and values which provide a foundation for future decision making.

Culture is the term used to describe the values, attitudes, and patterns of behavior which are transmitted to all individuals in a particular social environment. Social scientists have defined culture in many ways, but most of these definitions have three central themes: (1) beliefs, values, and patterns of behavior are learned and passed on from one generation to the next; (2) culture provides a prescription for daily living and decision making; and (3) the components of a culture are valued by members of the culture and are considered to be right and not open to questioning.

Every culture has a schema, composed of specific components, which shapes such things as family structure, dietary habits, religious practices, the development of art, music, and drama, ways of communicating, dress, and health behavior (see Figure 6-2). A culture schema, for instance, affects how one perceives health and illness and when and from

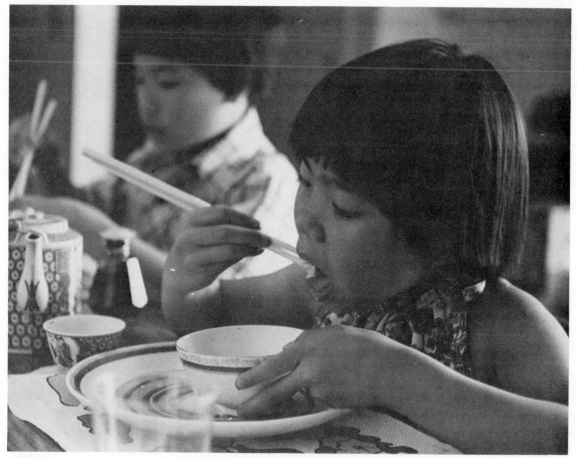

FIGURE 6-2 Cultural values and attitudes provide a foundation for activities of daily living.

whom one seeks health care. Because the Jewish culture believes in the sacredness of human life and health, members of this particular cultural group have traditionally respected health care providers and have engaged in activities, regardless of the expense, to restore health. The value the Jewish culture places on health is reflected in a favorite Yiddish parting phrase, *Sei gesund,* "be well" (Kensky, 1977, p. 197). In contrast to the health values held by the Jewish culture are the beliefs and values transmitted by the Mexican-American culture. Many individuals from this culture are influenced by a folk system which encourages the use of folk medicine and supports the belief that one has very little control over one's life; it is felt that supernatural forces cause disease and that one can do very little to prevent illness. Mexican healers, *curanderos(as),* rather than health care professionals are used by some Mexican-American families when health care services are needed (Baca, 1973; Prattes, 1973; and Samora, 1978).

A rich diversity of cultural values and attitudes exists in our nation. In community health nursing practice, encountering clients who have beliefs which differ from those of the health care professional is a common occurrence. In order for community health nurses to work effectively with such clients, they must develop an appreciation for the inherent worth of different cultural patterns. This involves a process which not only increases one's knowledge about various cultural schemata but also increases one's acceptance of all human beings and their cultures.

When learning about specific cultural beliefs, it is best to seek information about these beliefs from members of the particular culture being studied. Many cultural patterns are not written or recorded. Most, in fact, are transmitted from one generation to another through oral communication and behavioral transactions. When one is receiving input from individuals who represent a given cultural group, it is extremely important to remember that diversity exists within cultures as well as between cultures. Knowledge about cultural values and attitudes helps one to identify the parameters to consider when collecting data about family functioning. This knowedge, however, never replaces the need to obtain specific data from individual families during the assessment process.

Developing cultural sensitivity in clinical practice is not an easy task. Health care professionals, like clients, are influenced by their own social conditioning, which has a long-lasting effect on everything they do. It is often difficult to recognize the effects of earlier influences, because patterns of functioning derived from social conditioning become a way of life. These patterns subtly influence behavior even when they are no longer recognized on a conscious level. Hence, health care professionals need to examine carefully how their values and attitudes are affecting their clinical judgments. This process can be painful, especially when it is identified that one's interventions are not therapeutic because the client's health beliefs have been discounted. Remember, if this happens, that all practitioners have at one time or another experienced professional situations in which they have not been effective because of value conflicts. Being able to identify that one's behavior is adversely affecting professional interactions and to take action to alter nontherapeutic intervention is one of the characteristics of a sensitive professional.

Religious Beliefs

Cultural values and attitudes are often shaped and maintained by our religious systems. From earliest times, religious systems have preserved and transmitted traditions from one generation to another and have greatly influenced the development of norms for social behavior. Spiritual beliefs valued by these systems have provided a foundation for moral behavior in societies; they have also helped to maintain order and cohesiveness in social groups.

Despite major changes in our religious systems in the past two decades, spiritual beliefs still affect the lives of most individuals. They influence such things as contraceptive practices, dietary habits, developmental transitions through rites of passage, selection of marriage partners, and reactions to health and illness.

Spiritual beliefs of clients are often not addressed in the clinical setting. This is unfortunate, because their beliefs frequently bring comfort to distressed individuals and help them to cope with illness and crisis. Involving spiritual leaders in a client's care and allowing clients to verbalize their feelings about their religious values can strengthen the relationships between health care professionals and clients and can promote effective decision making about needed health care services.

Process Parameters for Family Assessment

Basic to the understanding of family functioning is the analysis of family processes. Family processes are methods used by families to determine how their structure evolves, how decisions are made, and how the family carries out its functions to maintain itself.

There are several parameters to consider when assessing family processes:

1. How the family integrates its role relationships

2. How the family utilizes information from the environment

3. How the family adapts to changes occurring within the family system and its environment

4. How the family makes and implements decisions

5. How the family deals with conflict or disagreement

6. How the family maintains the integrity of the family unit, as well as the personal autonomy of family members.

Family health is a function of process rather than outcome. It is family process which helps the family to manage stress, to survive crises, to deal with conflict, and to organize itself so that it can achieve its goals. Usually, however, a family comes to the attention of the health care professional because its outputs are inadequate or because the family perceives it is having difficulty meeting its goals. When one is assessing family functioning, it is extremely important to examine process variables as well as outcomes desired by a family; family processes frequently need to be altered before desired outcomes can be reached.

Direct observation of the family system is the best way to gain an understanding of family processes. This is especially true during times of crisis, because it is during these periods that functional or dysfunctional behaviors become more evident. Decision-making as well as communication patterns should be analyzed carefully in an assessment of family processes. Chapter 7 presents the concepts of stress and crisis and examines some of the factors which affect decision making when people are distressed. Parameters to observe when one is looking at family communication patterns have been discussed previously in this chapter. Publications by Ackerman (1959, 1970), Bowen (1973), Haley (1971), Jackson (1968), Minuchin (1974), Satir (1967, 1972), and Watzlawick (1967) provide an in-depth analysis of family processes and are very useful references for practitioners who view the family as their unit of service.

TOOLS WHICH FACILITATE THE FAMILY ASSESSMENT PROCESS

There are a variety of tools a community health nurse can use to facilitate family assessment. Some of these tools will be discussed below. They are designed to help the practitioner elicit data about certain aspects of family structure, function, and process and aid the health professional in determining major family concerns, needs, and strengths. Assessment tools, however, are only guides, and before using them, one needs to have an understanding of family theory and of communication processes that enhance effective nurse-client relationships.

Family Assessment Guides

Many community health agencies have developed family assessment guides so that staff members can focus attention on family functioning as well as on the health status of individual family members. The Appendix to this chapter is an example of such a tool. When completed, it provides a quick visual summary of family strengths, family behaviors which need to be altered, and anticipated guidance needs.

Generally, family assessment guides examine both the family's relationships with its environment and its internal functioning. It is extremely important when designing guides to facilitate the data collection process to take into consideration the need to identify both functional and dysfunctional behaviors within a family system. It is very easy to focus only on family problems. When this is done, areas of family dysfunctioning may be overemphasized. This, in turn, can have a devastating affect on the family and the nurse and lead to frustration, discouragement, and a feeling of hopelessness for all. Nurses who are unable to see family strengths "burn out" quickly; families who never receive positive feedback for

what they are handling well question their ability to adequately maintain themselves and often become dependent on others for decision making.

Before constructing a family assessment guide, an agency needs to make a careful analysis of its philosophy of nursing practice, so that it is reflected in the assessment tool being developed. For instance, a belief in preventive health behavior would be operationalized if staff members were encouraged to discern anticipatory guidance needs and then to plan nursing intervention strategies which might prevent future health problems. Perhaps hazards in the environment have not yet caused an accident; however, if hazards such as medications left where small children can reach them are not eliminated, a serious health problem may result. Health counseling assists parents in realizing how much of a threat medication might be to small children, and it may be the impetus which influences preventive health changes in a family's environment.

The community health nurse should be allowed to use a variety of assessment methodologies when implementing an agency's philosophy of practice. If a tool interferes with a practitioner's clinical style, it is highly unlikely that it will be used. Or, if the practitioner does attempt to use it, even though it does not relate to the practitioner's frame of reference, the nurse-client relationship may be distorted. Family assessment tools should be used to provide guidelines for data collection only. They should not tie a nurse into a particular interactive style or theoretical framework for family assessment.

A family assessment tool must be easily utilized by the practitioner. Tools which take a minimal amount of time to complete and which provide a composite picture of family strengths and needs are most beneficial. Many community health nurses have heavy caseload demands and become frustrated if they are asked to fill out a lengthy assessment form.

Family assessment tools are only useful when the practitioner has the theoretical background to handle them. Having knowledge about such things as role theory, cultural values and attitudes, family decision making, and concepts of stress and crisis is essential before an assessment guide can be used effectively. Assessment tools can never replace a genuine understanding of theories which analyze family functioning or which describe how nurse-client interactions affect the therapeutic process.

Genograms

A genogram is a tool which aids the community health nurse in collecting generational information about family structure and processes. It visually portrays to the nurse and the family how the family has evolved. It very quickly helps the community health nurse to identify the relationships between significant family members, the health status of individual family members, and the family's reactions to sociocultural and spiritual variables which have affected their lives.

Illustrated in Figure 6-3 is a partial genogram constructed by a community health nurse during her sixth home visit to the Z. family. Prior to doing the genogram, the nurse had been helping the family members deal with their feelings about the son's recent diagnosis of allergies. She identified that there was a discrepancy in how each parent viewed the son's health status. Wondering whether this was related to previous life experiences, the nurse completed a genogram with the family. By doing this, the nurse was able to trace each parent's attitudes about health and illness. She was also able to identify that the family lacked a significant support system, that both parents had had an unhappy childhood, and that they

were afraid that they were "going to raise their son wrong." In addition, it was discovered that the family was having difficulty adjusting to recent role changes and that all family members had unresolved feelings about the death of two children in the family. The community health nurse who constructed the genogram in Figure 6-3 found that this tool helped both her and the family to focus more clearly on current significant events as well as to gain an appreciation for how past happenings were influencing present health behavior. The development of the genogram provided structure for the interviewing process and helped the community health nurse to obtain an extensive family history very rapidly.

Genograms schematically depict a family tree. Geneticists, physicians, and nurse clinicians have used them to trace genetic disorders in families. They are now being used by health care professionals to integrate health and sociocultural data. A family tree drawn by a professional differs from the one drawn by a family in that the professional uses theory as a basis to elicit data about family structure, function, and process. Normally a family tree done by a lay person illustrates only structural information.

The interview process is the most critical component to consider when one is completing a genogram. If information concerning child-rearing practices, health beliefs and attitudes, significant social data, and traditions passed on from one generation to another is not obtained, the genogram has very little meaning. Completing the actual drawing of a genogram takes minimal skill; focusing the conversation on relevant aspects of family functioning requires not only interviewing skill but also knowledge of family dynamics.

Eco-map

An eco-map is another tool used by health care professionals which schematically portrays fac-

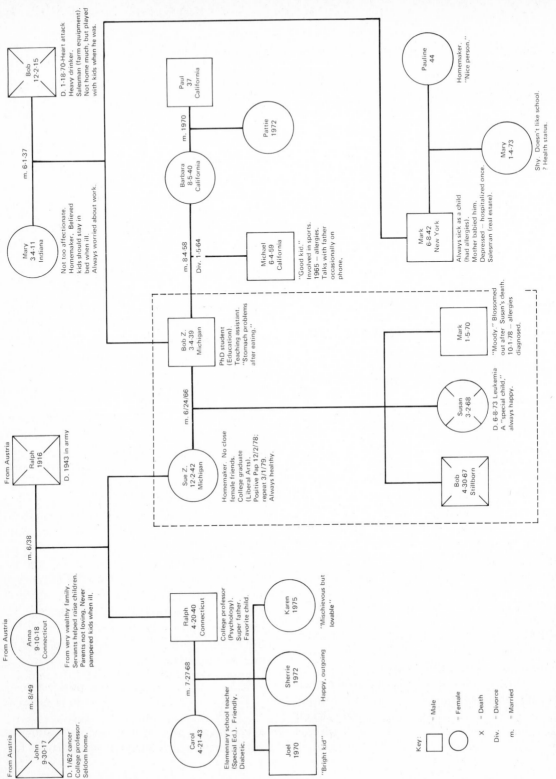

FIGURE 6-3 Sample genogram of the Z. family.

tual data about family relationships. It helps the family and the nurse to visually analyze a family's interactions with its external environment. Presented in Figure 6-4 is an eco-map developed by Dr. Ann Hartman for workers in a child welfare practice (Hartman, 1978, p. 466). Based on a systems theoretical framework, Hartman's tool examines boundary-maintenance aspects of family functioning. It dramatically illustrates the amount of energy used by a family to maintain its system as well as the presence or absence of situational supports and other family resources. By utilizing this tool, for example, families can be helped to identify that their energies are being used to handle stressful encounters with external systems rather than to enhance positive, supportive relationships with others. For instance, if a family's flow of energy as depicted on the eco-map reflects only an outward directional process ($\rightarrow \rightarrow \rightarrow$), the family may recognize why its goals are not being achieved.

Community health nurses have found the use of the eco-map beneficial because they are frequently involved with clients who have encounters with numerous health and welfare agencies, who have few support systems, or who "lack energy" to maintain their family system. An eco-map assists a family in visualizing how their relationships with external systems are affecting their state of well-being. One community health nurse decided to use this tool with a family because its multiple relationships with agencies were unclear and because the family members were having difficulty verbalizing their feelings about their "hopeless" family situation. "We have tried everything, and still our situation gets worse." The use of the eco-map increased the family's involvement in the therapeutic process and gave them something concrete to do, which relieved at least some of their anxiety about their "hopeless" state of affairs. When the eco-map was completed, it was obvious to both the nurse and the family that there were numer-

ous stressors that were affecting the family's feelings about itself. The family was allowing health and social agencies to take over its affairs, extended-family members gave only negative feedback, friends seldom visited, and the family had few leisure activities. The eco-map pointed out to the family the multiple problems they were encountering and assisted the nurse in planning her intervention strategies as well.

It is impossible to function effectively in the community health setting without looking at how the family interfaces with its external environment. The eco-map enhances the community health nurses's ability to gain this type of information. It is an especially useful tool because it summarizes, on one page, family strengths, conflicts, and stresses in relation to its interactions with individuals and agencies outside the family system.

Family-Life Chronology

Community health nurses may encounter families who are experiencing relationship problems, a situation which makes it difficult for them to concentrate on health concerns or to take needed health actions. These families can find it hard to examine objectively what is happening in their relationships or to make a decision about seeking counseling. Satir's (1967, p. 135) family-life chronology model (Figure 6-5) helps the community health nurse and the family to identify interactive processes that have evolved. Stresses are often related only to current family changes, such as a chronic health problem, an additional family member, or financial difficulties. Helping a family's members to look at how successful they have been in handling interpersonal interactions up to this point may provide the positive reinforcement they need to examine how they can alter their current behavior to reduce existing stresses. Sometimes, however, it will be found that a family has had long-standing relation-

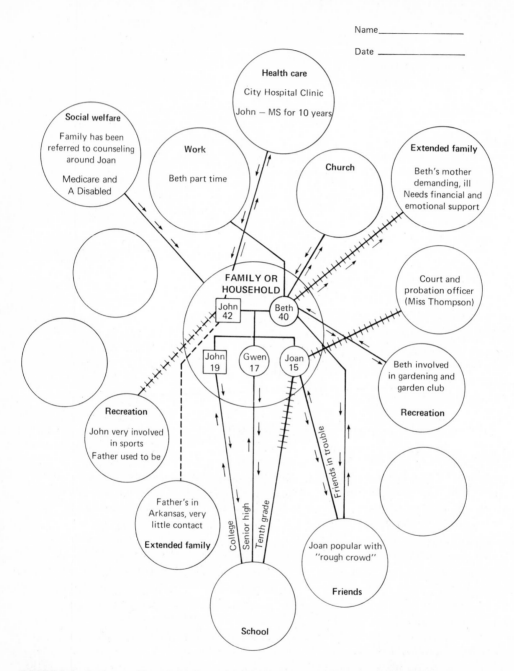

FIGURE 6-4 Eco-map. (*From A. Hartman. Diagrammatic assessment of family Relationships. Social Caseword, 1978, 59, p. 470.*) Fill in connections where they exist. Indicate nature of connections with a descriptive word or by drawing different kinds of lines:————— for strong; -------- for tenuous; –/–/–/–/ for stressful. Draw arrows along lines to signify flow of energy, resources, etc. (→ → →). Identify significant people and fill in empty circles as needed.

To mates

Asks about how they met, when they decided to marry, etc.

To wife	**To husband**
Asks how she saw her parents, her sibs, _____ her family life	Asks how he saw his parents, his sibs, his family life
Brings chronology back to when she _____ met her husband	Brings chronology back to when he met his wife
Asks about her expectations of _____ marriage	Asks about his expectations of marriage

To mates
Asks about early married life; comments on influence of past

To mates as parents
Asks about their expectations of parenting; comments on the influence of the past

To child
Asks about the child's views of the parents, how he or she sees them having fun, disagreeing, etc.

To family as a whole
Reassures family that it is safe to comment; stresses need for clear communication; gives closure, points to next meeting, gives hope

FIGURE 6-5   Main flow of family-life chronology. (*From V. Satir. Conjoint family therapy: A guide to theory and technique. Palo Alto, Calif.: Science and Behavior Books, 1972, p. 135.*)

ship problems. Helping family members to identify the chronic nature of their current difficulties may assist them in seeing the need for psychosocial counseling.

The process for collecting a family-life chronology is discussed in Satir's book, *Conjoint Family Therapy (1967)*. Community health nurse practitioners have found this book to be a valuable reference that helps them work more effectively with families who are experiencing distress in their relationships.

A community health nurse cannot ignore relationship problems when working with families in their homes. Such difficulties can disrupt all parameters of family functioning and are often the key factor in preventing a family from taking needed health action. If these difficulties are not addressed, nursing intervention strategies can be very ineffective. Dealing with the symptoms of distress, such as

physical health problems, complaints about lack of time for leisure activities, or feelings of depression, rather than with the relationship difficulties themselves, will not alter a family's functioning in any lasting way. One mother, for example, complained to the community health nurse that she had no time for herself and that she found caring for three children, 4, 6, and 8 years old, very restrictive. Suggestions by the community health nurse on how she might care for her children and still have time for leisure activities were ignored. The mother finally shared with the nurse that her husband felt that "a women's place was in the home. Even if I enrolled my 4-year-old son in a nursery school, I still could not get out of the house. My husband gets very upset if I am gone from home without him." This woman was depressed and discouraged. She loved her children but also wanted to explore adult interests; the only way she was able to accomplish this was to deal with the conflicts between herself and her husband.

The above situation illustrates that in working with individual family members, a nurse must determine how other members of the family view the issues being raised. Otherwise, significant data will be missed and interventions will be planned that are inappropriate to the needs of the family. It is best to obtain the ideas and opinions of all family members by seeing them together. If this cannot be arranged, asking questions such as "How does your husband react when you talk about getting a job?" provides clues about family interactions and differing value systems. It must be emphasized that family meetings can be arranged more frequently then they are; often nurses do not suggest this strategy because they do not feel comfortable in dealing with family dynamics.

Schedule of Recent Experience (SRE) Life Changes Questionnaire

Research since the early sixties has documented that significant life changes can adversely affect the health status of individuals (Rahe, 1972, p. 62). The Life Changes Questionnaire (see Table 6-3) developed by Holmes, Rahe, Masuda, and others, has been used throughout the United States and in foreign countries to demonstrate the relationships between a cluster of events requiring life changes and illness. It has been shown that individuals whose life change units (LCU) are greater than the value of 150 in a year's time are more susceptible to illness than individuals whose life change units are below this value. Studies conducted by Rahe while at the University of Washington in Seattle, for instance, demonstrated that 50 percent of the individuals whose life change units ranged from 150 to 300 LCU had an illness within the following year. In addition, 70 percent of those individuals whose LCU values exceeded 300 had an illness the following year (Rahe, 1972, p. 68).

Practitioners as well as researchers have used the Life Change Questionnaire to identify persons at risk for illness. When they discover individuals who have high LCU values, they discuss the impact of several life changes on one's health status and the importance of not making other major life changes at this time.

The Life Changes Questionnaire can easily be used in community health nurse practice, both in the home and in the clinic setting, to quickly discern individuals who are experiencing multiple stressors. Practitioners who have used this tool have often seen clients experience a sense of relief when they find out that it is normal to be distressed by multiple changes occurring in a short time period. Frequently, clients who have encountered several major life changes do not recognize that this has happened. The Life Changes Questionnaire can help them to visualize the relationship between their feelings of distress and the events that have occurred in their lives within a year's time.

Videotaping

Videotaping is another tool which has helped the community health nurse to identify family dynamics. It has been used in some community health nursing settings to assess family interactions when a handicapped child is performing activities of daily living. Community health nurses have used videotaping in these situations to observe simultaneously the interactions of a child and family, as well as the functional capabilities of the client being assessed. It is important to observe both the client and significant others during a functional assessment, because behavior of significant others either inhibits or enhances functional capabilities.

Videotaping provides specific data about

TABLE 6-3 Life Change Events

Events	LCU values	Events	LCU values
FAMILY		Major revision of personal habits	24
Death of spouse	100	Changing to a new school	20
Divorce	73	Change in residence	20
Marital separation	65	Major change in recreation	19
Death of close family member	63	Major change in church activities	19
Marriage	50	Major change in sleeping habits	16
Marital reconciliation	45	Major change in eating habits	15
Major change in health of family	44	Vacation	13
Pregnancy	40	Christmas	12
Addition of new family member	39	Minor violations of the law	11
Major change in arguments with wife	35		
Son or daughter leaving home	29	WORK	
In-law troubles	29	Being fired from work	47
Wife starting or ending work	26	Retirement from work	45
Major change in family get-togethers	15	Major business adjustment	39
		Changing to different line of work	36
		Major change in work responsibilities	29
PERSONAL		Trouble with boss	23
Detention in jail	63	Major change in working conditions	20
Major personal injury or illness	53		
Sexual difficulties	39	FINANCIAL	
Death of a close friend	37	Major change in financial state	38
Outstanding personal achievement	28	Mortgage or loan over $10,000	31
Start or end of formal schooling	26	Mortgage foreclosure	30
Major change in living conditions	25	Mortgage or loan less than $10,000	17

SOURCE: From R. H. Rahe. Subjects' recent life changes and their near-future illness reports. *Annals of Clinical Research,* October 1972, *4,* 250–265. This study report was supported by the Bureau of Medicine and Surgery, Department of the Navy, under Research Work Unit MF51.524.002-5011-DD5G (Report No. 72-31). Opinions expressed are those of the authors and are not to be construed as necessarily reflecting the official view or endorsement of the Department of the Navy.

family dynamics and a child's functional abilities which are often missed during a home visit. It is easy to overlook small accomplishments of a child when other things are occurring in the environment. It is equally easy to miss nurse or family behaviors which negatively affect a child's performance. For instance, use of videotaping enabled one nurse to identify that she had not given the 4-year-old child she was assessing sufficient time to complete the tasks she asked him to perform. A repeat assessment on her next home visit provided her with more accurate data in relation to the child's level of functioning. Without videotaping, this child's level of performance would have been assessed inappropriately.

Families are usually receptive to videotaping, especially when the community health nurse explains that a more accurate evaluation of a child's abilities may be obtained through the use of this tool. Assuring them that confidentiality will be maintained also relieves their anxiety.

A videotaped child assessment can be very motivating to families because it dramatically illustrates a child's strengths and needs.

Videotaping helps a family to identify positive and negative behaviors which are promoting or inhibiting a child's growth. The impact of seeing actual behaviors is not quickly forgotten.

SUMMARY

Despite its changing nature, the family is still considered the basic unit of service in community health nursing settings. Historical evidence from clinical practice has sufficiently demonstrated that family-centered nursing services more effectively meet the needs of individuals, families, and communities than do services delivered only to individual clients. Viewing the family from the traditional perspective, however, is no longer appropriate because alternative family life-styles are becoming more evident in our culture. The nuclear family unit is no longer the only acceptable form of family life.

It is essential for community health nurses to have an understanding of family theory in order to implement a family-centered preventive health approach to nursing care. Theory helps the practitioner to assess family structure, function, and process in an organized and logical fashion. It provides parameters to consider when one is collecting data about client situations. It assists in explaining the phenomena that are occurring within a family, which in turn helps one to plan effective intervention strategies.

Tools such as the genogram, the eco-map, and the Life Change Questionnaire are available for facilitating the family assessment process. These tools do not, however, take the place of a genuine understanding of family dynamics. They only provide guidelines for the organization and collection of data.

Appendix 6-1
Family Assessment Guide
Family name _____ Family ID no._____
Source of referral _____
Reason for referral _____
Occupational status _____
Health insurance _____
Medical emergency plan _____
Preventive health care _____

Family composition: Map family constellation; include health problems of individual members.

Date		Assessment parameters	Rating		Significant data
1st	*2d*		*1st*	*2d*	
		1. *Structural characteristics*			
		a. Financial resources			
		b. Educational experiences			
		c. Allocation of family and personal roles			
		d. Division of labor			
		e. Distribution of power and authority			
		f. Cultural influences			
		(1) Health beliefs and attitudes			
		(2) Family goals			
		(3) Norms for social behavior			
		(4) Spiritual beliefs			
		(5) Beliefs about folk diseases and medicine			
		g. Activities of daily living			
		(1) Dietary habits			
		(2) Child-rearing practices			
		(3) Housekeeping			
		(4) Sleeping arrangements			
		(5) Laundry facilities			
		(6) Transportation			
		(7) Care of ill family members			
		(8) Knowledge of health problems			
		(9) Understanding of health promotion practices			
		2. *Process characteristics*			
		a. Atmosphere of home			
		b. Communication patterns			
		c. Decision-making processes			
		(1) How decisions made			
		(2) How decisions implemented			
		d. Conflict negotiation			
		e. Achievement of developmental tasks			
		f. Adaptation to change			
		g. Autonomy of individual family members			
		3. *Relationships with external systems*			
		a. How family boundaries established			
		b. Utilization of information from environment			
		c. Contact with extended families			
		d. Interactions with friends and neighbors			

Date		Assessment parameters	Rating		Significant data
1st	*2d*		*1st*	*2d*	
		e. Attitudes about community systems			
		(1) Health			
		(2) Welfare			
		(3) Educational			
		(4) Others (describe)			
		f. Use of the referral process			
		(1) Ability to seek assistance			
		(2) Level of independence			
		4. *Environmental characteristics*			
		a. Neighborhood			
		(1) Accessibility of facilities to meet basic needs			
		(2) Availability of recreational, educational, religious, and other resources			
		(3) Safety (physical and psychosocial)			
		b. Housing			
		(1) Suitability in relation to family needs			
		(2) Condition of structural components			
		(3) Suitability of home furnishings			
		(4) Sanitation (water source and sewage and garbage disposal and housekeeping practices)			
		(5) Accident hazards			
		(6) Barriers to family mobility			

Date		
1st	*2d*	
		Professionals and volunteers working with family (identify person and agency)
		Summary of family strengths (based on categories rated No. 1)
		Description of family priorities and assistance desired

Date		Specific factors to consider when developing and implementing a management plan
1st	*2d*	

Assessor_____ Date_____
Assessor_____ Date_____
Assessor_____ Date_____

NOTE: Code for recording assessment data—use a different-color ink for the first and second assessment or rating (generally it takes several home visits to complete a family assessment). Rating scale: 1 = strength; 2 = problem; 3 = anticipatory guidance warranted; 4 = problem—family does not wish to change this area of functioning at this time; 5 = not applicable. Family functioning should be rated every 4 months to assist in evaluating family progress and nursing intervention strategies.

REFERENCES

Ackerman, N. W. (Ed.). *Family process.* New York: Basic Books, 1970. *The psychodynamics of family life: Diagnosis and treatment of family relationships.* New York: Basic Books, 1959.

Baca, J. E. Some health beliefs of the Spanish speaking. In A. Reinhardt and M. Quinn (Eds.), *Family-centered community nursing: A sociocultural framework.* St. Louis: Mosby, 1973.

Bane, M. J. *Here to stay—American families in the twentieth century.* New York: Basic Books, 1976.

Beavers, W. R. *Psychotherapy and growth: A family systems perspective.* New York: Brunner/Mazel, 1977.

Bernard, J. The adjustments of married mates. In H. T. Christensen (Ed.), *Handbook of marriage and the family.* Chicago: Rand McNally, 1964, pp. 675–739.

Bowen, M. Toward the differentiation of a self in one's own family. In J. L. Framo (Ed.), *Family interaction: A dialogue between family researchers and family therapists.* New York; Springer, 1973.

Bredemeir, H. C., & Stephenson, R. N. *The analysis of social systems.* New York: Holt, 1965.

Briar, Scott. The family as an organization: An approach to family diagnosis and treatment. *The Social Service Review,* September 1964, *38,* 247–255.

Broderick, C. B. Beyond the five conceptual frameworks: A decade of development in family theory. *The Journal of Marriage and the Family,* February 1971, *33,* 139–159.

Castles, M. R. Game theory as a conceptual framework for nursing practice. In D. P. Hymovich & M. U. Barnard (Eds.). *Family health care.* New York: McGraw-Hill, 1973.

Christensen, H. T. (Ed.). *Handbook of marriage and the family.* Chicago: Rand McNally, 1964.

Churchman, C. W. *The systems approach.* New York: Dell, 1968.

Clemen, S. J. *Introduction to health care facility: Food service administration.* University Park: The Pennsylvania State University Press, 1974.

Duvall, E. M. *Marriage and family development,* (5th ed.) New York: Lippincott, 1977.

Eshleman, J. R., & Clarke, J. N. *Intimacy, commitments, and marriage: Development of relationships.* Boston: Allyn & Bacon, 1978.

Flanzraich, M., & Dunsavage, I. Role reversal in abused/neglected families. *Children Today,* November–December 1977, *6,* 13–15.

Hacker, S. Sexual values for teachers and administrators. Presented for the Comprehensive Youth Services for Teachers, Oakland University, Pontiac, Mich., July 25, 1979.

Haley, J. (Ed.). *Changing families.* New York: Grune & Stratton, 1971.

Hartman, A. Diagrammatic assessment of family relationships. *Social Casework,* October 1978, *59,* 465–476.

Hill, R., & Hansen, D. A. The identification of conceptual frameworks utilized in family study. *Marriage and Family Living,* November 1960, *22,* 299–311.

Howe, L. K. *The future of the family.* New York: Simon and Schuster, 1972.

Jackson, D. D. (Ed.). *Communication, family and marriage,* vol. 1. Palo Alto, Calif.: Science and Behavior Books, 1968.

Kensky, A. D. Cultural influences on the Jewish patient. In S. A. Clemen and M. Will (Eds.), *Family and community health nursing: A workbook,* Ann Arbor: The University of Michigan Press, 1977.

Lewis, J., Beavers, R., Gossett, J. T., & Phillips, V. A. *No single thread: Psychological health in family systems.* New York: Brunner/Mazel, 1976.

Linton, R. The natural history of the family. In R. N. Anshen (Ed.), *The family: Its function and destiny* (rev. ed.). New York: Harper & Row, 1959.

Minuchin, S. *Families and family therapy.* Cambridge, Mass: Harvard University Press, 1974.

Nye, F. I. *Role structure and analysis of the family.* Beverly Hills: Sage, 1976.

Otto, H. Criteria for assessing family strengths. *Family Process,* September 1963, *2,* 329–338.

Peterson, R. What are the needs of the chronic mental patients? Presentation for the APA Conference on the Chronic Mental Patient, Washington, D.C., Jan. 11–14, 1978.

Pratt, L. *Family structure and effective health behavior: The energized family.* Boston: Houghton Mifflin, 1976.

Prattes, O. Beliefs of the Mexican-American family. In D. Hymovich and M. Barnard (Eds.), *Family*

health care. New York: McGraw-Hill, 1973.

Rahe, R. H. Subjects' recent life changes and their near-future illness reports. *Annals of Clinical Research,* October 1972, *4,* 250–265.

Samora, J. Conceptions of health and disease among Spanish-Americans. In Martínez, R. A. *Hispanic culture and health care: Fact, fiction, folklore.* St. Louis: Mosby, 1978.

Satir, V. *Conjoint family therapy: A guide to theory and technique.* Palo Alto, Calif.: Science and Behavior Books, 1967.

———. *Peoplemaking.* Palo Alto, Calif.: Science and Behavior Books, 1972.

———. You as a change agent in helping families to change. In V. Satir, J. Stachowiak, & H. Taskman, *Helping families to change.* New York: Jason Aronson, 1975.

Stryker, S. The interactional and situational approaches. In H. T. Christensen (Ed.), *Handbook of marriage and the family.* Chicago: Rand McNally, 1964, pp. 125–170.

Sussman, M. B. (Chairperson). Changing families in a changing society. In *1970 White House Conference on Children, Forum 14 report.* Washington, D.C.: Government Printing Office, 1971.

Von Bertalanffy, L. *General systems theory.* New York: George Braziller, 1968.

Watzlawick, P., Beavin, J. H., & Jackson, D. D. *Pragmatics of human communication: A study of interactional patterns, pathologies, and paradoxes.* New York: Norton, 1967.

White House Conference on Families, 1978. Joint hearings before the Subcommittee on Child and Human Development of the Committee on Human Resources, U.S. Senate and the Subcommittee on Select Education of the Committee on Education and Labor, House of Representatives, Ninety-fifth Congress. Washington, D.C.: Government Printing Office, 1978.

Wiener, N. Cybernetics in history. In W. Buckley (Ed.), *Modern systems research for the behavioral scientist.* Chicago: Aldine, 1968.

Yorburg, B. *The changing family.* New York: Columbia University Press, 1973.

SELECTED BIBLIOGRAPHY

Allen, W. R. The search for applicable theories of black family life. *Journal of Marriage and the Family*, February 1978, *40*, 117–129.

Barbeau, C. (Ed.). *Future of the family.* New York: Bruce, 1971.

Cooper, D. G. *The death of the family.* New York: Pantheon, 1970.

Crawford, C. O. *Health and the family.* New York: Macmillan, 1971.

Duhl, F., Grey, W., & Rizzo, N. D. *General systems theory in psychiatry.* Boston: Little, Brown, 1969.

Erickson, P. M., & Rogers, L. E. New procedures for analyzing relational communication. *Family Process*, September 1974, *13*, 245–267.

Farber, B. *Family and kinship in modern society.* Glencoe, Ill.: Scott, Foresman, 1973.

Fedman, H., & Feldman, M. The family life cycle: Some suggestions for recycling. *Journal of Marriage and the Family*, May 1975, *37*, 277–284.

Fogarty, M. P., Rapoport, R., & Rapoport, R. N. *Sex, career and family: Including an international review of women's roles.* London: Allen & Unwin, 1971.

Frederick, R. F., & Herrick, J. Family rules: Family life styles. *American Journal of Orthopsychiatry.* January 1974, *44*, 61–69.

Freedman, M. (Ed.). *Family and kinship in Chinese society.* Stanford, Calif.: Stanford University Press, 1970.

Geismar, L. *555 Families, a social-psychological study of young families in transition.* New Brunswick, N. J.: Transaction Books, 1973.

Handel, G. (Ed.). *The psycho-social interior of the family.* Chicago: Aldine-Atherton, 1967.

Hardy, M. E., & Conway, M. E. *Role theory: Perspectives for health professionls.* New York: Appleton-Century-Crofts, 1978.

Hareven, T. R. (Ed.). *Transitions: The family and the life course in historical perspective.* New York: Academic, 1978.

Heiss, J. *Family roles and interaction: An anthology.* Chicago: Rand McNally, 1968.

Hernandez, C. A., Haug, M. J., & Wagner, N. N. (Eds.). *Chicanos: Social and psychological perspectives.* St. Louis: Mosby, 1976.

Hill, R. A. *The strengths of black families.* New York: Emerson Hall, 1972.

Hopkinson, A. *Families without fathers.* London: Mother's Union, 1973.

Knafl, K. A., & Grace, H. K. *Families across the life cycle: Studies for nursing.* Boston: Little, Brown, 1978.

May, J. T. *Family health indicators: Annotated bibliography.* Rockville, Md.: U.S. National Institute of Mental Health, 1974.

Maurer, B. (Ed.). *Mountain heritage.* Morgantown, W.Va.: Morgantown Printing and Binding, 1974.

Miller, J. R., & Janosik, E. H. *Family-focused care.* New York: McGraw-Hill, 1980

Morey, S. M., & Gillian, O. L. (Eds.). *Respect for life: The traditional upbringing of American Indian children.* Garden City, N.Y.: Waldorf Press, Adelphi University, 1976.

Partridge, W. L. *The hippie ghetto: The natural history of a subculture.* New York: Holt, 1973.

Putt, A. M. *General systems theory applied to nursing.* Boston: Little, Brown, 1978.

Queen, S. A., & Habenstein, R. W. *The family in various cultures.* Philadelphia: Lippincott, 1974.

Rodgers, R. *Family interaction and transaction: The developmental approach.* Englewood Cliffs, N.J.: Prentice-Hall, 1973.

Samovar, L. A., & Porter, R. E. *Intercultural communication: A reader* (2d ed.). Belmont, Calif.: Wadsworth, 1976.

Sedgwick, R. The family as a system: A network of relationships. *Journal of Psychiatric Nursing and Mental Health Services*, March–April 1974, 17–20.

Skolnick, A. S., & Skolnick, J. H. *Intimacy, family and society.* Boston: Little, Brown, 1974.

Snow, L. F. Folk-medical beliefs and their implications for care of patients. *Annals of Internal Medicine*, July 1974, *81*, 82–86.

Staples, R. (Ed.). *The black family: essays and studies.*

Belmont, Calif.: Wadsworth, 1971.

Streib, G. F. (Ed.). The changing family: Adaptation and diversity. Reading, Mass.: Addison-Wesley, 1973.

Toman, W. *Family constellation: Theory and practice of a psychological game.* New York: Springer, 1961.

Turner, R. H. *Family interaction.* New York: Wiley, 1970.

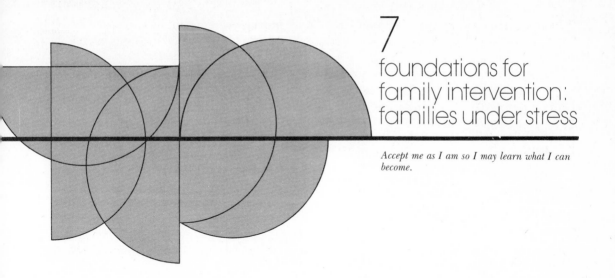

Accept me as I am so I may learn what I can become.

A major preventive responsibility of the community health nurse is to help individuals and families handle stressful life events so that their energies can be used to achieve self-fulfillment and to develop a capacity to extend themselves to others. Some stress is normal and essential for life and growth. Stress provides the stimulus needed to adapt to the ever-changing conditions of life. Too much stress, however, prevents people from seeing what "they can become."

Selye (1975, p. xv), has found that any emotion or activity, whether it produces joy or sadness, causes stress. He believes that stressful life events (see Table 6-4) will more likely result in disease and unhappiness when individuals and families are not prepared to deal with them. Persons who are not prepared to handle the pressures and experiences encountered throughout life often do not recognize signals of distress that reflect a need to mobilize different coping mechanisms.

Community health nurses are in a key position to help individuals and families adapt to new or threatening life changes. Daily in their work in the home and other settings, they encounter clients who are experiencing various degrees of stress. Many times these clients have not had life experiences or exposure to knowledge that would assist them in altering patterns of functioning that intensify stress. Most parents, for instance, have not been prepared to handle children whose growth and development significantly deviate from normal patterns of functioning. Hence, they experience heightened distress and are frequently open to professional intervention. Illustrative of this is the situation encountered by a community health nurse when she visited the Slavovi family for the first time:

The Slavovi family was referred to the community health nurse for health supervision follow-up after the birth of their fourth child, Stephanie, who had multiple handicaps. Even though this was the family's first exposure to community health nursing service, Mr. and Mrs. Slavovi talked freely when the nurse visited. Both manifested high levels of anxiety and confusion about how to care for their newborn infant. Angel and Maria Slavovi had always taken great pride in being good parents. Stephanie's physical and mental handicaps were particularly distressing to them: "We don't know how to help her. She continues to cry even when we hold her and seems to hurt all the time. Children need loving.

Why doesn't Stephanie want us to hold her? We must be doing something wrong."

Having an understanding of the concept of stress helps the community health nurse to intervene more effectively with clients like the Slavovis. Stress theory provides the foundation for identifying signs and symptoms of distress and for recognizing potential stressors. It also provides clues about how to bring about change when a client's usual methods of coping are no longer effective.

Hans Selye has written extensively about the concept of stress. Since only a very brief overview of this concept will be presented in this text, the reader may wish to refer to Selye's works to obtain an in-depth understanding of the stress phenomenon.

THE STRESS PHENOMENON

Selye (1975, p. 1) has defined stress "as the non-specific response of the body to any demand." It is a dynamic state triggered by stressors which help to maintain an internal balance within human systems. Stressors are "anything which produce stress" (Selye, p. 78).

Stress theory is based on the concepts of homeostasis (state of balance) and adaptation. Because stress is an inherent and integral part of life, individuals and families must constantly readjust to maintain themselves. One's state of balance is maintained when one learns to recognize the signals of distress and then adapts or changes functioning to meet the demands of the stress encountered. *Distress,* as defined by Selye, "is unpleasant or disease-producing stress" (Selye, p. 465). In contrast, "eustress is seen as good, pleasant, or curative stress" (Selye, p. 466).

Physiological responses (Figure 7-1) in the nervous and endocrine systems alert individuals to the occurrence of distress or eustress. These responses produce feelings such as joy, fatigue, or uneasiness. They help individuals to identify that their steady state is being threatened.

The physiological changes that occur in response to stress are nonspecific. They produce changes that affect a person's entire body and that happen any time an individual is experiencing stress, no matter what the cause. According to Selye (p. 163), the nonspecific responses to stress evolve in three stages, which he has labeled the *general adaptation syndrome* (GAS):

1. The *alarm reaction,* during which defense mechanisms are mobilized

2. The *stage of resistance,* when adaptation is acquired because optimum channels of defense were developed

3. The *stage of exhaustion,* which reflects a depletion of adaptation energy necessary to cope with prolonged and intensified stress

Although stress is essential for life and growth, every individual has limits beyond which stress is no longer healthy. When these limits are reached, exhaustion occurs and energies needed to deal with activities of daily living become depleted. All individuals have the capacity to deal with distress; however, they need to learn the limits of stress they can tolerate and adaptive mechanisms that will help them to maintain homeostasis.

Our bodies provide numerous physiological and psychological signals that reflect disruption of our homeostasis. An outline of these signals, as identified by Selye (pp. 174–177), is presented below:

1. General irritability, hyperexcitation, or depression. This is associated with unusual aggressive-

ness or passive indolence, depending upon our constitution.

2. Pounding of the heart, an indicator of high blood pressure (often due to stress).

3. Dryness of the throat and mouth.

4. Impulsive behavior, emotional instability.

5. The overpowering urge to cry or run and hide.

6. Inability to concentrate, flight of thoughts and general disorientation.

7. Feelings of unreality, weakness, or dizziness.

8. Predilection to become fatigued, and loss of the "joie de vivre."

9. "Floating anxiety," that is to say, we are afraid although we do not know exactly what we are afraid of.

10. Emotional tension and alertness, feeling of being "keyed up."

11. Trembling, nervous ticks.

12. Tendency to be easily startled by small sounds, etc.

13. High-pitched, nervous laughter.

14. Stuttering and other speech difficulties which are frequently stress-induced.

15. Bruxism, or grinding of the teeth.

16. Insomnia, which is usually a consequence of being "keyed up."

17. Hypermotility. This is technically called "hyperkinesia," an increased tendency to move about without any reason, an inability to just take a physically relaxed attitude, sitting quietly in a chair or lying on a sofa.

18. Sweating. This becomes evident only under considerable stress by inspection of the skin.

19. The frequent need to urinate.

20. Diarrhea, indigestion, queasiness in the stomach, and sometimes even vomiting. Also, all signs of disturbed gastrointestinal function which eventually may lead to such severe diseases of

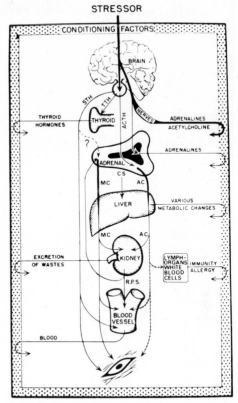

FIGURE 7-1 Physiological responses to stress. *(From H. Selye, The stress of life. New York: McGraw-Hill, 1976, p. 15.)*

adaptation as peptic ulcers, ulcerative colitis, the "irritable colon."

21. Migraine headaches.

22. Premenstrual tension or missed menstrual cycles, both of which are frequently indicators of severe stress in women.

23. Pain in the neck or lower back. In conversational English, the expression "this is nauseating," "he gives me ulcers," "this business is an awful headache," or "he gives me a pain in the neck" are not merely colorful expressions, but based on actual experience. For example, the pain in the neck or back is usually due to increases in muscular tension that can be objectively measured by physicians with the electromyogram (EMG).

24. Loss of or excessive appetite. This shows itself soon in alterations of body weight, namely excessive leanness or obesity. Some people lose their appetite during stress because of gastrointestinal malfunction, whereas others eat excessively, as a kind of diversion, to deviate their attention from the stressor situation. Besides, a well-filled stomach and intestine shift a great deal of blood to the abdomen, resulting in a relative decrease in brain circulation which tranquilizes by decreasing mental alertness.

25. Increased smoking.

26. Increased use of legally prescribed drugs, such as tranquilizers or amphetamines.

27. Alcohol and drug addiction. Like the phenomenon of overeating, increased and excessive alcohol consumption or the use of various psychotropic drugs is a common manifestation of exposure to stressors beyond our natural endurance. Here again, we are actually dealing with flight reactions, known as diversion or deviation, to which we resort presumably because they help us to forget the cause of our distress and tend to temporarily replace it by the eustress of psychic elation, or at least tranquilization.

28. Nightmares.

29. Neurotic behavior.

30. Psychoses.

31. Accident proneness. Under great stress (eustress or distress) we are more likely to have accidents at work or while driving a car. This is also a very important reason why pilots and air traffic controllers must be carefully checked for their stress status.

In terms of the family, stress is manifested by dysfunctional family patterns, as well as by the occurrence of the above signs and symptoms in its individual family members. Child abuse and neglect, domestic violence, strained communication patterns and decision-making conflicts are a few such dysfunctional patterns that may result when a family is under stress.

Individuals and families who learn that the above signs and symptoms result when they are experiencing stress beyond tolerable limits may be able to mobilize or adjust their coping mechanisms in a way that increases their resistance to stress. Persons who ignore signals of distress or who do not initiate appropriate defense mechanisms experience crisis.

THE CRISIS PHENOMENON

Crisis, like stress, is an elusive concept which can only be identified by recognizing the manifestations or characteristic signs and symptoms of the crisis state. That is why it is so important for nurses to have a firm understanding of the crisis sequence. Concepts of crisis help the practitioner to quickly recognize clients who need to adjust their coping mechanisms. It is especially critical for community health nurses to be well-grounded in crisis theory, because they frequently encounter clients in the home environment who are dealing with new, different, or threatening stressful events. Early identification of those clients who are

having difficulty coping with these events could prevent an intensified crisis state.

A preventive health philosophy stimulated the development of crisis theory and intervention. Erich Lindemann (1944), through his classic study of grief reactions, identified the need for *preventive counseling* with clients experiencing loss through death or separation. After investigating the responses of clients who had lost a relative in the famous Coconut Grove fire in Boston, he concluded that appropriate psychiatric intervention with clients who were experiencing grief could prevent prolonged and serious social maladjustment

(Lindemann, p. 147). He further concluded, after observing clients who experienced an "anticipatory grief reaction," that prophylactic counseling could prevent family crisis (Lindemann, p. 148). Anticipatory grief reactions occur when there is a threat of death, such as when soldiers engage in war activities. Clients in these situations go through all the stages of grief. It has been found in some cases that wives of soldiers in the war handled the grief process so effectively that they emancipated themselves from their spouse. This precipitated a crisis if husbands returned from the war, because their wives needed to reestablish marital relationships before they could express feelings of love and caring. Husbands in these situations felt that their wives no longer loved them and frequently asked for a divorce (Lindemann, pp. 147–148).

Crisis reactions, such as those described by Lindemann, can be predicted and often prevented. Lindemann, Caplan, and other crisis theorists have delineated a sequence of events that occur when a client is experiencing a crisis, as well as factors that intensify the crisis state. In addition, these theorists have identified situations that frequently precipitate a crisis during the developmental life cycle of a family and therapeutic processes that have a positive influence on client functioning when the family is experiencing a crisis.

The Crisis Sequence

Gerald Caplan (1961, p. 18), the father of preventive psychiatry, describes *crisis* as a state "provoked when a person faces an obstacle to important life goals that is, for a time, insurmountable through the utilization of customary methods of problem solving. A period of disorganization ensues, a period of upset, during which many different abortive attempts at solution are made. Eventually some kind of adaptation is achieved, which may or may not be in the best interests of that person and his fellows."

When describing the normal sequence of events that occur during a crisis, Caplan (1964, pp. 40–41) identifies four characteristic phases:

1. An initial phase when an individual's tension rises as he or she uses habitual problem-solving responses to achieve emotional homeostasis.

2. A second stage in which tension increases and the individual becomes ineffective and upset because normal coping mechanisms were not effective in resolving the state of crisis.

3. A third threshold when tension mounts and stimulates the mobilization of new and emergency problem-solving mechanisms. The problem may be resolved if an individual can redefine the situation in order to cope with it and can adjust to role changes that have occurred.

4. A final phase when tension mounts beyond the limits an individual can tolerate; major disorganization results.

Inherent in Caplan's description of a crisis are several key ideas: (1) change which threatens an individual's ability to meet life goals disrupts the individual's homeostasis; (2) crisis results when an individual's customary methods of adaptation are ineffective in handling change; (3) disorganization occurs during the crisis state; (4) crisis is self-limiting, with a subsequent reduction of emotional tension (adaptation); (5) biopsychosocial homeostasis following a crisis may be at a level the same as, better than, or worse than the precrisis level. The goal of crisis intervention is to help the client to maintain a level of functioning equal to or better than the precrisis level.

It is not uncommon for community health nurses to work with families who have been unable to return successfully to their precrisis level of functioning after experiencing a crisis. When first encountered by the community health nurse, these families often present multiple difficulties, ineffective problem-solving methods, and feelings of helplessness and hopelessness.

Community health nurses also encounter families who not only return to precrisis levels of functioning but, in addition, experience growth during crisis situations. Many families develop new methods of coping which provide alternative ways for handling future stresses. Many also develop a cohesive family unity which increases the supportive and nurturing aspects of their family life-style and which encourages risk taking. Risk taking may expose individuals and families to other growth-producing opportunities.

There are several factors that affect how well a family handles stress and deals with crises. Community health nurses who understand these variables are better able to help families achieve successful resolution and growth during a crisis state.

Factors Affecting the Outcome of a Crisis

Aquilera and Messick (1978, p. 67) contend that there are three balancing factors that relate to the precipitation and successful resolution of a crisis. These are *perception of the event, available support systems,* and *adequate coping mechanisms.* Figure 7-2 presents the paradigm developed by Aquilera and Messick (p. 68) to study the influence of these balancing factors during times of stress. It illustrates that clients must achieve a realistic perception of the event, develop adequate situational supports, and mobilize coping mechanisms to achieve successful adaptation during periods of disequilibrium.

Aquilera and Messick's paradigm provides a logical and useful model for analyzing a

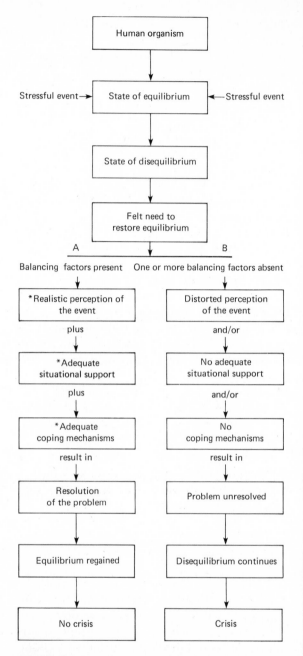

FIGURE 7-2 Paradigm: effect of balancing factors in a stressful event; * = balancing factors. [*From Donna C. Aquilera & Janice M. Messick. Crisis intervention: Theory and methodology (3d ed.). St. Louis: Mosby, 1978, p. 68.*]

client's ability to adjust when experiencing stress. Their paradigm provides a framework for identifying significant parameters to assess when working with persons who have encountered threatening life events. A data base relative to each of Aquilera and Messick's balancing factors should be obtained when working with such persons. In their text, *Crisis Intervention: Theory and Methodology*, Aquilera and Messick have shared several case situations which illustrate the significant influence these balancing factors have during times of stress.

Perception of the event. Crisis is the emotional reaction that occurs in relation to a new, different, or threatening event, not the event itself. Basically, the extent of this emotional reaction is determined by how the client (individual, family, population group) defines his or her particular circumstances (Aquilera and Messick, 1978; Burr, 1973; Caplan, 1964; Hansen and Hill, 1964; Rahe, 1974).

There are a number of factors that influence how a client perceives a hazardous situation. Specifically, the practitioner should analyze the following variables when working with clients who have intensified stress:

1. Number of stressors client is experiencing

2. Client's past experiences in handling current stressor(s)

3. Biopsychosocial status of the client prior to encountering hazardous event(s)

4. Duration of exposure to current stressor(s)

5. Magnitude or seriousness of current event(s)

6. Suddenness of the event

7. Client's understanding of the stressor event(s)

Even though the responses of individuals to hazardous events are highly variable, there is evidence which supports the theory that distress increases when one encounters multiple stressors (Rahe, 1974), experiences the stressor or stressors for a prolonged length of time (Selye, 1975), is exposed to a stressor with little or no time for anticipating problem solving (Hansen and Hill, 1964), faces an event that is highly ambiguous (McHugh, 1968), or encounters a situation that presents hardship or has serious consequences, such as death (Hill, 1949). When distress heightens, clients are more likely to have a distorted view of the current stressor. They may experience such feelings as helplessness, hopelessness, anxiety, fatigue, or depression. It must be emphasized, however, that even when one or more of the above factors exist in stressful occurrences, the perceived meaning of occurrences varies from one individual to another. The above factors only place individuals more at risk for developing crisis.

Caplan (1964, pp. 42–43) has found that for a stressor to become problematic, "it must be perceived as a threat or loss to need satisfaction or as a challenge." He believes that two major variables, personality and sociocultural factors, significantly affect how one perceives life events. These variables determine the type of life experiences one has, prescribe the limits of acceptable behavior when dealing with stress, and influence how one feels about one's abilities to handle changes in life. Case situations can best illustrate how the variables of personality and sociocultural influences affect one's perception of an event.

Mrs. Farias was 34 years old and left with two sons, 8 and 10 years old, and one daughter, age 14, when her husband was killed in a car accident. The community health nurse had encountered the Farias family prior to Mr. Farias's death, because Carmelina, their 14-year-old daughter, needed orthopedic follow-up for a scoliosis problem discovered through health screening at her high school. During a home visit 8 months after Mr. Farias's death, the community health nurse became concerned about Mrs. Farias's physical and psychological health. She looked uncared for, her home was untidy, and she had no interest in talking about Carmelina's health problems. Weeping, Mrs. Farias shared with the nurse that "nothing was going right lately; the children don't obey, I can't get my husband's life insurance, and my friends haven't visited lately." She became particularly distressed when she talked about how she was going to feed her family in the future. "Our savings are almost gone. I can't get a job. What will I do? I have never worked, because Julio thought that a wife should stay at home. My folks thought that girls should marry and raise a family. I never was good at much except maybe cooking, housekeeping, and loving the kids. My family thinks it is wrong to take money from the welfare department. They say they will help me until I remarry, but I know they don't have anything extra. Besides, I am too old to remarry. Most men I know want their own children, not someone else's. You can't meet men when you are my age."

Another case situation illustrates different family reactions to the death of its male provider.

Mrs. Ulisses was a 33-year-old widow with two daughters, 2 and 6 years of age, and two sons, ages 8 and 11. Her husband was killed while hunting. The community health nurse started visiting Mrs. Ulisses after she brought her 2-year-old to the well-baby clinic, 6 weeks after her husband's death. At that time, she expressed a desire to obtain information about day-care centers. The nurse visited regularly for a year to help Mrs. Ulisses sort out what she would like to do in the future. She and her husband were never able to save much, so Mrs. Ulisses applied for financial assistance from the Department of Social Service. She did not like receiving Aid to Dependent Children and Family monies, but felt that she needed time to make child-care arrangements before she went back to work. Seven and a half months after her husband's death, Mrs. Ulisses enrolled in college. "I know I can find a job, because I have worked off and on since age 15. If I had some training, however, I would be more secure in the future. I am still not sure if I want to get married again, so I better prepare myself to care for my family."

Both Mrs. Farias and Mrs. Ulisses were facing similar situations. They experienced the loss of a significant other who had assumed the provider role in their family system when he was living. Mrs. Farias, however, was more threatened by her circumstances because past and current cultural influences affected her ability to be flexible when role changes were needed. In addition, Mrs. Farias lacked confidence (personality factor) in her abilities to succeed in work and social settings. Her life experiences were focused on preparing her for traditional female roles only.

Mrs. Ulisses, on the other hand, was discouraged at times, but was actively involved in planning for a future career. She was better prepared to assume the provider role, having worked off and on since her teenage years, and felt more confident about her abilities to succeed outside the home setting. Her life experiences provided her with a different perception of her female role.

Situational supports. It has long been recognized that people need meaningful human relationships in order to cope with the stresses of life. Sensory-deprivation experiments, psychological case studies, and anthropological research have clearly demonstrated that lack of human support and caring result in maladaptive behaviors which are harmful to individuals and at times to others in their social environment. The true story of Sybil (Schreiber, 1973), for instance, dramatically portrayed how significant others affect the manner in which people respond to stress. Sybil developed multiple, crippling personalities to ward off the traumas she was experiencing because adequate situational supports were lacking. When she was able to engage in a trusting relationship with her analyst, however, growth-producing adaptive mechanisms emerged.

Significant others (family, friends, relatives, professionals, and others) can increase or decrease an individual's vulnerability to crisis during times of stress. That is why it is so important to ascertain information about the *quality* of the interactions clients have with others, along with the amount of contact they have with them. During periods of disequilibrium, persons need supportive relationships that allow them to verbalize feelings and encourage them to sort out the realities of their situation. Clients also need assistance with problem solving. In addition, concrete help is frequently needed to facilitate their ability to obtain resources, such as financial assistance, from their environment (see Chapter 9). Behaviors that support a client's distorted perception of the event are not helpful. A friend, for example, who reinforces a client's blaming behaviors inhibits client growth and successful resolution of a crisis; this type of behavior supports the client's current ineffective coping style, which in turn prevents the client from mobilizing more effective coping mechanisms.

When working with clients who are experiencing a crisis, it is extremely important to remember that their significant others may also be in crisis. Often the practitioner finds that others in a client's social network are experiencing as much or more distress than the client. Thus, they are unable to provide the assistance needed by the client to achieve healthy adaptation and may, in fact, be reinforcing maladaptive behaviors. Because of this, there is a trend toward involving significant others in the therapeutic process so that they do not inhibit a client's growth and so that they receive the help they themselves need to cope with the stressful changes being experienced.

Adequate coping mechanisms. The stress-crisis sequence evolves when an individual's usual coping mechanisms or ways of reducing stress are inadequate to deal with the threatening event(s) being encountered. If the client becomes im-

mobilized, he or she will probably emerge from the crisis functioning at a level lower than the precrisis state. On the other hand, if the client is able to mobilize untapped, inner strengths or resources, positive outcomes may result; the client could resolve problem(s) and learn new ways of coping with stress in the future.

During the crisis sequence, clients generally experience heightened anxiety, which often results in two types of behavior. First, the client will attempt, sometimes frantically, to use previously learned patterns of coping to alleviate discomfort. Clients usually cling to the familiar during a state of anxiety because it provides a sense of stability, even if real stability does not exist. Second, because a high level of anxiety is accompanied by feelings of helplessness and hopelessness, clients are frequently more amenable to outside influence and assistance. This is especially true during the period of disequilibrium. When reorganization and equilibrium begin to occur and new adaptive or maladaptive defense patterns evolve, this is less true. That is why crisis theorists stress the importance of high-quality therapeutic intervention during the time the person in crisis is establishing new coping mechanisms. Caplan (1964, p. 53) has found that intervention at this time can be the critical balancing factor in helping clients to achieve positive outcomes during crisis states.

The major task for an individual who is experiencing a crisis is to recognize that customary coping mechanisms are ineffective and that new patterns for coping must be established. Some clients, particularly those who have adequate situational supports and who have been flexible in the past, are able to accomplish this task with little or no assistance. Other clients, especially those who have few or no situational supports, who rigidly define role patterns, and who lack maturity because of past experiences, will need help from others in developing new ways for handling stress. These persons are frequently unable to identify the nature of the stress they are experiencing or why their patterns of functioning are ineffective.

It should be obvious at this point that the balancing forces in Aquilera and Messick's paradigm (Figure 7-2) are interrelated and must be viewed as a composite of forces rather than isolated elements. If this view is not taken, nursing interventions may be inappropriate to meet the needs of the client. Ms. Himes's case situation is a good example. She called the county health department and requested nursing service for her mother. Without emotion she stated that "someone needs to show me how to care for her. I don't know what to do any longer."

Sally Himes was a 50-year-old single woman. She lived with her 85-year-old mother, who had had a CVA 15 years ago which left her paralyzed and unable to speak. Before her father's death, Ms. Himes had promised him that she would always take care of her mother. When the community health nurse arrived at the Himes's home, Sally immediately took her into the bedroom to see her mother, who appeared very comfortable in her current surroundings. Sally insisted, however, that the nurse check her over. "I am doing something that is not right. The doctor needs to visit more frequently to give mother shots for water in her lungs." The nurse examined Sally's mother carefully and, finding nothing seriously wrong, decided to spend the rest of the visit talking with Sally.

After the nurse provided positive reinforcement for how well Sally was caring for her mother, Sally replied, "The mailman came today." It took several probing questions like, "Was there something special about the mailman's visit?" before Sally identified that she had received an invitation to her niece's wedding. She was distressed because her mother had not also been invited. "They don't care about her anymore." Further interviewing revealed that for the past 2 years Sally had isolated herself from family and friends because she felt her mother's condition was deteriorating and that significant oth-

ers were too busy. "I can't leave her. No one else knows what to do. Besides, my family has lots of other responsibilities. I always thought they cared about mother, but now I wonder. If they really cared, they would have invited her to Sue's wedding. Sometimes I really get discouraged. I wonder if my family and friends care about me."

The invitation Sally had received from her family challenged her thought processes. It brought to a conscious level feelings of noncaring, which was fortunate because Sally had been coping with these feelings by withdrawing. She was no longer able to ask for assistance from her family and friends and increasingly limited most of her social contacts. With the help of the community health nurse, she was able to identify why she had become so upset when the invitation was delivered. She was also able to recognize that she needed to make changes in her situation so that her own needs could be met. One nursing intervention strategy, arranging a conference with the entire family, resulted in a plan in which all family members would share the responsibility for the care of Sally's mother. This would not have happened if the community health nurse had focused only on helping Sally to see that her perceptions about how well she was caring for her mother were distorted. Changes in Sally's situation would also not have occurred if emphasis had been placed on examining only Sally's feelings about who was invited to Sue's wedding. Helping Sally to recognize that she needed situational supports was critical to the successful resolution of her crisis.

When nurses work with clients who are experiencing heightened stress, they find that a triggering event (e.g., the invitation to Sue's wedding) stimulates the development of a crisis. This event produces additional stress to the point where the client is no longer able to adapt. The triggering event must be recognized as a signal of distress, otherwise clients will not be helped to develop new ways of coping. At times it is easy to miss symptoms of distress because the triggering event is a very minor occurrence. For example, a child who comes sobbing into the health clinic at school because of a shove by peers on the playground could need just a little extra attention. On the other hand, if this child perceives the push to mean that he or she is not liked, the child may be having difficulty developing social relationships. The sobbing could be a cry for help. Taking time to collect sufficient data helps a nurse to discriminate between simple and serious difficulties such as those described above. It is usually wise for a community health nurse to obtain information about the client's daily functioning and support systems when she or he believes that an emotional reaction to an event is disproportionate to what one would expect.

It will also be found when working with clients, particularly those who tend to perceive all difficulties as crises, that problems from the past are reactivated during the crisis state. This happens because they had been unsuccessful in dealing with these problems (Caplan, 1964, p. 41). This can compound the effects of the current threatening event but can also provide an opportunity for growth. Clients, during times of crisis, can be helped to resolve old as well as new problems.

Types of Crisis

Although crisis is basically an individual perceptual matter, certain life events have frequently been found to produce or increase the potential for crisis. These events are viewed as developmental, situational, or a combination of the two. They encompass change, either internally or externally produced, which necessitates altering one's thinking, feelings, and coping style.

Developmental or maturational crises occur across the life spectrum. They relate to critical transition points in the course of normal human development which involve many physical, psychological, and social changes. These transition stages, such as entry into school, puberty, starting a career, leaving home, marriage, parenthood, middlescence, retirement, and facing one's own death and that of others due to aging, require many role changes and produce heightened stress. The role changes that occur during these anticipated crises are discussed in Chapters 13 through 18.

Situational crises also occur across the lifespan, but they are usually not anticipated and do not relate to normal maturational processes. They are precipitated by such things as divorce, illness, accidents, changes in social status, cultural relocation, and early death of a significant other. Since situational crises are frequently sudden and unexpected, an individual or family faces this type of crisis situation without benefit of anticipatory problem solving. This puts the individual or family more at risk for developing distress, because they are unprepared to deal with the changes that accompanied these life events.

Sometimes situational and developmental crises occur simultaneously. When this happens, an individual's or a family's adaptive energies are seriously overtaxed. Multiple stressors make it more difficult for these persons to evaluate realistically the changes that are occurring and to adjust their coping style to accommodate them. For example, a 5-year-old child who has recently changed cultural settings must deal with stresses related to school entry as well as those related to living in a new environment. School entry is in itself often very traumatic. This, coupled with the pressures that result from relocation, such as learning a different language, developing all new friendships, and adjusting to an unfamiliar life-style, can be overwhelming.

Because community health nurses are frequently present when crisis-producing events are occurring, they are in a favorable position to initiate supportive interventions that will enhance a client's ability to adapt. In order to do so, they must know about life events which can precipitate crisis, must recognize signs and symptoms which signal distress, and must develop skill in utilizing several types of intervention strategies with clients who are experiencing stress or crisis.

NURSING INTERVENTION STRATEGIES

Community health nurses use a variety of intervention approaches to facilitate adaptation during times of stress and to enhance successful resolution of crisis. Some of these approaches will be briefly summarized under two major categories: educative and problem-solving. Separating strategies into categories is an artificial technique which is used here only to focus discussion about ways to effect client change. In reality, community health nurses find that often they must integrate several intervention approaches in order to intervene effectively with clients.

Establishing rapport and collecting adequate data to identify the task to be accomplished are the essential first steps in any intervention process. These steps are discussed in Chapters 6 and 8 and will not be repeated here. They should, however, be kept in mind when one is selecting a particular intervention modality.

Educative Approach

Health education has traditionally been a function of the community health nurse. Lillian Wald cared for the sick in the home and also provided instruction so that families were better equipped to assist their ill members. Lina Rodgers taught personal hygiene to school-age children and their families and as a result the spread of disease was reduced and wellness was promoted. Funds were made available through Federal Maternal and Child Health Grants in the twenties and thirties so that community health nurses could be hired to provide health teaching in relation to child care, nutrition, and family-life education. Monies were also allocated at this time for preventive health teaching services aimed at combating communicable diseases such as tuberculosis and childhood illnesses.

The health education function of nurses in the community setting has remained viable over the years. It is still a major focus of all community health nurses, regardless of the setting in which they practice, because practitioners in the field have clearly demonstrated the value of this activity.

Health education activities are designed to promote wellness and to prevent illness. They are used to prepare clients to deal with maturational and situational events that produce stress. They are also used to promote personal habits that foster optimal health, including obtaining immunizations to prevent communicable disease, eating balanced meals, and seeking medical care when ill. Psychosocial as well as physical aspects of health and disease are taken into consideration when the community health nurse utilizes this intervention strategy.

The educative strategy has two major components: (1) increasing the learner's understanding of new events and his or her healthy functioning through the acquisition of knowledge and (2) helping the learner to apply the new information. Readiness of the learner must be assessed and established before either of these components can be implemented successfully. Sharing information the client does not wish to assimilate does not increase client understanding. In fact, when this happens clients frequently do not hear what is being shared.

Use of the nursing process (see Chapter 8) combined with an understanding of the principles of teaching and learning aids the community health nurse in assessing learner readiness. These factors also help to individualize educational plans based on client needs and circumstances. Writings by Brill (1978), Pohl (1978), and Redman (1976) are valuable resources if one wants to review or expand knowledge in relation to the principles of teaching and learning.

After community health nurses establish learner readiness, they and their clients develop teaching and learning goals. Together they also select from a variety of alternative intervention options a teaching strategy which best fits the client's needs and circumstances. Frequently a combination of two or more teaching methods is used. For example, a community health nurse might combine discussion, demonstration, and use of pamphlets to teach new parents how to bathe a baby. Or the nurse might use group process, audiovisual aids, self-instructional materials, and a baby bath demonstration to teach this same procedure. Whatever techniques are selected, however, the learner should have the opportunity to obtain new knowledge as well as to apply the knowledge gained. Understanding how to bathe a baby, for instance, does not always increase a new parent's level of comfort when doing so. Being allowed to demonstrate what has been learned when assistance is available is more likely to promote ease with such a procedure.

Developing specific measurable, client-centered goals for the teaching and learning process is essential for several reasons. Specific goals help to determine what content or information is needed by the client. They also aid in developing and implementing teaching techniques that are relevant to the client's needs. In addition, they facilitate evaluation of the learning process because they define what the client desires to learn. A global goal such as "learning about growth and development" does none of these things. It does not define what information parents need in order to handle the developmental needs of their child more effectively. A goal which states that "Jean will verbally identify the developmental tasks of a 1-year-old" is much clearer.

Individualizing teaching and learning plans is crucial because client needs vary even when different people encounter similar situations. Some parents, for instance, understand normal growth-and-development processes very well but have difficulty handling the physical aspects of child care. Others are at ease with feeding, bathing, and clothing their infant but become frustrated when the child does not achieve developmental tasks, even if it is too soon for him or her to accomplish them. Differences like these are not uncommon among clients who are experiencing similar situations.

Opportunities to use the educative strategy in the community health setting are endless. Teaching a child at school how to prevent infection when hurt, discussing sexuality issues with a mother who has preadolescent children, and sharing information about the hereditary aspects of diabetes when a family history reflects a need are a few examples of when a community health nurse uses the educative strategy. Education is not always needed, however, and can be misused. This happens particularly when the nurse makes an assumption about what the client needs to learn without first collecting data, or when the nurse imposes information on the client because of value conflicts. Some parents who have several children, for example, desire to have more. Continuing to teach about family planning after it has been validated that the parents know how to prevent pregnancy and understand the pros and cons of increasing their family size is meeting the nurse's needs, not the family's needs.

Problem-Solving Approach

In the community health setting, nurses encounter clients who are having difficulty making decisions about a variety of personal life events. Specifically, community health nurses help clients to make decisions about such things as career choices, maintaining or establishing intimate relationships with others, when and where to obtain preventive and curative health care services, how to deal with family conflicts, how to handle financial crises, or how to provide needed care for aging family members. At times, when clients are dealing with situations such as these, they have difficulty identifying why they cannot make a decision about what to do. They know that something is wrong because symptoms of anxiety are present, but they are unable to take action to reduce their stress.

There are various reasons why clients are unable to alter their behavior in a way that will help them to resolve their stress appropriately. Some reasons, and case situations to illustrate when they might occur, are shared below:

Client Has Not Specifically Identified the Nature of the Problem

Barb Lehi, a 28-year-old wife and the mother of two children, returned to work when her youngest child entered school. Her family adjusted well to her role change because joint decision making occurred prior to Barb's employment. Barb was enjoying what she was doing but began to have tension headaches 2 months after she started her new job. She felt her headaches were related to the adjustments she had to make in her daily routine, and assumed that they would go away shortly. They did not, however, until she was able to identify that she was having guilt feelings about being a working mother.

Client Has a Vested Interest in Not Identifying the Problem

Mrs. Jackson, a 68-year-old widow living by herself, kept finding reasons why she should not see a physician after she started having "fainting spells." Her family became frustrated and worried and asked the community health nurse to visit. Referral for medical evaluation was successfully implemented only when Mrs. Jackson was able to verbalize that being ill was the only way she could get attention from her family. Her family visited very sporadically when she was well but daily when she was ill.

Client Is Unable to Acknowledge Feelings

Gail Hayes, a 31-year-old mother and wife, provided no stimulation for her 2-year-old daughter who was retarded due to rubella exposure in utero. The community health nurse became involved after hearing from a neighbor that Gail left her daughter alone in the house when she visited friends and neighbors. After several home visits, the nurse discovered that Gail did so because "I can't stand to be with her. She is such a fussy child and wants attention all of the time. I hate seeing her so deformed and feel guilty because if I hadn't gotten measles while pregnant, she would be all right." Gail had never before acknowledged these feelings. When she did, she was able to use the help offered by others and to relate more effectively to her daughter.

Client Does Not Assume Accountability for Feelings

Bob Woodrow, a 40-year-old construction worker, was referred to the health department for rehabilitative services after a myocardial infarction. Due to the strenuous nature of construction work, it was recommended that he seek other employment. He verbalized an interest in obtaining job training through the Division of Vocational Rehabilitation but took no action. When the community health nurse questioned why, he responded by placing the blame on others. "My wife thinks it is too soon and nags me about not going back to work. I am not sure if my physician thinks I should, because he is always so vague about what is happening with my heart. My car needs fixing before I can use it regularly, and we don't have the money to get it fixed." It took several months for Bob to see that he was not taking action because of his own fears about having another heart attack and about not being able to succeed in a new line of work.

Client Cannot Distinguish between Feelings and Facts

Carol Strang, a 17-year-old junior, repeatedly visited the school nurse for minor physical concerns. Assessments made by the nurse revealed that this occurred when Carol felt that she was not performing well academically. In reality, Carol was very successful in her schoolwork, ranking in the top 5 percent of her class. In addition, she had several close friends who provided praise for her academic achievements. Carol, however, only perceived that she was achieving satisfactorily when she received straight As. When she received anything less than an A, she expressed feelings associated with failure.

Client Lacks Experience with Problem Solving

Mrs. Raabe, a 71-year-old widow, became confused and severely upset after her husband's death. All her life she had been cared for by others. Her parents and her brothers anticipated her needs because she was the "baby" of the family and "helpless." Because her husband assumed the same role as her family, Mrs. Raabe felt lost when he died. She found managing her finances particularly stressful since she had never taken care of the family budget. She needed help with such basic things as writing a check, how to deposit money in the bank, and how to balance her income and her expenses.

Client Has Undetected Physical or Perceptual Problems

Mrs. La Rosa, a 37-year-old divorced mother of six children, was referred to the health department by her caseworker from the Department of Social Service. Her caseworker believed that Mrs. La Rosa was neglecting her children and felt that environmental conditions were dangerous to the family's health. Mrs. La Rosa told the community health nurse that "I know I should keep my home more tidy, but I am just too tired to keep up with things that need to be done around the house. Sometimes all I want to do is sleep." The community health nurse assisted her in obtaining a medical evaluation. It was found during this evaluation that Mrs. La Rosa had hypertension and diabetes. When both of these conditions were under control, home management and child care skills improved.

Client Missed Essential Steps in Skill Development

Mrs. Lueck was extremely upset when her 10-year-old retarded son was sent home from camp because he could not handle activities of daily living such as bathing and toileting. "Tommie always does these things at home. They just don't know how to work with retarded kids." Upon talking with Mrs. Lueck, the community health nurse discovered Tommie did wash himself when bathing at home, but that family members helped him with most of the activities necessary for completing a bath. For example, the family ran his bath water for him; assembled the materials he needed to take a bath, including soap, washcloth, and towel; and selected the clothing he would wear afterward. It was obvious to the nurse, but not the mother, that Tommie never really learned how to handle his personal hygiene needs. He had skill in washing body parts, but lacked decision-making skill about how and when to carry out these activities.

Client Is Unable to Generate Alternative Options during Problem Solving or Fears the Consequences of a Newly Generated Alternative

Amy Schmidt, wife and mother of two preschoolers, was physically abused by her husband regularly and expressed a desire to leave him. She found it difficult to take this action because she thought that it was impossible for her to do so. She felt trapped because she had no job skills and her family and friends were unable to assist her financially. In addition, she felt that the abuse would not stop, even if she left home, because her husband could always find her. The community health nurse assisted Mrs. Schmidt in identifying ways to obtain financial aid as well as legal assistance to control her husband's behavior. Mrs. Schmidt was also helped to see that living alone could be less frightening for her and her children than being physically abused.

The situations presented above are far more complex than indicated by the discussion. They are briefly summarized to illustrate that there are many reasons why established problem-solving patterns are ineffective during times of stress and crisis. Identifying the specific reason(s) for each client's stress is the essential first step when the community health nurse utilizes the problem-solving approach to enhance client growth.

A community health nurse has two major goals when using the problem-solving approach: (1) to assist the client in solving immediate problem(s) and (2) to help the client increase independent problem-solving abilities. Implicit in these goals is the belief that clients *can learn* skills which will help them to make decisions wisely and to alter behavior accordingly. A community health nurse who has difficulty *internalizing* this belief will find it hard to move a client toward independence. This nurse is more likely *to do for* the client than *to work with* the client.

A variety of techniques can be used to help a client enhance his or her problem-solving abilities, including such things as individual counseling, group work, role modeling, and behavioral programming. When using any one of these techniques, the community health nurse should focus on helping the client to identify the nature of the problem(s), to discover alternative options for problem solving, to make decisions about which option is most appropriate, and to take action to resolve the problem(s). The community health nurse should not assume that the client will take action after making a decision about the most appropriate option and prematurely close the family to service. Taking action is often the most difficult step in the problem-solving process because it is at this point that the client is giving up the "secure" familiar for the "threatening" unknown.

Clients must be allowed to make decisions and to take action for themselves before they are able to achieve independent problem-solving abilities. It is natural to want to "rescue" clients when they are experiencing pain. *Rescue behavior, such as giving advice and doing for the client, reduces anxiety only temporarily, because* *the client is not prepared to handle stress in the future.* It can be helpful for the community health nurse to share alternative ways for handling stresses, but the client should be encouraged to evaluate suggestions in terms of his or her own circumstances. The client should be given the message that no one way is being advocated but that these options have worked with others in the past.

When clients are experiencing crisis, they often desperately want others to make decisions for them. Cadden (1964, pp. 293–296) has delineated several principles of crisis intervention that help a community health nurse avoid rescue activities and provide constructive aid to the family. These are:

1. *Help the client confront the crisis* by supporting expression of feelings and emotions such as fear, guilt, and crying.

2. *Help the client confront the crisis in manageable doses* without dampening the impact of the crisis to a point where the client no longer recognizes the need to alter coping mechanisms. Drugs and diversional activities are helpful when they are used to decrease unmanageable stress. They are harmful when they prevent the client from looking at the realities of his or her situation.

3. *Help the client to find the facts,* because truth is less frightening than the unknown. Clients may need frequent visits during periods of crisis because they may not have the energy to analyze all the stresses they are experiencing during one home visit.

4. *Do not give the client false reassurance* because this leads to mistrust and maladaptive coping behaviors. To succeed in resolving a crisis, a client needs reassurance which supports his or her ability to handle the crisis situation.

5. *Do not encourage the client to blame others,* because blaming only reduces tension mo-

mentarily and can help the client to suppress feelings. This can result in maladaptive behaviors that decrease the client's level of functioning after crisis resolution.

6. *Help the client to accept help* because some clients avoid confronting a crisis by denying that they need help and that a problem exists. If the client does not face the crisis, he or she will not mobilize coping mechanisms that will enhance growth.

7. *Help the client with everyday tasks* in a manner that reflects kindness and thoughtfulness rather than one that gives a message that the client is weak or incompetent. Clients need help with everyday tasks because it takes considerable energy to resolve a crisis; thus, clients often lack sufficient energy to handle daily activities as well.

Problem solving takes time. Both the client and the community health nurse must guard against expecting change too rapidly. When progress is slow, a client may question if the nurse can really help, and the nurse often begins to wonder whether or not the client really wants to change. At times, both of these feelings are justified. More frequently, however, the need is for the client and nurse to recognize that well-established patterns of behavior cannot be changed immediately.

Community health nurses cannot help all clients to learn to make decisions wisely. Some situations are beyond their competence and must be referred to others who are better qualified. Because competence varies from one community health nurse to another as a result of differences in academic preparation and work experiences, nurses must learn how to discriminate between situations that they can and cannot handle. Peer and supervisory conferences will assist a new nurse to objectively evaluate her or his skills.

Underestimating one's ability to help a client, rather than overestimating competency, is often more of a problem when nurses begin practice in the community health setting. Most clients experiencing stress and crisis do not need psychotherapy. Instead, they need someone who cares and who will provide supportive guidance and positive reinforcement for the strength they have.

SUMMARY

The community health nurse is often the primary source of assistance when a family is experiencing stress. Stress is a normal, human phenomenon necessary for survival and growth. It triggers the general adaptation syndrome which helps people to adapt to the demands and pressures of life. Although stress is essential for survival and growth, every individual has limits beyond which stress is no longer tolerated. Prolonged and intensified stress results in crisis, especially when an individual's coping mechanisms are inadequate to reduce disequilibrium.

A person in crisis experiences disorganization and heightened stress. Crisis is self-limiting but biopsychosocial homeostasis following a crisis may be at a level equal to, better than, or lower than the precrisis level. Timely supportive intervention may be the critical factor that determines if an individual or family has a positive or negative outcome during periods of crisis.

REFERENCES

Aquilera, D. C., & Messick, I. M. *Crisis intervention: Theory and methodology.* Saint Louis: Mosby, 1978.

Brill, N. I. *Working with people: The helping process.* Philadelphia: Lippincott, 1978.

Burr, W. R. *Theory construction and the sociology of the family.* New York: Wiley, 1973.

Cadden, V. Crisis in the family. In G. Caplan (Ed.), *Principles of preventive psychiatry.* New York: Basic Books, 1964, pp. 228–296.

Caplan, G. *An approach to community mental health.* New York: Grune & Stratton, 1961.

———. *Principles of preventive psychiatry.* New York: Basic Books, 1964.

Hansen, D. A., & Hill, R. Families under stress. In H. T. Christensen (Ed.), *Handbook of marriage and the family.* Chicago: Rand McNally, 1964, pp. 782–819.

Hill, R. *Families under stress.* New York: Harper & Row, 1949.

Lindemann, E. Symptomatology and management of acute grief. *American Journal of Psychiatry,* September 1944, *101,* 141–148.

McHugh, P. *Defining the situation: The organization of meaning in social interactions.* Indianapolis: Bobbs-Merrill, 1968.

Pohl, M. L. *The teaching function of the nursing practitioner.* Dubuque, Iowa: Wm. C. Brown Company Publishers, 1978.

Rahe, R. H. The pathway between subjects' recent life changes and their near-future illness reports: Representative results and methodological issues. In B. S. Dohrenwend & B. P. Dohrenwend (Eds.), *Stressful life events.* New York: Wiley, 1974.

Redman, B. K. *The process of patient teaching in nursing.* Saint Louis: Mosby, 1976.

Schreiber, F. R. *Sybil.* New York: Warner Books, 1973.

Selye, H. *The stress of life.* New York: McGraw-Hill, 1975.

SELECTED BIBLIOGRAPHY

Ader, R. The role of developmental factors in susceptibility to disease. *International Journal of Psychiatry in Medicine,* 1974, *5,* 367–376.

Bould, S. Female-headed families: Personal fate control and the provider role. *Journal of Marriage and the Family,* May 1977, *39,* 339–348.

Burkhalter, P. *Nursing care of the alcoholic and drug abuser.* New York: McGraw-Hill, 1975.

Burr, W., Hill, R., Nye, F. I., & Reiss, I. L. (Eds.). *Contemporary theories about the family. Volume I: Research-based theories.* New York: The Free Press, 1979.

Butehorn, L. A plan for identifying priorities in treating multiproblem families. *Child Welfare,* June 1978, *57,* 365–372.

Cannon, W. B. *The wisdom of the body.* New York: Norton, 1932.

Clark, C. C. *Mental health aspects of community health nursing.* New York: McGraw-Hill, 1978.

Fassler, T. *Helping children cope.* New York: The Free Press, 1979.

Fink, S. L. Crisis and motivation: A theoretical model. *Archives of Physical Medicine and Rehabilitation,* 1967, *48,* 592–597.

Glasser, P., & Glasser, L. *Families in crisis.* New York: Harper & Row, 1970.

Gordon, A. K., & Klass, D. *They need to know: How to teach children about death.* Englewood Cliffs, N.Y.: Prentice-Hall, 1979.

Guest, J. *Ordinary people.* New York: Ballantine Books, 1976.

Hall, J., & Weaver, B. *Nursing of families in crisis.* Philadelphia: Lippincott, 1974.

Hill, R. *Families under stress.* New York: Harper & Row, 1949.

Janken, J. The nurse in crisis. *Nursing Clinics of North America,* March 1974, *9,* 17–26.

Lawson, B. Chronic illness in the school aged child:

Effects on the total family. *Maternal-Child Nursing,* January–February 1977, 49–56.

Lazarus, R. S. *Psychological stress and the coping process.* New York: McGraw-Hill, 1956.

Loomis, M. E., & Horsley, J. A. *Interpersonal change: A behavioral approach to nursing practice.* New York: McGraw-Hill, 1974.

Martin, E. P., & Martin, J. M. *The black extended family.* Chicago: The University of Chicago Press, 1978.

McCubbin, H. I. Integrating coping behavior in family stress theory. *Journal of Marriage and the Family,* May 1979, *41,* 237–244.

McGrory, A. *A well model approach to care of the dying client.* New York: McGraw-Hill, 1978.

Minuchin, S., & Montalvo, B. Techniques for working with disorganized low socioeconomic families. In J. Haley, *Changing families.* New York: Grune & Stratton, 1971, pp. 202–211.

Olshansky, S. Chronic sorrow: A response to having a mentally defective child. *Social Casework,* April 1962, *43,* 421–424.

Parad, H. J. (Ed.). *Crisis intervention: Selected readings.* New York: Family Service Association of America, 1965.

Roy, M. (Ed.). *Battered women: A psychosociological study of domestic violence.* New York: Van Nostrand Reinhold, 1977.

Rueveni, U. *Networking families in crisis.* New York: Human Sciences Press, 1979.

Savino, A., & Sanders, R. W. Working with abusive parents: Group therapy and home visits. *American Journal of Nursing,* March 1973, *73,* 482–484.

Selye, H. *Stress without distress.* New York: Lippincott, 1974.

Sprey, J. The family as a system in conflict. *Journal of Marriage and the Family,* November 1969, *31,* 699–706.

Walker, K. N., & Messinger, L. Remarriage after divorce: Dissolution and reconstruction of family boundaries. *Family Process,* June 1979, *18,* 185–192.

Watzlawick, P., Weakland, C. E., & Fish, R. *Change principles of problem formation and problem resolution.* New York: Norton, 1974.

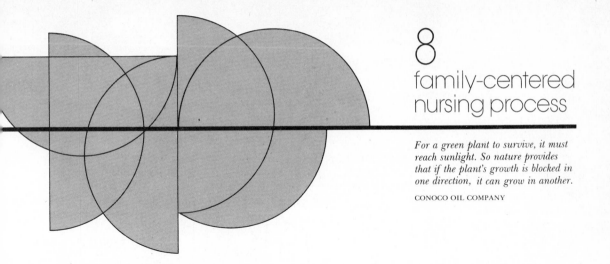

For a green plant to survive, it must reach sunlight. So nature provides that if the plant's growth is blocked in one direction, it can grow in another.

CONOCO OIL COMPANY

People, like green plants, can grow in multiple directions. Stumbling blocks along the way do not necessarily stop growth. Caring, support, and assistance from significant others can help humanity to change the course of its development when barriers are inhibiting the growth process.

Although human growth follows a predictable pattern, all individuals are still unique. As they develop, they make choices about pathways to take to reach sunlight and to achieve happiness. Although physiological, psychosocial, cultural, and spiritual forces influence individual decision making about what brings a rich and satisfying life, every human being also needs the opportunity to define which pathways lead to personal growth and self-fulfillment. Individuals who encourage others to make independent decisions about life choices are more likely to facilitate growth than individuals who impose on others their beliefs about appropriate life pathways.

Community health nurses can facilitate the human growth process. They work to develop trusting, supportive relationships so that clients can reach out and use their help when needed. Some clients will not seek assistance from community health nurses because they have found other support systems more relevant to them.

However, when a client does accept the help offered by a community health nurse, it is extremely important for the nurse to recognize that her or his role is to help the client determine which pathways to brightness are appropriate for that individual. The nurse cannot know what is best for other human beings. Taking away an individual's independence leads to darkness, not light.

Increasingly, nurses and other health care professionals have accepted the client's right of self-determination in relation to decision making and change. They have identified that doing *for* the client instead of working *with* him or her can result in client dependence and other modes of limited behavioral action. Clients must internalize the need for change before they will alter their behavior. Take, for example, a 40-year-old man with a cardiac problem who has been advised to modify his diet. In the hospital he was served low-sodium food. If this client does not understand his diet, or why it is necessary, he is likely to resume his previous eating patterns once he returns home. In his own environment, the client makes decisions about what he will eat. Nurses can influence client change but only the client can alter his behavior.

At times, the concept of individual self-de-

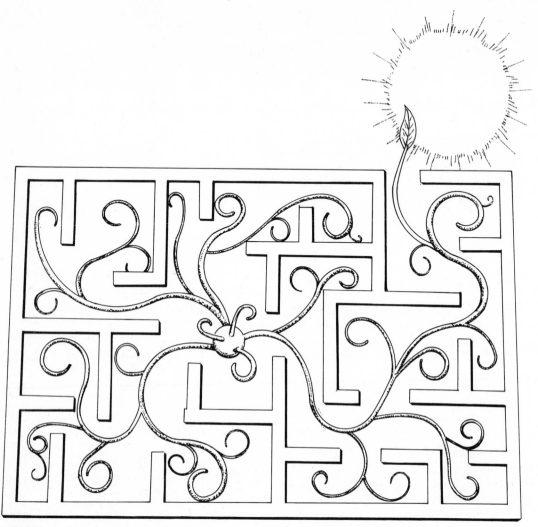

FIGURE 8-1 Nature doesn't explore just one path to reach a goal. Neither should man. (*Conoco Oil Company.*)

termination is difficult to operationalize, because a professional's personal feelings can influence the interactions between the community health nurse and the client. It is easy for a nurse to feel like a failure when a client does not alter health actions, especially when this behavior is adversely affecting the client's health status. Viewing oneself as a client often helps. Stop and think for a while how you make changes in your life-style. For most people, being ordered to change produces feelings of resentment and increases resistance. People want to believe that they are capable of making decisions about their lives, and they want the freedom to make choices even if the choices have negative consequences. Depending on the situation, clients may want or need varying degrees of guidance and support, but at all times they should be given a message that they are capable of independent decision making.

To function effectively in the community setting, a nurse must accept the fact that clients are responsible for their health behavior, even when they choose a plan of action that the nurse would not choose. Nurse-defined goals for clients are seldom achieved. Goals defined by the client are more frequently accomplished. The nurse who takes over for clients quickly becomes frustrated with the lack of client response and may "burn out."

The nursing process helps the community health nurse to facilitate client goal setting. This therapeutic process is used by nurses in all settings. However, it is labeled the *family-centered nursing process* in the community health setting because community health nurses use it to analyze family functioning and to extend services to all family members. This focus is based on the belief that the family is the basic unit for nursing service: family functioning affects the health of all family members by inhibiting or facilitating the growth process and by influencing when family members will accept help from community systems.

FAMILY-CENTERED NURSING PROCESS DEFINED

The family-centered nursing process is a systematic approach to scientific problem solving, involving a series of circular dynamic actions—assessing, analyzing, planning, implementing, evaluating, and terminating—for the purpose of facilitating optimum client functioning. There are four key elements in this definition:

· *A systematic approach:* This process enables the community health nurse to function in an orderly, logical manner. The nurse *plans* her or his actions to achieve specific goals and recognizes that time and efforts are often wasted if a "hit-or-miss" approach is used.

· *Scientific problem solving:* Decisions made about client needs and appropriate nursing interventions are based on scientific principles. The problem-solving approach is used in everyday life. The nursing process differs from simple problem solving: scientific knowledge gained from advanced study assists the nurse in refining the data analysis process in relation to health, illness, and pre-vention, and in expanding intervention options which aid clients in maximizing their self-care capabilities. The nursing process helps nurses to function in a deliberative rather than an intuitive way (McCain, 1965, p. 82).

· *A series of circular, dynamic actions:* No one action alone helps the community health nurse to enhance client growth. All phases of the nursing process must be carried out in order for sound decision making and effective nursing intervention to occur. Dynamic implies that care plans are revised when assessment and evaluation data reflect needed change. The nursing process is circular in nature because each phase provides data which either validate or alter original nursing diagnoses, goals, and plans.

· *Purpose of facilitating optimum client functioning:* Nursing interventions should help the client to resolve his or her health care needs and to achieve specific, client-defined goals and objectives. A helping interactive process whereby the *client* and the nurse share data for the purpose of identifying ways to make things less difficult for the client facilitates this process. To effectively facilitate client functioning, the nurse must individualize nursing actions, since clients define optimum functioning differently.

A community health nurse using the nursing process is much like a master chef using a recipe to bake a cake. The master chef does not just throw things together, as can be seen in Figure 8-2. The chef, unlike his juggler friend, knows that the right ingredients in correct proportion must be thoroughly mixed and baked at the proper time and temperature. Through knowledge and experience, he has learned how to adjust his ingredients to add a special flavor to his cake.

An effective nurse, like a master chef, learns that by using a systematic process, more satisfying results can be obtained. The nurse knows that it is necessary to have guidelines to follow (scientific knowledge), the right ingre-dients in correct proportion (adequate data), thorough mixing (analysis of data), a specific cake form (specific client goals and nursing interventions), and testing of the finished product (evaluation). Illustrative of this are the factors the nurse takes into consideration when working with a child who has juvenile diabetes. Based on scientific information, it is known that this child needs such things as:

· Adequate nutrition

· Proper hygiene

· Insulin injections

· Regular urine testing

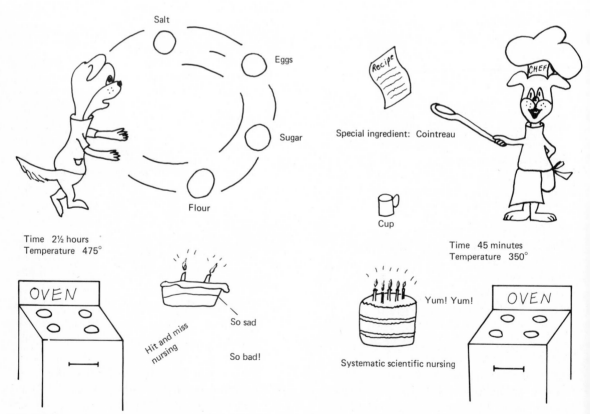

FIGURE 8-2 The juggler and master chef at work. (*Courtesy of Leslie Davis.*)

· Adequate exercise

· Socializing experiences like interactions with peers

Teaching about these needs could lead to a jumbled mess, just like the juggler's cake, unless the nurse considers the:

· Family's financial situation

· Family's daily living patterns and how these patterns may need to be altered to provide adequate nutrition, proper hygiene, and appropriate medication for the child

· Family's perceptions of the child's health and knowledge about his or her health condition

· Child's emotional reaction to the diabetic condition and knowledge about his or her health status

In order to achieve desired goals relative to the child's needs, the nurse must take all the knowledge available about diabetes and mix it well within the framework of the child's family situation. All good cooks know how to adjust their actions to fit individual situations, and so must a community health nurse. The family's perceptions of their child's health, along with the child's emotional reaction to his or her condition, are two critical factors that nurses consider when individualizing management plans. Intervention strategies are often ineffective until these variables are analyzed. One community health nurse, for instance, visited intensively the family of a 6-year-old child who had brittle diabetes. The child did not follow her prescribed diabetic regimen and one consequence was frequent hospitalizations for treatment of diabetic coma. When the nurse finally questioned the parents about their perceptions of their child's health condition, she discovered that they were not ready to accept the diagnosis as permanent. Denying the diagnosis was their way of coping with it. The nurse had to help the parents handle their feelings of guilt and anger before she could discuss treatment plans with them.

The family-centered nursing process facilitates the analysis of psychosocial influences as well as physiological ones. Looking more closely at the nursing process, the reader can find that it consists of the following six phases:

· Assessing

· Analyzing

· Planning

· Implementing

· Evaluating

· Terminating

Although each phase will be discussed separately, it should be remembered that they interrelate and overlap. The interrelated nature of these phases, along with nursing activities during each phase, is presented in Table 8-1. When examining this diagram, it is important to note the relationships between the data-collection phase and the triangle of family health. Collected data should always be validated with the family before nursing diagnoses, goals, and intervention strategies are formulated. The family-centered nursing process is a client-oriented process, not a nurse-oriented process.

PHASES OF THE FAMILY-CENTERED NURSING PROCESS

It may be found that phases and terms within the nursing process are labeled differently from what the reader has seen before. There are hundreds of books and articles written on the nursing process, and terminology varies from one author to another. The dispute over terminology serves to confuse practitioners and makes it difficult to recognize that it is the *process*, not the terminology, that is significant. Focusing on the process aspects of the phases as they are discussed will allow the reader to effectively implement the family-centered nursing process regardless of the terminology used in different practice settings.

Assessing

The assessment phase involves a systematic data collection process which provides the foundation for making nursing diagnoses. During this phase, the community health nurse places emphasis on collecting specific data about client (family) functioning so that objective conclusions regarding the client's health status can be made. Inferences about a client's level of functioning should only be made after a sufficient data base has been obtained.

The primary responsibilities of the community health nurse during the assessment phase are threefold: (1) developing a trusting, therapeutic relationship; (2) using a variety of data collection methods to obtain client information from all available resources; and (3) assessing all parameters of family health, including family dynamics and the health status of individual family members. Careful attention given to all three of these activities helps the community health nurse to clearly delineate client needs and goals and intervention strategies which may enhance client growth.

Relationship Building

The type of relationship established during the assessment phase can be the critical factor in helping the client determine whether or not to accept the assistance offered by the community health nurse. It is natural for clients to evaluate their interactions with community health nurses during the assessment phase. Most people take time to assess how others respond to them before they develop a trusting relationship which allows disclosure of personal thoughts, feelings, and problems.

Explaining the purpose of community health nursing visits, describing services the community health nurse can provide, and fostering a nonthreatening atmosphere which allows the client to share data at his or her own pace often promote trust between the nurse and the client. Mayers (1973, p. 330) found when conducting a study in which she observed 16 staff community health nurses making 30 home visits, that in roughly one-half of the situations, the client did not know the purpose of the visit. Mayers's findings are not atypical. The authors have found similar results when they have requested students or staff to ask their clients why they thought the nurse was visiting. Frequently, clients have stated, "I don't know." This can happen for several reasons, including the nurse not adequately explaining his or her role, the client not hearing what was shared, or the nurse developing goals unrelated to the initial purpose after assessment data were collected.

Clarifying why the community health nurse is visiting is essential. When clients do not understand the purpose of nursing visits, it is hard for them to become involved in the therapeutic process. Lack of clarity in the therapeutic relationship can result in frustration and mistrust and inhibit the expression of thoughts, feelings, and data. Clients usually do not share information freely until they understand why the information is needed.

Clients are more likely to develop a trusting relationship with professionals who are open and honest and who show a genuine concern for their welfare than with professionals who do not demonstrate these characteristics. An interview style which reflects sensitivity, a nonjudgmental, accepting attitude, and a respect for the client's right of self-determination facilitates the development of a trusting relationship. A skillful interviewer avoids barriers to communication such as false reassurance, ad-

TABLE 8-1　Relationships between the Phases of the Family-Centered Nursing Process

Assessing	Analyzing	Planning	Implementing	Evaluating	Terminating
Process for obtaining a data base	A cognitive data ordering process for the purpose of identifying nursing diagnoses	Formulation of desired family outcomes (goals) and identification of actions (intervention strategies) to achieve goals	A systemic approach to action used by the family and nurse to achieve desired family outcomes	A continuous, concurrent process used to critique each component of the nursing process	A therapeutic process which helps the client and the nurse to end their relationship

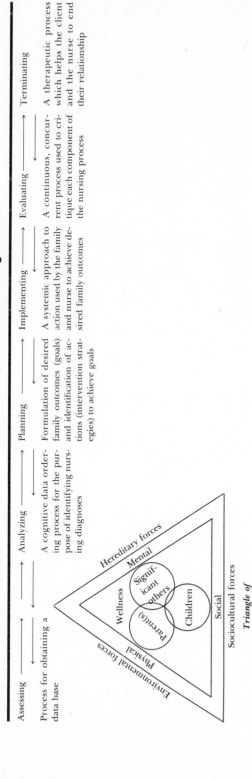

Triangle of
family health

Assessing	Analyzing	Planning	Implementing	Evaluating	Terminating

1. Develop a trusting relationship
  a. Explain purpose of community health nursing visit
  b. Describe what community health nurse has to offer
  c. Facilitate the sharing of thoughts, feelings, and data
  d. Set time parameters for evaluation and frequency and length of visits
	1. Make differential conclusions about family needs by:
	  a. Using theoretical knowledge to identify significant signs and symptoms
	  b. Grouping data to show relationships between assessment categories and to identify patterns of behavior
	  c. Relating family data to relevant clinical and research findings
		1. Consider three key principles:
		  a. Individualization of client care plans
		  b. Active client participation
		  c. Client's right of self-determination
		2. Formulate client-centered goals and objectives
		  a. Establish realistic goals consistent with the data base and nursing diagnoses
			1. Base nursing actions on data obtained during the assessment phase; family needs, knowledge, receptivity, and level of understanding
			  a. Demonstrate awareness of proper timing when carrying out intervention activities
			  b. Adapt or modify intervention strategies when client situation changes
			  c. Modify activities to accommodate factors in the home
				1. Elicit ongoing feedback from client to determine if goals, plans, and interventions are appropriate
				2. Identify the results of intervention activities taken by:
				  a. Client
				  b. Community health nurse
				  c. Other health care professionals
				3. Determine why intervention activities have been ineffective, if warranted
					1. Deal with feelings associated with termination
					2. Review client achievements
					3. Discuss what the therapeutic process has meant
					4. Plan carefully the termination of visits
					5. Share with client how to reestablish contact if needed

TABLE 8-1 · Relationships between the Phases of the Family-Centered Nursing Process (Continued)

Assessing	Analyzing	Planning	Implementing	Evaluating	Terminating

2. Collect data in a variety of ways
  a. Observation
  b. Interview
  c. Inspection
  d. Contact with secondary sources
  e. Review of records
3. Assess all parameters of family functioning
  a. Family dynamics
  b. Physiological data
  c. Psychosocial data
  d. Sociocultural data
  e. Environmental data
  f. Preventive health practices
4. Obtain data from multiple sources
  a. Client, family
  b. Health team members
  c. Community agencies
  d. Significant others
  e. Relevant records
5. Use standards of care to focus the interviewing process (see Chapter 21)
	d. Comparing nursing diagnoses with diagnoses of other health professionals
	2. Formulate specific nursing diagnoses
	  a. Base diagnoses on a strong data base
	  b. Identify the functional aspects of a client's current health status
	  c. Determine various levels of family functioning
	    (1) Strengths
	    (2) Needs
	    (3) Anticipatory guidance warranted
	  d. Identify when data are insufficient to make a nursing diagnosis
		b. State goals and objectives in specific, achievable, and measurable terms
		c. Develop goals and objectives in collaboration with the family (contracting)
		d. Identify family as well as individual goals and objectives
		e. Formulate cognitive, affective, and psychomotor objectives when appropriate
		f. Distinguish between nurse-focused goals and client-focused goals
		3. Identify alternative intervention strategies
		  a. Identify various intervention activities based on assessment data, nursing diagnoses, and client goals and objectives
			2. Recognize social, cultural, economic, and environmental barriers, and work within these limitations (see Chapter 9)
			3. Carry through with planned interventions
			  a. Administration of nursing care activities
			  b. Engaging the family in the referral process
			  c. Implementing teaching, learning plans
			  d. Helping family to problem-solve
			  e. Keeping appointments with the family
			4. Base intervention activities on scientific principles and knowledge
			  a. Review literature to obtain knowledge in relation to content being taught or situation being encountered
				4. Modify the management plan when appropriate
				5. Use a variety of methods to evaluate
				  a. Obtain feedback from client
				  b. Consult with peers, supervisors, and other health care professionals
				  c. Summarize records
				  d. Conduct nursing audits (see Chapter 21)	

b. Consult with peers, supervisor, and other health care professionals to expand knowledge and to evaluate appropriateness of nursing interventions

b. Determine activities which the client, the nurse, and other health professionals might carry out to help the client to achieve desired goals and objectives

c. Identify pros and cons of each intervention strategy

d. Assist the client in identifying alternative courses of action and in making decisions about actions to be implemented

4. Establish priorities in relation to client goals and intervention strategies

a. Differentiate between problems that need immediate action and those that can wait

b. Consider the health and safety of the client

c. Use theory and the family data base to identify potential crisis situations

5. Identify criteria for evaluating goal attainment

vice giving, excessive talking, and the showing of approval or disapproval. At times, this is not easy. For example, when families are under stress they may press for advice. Frequently a family member will say, "What would you do if you were me?" An empathic interviewer responds to the family's feelings of distress but supports its ability to make its own decisions. Advice giving can lead to an unhealthy dependency.

The community health nurse needs to be careful not to foster unnecessary dependency. However, dependency is not always negative. In fact, an inability to accept help when one needs it can be as dysfunctional as not doing anything for oneself. A mature adult *recognizes* and acts on the need for support, caring, and concern from others while maintaining decision making independent from them. Too often a client's need for support, encouragement, and assistance with problem solving is viewed negatively and labeled "overdependent" and "immature." Sable (1979) differentiates between attachment and dependency because he believes a counselor's fear of dependency can be detrimental to the client-worker relationship. He believes workers may feel inappropriately restrained from providing a secure base for some clients who are attempting to achieve a healthy attachment to others if they are inaccurately labeled "overdependent." Attachment is a natural instinctive process in which an individual strives to develop affectional bonds with significant others. Often clients are distressed because they lack this meaningful relationship, not because they have unresolved dependency needs. They seek, through the professional worker, to obtain the comfort they naturally need from enduring interactions with significant others. *Helping these clients to recognize they need significant relationships is far more beneficial than discouraging dependency* (Sable, 1979, pp. 140–141).

Warmth, caring, and a genuine interest in helping demonstrate to clients that they can develop significant relationships with others. These professional attributes assist clients in mobilizing inner strengths necessary to effect change. These behaviors also encourage clients to share data pertinent to the understanding of *their perceptions* of their needs.

Numerous books discuss interviewing techniques that promote a therapeutic relationship. Readers are encouraged to examine various theoretical viewpoints of counseling in order to determine which style fits their needs. Whatever interviewing or counseling style is used, however, it must be individualized for each unique client. For example, some individuals do not verbalize spontaneously: they share what they feel is important to share and then are silent until further information is requested. A nurse who firmly believes in a nondirective approach would have difficulty relating to such clients, if he or she did not adjust the interviewing style.

Working with families presents special interviewing challenges for the community health nurse because families are composed of several "unique" individuals who have varying needs, concerns, and communication styles. Since the goal of community health nursing service is to help the family as a unit, rather than to help each individual family member separately, the nurse must become a "third ear of the family, listening for the effect of a person's statements on other people" (Haley, 1971, p. 281). The nurse needs to facilitate effective interaction between all family members in order to promote the family's nurturing and decision-making processes. At times this can be difficult, especially when there are conflicting interests that need to be negotiated between individual family members.

When a nurse is allowed to cross the family boundaries and is accepted by the family system, what influences the nurse has on that system must be examined carefully. The nurse needs to watch closely her or his interactions with the family, as well as interactions between individual family members. Haley suggests that counselors (nurses) should view themselves as part of the "diagnostic unit because the way the family is behaving is influenced by the ways the counselor [nurse] deals with them" (Haley, 1971, p. 282). Nurse bias in family counseling can disrupt the family system. Sills (1975, p. 16) believes "bias occurs when there is unwitting or unintentional and unwanted social influence introduced into the family therapy session by the therapist." From clinical practice she has developed three categories of bias which negatively influence family functioning. These are "coalition biases, dynamic biases, and social biases" (Sills, 1975, p. 17).

Coalition biases occur when a nurse unknowingly forms an alliance with one family member and closes out other family members. Age and sex of the nurse and identification with the labeled client can influence the development of such coalitions within the family system (Sills, 1975, p. 18). A nurse, for instance, who firmly believes that all women need a career outside the home may strongly support a female client's desires to work without allowing her husband to verbalize his concerns. This may disrupt joint decision making for the couple.

It is particularly easy for community health nurses to form coalition biases because they are not always able to see the entire family unit together. When interviewing only one family member, it can be difficult not to take sides. Taking sides is not therapeutic, however, because it may reinforce dysfunctional family patterns. If, for example, the family is having difficulty negotiating conflicting issues, it does not help the family to deal with these issues when the nurse supports one member's viewpoint. This type of behavior by the nurse only serves to give one family member ammunition to use against other family members, which in turn discourages analysis of all viewpoints and family decision making. If communication, de-

cision-making, or relationship difficulties are presented as the major family concern, every effort should be made by the community health nurse to see all family members together.

Dynamic biases may result when a nurse attempts to change his or her theoretical orientation about family counseling. For example, in moving from a concept of a "problem" family member to a concept that views the family system as the "problem," a nurse may unintentionally focus on a "problem" family member before becoming comfortable with the systems approach. In addition, a nurse who acts on intuitive diagnoses without confirming them by collected data from the family is engaging in a dynamic bias (Sills, 1975, p. 20). Inappropriate methods of professional intervention result from this type of action. One community health nurse, for instance, felt a mother needed nutritional counseling after she observed one family meal and discovered that a child in this family had severe nutritional anemia. She later found out that this child refused to eat solid foods. The mother had a good understanding of the "basic four," but needed assistance with feeding techniques and child discipline.

Social biases stem from the "social positions and social roles that the therapist occupies in addition to his professional role" (Sills, 1975, p. 21). Nurses who are wives and mothers or husbands and fathers, for example, develop perceptions of how these roles should be implemented. Unconsciously, they may label behavior as dysfunctional if it does not correspond with their role perceptions.

Values, attitudes, and beliefs can and frequently do influence the dynamic interactive processes that occur between people. Use of peer collaboration, professional supervision, and self-scrutiny helps the professional nurse to identify when personal values, attitudes, and beliefs are adversely affecting the therapeutic process. It is not uncommon for families to be viewed as "hopeless" because they do not change in the way professionals would like them to change. When this happens, both nurses and clients become frustrated. An objective third party (colleague, supervisor, or consultant) can often help professionals to identify why frustration occurs in the therapeutic process and how to alter their perceptions of the situation.

Sources and Methods for Collecting Data

During the assessment phase, both primary and secondary data are collected from all available sources to determine how well the client is coping with the encountered stressors. Primary data are those data which the community health nurse actually obtains from the client or sees, hears, feels, or smells in the client's environment. An astute community health nurse carefully notes observations as well as verbal information received from the client because it is often found that significant clues about a client's level of functioning are obtained by observing how the client interacts with the environment. For example, it is not unusual for the community health nurse to discern a child discipline problem by repeatedly watching parents interact with their children during home visits. When a nurse observes client functioning, it is important to remember that inferences about client problems should be based on *patterns* of behavior rather than isolated incidents of behavior. Labeling behavior dysfunctional after one observation is a dangerous practice and can adversely affect the nurse-client relationship.

In the community health setting, secondary data are obtained from a variety of sources such as significant others, personnel from health and social agencies, the family's physician, spiritual leaders, and health records. When these data are recorded, the source of the information should also be recorded. Generally, the community health nurse receives

either verbal or written permission from the client before making contact with secondary sources of data outside the family system. This practice not only protects the client's right of privacy, but also promotes honesty and trust in the therapeutic relationship. In addition, seeking a client's permission to obtain information from others demonstrates to the client that the nurse does respect the client's rights of self-determination.

When using secondary data, the nurse must recognize that this type of data may not accurately reflect *clients' perceptions* of themselves or their needs. Instead, secondary data may reflect what others perceive about clients and their needs. This point is particularly significant for a community health nurse to keep in mind, because frequently secondary data about the problems of family members are obtained when these individuals are not present. When this occurs, the community health nurse often finds it necessary to make arrangements to obtain primary data. She or he may, for instance, visit a child in school or schedule a home visit after school hours in order to identify how this child is reacting to a newly diagnosed health problem.

Various assessment methodologies should be used to collect primary and secondary data. Interview, observation, direct examination (auscultation, percussion, palpation, inspection, and measurement), contact with secondary sources of data, and review of relevant records are methods used by the community health nurse to obtain an accurate and a complete profile of a client's situation. These methods are used to identify client *strengths* as well as client needs.

The significance of utilizing a variety of methods to collect data about family functioning cannot be understated. No one data collection method provides the community health nurse with all the information needed to formulate accurate nursing diagnoses. The Daniels family case situation which follows illustrates this fact by showing the difference between the type of data one nurse obtained from inverview and from direct observation.

Following hospitalization of Mr. Daniels for an acute exacerbation episode of multiple sclerosis, the Daniels family was referred to the health department for health supervision follow-up. Ms. Garitt, hospital social worker, requested that a community health nurse assess this family's needs in relation to their understanding of multiple sclerosis, their ability to handle activities of daily living, and their knowledge of community resources. While Jane Mathews, CHN, was interviewing the family and collecting data on the entire family situation, she asked Mr. and Mrs. Daniels how they were managing Mr. Daniels's exercises. Both related that they were doing them regularly. Mrs. Daniels accurately described how the exercises should be done and verbalized that she felt comfortable handling them, since she was instructed how to do so by hospital staff. While Mrs. Daniels was demonstrating what she had learned, it was found that she did have an understanding about the proper exerises for her husband. However, her body mechanics were inappropriate and this caused severe backache which she failed to mention during the interviewing process. In addition to Mrs. Daniels's poor body mechanics, the nurse also discovered that Mr. Daniels was very demanding of his wife, expecting her to do exercises for him that he could do independently. Further exploration revealed that Mr. Daniels was doing very little for himself. Before his illness he had been the "man of the house." "Now I can't do anything." Through demonstration and return demonstration, the nurse showed Mr. Daniels that he was not helpless and assisted Mrs. Daniels in learning how to position herself appropriately when helping her husband.

If the community health nurse, in the above situation, had not observed Mr. and Mrs. Daniels's functioning, it could have taken her a considerable length of time to collect the data needed to accurately identify the real concerns in this family situation. Observing family interactions provided this nurse with data about family functioning that were not obtained through interview.

Assessing All Parameters of Family Health

The family-centered approach to nursing care focuses on the family as a "unit of people," rather than a collection of individual family members. This implies that the family is viewed as a system, where the actions and health status of one family member always affect the behavior and health status of all other family members. Thus, when community health nurses assess family health, they not only examine the health status of individual family members but look at *family dynamics* as well (Figure 8-3).

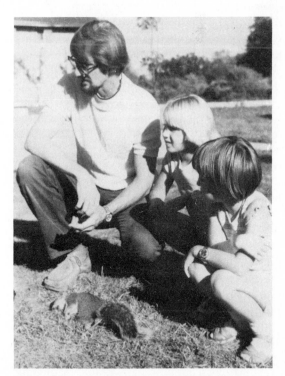

FIGURE 8-3 Family dynamics influence how well individual family members handle critical life events. The ability to provide support and security during times of stress (exposure to death) is a family strength which should be reinforced.

Family dynamics. To discern functional and dysfunctional characteristics of family dynamics, a community health nurse must establish criteria for evaluating family health to use for comparison purposes. In addition, a community health nurse must identify what type of data are needed for analyzing family functioning in order to focus assessment procedures. Parameters that must be considered when one is examining family dynamics are discussed in Chapter 6 and will not be repeated here. As previously mentioned, a conceptual framework should be used to organize the collection of family functioning data. It is also important to remember that if major emphasis is placed on the biological aspects of a family's health status during the beginning phase of a relationship, it may be difficult to refocus the family when the nurse wants to assess other parameters of family functioning. Explaining early in the therapeutic process why data about family dynamics are needed facilitates the collection of this type of information.

Identifying criteria for evaluating "family health" involves a process where one examines one's conceptual beliefs about health and about people and then delineates specific behaviors which reflect healthy functioning in relation to the family. Throughout this text, emphasis has been placed on viewing health "not merely as the absence of disease, but as a state of complete physical, mental, and social well-being" (WHO, 1947, p. 100). Dunn (1961) believes that implicit in this definition is the concept of high-level wellness which he defines as "an integrated method of functioning which is oriented toward maximizing the potential of which the individual is capable, within the environment where he is functioning." He sees wellness as being influenced by variables which are both internal and external to individual systems. "Well being both in body and mind and within the family and within community life should be interrelated in order for the individual to achieve a zest for life." Wellness,

according to Dunn, is a dynamic state, "ever-changing in its characteristics." "What is complete today, may be incomplete tomorrow" (Dunn, 1961, pp. 2–4). This implies that one always has the potential for growth, a philosophy which promotes a humanistic or caring approach to all humankind. It is believed by the authors that all clients should be approached in this way.

Inherent in Dunn's concept of "high-level wellness" for an individual is a conceptualization of family health. He sees the individual being influenced by his 'inner and outer [family] worlds" (Dunn, 1961, p. 25). Because families are responsible for meeting the needs of their individual family members, as well as for maintaining a functional family unit, family health can be defined as:

"An integrated method of functioning which is oriented toward maximizing the potential" (Dunn, 1961, p. 4) of individual family members throughout the life span and maintaining the integrity of the family as a system.

To be useful for comparison purposes, this global definition of family health must be translated into criteria which identify growth-producing family behaviors. Potential for growth is unique for each individual and each family unit. Client behavior must be analyzed from the client's perspective, because dysfunctional or maladaptive behavior in one family can be functional or adaptive in another. The family's perceptions about how well it is functioning must be the key factor which helps a nurse to determine whether or not a family is reaching its potential. If the family's perceptions are not understood, the community health nurse cannot influence a family to alter these perceptions.

Reviewing writings by Beavers (1977), Lewis, Beavers, Gossett, and Phillips (1976), Otto (1963), and Pratt (1976), and examining the Family Coping Index, a tool developed by the Richmond-Hopkins Cooperative Nursing Study

(Freeman and Lowe, 1964), will help the reader to delineate criteria for evaluating family health. The similarities between these authors' findings are striking. Flexible role patterns, responsiveness to the needs of individual members, active problem-solving mechanisms, ability to accept help, open communication patterns, and the provision of a warm, caring atmosphere were some of the main commonalities found in healthy families in these authors' studies. Table 8-2 presents an outline of the specific variables identified by Otto and Pratt. Although these variables are not in-tended to be normative, they do provide guidelines for data comparison purposes.

Individual functioning. The purpose of a family health assessment is to obtain pertinent data about the functioning of individual family members as well as the family system. In keeping with the view of health presented above, family members are viewed from an integrated, holistic, individual perspective. Biological, psychological, sociocultural, developmental, and environmental parameters of functioning are assessed in order to determine

TABLE 8-2   Criteria to Consider When Assessing "Healthy" Family Functioning: Two Authors' Viewpoints

Assessment parameters	Authors	
	Otto (1963) *Family strengths*	Pratt (1976) *Family structure and health behavior characterizing the energized family*
Adaptive abilities	The ability to provide for the physical, emotional, and spiritual needs of a family	Combined health behaviors of all family members are energized; all family members tend to care for their health
	The ability to use a crisis or seemingly injurious experience as a means of growth	Actively and energetically attempt to cope with life's problems and issues
	Ability for self-help and the ability to accept help when appropriate	Flexible division of tasks and activities
	An ability to perform family roles flexibly	
	The ability to communicate effectively	
Atmosphere and affect	The ability to be sensitive to the needs of family members	Responsive to the particular interests and needs of individual family members
	The ability to provide support, security, and encouragement	Regular and varied interaction among family members
Individual autonomy and integrity of family system	Mutual respect for the individuality of family members	Egalitarian distribution of power
	A concern for family unity, loyalty, and interfamily cooperation	Provide autonomy for individual family members
Relationships with others	The ability to initiate and maintain growth-producing relationships and experiences within and without the family	Provide regular links with the broader community through active participation in community activities
	The capacity to maintain and create constructive and responsible relationships in the neighborhood, the school, town, and local and state government	

SOURCE: Adapted from H. Otto. Criteria for assessing family strength. *Family Process*, September 1963, *2*, 333–336; and L. Pratt. *Family structure and effective health behavior: The energized family*. Boston: Houghton Mifflin, 1976, pp. 84–92.

the client's perception of his or her health status.

In general, clients do not think systematically about all the variables that affect their health. A major role of the community health nurse when completing an individual health assessment is to increase the client's awareness of all the factors that influence healthy functioning. A health assessment should be purposeful, meaningful, and goal directed and should provide the client with an opportunity to identify both personal strengths and needs in relation to the individual's current level of functioning. Data about preventive health practices and healthy aspects of coping along with information about ways in which the client handles illness should be elicited.

The vehicles used for organizing an individual functional assessment are the health history and the physical examination. Exploring the techniques of physical appraisal is beyond the scope of this text. Writings by Alexander and Brown (1974), Bates (1978), Burns and Johnson (1980), Sana and Judge (1975), and Sherman and Fields (1974) discuss extensively the physical examination process. It is essential for community health nurses to have skill in completing a gross physical appraisal, since clients may not have a regular source of medical care even though they may have health problems. Thus, community health nurses must have the ability to distinguish between *abnormal* and *normal* health findings. In addition, they need skill in the use of the referral process (see Chapter 9) in order to help clients obtain needed health care services when abnormal findings are identified.

"A nursing health history differs from a medical health history in that it focuses on the meaning of illness and hospitalization [health care] to the patient [client] and his family as a basis for planning nursing care. The medical history is taken to determine whether pathology is present as a basis for planning medical care" (McPhetridge, 1968, p. 68). When com-

pleting a health history, the community health nurse explores carefully the client's perceptions of his or her health status and how current stressors are affecting functioning; emphasis is placed on identifying the client as a *unique individual* rather than as a person who has a specific disease process.

Components included in a health history vary slightly from one author to another. Basically, the goal of a health history is to determine how well the client is meeting health needs and how activities of daily living have been altered to meet these needs. A comprehensive review of the client's past and current health status is elicited to identify an accurate and complete composite of the client's health functioning. With this information, the client and the nurse can explore ways for increasing the client's self-care capabilities.

Mahoney, Verdisco, and Shortridge (1976, p. 6) identify the following seven components of an individual health history:

1. *Reason for contact:* Why the client is seeking help at this time.

2. *Biographical data:* Structural variables common to all clients such as name, age, sex, marital status, religious preference, ethnic background, educational level, occupational status, health insurance, and social security information.

3. *Current health status:* The client's perceptions of his or her health, with a specific delineation of current complaints and activities of daily living.

4. *Past health history:* Data relative to the previous health or illness state of the client and contact with health care professionals, including a description of developmental accomplishments, health practices, known illnesses, allergies, restorative treatment, and social activities such as foreign travel which might be related to the client's current health status.

5. *Family history:* A description of the current health status of each family member, relationships among family members, and a genetic history in relation to health and illness.

6. *Social history:* An accounting of intrapersonal and interpersonal factors which influence the client's social adjustment, including environmental stressors which may be increasing or decreasing the client's vulnerability to crisis during times of stress.

7. *Review of systems:* A systematic assessment of biological functioning from head to toe.

When one is completing a health history, it is extremely important to elicit the client's expectations of the health care provider. If the client's and the professional's expectations are inconsistent, frustration results for all parties involved. A client, for instance, who has diabetes and is expecting a cure will likely have difficulty working with a health care professional whose goal is to help the client live a normal life within the limitations of his or her condition. If the discrepancy between these two goals is not resolved, neither of these goals will be reached.

Every nurse must decide on a format which will facilitate data collection. Although formats may vary, it is crucial to collect data in an *orderly* fashion on all parameters of client functioning before a nursing care plan is developed. There are times when a crisis situation warrants dealing with the immediate concerns of the client before all data are collected. However, in order to intervene effectively during times of crisis, the health care professional needs an *adequate* data base. Without this data base, it is impossible to help the client to make appropriate choices about solutions for resolving current health stresses.

Assessment guides can help the community health nurse collect health data in an orderly fashion. Assessment tools designed to collect information about the health status of individual family members should help the nurse to examine multiple aspects of a client's functioning. Appendixes 8-1, 8-2, and 8-3 are three assessment forms (antepartum, postpartum, and newborn) developed by community health nurses at the Seattle King County Department of Public Health. These tools aid the nurse in identifying psychosocial as well as physical components of a client's health status. In addition, they help a nurse to integrate individual and family functioning by raising issues pertinent to the needs of all family members.

Assessment tools have limitations and must be used only as guides to focus a nurse's attention on significant parameters to assess during the health interview and the physical examination process. Spontaneous interchange between the nurse and the client must always be allowed so that the client can fully express needs and can determine priorities which relate to her or his life-style. A barrage of questions from an assessment form stifles communication.

Analyzing

Once individual and family data are collected, the analysis phase of the nursing process begins. This phase encompasses a cognitive data ordering process, which results in the formation of nursing diagnoses. Nursing diagnoses are inferences made about a client's health status based on patterns reflected in assessment data (Durand and Prince, 1966, p. 52). Nursing diagnoses identify actual or potential client problems and their underlying causes, which are amenable to *nursing interventions* (Gordon, 1976, p. 1299). They also delineate client strengths which should be reinforced when the nurse is helping the client to enhance his or her self-care capabilities. In the community health setting, nursing diagnoses examine the needs and strengths of family units as well as the needs and strengths of individual clients.

In order to formulate nursing diagnoses, the community health nurse must group data so that relationships between assessment categories can be analyzed and patterns of behavior can be identified. Establishing relationships between assessment categories involves looking at all parameters of individual as well as family functioning. It requires a synthesis of data to determine the unique combination of biological, psychosocial, developmental, and environmental factors that are making an impact on a specific family unit. It is important to synthesize data collected from a family, as client needs vary even when clients are experiencing similar situations. For example, one community health nurse was visiting two families who were both expressing concern about a child who cried when preparing to leave for school. In one family situation, the nurse's diagnosis of this behavior was that "Susie is distressed due to family illness," because assessment data revealed that (1) Susie had enjoyed school until her father had a heart attack; (2) Susie's father had his heart attack while she was at school; and (3) Susie had been asking lately if her father was going to die. In the other family situation, the nursing diagnosis in relation to the child's crying was quite different. It read, "Bonnie's dependency on her mother is inhibiting her psychosocial development." The community health nurse came to this conclusion after the parents shared that (1) Bonnie started school a year late because she was "immature" for her developmental age; (2) Bonnie had never enjoyed school; (3) Bonnie spent most of her free time with her mother, even when children her own age were around; and (4) Bonnie would cling to her mother when baby-sitters came to the house.

Nursing diagnoses must be based on a strong data base validated by the client and data must be synthesized before nursing diagnoses are established. Formulating diagnoses without adequate information or in relation to fragmented pieces of data leads to invalid diagnoses and inappropriate client goals and nursing interventions. A nursing diagnosis, for instance, which is based only on environmental observations (fragmented data) and which reads "unsafe housekeeping practices," provides very little direction for client and

nursing intervention. Unsafe housekeeping practices can result from several factors, including lack of home management skill, energy depletion due to maturational and situational crises, and differing values about environmental safety. How a community health nurse would intervene when unsafe housekeeping practices are encountered is greatly influenced by the data base obtained and the nursing diagnosis developed. For example, an educative strategy is used when a client lacks home management skill, whereas a crisis intervention approach is initiated when a client's energies are depleted because of crisis.

Use of scientific knowledge such as Maslow's hierarchy of needs, theories of growth and development, and concepts of stress and crisis enhances a community health nurse's ability to synthesize data and to formulate an appropriate nursing diagnosis. Scientific knowledge helps a nurse to identify significant signs and symptoms of distress and to organize collected data into a meaningful whole. Grouping the symptoms presented by a client and then comparing them to clinical and research findings such as those presented in Chapter 7 aids the nurse in determining when a client may be in a state of crisis or vulnerable to crisis.

When comparing collected data with relevant clinical and research findings, it is important to identify nursing diagnoses in relation to client strengths as well as client needs. Discerning client strengths helps the community health nurse to reinforce self-sufficiency skills, which in turn aids the nurse in avoiding dependency-building nursing activities. In the community health nurse setting, special emphasis is placed on identifying nursing diagnoses that relate to situations or potential problems which warrant anticipatory guidance counseling. This emphasis is based on the belief that primary prevention should be a major focus in community health nursing practice. Situations throughout one's life-span that warrant anticipatory guidance are covered in Chapters 13 through 19.

Synthesizing data and formulating nursing diagnoses can be difficult when the nurse works with clients in the community health setting because data about several individuals as well as family dynamics must be integrated. Peer consultation, supervised clinical practice, and comparison of nursing diagnoses with diagnoses of other health professionals can help practitioners to increase their diagnostic abilities. Knowing when to seek assistance from others is one earmark of a professional nurse.

A National Group on Classification of Nursing Diagnoses is currently working on developing a common diagnostic classification for nursing. The efforts of this group will help nurses in all settings to refine their diagnostic skill and to document the effectiveness of nursing services. Any professional nurse interested in identifying and classifying nursing diagnoses can seek membership in this group by registering with the Clearinghouse for Nursing Diagnosis at St. Louis University (Gordon, 1979, p. 488).

Planning

After nursing diagnoses are established and *validated with the client,* the community health nurse and the client move into the planning phase of the nursing process. Two major activities occur during this phase: (1) client-centered goals and objectives (criteria) for evaluating goal attainment are formulated and (2) alternative interventions are identified and evaluated. A goal is a broad desired *outcome* toward which behavior is directed, such as "the family will value preventive health care services." An objective delineates *client behaviors* which reflect that a goal has been reached. "The family will obtain a regular source of medical care by September" might be one objective established to determine if the above goal has been accomplished. Alternative inter-

ventions are *activities* which may be implemented by the client, the nurse, and other health care professionals to help the client achieve the desired goals. For example, in relation to the above objective, the nurse might discuss with the client the services of all the available medical resources in the community and assist the client in obtaining transportation if necessary.

All goals and objectives should be stated in specific and realistic terms and relate to the nursing diagnoses that have been established. They should not include expectations that are beyond the professional's or client's resources or capabilities. A goal, for instance, of a severely retarded child achieving normal growth and development is extremely unrealistic. It is very appropriate to work toward maximizing this child's potential but inappropriate to expect that this child will reach normal growth and development parameters.

Goal statements and objectives that are written in positive terms provide direction for nursing interventions more effectively than those that have a negative orientation. Negative goal statements such as "parents will not use harsh disciplinary measures with their children" tend to focus on family weaknesses rather than on family strengths, which can be mobilized to reduce current stresses. Positive goal statements, such as "parents will talk with their children when the children act out," lead to the development of more positive interventions for achieving goals.

The nurse may find after client-centered goals are developed that the client finds it impossible to work on all of them immediately. When this happens, the nurse and the client should work together to differentiate between problems that require immediate action and those that are of less concern to the client. When establishing priorities in relation to client goals, the nurse must keep in mind that the client has the right to make the final decision about goals to focus on. The nurse does have a responsibility, however, to share concerns when she or he believes that client actions are unsafe or are precipitating a crisis situation.

After client-centered, positively stated goals have been established and priorities determined, behavioral objectives that can be measured should be written. Behavioral objectives, sometimes labeled subgoals, help the client and the nurse to identify intervention strategies that will facilitate goal attainment. Bloom (1956), Krathwohl, Bloom, and Masia (1964), Mager (1975), and Reilly (1975) discuss extensively the process for formulating behavioral objectives. Practitioners regularly refer to writings by these authors when they want to develop meaningful, cognitive, affective, and psychomotor behavioral objectives.

The importance of formulating specific objectives for evaluating goal attainment must be stressed. Broad, general goals do not provide sufficient direction for planning intervention strategies. "Maximizing the potential" of a child who has a developmental lag, for example, does not specifically identify needed areas of improvement. Objectives such as those listed below more appropriately facilitate the development of intervention strategies because they focus on specific developmental needs of the client:

· Joel will achieve daytime bladder and bowel control by December.

· Joel will eat solid foods by October.

· Joel's family will share their feelings about Joel's condition and will verbally identify how their feelings may be adversely affecting his growth and development.

Interventions, like objectives, should be specific and based on sound scientific knowledge. "Teaching about growth and development" is not a specifically stated intervention. It is extremely global and does not take into account the individual needs of a particular family. A community health nurse could better prepare for family visits if the above intervention were stated as follows: "discuss various ways to achieve daytime bladder and bowel control."

When delineating a plan for intervention, both family and nurse activities should be identified. If only nursing actions are established, the client cannot be an active participant in the therapeutic process. Unfortunately, family resources are frequently overlooked when intervention strategies are developed. For instance, plans are too often made to involve community resources in the client's care even though friends or family members are available and would be more than willing to assist the client in achieving his or her goals.

When intervention strategies are discussed, it may be found that referral to other health care professionals can best help the client to meet his or her needs. In these instances, the community health nurse should discuss with the family how essential data about their situation can be shared. The family's permission should be obtained before releasing any information to other health care agencies. The client has the right to determine what data shared in confidence with the nurse should or should not be shared with others. Indiscriminate exchange of client information among professionals violates the client's right to confidentiality and usually promotes mistrust and resistance to professional intervention. The principle of confidentiality is most often violated when goals are not mutually established and the nurse shares or seeks data to validate nurse-focused goals.

Interdisciplinary collaboration is appropriate and often essential. The family must, however, support the need for such an approach before it can be fully successful. Application of the principles of the referral process which are discussed in Chapter 9 usually help a nurse to reduce resistance to interdisciplinary collaboration.

Three key principles must be taken into

consideration during all phases of the planning process. These are (1) individualization of client care plans; (2) active client participation; and (3) the client's right of self-determination. The family-centered nursing process is a scientific process designed to meet the needs of *clients*. Inherent in this concept is the belief that clients have unique needs and, thus, care cannot be standardized. Unique needs of clients can only be discovered by actively involving the client in the therapeutic process. Active client participation also promotes client commitment to goal attainment and decreases resistance to change. Taking over for a client, on the other hand, may reinforce a client's feelings of inadequacy or increase the client's resentment of authority figures. These types of feelings can foster dependency or rejection of aid offered by the community health nurse.

For clients to fully participate in the therapeutic process, they must have the right to refuse any course of action they deem inappropriate for them. The community health nurse can help a client to examine the pros and cons of certain health actions or the consequences of continuing a particular pattern of functioning. The nurse should not, however, make decisions for the client or expect the client to make decisions in the way the nurse would make them. This is not meant to imply that the nurse should reinforce behavior which could be harmful to the client. Rather, it emphasizes that clients are responsible for the decisions they make and that they should not be rejected (i.e., viewed as "hopeless" or "resistant to change") if they do not make decisions in the way the health care professional would make them. Occasionally the community health nurse does intervene without a client's consent because the client is a threat to others (i.e., child abuse, spread of communicable disease) or to herself or himself (suicidal). Even in these situations the community health nurse works with the client, if possible, to help reduce the distress being experienced and to develop new patterns of coping.

To effectively apply the principles of individualization, active participation, and self-determination, the community health nurse must *internalize* the belief that all clients are unique and capable of making decisions about health care issues. Nurses must also consistently examine how personal attitudes, beliefs, motivations, and conditioning are influencing their professional relationships. Personal biases can and do subtly influence how professionals interact with clients. One community health nurse, for instance, found it difficult to maintain a therapeutic relationship with families when the male provider in the family had a "drinking problem." She would support the female's viewpoints without helping her to analyze how she might be reinforcing her husband's dysfunctional behavior. The nurse recognized that this was happening and was able to verbalize that she felt her sister died prematurely as a result of stress associated with her husband's drinking problem. When the nurse was conscious of her feelings, she was able to deal with them and better assist clients in these situations.

Professional Contracting

Contracting with clients is one way of consistently monitoring professional biases and applying the principles of individualization, active participation, and self-determination. A contract, a mutual agreement between two or more persons for a specific purpose, provides a framework for evaluating the interactions which are occurring between people. It does so because a contract clearly identifies what each person in the relationship can expect from the other person in the relationship.

Contracts are used for a variety of reasons. They may be formal, legally binding, long-term agreements, such as when a couple buys a home, or they may be casual, short-term commitments, such as when a friend consents to dog-sit while the dog's owner is gone on vacation. Contracts are also being used effectively by health care professionals to encourage their clients to participate more actively in dealing with their own health care needs. In these situations, the contract assumes a different purpose. It becomes a method of professional intervention that facilitates the helping relationship with clients. Contracting has been used by health care professionals more frequently in recent years, because there is a growing interest in promoting a philosophy of professional practice which supports the client's self-care capabilities. Increased use of contracting has also occurred because it has been found that clients who are actively involved in identifying their own health needs and in formulating health care goals are more likely to change their health behaviors than clients who have no voice in these decisions.

A professional contract may be defined very simply as a mutually agreed upon working understanding that relates to the terms of treatment and is continuously negotiable between the nurse and the family (Maluccio and Marlow, 1974; and Seabury, 1976). The contract may be either written or oral, but it must be clear and explicit to all parties involved. When methods for *reinforcing* clients' actions are explicitly spelled out, the contract is labeled a *contingency contract*. The contingency contracting process is based on theories of behavior modification, which postulate that reinforcers or rewards increase the probability that a desired response will occur. Before implementing contingency contracting, the professional should have a firm understanding of the principles of behavior modification.

The professional using the contracting method of intervention must feel comfortable with the philosophy that all individuals have the potential for growth and that they are capable of effective decision making. The professional must also believe that the client has the right to determine which course of action will best meet his or her health care needs. In essence, contracting is a *philosophy of practice*

that governs how the community health nurse implements the family-centered nursing process. The nurse who believes in contracting involves the client in all aspects of care. She or he makes an agreement with the client which spells out explicitly the responsibilities of both the nurse and client in achieving mutually defined, client-centered goals. The quality of explicitness implies that terms of intervention are known to both the client and the nurse. When contracting occurs, all involved parties have a mutual understanding about:

1. Purpose of client-nurse interactions

2. Nursing diagnoses

3. Desired outcomes (goals) toward which behavior is directed

4. Priority needs in relation to client goals

5. Methods of intervention

6. Specific activities each party will carry out to achieve stated goals

7. Established time parameters for evaluation and the frequency and length of visits

Contracting increases the clarity in nurse-client interactions. Specific commitments are made orally so that each party is aware of its role in the therapeutic process. Increased clarity often enhances the therapeutic relationship. This is especially true when clients have multiple problems or are unable to identify the nature of their problems. A case situation can best illustrate this point.

The Beech family, two parents with five children, had been visited by community health nurses for years. The family folder reflected many problems; marital stress, financial difficulties, poor nutrition, lack of preventive health care for family members, irregular school attendance, and frequent childhood infections were the primary problems with which the family was dealing. Infrequent visits were made by the community health nurse because the family continually failed to deal actively with health care needs. Because they moved frequently, the Beech family never had consistent contact with one nurse for any length of time. Finally the community health nurse decided to talk with Mrs. Beech about terminating nursing service because she believed that the family did not desire assistance. To her surprise, Mrs. Beech verbalized that her family did need help and that she really wanted the nurse to continue visiting. She further shared that she had difficulty concentrating on anything because the family had so many problems to handle. The nurse agreed with Mrs. Beech that it was an impossible task to solve all the family problems at once. She proposed that it might be helpful if the family and the nurse could work together to resolve the one health problem Mrs. Beech felt was most distressing at that time. Mrs. Beech had trouble focusing on one particular concern, because she had never before attempted to do so. Because she spent a considerable amount of time talking about Mary, her 10-year-old who had recently failed a hearing test at school, the nurse questioned if Mrs. Beech might want to explore ways to resolve this health care problem. The nurse also suggested that it might be helpful to order the family's health problems from most significant to least significant. Since these suggestions were acceptable to Mrs. Beech, the following contract was established:

· *Purpose of client-nurse interactions:* The community health nurse will help the family to establish priorities in relation to their health problems and to handle their problems in manageable doses.

· *Priority need:* Mary's failure of hearing test at school.

· *Mutual goal:* Mary's hearing problem will be evaluated by a physician.

· *Method of intervention:* Family will take Mary to the hearing specialist she had seen before. (This decision was made after the nurse discussed all the possible resources where Mary could obtain care and Mrs. Beech shared that Mary had had hearing problems in the past.)

· *Responsibilities of family:* (1) Make appointment with the doctor; (2) arrange for child care for their two preschoolers for the afternoon of the appointment; (3) arrange for transportation; (4) together with the nurse, make list of questions to ask the doctor during the visit.

· *Responsibilities of nurse:* Contact the physician to share the results of Mary's hearing test and Mrs. Beech's fears about health care professionals. (Mrs. Beech had been frequently criticized by health care professionals in the past for waiting too long before she sought medical help.) Visit weekly to evaluate how plans for Mary's care are progressing and to help the family establish priorities for health care action.

· *Time limits:* Mary to see the physician by the end of the month.

Mary saw the physician within the appropriate time frame; it was determined that she would need ear surgery. Since the contracting method of intervention helped Mrs. Beech to achieve her first goal, Mrs. Beech and the nurse agreed to renegotiate for follow-up based on the doctor's recommendation. Many other contracts were made before this family case record was closed. Accomplishing resolution of one problem helped the family to see that their situation was not hopeless. Setting priorities in relation to goal attainment decreased the family's anxiety about all the problems they had to handle.

Contracting is a dynamic, complex process which gradually evolves as the therapeutic relationship is strengthened. It should not be viewed as a simple procedure, involving only a discussion about goals, intervention strategies, and time limits. To successfully engage a family in the contracting process, the community health nurse must help the family to gain a clear understanding of its needs. The nurse must also explain the nature of a therapeutic relationship and explore with the client the range of alternative interventions that are available.

It is important to remember when thinking about contracting with clients that clients may not know about all of the available resources.

They also may not know why they are experiencing distress at this time. A new mother, for example, may recognize that she is concerned about the physical aspects of child care, but she may not realize that some of her stress is related to role changes associated with parenthood.

Initially a contract may be very general and only include an agreement to explore the nature of the client's problems and the meaning of a therapeutic relationship. The terms of a contract become more inclusive as specific data are obtained. Establishing time parameters is important even when a general contract is developed, because they emphasize the need for reviewing progress made in relation to goal attainment.

Contracting is an effective way to involve families in their own health care. Contracting can reinforce dysfunctional family patterns, however, if the nurse does not analyze carefully family dynamics. When a contract supports unhealthy family functioning, it is labeled a *corrupt contract* (Beall, 1972, p. 77). A corrupt contract might evolve, for instance, when a community health nurse is working with a family who would like their aging parents to move to a nursing home. Sometimes families push for nursing home placement to meet their own needs rather than the needs of their aging parents. If the community health nurse supports the family's decision and encourages the parents to move without talking to them about their needs and desires, he or she is violating the rights of the aging parents and the principles of contracting.

During the contracting process, a community health nurse may identify problems such as lack of protection against communicable diseases or inadequate dental care that do not seem to be of concern to the family. In these situations, a nurse-centered goal rather than a client-centered goal is formulated. A nurse-centered goal should be stated as such and should not emphasize family action like the

"family will make an appointment at the immunization clinic." Instead, it should focus on increasing the family's awareness of the problem and be stated in such terms as "the family will verbalize the need for immunizations." Distinguishing carefully between nurse goals and family goals helps the community health nurse to prevent imposing personal values on clients and helps the nurse to focus on the problems and goals important to the family. Generally, families do not explore problems identified by the nurse that they do not see as problems until they have achieved their own client-centered goals.

Throughout the contracting process, the community health nurse must clearly document on the family record assessment data, goals, objectives, intervention strategies, and evaluation findings. Written data are retrievable, whereas oral information can be easily lost or misinterpreted. The family service record should provide concrete data, organized in such a manner that they can be easily analyzed. Lack of documentation discourages effective evaluation of nursing care and client goal attainment. It is often indicative of inadequate data analysis and insufficient planning. In Chapter 21, the significance of accurate recording in relation to the development of a sound quality assurance program is discussed. The record system used in the community health setting is extremely important, and a variety of formats can be effectively used to document all aspects of the nursing process.

It is crucial that the record format represents and shows the flow between all aspects of the nursing process presented in Table 8-1. This is not an easy task, but it must be addressed. The quality of the record system will affect the quality of care given to a client, especially in relation to continuity of care. It is often helpful to place diagnoses, goals, plans, interventions, and evaluation findings on one sheet in the record so that the relationship between each phase can be easily identified. If the phases of the nursing process are on different pages of the record, it is difficult to coordinate diagnoses, goals, plans, interventions, and evaluations findings.

Implementing

The implementation phase of the nursing process deals specifically with how activities are carried out to achieve client goals. Together, the client and the nurse select and test intervention strategies to determine their appropriateness in helping the client move toward problem resolution. Priorities concerning when actions will be taken are established so that the client can deal with his or her problems in manageable doses. If needed, other resources are mobilized to help the client handle the change process.

Because change is often threatening, a warm, caring, supportive atmosphere which reinforces client accomplishments should be fostered. Focusing on what remains to be accomplished rather than emphasizing positive results that have already occurred only serves to discourage the client. Honest, positive feedback can be the motivating factor that promotes client involvement in the therapeutic process. Positive feedback can also help to increase clients' self-esteem and confidence in their ability to assume responsibility for maintaining and promoting their health status.

There are a variety of intervention strategies that the community health nurse utilizes to help clients alter those aspects of life they desire to change. Some of these are discussed in Chapter 7, where the educative and problem-solving strategies were explored. Nursing actions should be based on sound scientific principles and knowledge. If a planned intervention, for instance, is to increase the client's understanding of how to prepare nutritious meals, the teaching methodology chosen should take into consideration specific client characteristics, such as financial resources, demands on the homemaker's time, nutritional needs of all family members, and cultural preferences in relation to food likes and dislikes. It should also reflect current knowledge about nutritional requirements and appropriate application of the principles of teaching and learning.

All other phases of the nursing process are usually carried out during the implementation phase. While clients are actively participating in the intervention process, they share data verbally or nonverbally through action taken or not taken. The community health nurse must analyze this new data carefully to determine if care plans need to be revised. Nursing care plans should never be static. Rather, they should be continuously open to renegotiation as the client's situation changes or new data are discovered.

The community health nurse must be *flexible* when implementing intervention strategies, since new data are often generated which alter original nursing diagnoses and client goals. Some clients are unable to identify the nature of their problems until they attempt to change their behavior and find that change does not relieve their discomfort. This was illustrated in Chapter 7, when Mrs. Lehi discovered that her headaches were related to guilt feelings about being a working mother rather than to excessive demands on her time. In this situation the nurse and Mrs. Lehi revised their original goal, "Mrs. Lehi will discover ways to adjust her daily schedule to reduce stress," to "Mrs. Lehi will identify ways to achieve her self-fulfillment needs without distress." Intervention strategies were altered accordingly. Instead of discussing Mrs. Lehi's daily activities and support systems, the nurse and Mrs. Lehi explored issues such as Mrs. Lehi's feelings about motherhood, the needs of school-age children, and an individual's need for self-fulfillment.

Both the client and the nurse should have responsibilities to meet when interventions are planned and mutually agreed upon. If either the client or nurse is unable to meet these responsibilities, this must be discussed and interventions revised as necessary. The family-centered nursing process is a collaborative process, and the client must be involved in its implementation. A nurse who assumes responsibilities for the client when he or she can independently handle them instead of talking about why planned interventions are not being implemented is not helping the client to achieve goals.

During the implementation phase, it is not unusual to discover that clients do not wish to pursue a particular goal, even though they expressed a desire to do so during the planning phase. Sometimes clients verbalize an *awareness* that a problem exists but are not ready to change their behavior in the way that is necessary to resolve that problem (see Chapter 9). Clients may not recognize the difference between awareness and readiness until concrete plans have been made to alter their current situation. If this happens, it can be difficult for these clients to verbally convey to the nurse that they are not ready for change. Frequently they share this message nonverbally by not taking action. That is why it is so important for the community health nurse to find out why clients are not meeting commitments which had been mutually agreed upon. Goals and plans should be modified if clients are not ready to alter their behavior.

Some clients are resistant to change because all their alternatives for change have negative consequences. A woman, for example, who has limited financial resources, no preparation for a job, and few support systems may be very hesitant to divorce her husband, even though their marital relationship is destructive to her emotional health. The fear of not being able to support herself and being alone might be far more stressful to her than the emotional pain she is experiencing in the marital relationship. When a community health nurse encounters such a situation, she must remain *empathetic* and guard against feeling that the woman has no options. Community health nurses do find it difficult to handle situations when all the alternatives for change have some negative consequences, and they may find that feelings of sympathy rather than empathy evolve. If such feelings emerge, nurses should seek assistance from their peers and nursing supervisor in order to objectively evaluate what is happening in the therapeutic process.

Evaluating

Evaluation is the continuous critiquing of each aspect of the nursing process. Although it is discussed as a separate phase, it must take place concurrently with all phases of the nursing process. Ongoing feedback should be elicited from the client to determine whether goals, plans, and intervention strategies are appropriately focused. When objectives are established, defining how they will be evaluated is a necessity. A well-written objective will contain the potential for evaluation. For example, "John will learn how to give his own insulin injection by the end of the month" is a concise statement which can be used to determine whether John has or has not achieved a desired goal.

Although evaluation is one of the most significant aspects of the nursing process, it is the one most frequently neglected or haphazardly done. When developing the nursing care plan, intervals should be established for the systematic review of all aspects of the nursing process. Some community health agencies have a policy which states that all records should be summarized and analyzed after a given number of visits have been made or when the family case is being transferred to another nurse. Even if such a policy does not exist, summarization of records must be done on a regular basis because it facilitates evaluation of client services and outcomes. A well-written summary helps the community health nurse to synthesize data and to vividly identify what has or has not been accomplished in a specified period of time.

Summarizing records is one way to ensure that a systematic evaluation of family progress is done. Consulting with peers, supervisors, and other health care professionals can also help a community health nurse to review progress or lack of progress in family situations. Evaluation is absolutely essential and it must be carefully planned; lack of evaluation often prolongs the therapeutic process.

When evaluating the effectiveness of intervention strategies implemented by the client, the nurse, and other health care professionals, it is not sufficient just to identify that the family is participating in the therapeutic process. The *outcome* of actions taken by the family and health care professionals must also be examined. Noting only that the family has kept an appointment at a clinic, for example, provides very little data about the effectiveness of this intervention strategy. Identifying what happened when the family went to the clinic and what motivated them to do so is far more significant. This type of data provides the key for future interventions. Finding out, for instance, if the family was satisfied with the care they received or if the family understood the recommendations for follow-up can help the nurse to identify barriers to the utilization of health care services. Data obtained from these types of questions can also assist the nurse in planning interventions *specific* to the current needs of the family.

When evaluating the effectiveness of intervention strategies, the nurse may find that clients are not reaching their goals. This happens for a variety of reasons that are not always obvious to either the client or the nurse. Outlined below are some factors for the nurse to consider as guidelines when examining why client goals have not been achieved:

1. Data base inadequate to identify the actual needs of the family.

2. Goals and objectives too broad and general.

3. Goals and objectives not mutually established; nurse's goals being imposed on the family.

4. Family priorities in relation to goals and objectives not ascertained.

5. Family attempting to deal with too many problems at once.

6. Family energies depleted as a result of maturational and situational crises.

7. Barriers to care not identified because follow-up on client and nurse actions is neglected.

8. Nursing diagnoses, goals, and objectives not revised as the family situation changes.

9. Intervention strategies inappropriate.

10. Family lacks the support they need to reduce anxiety during the change process.

11. Coordination of care among all health professionals neglected; family receiving inconsistent messages about appropriate intervention actions; gaps in services.

The coordination of services among all professionals is crucial. It should not be assumed that particular services will be provided by an agency when a client is referred to that agency. When multiple agencies are working with a family, clearly defined mechanisms for deciding who will do what and for evaluating the quality of the care being delivered by the health team should be established. The client must be involved in determining how interdisciplinary collaboration and coordination will evolve. Generally clients are more than willing to consent to an interdisciplinary approach to the delivery of health care when they understand why it is important and how it will help them.

When an interdisciplinary approach is used to provide services for clients, the community health nurse must carefully evaluate when nursing services are and are not needed. Referring a client to another community agency does not necessarily mean that all of the client's needs will be met by that agency. The community health nurse still has a responsibility to evaluate the effectiveness of the referrals that have been made (see Chapter 9) and to discern if the client has other needs that are amenable to nursing interventions. After the referral has been implemented successfully, it may be found that nursing services are no longer needed. When this happens, the client is prepared for termination and the family case is closed to service.

Use of the evaluation process helps the community health nurse to provide care to clients more effectively. It assists the nurse in determining which goals have been accomplished, either completely or partially, and helps the nurse to modify intervention strategies if goals are not being reached. It also aids the nurse in making sound decisions about when to terminate nursing services.

Terminating

Terminating is seldom identified as a separate phase in the nursing process. It is alluded to during the evaluation phase but very little attention is devoted to discussing what impact termination has on the nurse and the client in the community health setting. Frequently, feelings associated with the separation process are not handled by the client or the nurse. To effectively intervene with clients in the community health setting, a nurse must become *involved*. The inability to deal with feelings as-

sociated with the termination process can stifle the development of close, caring professional relationships. It is for this reason that the authors label terminating as a separate phase in the family-centered nursing process.

Terminating is the period when the client and nurse deal with feelings associated with separation and when they distance themselves (Kelly, 1969, p. 2381). Ending a meaningful relationship with a client should be carefully planned. Clients, as well as nurses, need time to deal with the strong emotions that are often evoked by separation. Anger, sadness, denial, and rejection are some normal feelings experienced by both the client and the nurse during the termination phase. The type of reaction which occurs depends, to a great extent, on how the nurse and client have dealt with separation in the past. In social situations the sense of sadness is verbalized when friends are leaving, but "denial, suppression and repression of feelings are encouraged." Because of this type of socialization process, clients and nurses have not learned how to talk freely about what separation means to them (Sene, 1969, p. 39).

In the community health setting, the nurse encounters termination issues frequently. Some clients are seen on a short-term basis, in three or four visits, whereas long-term relationships are established with other clients who have multiple problems to resolve. It is not uncommon to have a client move abruptly or to have a staff nurse's district changed. Clients who have experienced frequent changes in the nurse assigned to their case may have trouble becoming closely involved with any nurse. Talking about what these changes mean to the client and the nurse can be a learning process for both. A nurse, however, who uses denial to cope with feelings associated with termination will be unable to help the client deal with these feelings.

The authors' clinical experiences have demonstrated that the issue of termination is too often neglected in the community health setting. Family case situations are closed without prior notice to the family, or a nurse's district is changed without providing sufficient time for the nurse to handle the termination process with clients. At times, cases are not closed because the client regresses when it is discovered that the nurse believes her or his services are no longer needed. The client may verbalize the same belief but still regress because he or she is not given the opportunity to explore feelings associated with loss. One 40-year-old client who had multiple sclerosis, for instance, abruptly stopped doing his exercises when the nurse remarked how well he was progressing. He finally verbalized that he was afraid the nurse would no longer visit when he was able to care for himself. At other times, the nurse does not close a family case to service because of difficulty in ending the relationship with the family. The nurse may only visit monthly "just to see how they are doing," not recognizing that she or he is having difficulty ending a meaningful relationship.

The need to handle separation issues when terminating a nurse-client relationship is essential. Termination may not be an easy process, especially when the nurse and the client have had a long-term relationship. Clients need a supportive atmosphere which encourages them to express feelings and emotions. Often the nurse must initiate discussion about termination before the client will feel free to share feelings about this issue. This was dramatically illustrated when one of the authors ended a long-term relationship with a family because they were moving.

The Grostics had been visited weekly for approximately a year because they were dealing with both developmental and situational crises. Child neglect had been evident when the family case was first opened, but a year later both children were happy, thriving youngsters. Upon moving, Mrs. G. felt that the family still needed nursing services, so plans were made to refer the family for community health nursing follow-up in their new community. Both the client and nurse had shared positive feelings throughout their relationship, but neither verbalized these feelings when plans for referral were discussed. Mrs. G.'s mother altered this situation. She saw the nurse in the immunization clinic prior to the nurse's last visit to the family and stated that Mrs. G. was very upset about having a new nurse. "No one could be like you." Finally, during the last visit both the nurse and Mrs. G. hugged each other and openly discussed what they were feeling. The nurse even felt better when she heard that the family was doing well in their new location.

A client helped the nurse in the above situation see the value of dealing with feelings associated with termination and the rewards of involvement. Although termination may be difficult, it is a learning and growing experience for both the nurse and client. When properly implemented, both are able to see what has and has not been accomplished in the therapeutic process and the reason(s) for the termination. Often termination occurs because all the goals established for the relationship have been reached and there is no further need for nursing service. The client should be informed that if health needs arise in the future, the community health nurse can be contacted again. Keeping records open just for the sake of keeping them open when no health goals are being actively worked on is not a good use of nursing time, nor does it project a realistic picture to the client of what nursing services are about.

SUMMARY

The family-centered nursing process is a systematic approach to scientific problem solving, involving a series of circular, dynamic actions—assessing, analyzing, planning, implementing, evaluating, and terminating—for the purpose of facilitating optimum client functioning. Nurses in all settings use this process in order to practice in an orderly, logical manner. It enables the nurse to individualize care for each client.

The principles of individualization, active participation, self-determination, and confidentiality must be applied in all phases of the nursing process. Contracting is increasingly used with clients because health care professionals experience more positive results when they encourage it. *Contracting* is a term used to denote a process that involves the establishment of mutually defined goals and intervention strategies. It is a working agreement be-

tween the client and nurse, explicitly stated, in which all parties involved are working together to achieve a common goal.

Use of the family-centered nursing process is rewarding and challenging. The family-centered nursing process assists the nurse in helping the client to mobilize personal strengths that will enhance the client's self-care capabilities. It provides the nurse with a framework for facilitating client decision making about health care matters. It also enables the nurse to become truly involved with other human beings in a supportive, therapeutic way.

APPENDIX 8-1

King County Health Department, Seattle, Washington, Nursing Assessment Guide: Antepartum

Patient's name_____

EDC_____GRAV_____PARA_____ABORT_____DATE MED. CARE STARTED _____

M.D._____HOSP._____SIGNIFICANT MEDICAL HISTORY OF PREGNANCIES _____

Mother's opinion of previous pregnancy, delivery, and newborn (NB) _____

Current pregnancy	Yes	No	First assessment, comments Trimester 1 2 3	Date_____	Yes	No	Second assessment, comments Trimester 1 2 3	Date_____
MEDICAL SUPERVISION								
Medical appointments made								
Plans to keep								
Dental appointments made								
Plans to keep								
M&I dental care completed								

Pt understanding of doctor's orders is:

SIGNS AND SYMPTOMS								
Nausea								
Vomiting								
Heartburn								
Spotting								
Bleeding								

Current pregnancy	Yes	No	First assessment, comments Trimester 1 2 3 Date_____	Yes	No	Second assessment, comments Trimester 1 2 3 Date_____
Edema						
Leg cramps						
Varicosities						
Backache						
Dyspnea						
Constipation						
Hemorrhoids						
Dysuria						
Frequency						
Fetal Movements						
Braxton Hicks						
Other						

PERSONAL MANAGEMENT

Weight gain

   Normal

Diet—type_____

   Breakfast

   Lunch

   Dinner

   Snacks

   Dislikes

   Fluid intake pattern

   Comments

Sleep—No. of hours

   Naps

Physical activity

   Very active

   Moderately active

   Limited activity

Clothing

   Supportive

Nursing assessment—Antepartum—Page 2   Patient's name_____
Current pregnancy
Emotional (complete with patient's feelings towards)

	First assessment	Second assessment
	Trimester 1 2 3 Date_____	Trimester 1 2 3 Date_____
Pregnancy		
Motherhood		
Changes in self-image		
Mood swings		
Pregnancy and parenthood affecting personal family goals		
Husband-wife social and sexual relationships		
Stresses created by emotional and physical changes of this pregnancy		
Anxiety re labor and delivery		
Social and financial family stability re future plans for NB		
Past and present personality difficulties		
Fetus		
Father's awareness of, interest and attitude		

Nursing assessment—Antepartum—Page 3   Patient's name_____

	Yes	No	Trimester 1 2 3 Date_____	Yes	No	Trimester 1 2 3 Date_____
PLANS FOR DELIVERY						
Made plans for hospitalization						
Made arrangements for care of family at home						
Knows what to expect of hospital routine						
Knows signs of labor						
Knows what to expect during labor and delivery						
Knows what to expect PP						

	Yes	No	Trimester 1 2 3	Date____	Yes	No	Trimester 1 2 3	Date____
PLANS FOR NEWBORN								
Plans to breast feed								
Plans to bottle feed								
Adequate layette and equipment								
Plans to have help PP								
Knows what to expect of NB								
FAMILY PLANNING								
Knows methods of birth control								
Wants information on family planning								

What kind of help does family want from CHN?

_____

_____

_____

What kind of help does family want from CHN?

_____

_____

_____

SOURCE: Printed with permission from the Nursing Division, King County Health Department, 1000 Public Safety Building, Seattle, Washington.

APPENDIX 8-2

King County Health Department, Seattle, Washington, Nursing Assessment Guide: Postpartum

Patient's name_____

GRAV____PARA____ABORT____M.D._____

HOSPITAL____SIGNIFICANT MEDICAL HISTORY OF PREGNANCIES _____

Check items which best describe patient or complete with notation.

First assessment date____   Second assessment date____

Postpartum exam

Temp____

	Yes	No		Yes	No
BREASTS					
Physical appearance: Normal					
Engorgement					
Soreness					
Soft					
Cracked					
Redness					

Check items which best describe patient or complete with notation.

*First assessment date*_____   *Second assessment date*_____

Postpartum exam

	Yes	No		Yes	No
Caked					
Inverted					
Lactation: Leaking					
Filling					
Nursing					
Not nursing					
"Dry up" pills					

ABDOMEN

Fundus (firmness, position)

C-section (incision)

RECTOVAGINAL

Laceration					
Episiotomy: None					
Clean					
Healing					
Painful					
Hemorrhoids					
Other					

LOCHIA

Rubra					
Serosa					
Alba					
Clots					
No. pads per day					

VOIDING

No difficulty					
Anuria					
Dysuria					
Frequency					
Burning					

Check items which best describe patient or complete with notation.

*First assessment date*_____   *Second assessment date*_____

Postpartum exam

	Yes	No		Yes	No
BOWELS					
Constipated					
No difficulty					
Other					

*First assessment date*_____ *Second assessment date*_____

PERSONAL HEALTH PRACTICES (Describe what the patient is doing about the following.)

A. Care
   Bathing _____
   Peri-care _____
   Breast care _____
B. Rest _____
   Sleep _____
   Recreation _____
   Exercise and activity _____
C. Foundation garment _____
D. Diet—Type _____
   Breakfast _____
   Lunch _____
   Dinner _____
   Snacks _____
   Dislikes _____
   Fluid intake _____
   Comments _____

E. Sexual relations _____

PSYCHOSOCIAL (Describe mother's feeling or reaction to the following.)

Pregnancy _____

Labor _____

Delivery _____

Newborn _____

Motherhood _____

Family's reaction to labor, delivery, NB _____

Other _____

MEDICAL SUPERVISION	*Yes*	*No*		*Yes*	*No*
Medical appointments made					
Plan to keep					
Dental care up to date					

Patient's understanding of doctor's orders is _____

FAMILY PLANNING

Future family plans (method, problems) _____
What kind of help does family want from CHN? _____
_____
_____
_____
_____

SOURCE: Printed with permission from the Nursing Division, King County Health Department, 1000 Public Safety Building, Seattle, Washington.

APPENDIX 8-3

King County Health Department, Seattle, Washington, Nursing Assessment Guide: Newborn Assessment

_____ (Name of infant) _____ (Number) _____ (Birth weight) _____ (Birthdate)

Significant history of pregnancy _____

_____ (Name of doctor) _____ (Apgar score—time) _____ (Hospital)

Underline significant	*Date* SU check and make comments	*Date* SU check and make comments
GENERAL APPEARANCE		
Length____cm		
Cry, color, spontaneous activity, body symmetry, subcutaneous fat, skin tumor		
SKIN		
Jaundice, edema, rashes, petechiae, transparent, unusual pigmentation, bruises, desquamation, forcep mark, hematoma, hemangioma, milia		

Underline significant	Date SU check and make comments		Date SU check and make comments	
HEAD				
Circumference_____cm				
Bulging or nonpalpable fontanels, caput succedaneum, cephalhematoma, overriding suture, enlarged head				
EENT				
Low-set ears, cleft lip and palate, eye opacities, sunset eyes, epicanthus folds, thrush, nevus, asymmetry, discharge, patency of nose and ears, gross reaction to light and sound				
CHEST AND NECK				
Chest retracted, respiratory patterns, webbing or swelling of neck, engorged breasts, mastitis				
ABDOMEN AND NAVEL				
Distention, drainage from cord, umbilical hernia				
GENITALIA AND RECTUM				
Hydrocele, hypospadius, anal stenosis, phimosis, undescended testicle, clitoris enlargement, genital size, tags, milky or bloody vaginal discharge, pilonidal dimple, circumcision				
BACK				
Contour of spine, hip abduction, skin folds, dermal sinus				
EXTREMITIES				
Paralysis, symmetric creases, club feet, metatarsus varus, webbed toes, extra digits				
REFLEXES				
State quality of reflexes assessed:				

Underline significant	Date _____ SU check and make comments			Date _____ SU check and make comments		
Moro _____ Tonic _____ Grasp _____ Root and suck _____						
STOOLS AND VOIDING (Including caliber of urinary stream)						

_____   _____

(Name of infant)   (Number)

History and observation of family care of infant

Date_____

FAMILY INTERACTION

FEEDING

Breast and supplement

_____

Formula (amount, frequency, total 24-h intake and preparation)

_____

Solids

_____

SKIN CARE

_____

SLEEP PATTERN

_____

CRYING PATTERN

_____

MEDICAL SUPERVISION
Medical directions:
Appointment planned:
Appointment kept:

_____

UNDERSTANDING OF DOCTOR'S ORDERS (Nurse's perception)

SOURCE: Printed with permission from the Nursing Division, King County Health Department, 1000 Public Safety Building, Seattle, Washington.

REFERENCES

Alexander, M., & Brown, M. S. *Pediatric physical diagnosis for nurses.* New York: McGraw-Hill, 1974.

Bates, B. *A guide to physical examination* (2d ed.). Philadelphia: Lippincott, 1978.

Beall, L. The corrupt contract: Problems in conjoint therapy with parents and children. *American Journal of Orthopsychiatry,* January 1972, *42,* 1, 77–81.

Beavers, W. R. *Psychotherapy and growth: A family systems perspective.* New York: Brunner/Mazel, 1977.

Bloom, B. S. (Ed.), Englehart, M. D., Furst, E. J., Itill, W. H., & Krathwohl, D. R. *Taxonomy of educational objectives: Handbook I, cognitive domain.* New York: McKay, 1956.

Burns, K. R., & Johnson, P. J. *Health assessment in clinical practice.* Englewood Cliffs, N.J.: Prentice-Hall, 1980.

Dunn, H. *High level wellness.* Washington, D.C.: Mount Vernon Publishing Co., 1961.

Durand, M., & Prince, P. Nursing diagnosis: Process and decision. *Nursing Forum,* 1966, *5* (4), 50–64.

Freeman, R., & Lowe, M. (Directors). Richmond-Hopkins Cooperative Nursing Study. *The family coping index.* Richmond, Va.: Richmond Instructive Visiting Nurse Association and City Health Department and the Johns Hopkins School of Public Health, 1964.

Gordon, M. The concept of nursing diagnosis. *Nursing Clinics of North America,* September 1979, *14,* 487–495.

———. Nursing diagnoses and the diagnostic process. *American Journal of Nursing,* August 1976, *76,* 1298–1300.

Haley, J. Family therapy: A radical change. In J. Haley (Ed.), *Changing families: A family therapy reader.* New York: Grune & Stratton, 1971.

Kelly, H. S. The sense of an ending. *American Journal of Nursing.* November 1969, *69,* 2378–2381.

Krathwohl, D. R., Bloom, B. D., & Masia, B. B. *Taxonomy of educational objectives: Handbook II, affective domain.* New York: McKay, 1964.

Lewis, J., Beavers, R., Gossett, J. T., & Phillips, U.A. *No single thread: Psychological health in family systems.* New York: Brunner/Mazel. 1976.

Mager, R. *Preparing instructional objectives* (2d ed.). Belmont, Calif.: Fearon Publishers, 1975.

Mahoney, E. A., Verdisco, L., & Shortridge, L. *How to collect and record a health history.* New York: Lippincott, 1976.

Maluccio, A. N., & Marlow, W. The case for the contract. *Social Work,* January 1974, *19,* 28–36.

Mayers, M. Home visit—Ritual or therapy? *Nursing Outlook,* May 1973, *21,* 328–331.

McCain, F. Nursing by assessment—not intuition. *American Journal of Nursing,* April 1965, *65,* 82–84.

McPhetridge, L. M. Nursing history: One means to personalize care. *American Journal of Nursing,* January 1968, *68,* 68–75.

Otto, H. Criteria for assessing family strength. *Family Process,* September 1963, *2,* 329–338.

Pratt, L. *Family structure and effective health behavior: The energized family.* Boston: Houghton Mifflin, 1976.

Reilly, P. *Behavioral objectives in nursing: Evaluation of learner attainment.* New York: Appleton-Century-Crofts, 1975.

Sable, P. Differentiating between attachment and dependency in theory and practice. *Social Casework,* March 1979, *60,* 138–144.

Sana, J., & Judge, R. D. *Physical appraisal methods in nursing practice.* Boston: Little, Brown, 1975.

Seabury, B. A. The contract: Uses, abuses and limitations. *Social Work,* January 1976, *21,* 8, 39–45.

Sene, B. Termination in the student-patient relationship. *Perspectives in Psychiatric Care,* January 1969, *8,* 39–45.

Sherman, J., & Fields, S. *Guide to patient evaluation: History taking, physical examination and the problem-oriented method.* Flushing, N.Y.: Medical Examination Publishing Co., 1974.

Sills, G. Bias of therapists in family therapy. In S. Smoyak, *The psychiatric nurse as a family therapist.* New York: Wiley, 1975.

World Health Organization. Constitution of the world health organization. *Chronicle of the World Health Organization,* January 1947, *1,* 29–43.

SELECTED BIBLIOGRAPHY

Bailey, J. T., & Claus, K. E. *Decision making in nursing.* St. Louis: Mosby, 1975.

Bermosk, L. S., & Mordan, M. J. *Interviewing in nursing.* New York: Macmillan, 1964.

Blair, K. It's the patient's problem—and decision. *Nursing Outlook,* September 1971, *19,* 587–589.

Bloch, D. Some crucial terms in nursing: What do they really mean? *Nursing Outlook,* November 1974, *22,* 689–694.

Burgess, A., & Burns, J. Why patients seek care. *American Journal of Nursing,* February 1973, *73,* 314–316.

Byrne, M., & Thompson, L. F. *Key concepts for the study and practice of nursing.* St. Louis: Mosby, 1972.

Chambers, W. Nursing diagnosis. *American Journal of Nursing,* November 1962, *62,* 102–104.

Crawford, C. *Health and the family: A medical-sociological analysis.* New York: Macmillan, 1971.

Daubenmire, M. J., & King, K. Nursing process models: A systems approach. *Nursing Outlook,* August 1973, *21,* 512–517.

Fielo, S. B. *A summary of integrated nursing theory.* New York: McGraw-Hill, 1975.

Francis, G. M., & Munjas, B. A. *Manual of social psychologic assessment.* New York: Appleton-Century-Crofts, 1976.

Hamdi, M. E., & Hutelmyer, C. M. A study of the effectiveness of an assessment tool in the identification of nursing care problems. *Nursing Research,* July–August 1970, *19,* 354–359.

Hilger, E. E. Developing nursing outcome criteria. *Nursing Clinics of North America,* June 1974, *9,* 323–330.

Hymovich, D. P., & Barnard, M. U. (Eds.). *Family health care: Developmental and situational crises.* New York: McGraw-Hill, 1979.

———— & ————. *Family health care: General perspectives.* New York: McGraw-Hill, 1979.

Kanfer, F. H., & Goldstein, A. P. *Helping people change: A textbook of methods.* New York: Pergamon, 1975.

Knight, J. H. Applying nursing process in the community. *Nursing Outlook,* November 1974, *22,* 708–711.

La Monica, E. *The nursing process: A humanistic approach.* Menlo Park, Calif.: Addison-Wesley, 1979.

Laros, J. Deriving outcome criteria from a conceptual model. *Nursing Outlook,* May 1977, *25,* 333–336.

Little, D. E., & Carnevali, D. L. *Nursing care planning.* Philadelphia: Lippincott, 1976.

Mayeroff, M. *On caring.* New York: Harper & Row, 1971.

Mayers, M. *A systematic approach to the nursing care plan.* New York: Appleton-Century-Crofts, 1978.

Meister, S. B. Charting a family's developmental status for intervention and for the record. *Maternal Child Nursing,* January–February 1977, 43–48.

Mundinger, M. O. N., & Jauran, G. D. Developing a nursing diagnosis. *Nursing Outlook,* February 1975, *23,* 94–98.

Nehring, N., & Geach, B. Patients' evaluation of their care: Why they don't complain. *Nursing Outlook,* May 1973, *21,* 317–321.

Riehl, J., & Roy, C. *Conceptual models for nursing practice.* New York: Appleton-Century-Crofts, 1974.

Roberts, S. *Behavioral concepts and nursing throughout the life span.* Englewood Cliffs, N.J.: Prentice-Hall, 1978.

Ryan, B. J. Nursing care plans: A systems approach to developing criteria for planning and evaluation. *Journal of Nursing Administration,* May–June 1973, *3,* 50–57.

Sobol, E., & Robischon, R. *Family nursing: A study guide.* Saint Louis: Mosby, 1975.

Tapia, J. A. The nursing process in family health. *Nursing Outlook,* April 1972, *20,* 267–270.

Yura, H., & Walsh, M. B. *Human needs and the nursing process.* New York: Appleton-Century-Crofts, 1978.

———— & ————. *The nursing process: Assessing, planning, implementing, evaluating.* New York: Appleton-Century-Crofts, 1978.

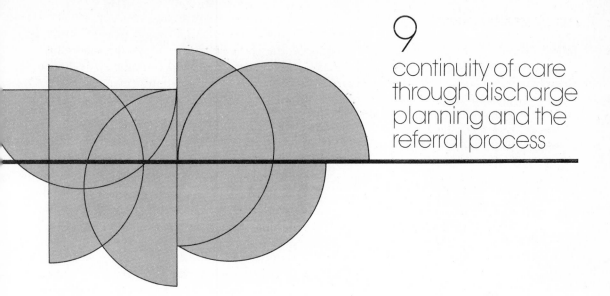

9
continuity of care
through discharge
planning and the
referral process

Continuity of care is a process through which a client's ongoing health care needs are assessed, planned for, and met. It necessitates comprehensive services, resource coordination, and close collaboration with the client and family. Integral components of continuity of care are discharge planning and referral.

Discharge planning is the preparation involved to ensure that a client's health care needs will continue to be met as he or she moves from one resource to another. Resource utilization is facilitated through the use of the referral process.

DISCHARGE PLANNING

Discharge planning takes into account the setting which the client is entering, the needs evidenced by the client, and resources that meet these needs. It is usually thought of in terms of a client being discharged from a hospital or an extended care facility. In this text, the term *discharge planning* is used in a broader sense and extends to clients leaving other health care settings, such as the home of a relative, group educational experiences, and clinics.

In planning for a client's discharge needs, the nurse looks at the resources and services that might help the client to function effec-

tively in the new environment. The setting will have a major impact on the health care needs evidenced by the client. Take, for example, 70-year-old Mrs. Flowers.

Mrs. Flowers's cooking, cleaning, laundry, medical, and personal needs were taken care of while she was in the hospital. Now she is ready to return home, where she is responsible for these activities of daily living but unable to handle all of them by herself. Options to assist her, such as homemaker services, transportation, friendly visitors, Meals-on-Wheels, the local Visiting Nurse Association, the help of a friend or relative, or a more supervised living situation, should be explored and planned for before Mrs. Flowers leaves the hospital setting.

The discharge planning needs of many clients are complex and long-term. Planning for discharge should start the day a client begins using a health care resource. Many health care resources, especially hospitals, are instituting multidisciplinary discharge planning teams and procedures and are developing mechanisms to evaluate client discharge needs. The discharge questionnaire in Figure 9-1 was designed to facilitate assessment of clients' needs prior to their leaving a formal health care environment, but it could be used in various settings. The information asked for on this questionnaire assists the nurse in identifying multiple client needs. It examines psychosocial as well as biological aspects of functioning and emphasizes preventive health care needs in addition to curative services. From the data obtained from this questionnaire, hospital personnel and community health nurses would have baseline information essential for determining further nursing interventions. Intervention strategies might include health education in the home setting, home care and rehabilitation services, or referral to other resources. When one is planning for client discharge needs, it is extremely important to discern if the client is already involved with other community agencies. Otherwise, there may be duplication of efforts and uncoordinated plans of action. The process through which the nurse assists the client to utilize resources and ensures coordination of care is labeled the *referral process*.

THE REFERRAL PROCESS DEFINED

The *referral process* is a systematic problem-solving approach involving a series of actions that help clients to utilize resources for the purpose of resolving needs. Clients may be either individuals or groups who require assistance from others in order to achieve their maximum level of functioning. The community health nurse's major goals for initiating a referral are to promote high-level wellness and to enhance self-care capabilities. Referral is a unique and important process; completing a form or telling a client to contact a community agency is only one small aspect of this process. The referral process demands knowledge, skill, and experience to be implemented effectively. Referral is an integral part of comprehensive, continuous client care and is essential to community health nursing practice (Coombs, 1976, p. 122).

A *resource* is defined as an agency, group, or individual that assists a client in meeting a need. Resources provide multiple services and have varying requirements for usage. The community health nurse needs to understand what community resources have to offer, as clients may or may not be aware of them or know how to use them.

Health care resources can be described as formal and informal. *Formal* health care resources exist primarily for the provision of health care services. They include hospitals, extended-care facilities, skilled nursing homes, health departments, and the offices of private health care practitioners. Increasingly, it is being found that coordination between these resources has improved the quality of care to clients, as well as reduced the amount of time spent in institutionalized, formal health care facilities (McCarthy, 1976; and Quinn, 1975).

Informal health care resources provide health services but do not exist primarily for this purpose. These resources can be relatives in the client's home, service organizations, and self-help groups. They are scattered throughout the community, are minimally coordinated, and are often more difficult to recognize than formal resources. An example of an informal health care resource is the local Lion's Club, which provides free ophthalmologic examinations and eyeglasses to children in the community who could not otherwise obtain them. It provides a health care service, but its primary function is not health related. There are many such organizations and individuals within the community; these resources are important to the provision of care for individuals, families, and populations at risk.

The community health nurse will make referrals to, and receive referrals from health care resources. Referrals may be categorized in many ways. In this text, referrals are discussed as (1) primary or secondary, (2) formal or informal, and (3) simple or complex. These categories give more specific information about the referral, including its initiator, the extent of contact made with the resource, and the level of difficulty.

Primary and Secondary Referrals

Referrals are either primary or secondary, depending on the referral initiator. *A primary referral* is initiated by the client. An example would be Mrs. Smith suggesting marriage counseling for herself and her husband. Community health nursing services are frequently initiated because the client requests the service. *A secondary referral* is initiated by someone other than the client. An example would be the community health nurse suggesting to Mrs. Smith that she and her husband may want to seek marriage counseling. Primary referrals are often readily accepted and implemented by clients because they perceive a need for assistance. However, secondary referrals are used extensively by the community health nurse with much success.

Formal and Informal Referrals

Referrals are categorized as formal or informal based on the extent of contact made with the resource. An *informal referral* involves discussion of a resource between two or more persons without contact being made on behalf of the client with the resource. An informal referral is usually the initial step to a formal one.

A *formal referral* involves contact being made with a resource, generally to initiate service procurement. The contact can be made by the client or someone on behalf of the client. Formal referrals are generally made only with client permission and are often processed through a system of standardized forms and procedures.

Simple and Complex Referrals

A *simple referral* is one in which the referral process reaches resolution on the initial attempt. A *complex referral* is one in which the process does not reach resolution of the need on the initial attempt. That is, if any step in the process must be redone, the process becomes complex. Even though many referrals are complex, it is not impossible to implement all of the actions needed to resolve client problems and concerns. It means that steps in the process will need to be reworked. The difference between simple and complex referrals becomes clearer when the referral process flow chart (see Figure 9-3) is examined.

Basic Principles of Referral

Wolff (1962) delineated some basic principles to take into consideration when one is helping clients to use the referral process. These principles are listed below:

1. *There should be merit in the referral.* The referral should meet the needs and objectives

The staff on (unit name) wants to make your return to the community as easy for you as possible. The nurse who is primarily responsible for helping you plan your discharge is _____. He or she will help you and your family reach any resources you may need for your health care at home. There are many agencies, including home care, which assist people in the community with health care problems.

Please complete the following questions with your family as soon as you feel able. Your discharge nurse will be in contact with you within a few days of your admission.

Data #1

When you get home

1. With whom will you live? _____

2. Will they be able to help with your care if needed? _____

3. Will you have difficulty getting around your home—stairs, small bathroom, low bed, safety problems, to the telephone, to shower, or bathtub? _____

4. Will you have any problems in getting any of the following—transportation, food, medicine, heat, place to stay, child care, pet care, water supply? _____

5. Will you need any of these to function at home—wheelchair, brace, cane, walker, crutches, special equipment? _____

6. How much of the following will you be able to do? (Please mark appropriate column.)

	Independent	*With family*	*Unable to do*
Turning in bed			
Bathing			
Dressing			
Eating			
Sitting			
Standing			
Transfers to tub			
Transfers to toilet			
Walking			

Data #2

1. Have you had a problem with any of these areas recently?
   a. Eyes/ears
   b. Mouth/throat/teeth
   c. Skin
   d. Lungs/breathing
   e. Breasts
   f. Heart/blood vessels
   g. Stomach/bowel
   h. Bladder/kidneys/urine
   i. Genitals
   j. Mental status
   k. Nerves/muscles

2. Will you have difficulty getting to your physician, nurse, or therapist often enough to have these checked?_____

Data #3

Please mark any of the following areas that you would like to know more about:

1. Your disease/illness/accident
   a. What caused it
   b. What can be done to prevent a repeat
   c. How to recognize a repeat
   d. How it will affect you later

2. Your medication
   a. What it does
   b. How much to take
   c. When to take it
   d. What side effects to be aware of

FIGURE 9-1 Discharge questionnaire. (*Adapted from M. Stone. Discharge planning guide. American Journal of Nursing, August 1979, 66, 1445–1447.*)

3. Your treatments, procedures, or exercises
   a. What they do for you
   b. How to do them
   c. How often to do them
   d. What difficulties to be aware of

4. Supplies or equipment you'll use at home
   a. What it does
   b. When to use it
   c. How to get more or to get repairs

5. Your nutrition
   a. How it affects you
   b. Special diets—how much to eat, when to eat, what to avoid
   c. How much and what to drink

6. Preventive health practices
   a. How to examine your breasts
   b. Pap smears
   c. Birth control
   d. Effect of cigarettes
   e. Effect of alcohol and drugs
   f. Dental health
   g. Seat belts
   h. Immunizations (yourself or children)
   i. Exercise

7. Other _____

Data #4
1. Which of these agencies are you involved with?
   a. VNA/Home Health
   b. Senior Citizens
   c. Vocational Rehabilitation
   d. Social Welfare
   e. Planned Parenthood
   f. Mental Health Agency
   g. Diet Club
   h. Alcoholics Anonymous
   i. Cancer Society
   j. Ostomy Club
   k. Meals-on-Wheels
   l. Diabetes Association
   m. Dialysis Association
   n. MS Society
   o. MD Society
   p. Association for the Blind
   q. Other_____

2. Please mark any of the areas that you would especially like to discuss with your discharge nurse.
   a. Finances, jobs
   b. Drugs, alcohol
   c. Caring for children or elderly relatives
   d. Emotional or nerve problem
   e. Sexuality
   f. Family or marital relationships
   g. Grieving
   h. School or work
   i. Problem, retirement
   j. Spiritual needs
   k. Legal problems
   l. Other_____

STOP HERE. YOUR DISCHARGE NURSE WILL HELP YOU COMPLETE THE FORM. Ask to see him or her if you haven't met yet, especially if you think you might go home soon.

Assessments (To be done by RN and patient)
1. Will there be a need for help with physical care at home?

2. Will there be a need for a nurse or therapist at home to assess physical status, disease process, or exercise and therapy?

3. Will the patient or family need more health education about any of the areas above (Data #3), either during hospitalization or at home?

4. Will the patient or family need more information or assistance with any of the psychosocial areas listed in Data #4?

Plan (To be done by patient and nurse together)
Consider the four assessments above. If there are *no* yes responses, proceed to section B and complete. If there are any yes responses, you *must* select either part 1 or part 2 of section A before completing section B.
A. 1. No referral necessary, but must have further education before discharge regarding _____

   2. Refer to: (see above list of agencies)

B. 1. Equipment or supplies to leave with patient _____

   2. Transfer plan _____

   3. Medical follow-up _____

   4. Surgical follow-up _____

of the client and should be necessary. Before referring the client to community resources, it is extremely important to assess what resources are available in the client's own environment. Often it will be found that family, friends, and neighbors can do as much or more for the client than can other community resources.

2. *The referral should be practical.* The client should be able to utilize the referral in an efficient, effective manner. It should not be a waste of time, money, and effort on behalf of the client, the resource, or the referral facilitator.

3. *The referral should be individualized to the client.* A referral that meets the needs of one client may not meet the needs of another. That is why it is essential to assess the individual needs and concerns of clients before decisions about the appropriateness of a referral are made. For example, some clients can learn very well in a group setting whereas others cannot.

4. *The client should have the right to say no to the referral.* This principle acknowledges the client's right to self-determination. The client has the right to refuse a referral, unless legal authority dictates otherwise. Cases of law are the exception and will vary from state to state. An example of a law that could require the community health nurse to refer a client without his or her consent is a child abuse law that mandates reporting suspected child abuse and neglect cases.

In order for the client's right to self-determination to be protected, the client must be aware of the referral. Referrals are sometimes made for clients without their knowledge or consent, as in the case of many postpartum clients who are referred by the hospital to the local health department for nursing service. This is not a wise practice and violates the client's right to self-determination. If the nurse makes contact with a client and finds out that the client was not aware of the referral and does not want it, the situation can be awkward. The nurse should explain the reason for the referral, the services she or he can provide, and apologize for any inconvenience to the client. Sometimes clients do not accept a referral only because they are not aware of the services offered by the resource.

At times, individuals are referred without their knowledge or consent because the referring agent considers them a threat to their own safety or the safety of others. Unless legal authority intervenes, the person still is not obligated to accept the referral.

Refusal of a referral may be difficult for the nurse to accept, especially if the referral appears to be helpful to the client. However, the client's right to self-determination must be respected. The nurse should not become discouraged or take the blame if the client does not accept a referral. If the client is aware of the services offered by a community resource, she or he may initiate a self-referral in the future. Imposing services on the client does not help; it only causes frustration for the nurse as well as the client.

Sources of Referral for the Community Health Nurse

Nurses initiate and receive referrals in the community health setting. Referrals may be interresource, intraresource, or self-referrals. *Interresource referrals* are referrals made from one resource to another. These referrals can involve either the community health nurse referring a client to a resource, or a resource referring a client to the community health nurse. Examples of interresource referrals are the community health nurse referring a client to a low-cost dental clinic for dental care, or a community mental health psychiatric nurse referring a client to the health department for nursing service. Interresource nurse-to-nurse referrals are common.

Intraresource referrals are made within the resource itself. These referrals may be nurse to nurse, nurse to other agency personnel, or agency personnel to nurse. Examples of intra-resource referrals are the health department clinic nurse referring a family to the community health nurse who makes home visits in the family's geographic area for nutritional teaching; the field community health nurse referring a family to the sanitarian for a concern they have about the safety of their well water; or the health department's chronic disease physician referring a family to the field nurse for teaching about tuberculosis control and follow-up.

Self-referrals involve the clients' referring themselves to a resource for service. The client may self-refer to most resources. However, some resources will request an agency referral on behalf of the client, because they do not consider self-referrals valid or because they require a needs assessment before monies are spent on health care. Service organizations frequently require that this assessment be done by the community health nurse because they believe that only nurses can identify physical health problems. At times, community health nurses suggest that these policies be changed because there are other health care professionals in the community, such as teachers, counselors, or social workers, who are just as qualified as the nurse to make decisions about some of the health care needs of clients. For example, it does not take a nurse to identify dental caries; teachers or school counselors can assess for dental problems and are often more aware of a family's financial difficulties than the nurse, who may only be in the school setting one day a week.

Answering a Referral

Answering referrals is an important part of the referral process. If referrals are not answered, or answered incompletely or tardily, the referral source may become discouraged and not send further referrals. Prompt, complete, and courteous answering of a referral helps to establish and maintain good working relationships and facilitates continuity of client care.

Referrals should be answered as soon as possible; ideally within a week after they have been received. The nurse should include in the communication with the referring agency comments on the needs that were recognized by the referring agency, as well as current assessment data, nursing diagnoses, and future actions and plans. If the client and nurse decide that nursing service should be continued, the referring agency should be given this information.

REFERRAL RESOURCES

The community health nurse must be familiar with both formal and informal health care resources in the community in order to work effectively with clients. Health professionals in the community and other community health nurses are good sources of information about area resources. Frequently, compilations of local resources are done by groups such as united community services, chambers of commerce, departments of social service, and health departments. Major service organizations, such as associations for retarded citizens, will compile resources specific to the groups they represent. City offices and planning commissions will also have local resource information. Various compilations should be sought out and utilized, but before referring a client, the nurse should independently explore the resource. An ongoing resource file in which resources are listed both alphabetically and by service should be maintained by the nurse. Resources that are frequently used, or used with success, may be colored-coded or tabbed for easy accessibility. It is necessary that resource information be clear, accurate, and concise.

The following information is essential for the nurse to know about a resource and is readily kept on file cards or in a loose-leaf notebook: (1) name of resource (include address, phone number, and name and title of person in charge), (2) purpose and services, (3) eligibility (who may use the resource), (4) application procedure, (5) fees, (6) office hours and days, and (7) geographic area served. Figure 9-2 is an example of what a compilation of this information could look like. In addition, data on client response to utilization of the resource should be kept.

The nurse should also be aware of specific information that a resource requests of a client when it provides service. Information frequently requested by resources includes the following:

National Foundation—March of Dimes
Payne County Office

    Address: 20100 Maplewood, Mio, MI 47235
    Phone: 811-2110 (Area 516)
    Person in charge: Mrs. Nellie Scott, Director

Purpose and services: Through referral and direct aid, assistance is provided in the areas of prenatal care, genetic counseling, diagnosis, and treatment. Offers prevention and treatment services for clients who have congenital malformations or birth defects through research, direct patient services, and public education. Sponsors scholarships in related health fields.

Eligibility: No restrictions.

Application procedure: Referrals by private physicians, public health clinics, or health departments.
Individuals are encouraged to contact the office for further information.

Fees: None

Office hours: 9 A.M. to 3 P.M., Tuesday–Saturday

Geographic area served: Payne County

FIGURE 9-2 Resource information.

TABLE 9-1   Resource Grid

Service needed	Types	Resource
Food	1. Emergency	1. Department of Social Services, Salvation Army, local churches, American Red Cross, Goodfellows, Women, Infants, and Children Program (WIC)
	2. Low-cost foods	2. Food stamps, food coops, school lunch programs
	3. Counseling	3. Expanded nutrition program, Health Department
Financial assistance	1. Emergency and short term	1. Department of Social Services, Salvation Army, Goodfellows, Lion's Club, Traveler's Aid, Volunteers of America, Kiwanis
	2. Long term	2. Department of Social Service, Social Security Administration, Veteran's Administration
Housing	1. Emergency	1. Catholic Social Services, Jewish Action League, Families United for Community Service, Department of Social Service, American Red Cross, Salvation Army, local churches, domestic violence facilities
	2. Public (low cost)	2. Housing Commission, Department of Social Service

SOURCE: Adapted from the University of Michigan School of Nursing, Family and Community Health Nursing. *Resource Grid.* Ann Arbor: University of Michigan School of Nursing, 1979.

1. Name, address, and telephone number of the client

2. Client age, sex, and marital status

3. Names and birthdates of family members and others living in the household

4. Medical care source and health history

5. Financial status and records

6. Resources with whom the client is presently working

7. Reason for seeking referral

A grid which shows frequently used resources can be a very valuable reference when one is visiting clients in the community setting. A grid that includes service areas and specific resources is especially helpful. An example of such a grid is presented in Table 9-1. It is not all-inclusive, and resources will vary from area to area, but it does illustrate how a service resource grid can be organized.

STEPS OF THE REFERRAL PROCESS

The referral process is a systematic, problem-solving approach which involves a number of client and nurse actions (Atwood, 1971). Figure 9-3 depicts the steps involved in successfully implementing a referral. These steps are also listed below. It will be found, when helping a client obtain needed assistance from community resources, that the process is circular. That is, as data are obtained in one step, other steps may need to be repeated. It is crucial to remember that these steps are interconnected and interrelated.

The following are the basic steps of the referral process:

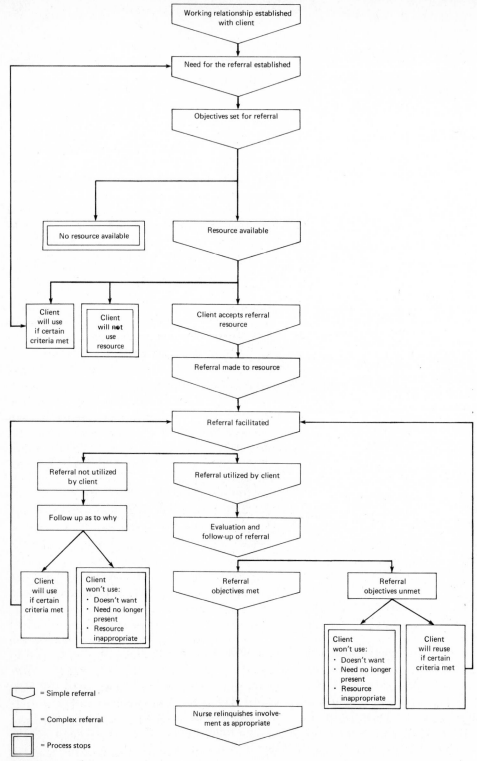

FIGURE 9-3 The referral process.

1. Establish a working relationship with the client

2. Establish the need for a referral

3. Set objectives for the referral

4. Explore resource availability

5. Client decides to use or not use referral

6. Make referral to resource

7. Facilitate referral

8. Evaluate and follow up

Client participation throughout the process is essential. The community health nurse guides the client through the process by facilitating informed decision making, determining client needs and objectives, exploring alternatives for need resolution, assisting the client to utilize resources, and evaluating the results of the entire process. The client is encouraged to be independent whenever possible.

Establish a Working Relationship with the Client

The referral process evolves after a working relationship with the client has been established. This relationship involves the formation of trust between the nurse and the client. This trust facilitates cooperation; it may be developed almost immediately or take place over a long period of time. While establishing the relationship, the nurse is able to gather data necessary for helping the client to make decisions about her or his health and welfare needs. Clients in crisis often initially establish a working relationship more quickly, because of the immediacy of their needs, than do other clients.

In many cases, the referral process will commence as this relationship develops to its potential. If referrals are necessitated early in the relationship, the nurse should proceed with

caution to be sure that sufficient data have been collected to determine if the referral is appropriate.

Establish the Need for a Referral

The community health nurse should utilize the nursing process to help the client to identify when health care needs necessitate referral. Often clients require assistance from the community health nurse to recognize referral needs. The nurse should aid the client in looking at referral alternatives; however, the client must recognize the need for the referral before it is made.

When establishing a need for referral, it is important to discriminate between problems the community health nurse can and cannot handle. For example, there are some budgeting problems that can be dealt with by a community health nurse and others that cannot. A community health nurse can help a family to analyze how its members can obtain the most for their food dollars by discussing such things as meal planning, low-cost meals, and inexpensive sources of protein. On the other hand, if the family is having difficulty with creditors, the family is usually referred to a credit-counseling resource.

The nurse needs to be honest with the client about what his or her needs appear to be. The client may not be aware of a need, such as immunizations to prevent communicable disease, until the nurse raises his or her consciousness about it. There may be situations in which the nurse finds it difficult to share perceived client needs, especially when the client is using denial to relieve anxiety. This is often the case when psychosocial problems such as marital crises exist. Frequently it helps in these situations to assist the client in seeing that symptoms of stress are evident and that stress will only be relieved when steps are taken to resolve the actual problem. Often, asking if the client wants to continue living as he or she is can facilitate discussion about real pressures being experienced. Making a referral in these situations with "a hidden agenda" is usually not helpful. Clients must be ready to deal with their problems before they will continue to use a referral resource. Often, honest confrontation can be very motivating when clients have difficulty taking action. This is particularly true when a caring relationship has been established between the client and the community health nurse.

The community health nurse and client should thoroughly assess the need for referral. Unnecessary or unwanted referrals are costly, often strain relationships between referring agencies, and can adversely affect nurse-client relationships. Once the need for a referral has been established, the nurse and client should establish objectives for the services required and should look at which resources in the community can best meet the client's needs.

Set Objectives for the Referral

What the client would like to see accomplished, tempered with what is realistically feasible, combine to determine the objectives for the referral. The nurse can help the client to be realistic in resource expectations, but the decision about specific objectives to be achieved should be made by the client. It is often helpful to write out objectives with the client in behavioral terms such as "Mrs. Black will contact the Department of Social Services in regard to obtaining food stamps by March 30, 1981." An integral part of setting objectives for the referral is deciding on what services are necessary from the referral source, as well as on a time frame for obtaining these services. The nurse should be careful when setting objectives not to set more than what is reasonable to be accomplished within a specified time period.

In this phase of the referral process, you may find that the client expects more than an agency can offer. An agency does not solve the client's problems, but it helps clients to help themselves. For example, Mrs. Quinn, a single mother, wanted counseling only for her 14-year-old daughter, who planned to drop out of school and marry her 21-year-old boyfriend. Mrs. Quinn thought a counseling agency could "talk some sense into her." The community health nurse assisted Mrs. Quinn in seeing that a family counseling agency helps a family to deal with its problems rather than assuming responsibilities for them. Joint counseling sessions arranged through the local Family and Neighborhood Counseling Center helped both mother and daughter to communicate together more effectively and to understand each other's concerns and needs. These sessions also helped the family to develop a pattern of functioning that facilitated family problem solving and decision making.

Explore Resource Availability

A source of aid must be available before a referral can be made. An appropriate resource is one that can meet the client's needs and objectives and is available, acceptable, and accessible to the client. If more than one appropriate resource exists, the client should be allowed to choose between them. If no resource is available, the referral objectives may need to be redefined or a resource developed. Many times, resources in the community will reconsider the services they provide to clients, especially if the community health nurse acts as an advocate for certain services.

Client Decides to Use or Not Use Referral

The client can say yes, no, or maybe when considering a referral. If the client says yes, the referral process continues. If the client says no or maybe, the nurse should explore with the client the reasons why. If the client does not want the referral under any condition, the right to self-determination must be respected. If the client would utilize a referral if certain criteria were met, the nurse may be able to assist the client in meeting these criteria. For example, a client might say that she would utilize a referral to the health department immunization clinic for her 2-year-old if transportation could be arranged to the clinic. The nurse may be able to help this client obtain transportation services from other community resources. If a client continues to place conditions on referral utilization, the nurse and client should take a close look at the reasons behind these conditions. It is possible that the client really does not want the referral but fears saying no.

It may be found that clients do not want to use one resource to meet a health care need but are willing to utilize another resource. An example of this is Mrs. Schlosser.

Mrs. Schlosser was an elderly client who was eligible for food stamps but would not apply for them. She viewed food stamps as charity and stated, "I do not accept welfare." The community health nurse was frustrated because Mrs. Schlosser's diet was inadequate, largely for financial reasons. Discussing the food stamp program with Mrs. Schlosser did not change her mind about using food stamps. Thus, the nurse explored alternatives with her. Because she wanted to eat better, she was receptive to learning about how to prepare low-cost, nutritious meals at home and was also interested in applying for a reduced cost, Meals-on-Wheels program in which she would pay for her meals. Mrs. Schlosser had refused a referral for food stamps, but she and the nurse were able to develop alternatives that helped to meet her nutritional needs.

Referral Made to a Resource

When the nurse is referring a client to a resource, the referral content should be specific, comprehensive, and reflect the client's objectives for the referral (Coombs, 1976, p. 126). The appropriate forms should be filled out

and procedures followed: referral information should be given out only with client consent, unless legally dictated otherwise. Clients usually do not hesitate to sign a release of information form when they have made a decision that they need a referral. The correct procedure for contacting the resource must also be followed. The referral is made formal at this point; if an appointment is necessary, it should be made. Either the client or nurse may be the contact person; the client should be encouraged, however, to be as independent as possible in contacting the resource.

An example of a referral form used by one local health department to refer clients to another resource is presented in Figure 9-4. This form includes essential referral information, such as data about the person making the referral, the individual or family being referred, the reason for the referral, summary of the client's situation, resources being used by the client, a statement on whether or not the client is aware of the referral, and a place for the receiving resource to share information with the referral agency.

Often, resources request that clients bring certain types of information with them to their first appointment. If clients are not aware of this requirement, they may have to return to the resource with the information or may be denied service. Returning to a resource takes additional time, effort, and money. It may present a barrier to the client in utilizing the referral.

Facilitate the Referral

Facilitating a referral involves preparing the client for the use of community services, as well as identifying and overcoming barriers to the utilization of these services. Throughout the process, the community health nurse evaluates the client's responses to the referral in order to determine if changes need to be made to effect client involvement. It is important to

OAKLAND COUNTY DEPARTMENT OF HEALTH

1200 North Telegraph Road
Pontiac, Michigan 48053
Telephone 858-1280

27725 Greenfield
Southfield, Michigan 48075
Telephone 424-7000

REFERRAL FORM

TO _____ FROM: _____

ADDRESS _____

☐ PONTIAC OFFICE

_____

☐ SOUTHFIELD OFFICE

Attention: _____ Telephone # _____ Date _____

REGARDING _____ Aware of referral? ☐ Yes ☐ No

ADDRESS _____ Telephone # _____

FAMILY ROSTER (Names, birthdate, relationship)

REASON FOR REFERRAL

SITUATION

(over)

KNOWN MEDICAL, AGENCY, COMMUNITY RESOURCES

REPLY REQUESTED: ☐ No ☐ Yes (see back)

Continuation of situation:

Agency reply to Oakland County Health Department

_____
(Signature)

Date _____

FIGURE 9-4 Sample referral form. *(Used by permission of the Nursing Division, Oakland County Health Department, Pontiac, Mich.)*

remember that client motivation is critical; if the client is not motivated to make the referral work, the referral process will probably not be successful. Barriers that decrease client motivation are discussed later in this chapter.

Evaluation and Follow-Up

Ongoing evaluation and follow-up is probably the most crucial step in the referral process. Effective evaluation of the referral process encompasses looking at how well client needs are being met, as well as the client's reactions to the services being received. In evaluating, the nurse must realize that there are times when a referral is not or was not effective. However, this judgment should not be made quickly. It will be found that some clients need support and encouragement, especially if their problems are not resolved immediately. The case of Mr. Connant is an example.

Mr. Connant decided that he was not going back to the mental health clinic for counseling after his first visit because the clinic counselor "did nothing but talk." In evaluating this situation, the nurse realized that she needed to discuss more specifically with Mr. Connant his expectations of counseling along with the need for him to share his feelings about his first session with the counselor at the clinic. Supportive assistance by the nurse facilitated Mr. Connant's return to the mental health center. Later, he expressed gratitude for the nurse's encouragement because the counseling was helping him to work through many of the issues that had been troubling him.

During evaluation, the client should be helped to look at why the referral was necessary and anticipatory guidance should be used in preparing the client to handle similar situations in the future. If it is seen that a client evidences the same problem over and over, the nurse and client should thoroughly assess why this is happening. Usually in these situations it is found that client problems are not being diagnosed completely. For example, repeated need for emergency food orders should be a clue that the client is having difficulty managing his or her budget. This could be a result of having a too-limited income or of not knowing how to allocate the funds that are available. Emergency food orders will not solve either of these problems on a long-term basis. If the client is not helped to explore other options, he or she may experience a crisis in the future which is difficult to resolve.

Probably the hardest part of the evaluation phase is realizing when it is time for the community health nurse to relinquish involvement with the client. This is an especially difficult task when the client and nurse have developed a strong, positive working relationship; termination in these situations provokes uneasy feelings within both the nurse and the client (see Chapter 8). Usually a client is ready to function independently when she or he can identify personal health care needs, take initiative to contact health care resources, and take action to resolve health care problems. If the client does not demonstrate these behaviors or demonstrates them only when the community health nurse is not available, the nurse-client relationship should be closely examined, as it may be fostering an unhealthy dependency.

BARRIERS TO THE UTILIZATION OF THE REFERRAL PROCESS

For each resource and each client, the nurse must identify the barriers that adversely affect the utilization of referral services. Barriers involve individual and resource components.

For example, an agency may have high fees for services (a resource barrier) which the client is unable to afford (a client barrier). In this case, fees are both a resource barrier and a client barrier. Some common resource and client barriers are briefly described below.

Resource Barriers

Attitudes of Health Care Professionals

Clients are quick to sense the attitudes of health care personnel in community resources. If clients are not treated with respect and courtesy, they are hesitant to use the resource again. Short, nonspecific answers given to a client's questions, minimal interchange with the client on an informal level, and conveying frustration when clients ask questions are a few examples of behaviors that foster negative reactions when clients are using community resources.

Physical Accessibility of Resource

Clients are less likely to use resources that are difficult to reach than those that are not. Once a resource is outside walking distance, other means of transportation must be found. Public transportation is sparse in this country. Even if the family has a car, the car may not be available at the time of the resource appointment. The problem is greatly magnified if the resource is at such a distance that the client must make arrangements for overnight stays in order to utilize the services it offers. Overnight stays often necessitate making arrangements for the care of small children or other members of the family, and they can be very costly to the client.

Cost of Resource Services

How much a client can or is willing to pay for a health service is an individual matter. Any cost at all may be more than a client can pay if income is minimal. If the service is not absolutely necessary or critical to the client's activities of daily living, the cost may be viewed as too high even if the client can afford the service. On the other hand, if the client places a high priority on receiving a given service, he or she may not object to paying even very high fees.

Client Barriers

Priorities

If the need is not of high priority for the client, he or she may not become actively involved in utilizing the referral services. If the client considers other needs to be higher priority, the nurse should assist him or her in meeting these needs first. For example, it may be more important for the family to care for an ill family member than to take a child to the well-baby clinic for immunizations; or if the family is having difficulty meeting its basic needs of food, clothing, and shelter, preventive health care serivces may not be viewed as a priority.

Motivation

If the client is not highly motivated to work on a need, it is not likely that much will be done by the client toward meeting that need. An integral part of client motivation is the concept of *awareness vs. readiness.* The fact that the client is aware of a need does not mean that he or she is ready to act on the need. If a differentiation is not made between awareness and readiness, the nurse may feel responsible for the failure of the client to follow through on a referral. Once it is established that the client is not ready to act on a need and the resultant referral, the nurse can help the client to prioritize the needs upon which he or she is ready to act. A good example of awareness vs. readiness is a client who acknowledges that his house needs to be cleaned, but after numerous nursing visits, much discussion, and ample time, the house is still not cleaned. The client is aware of the need but is not ready to act on it.

Previous Experience with Resources

If a client has not had a positive experience in utilizing a resource in the past, she or he may be hesitant to use this resource again or to utilize other community resources. In these situations, it is important to acknowledge the client's feelings as well as to explain ways to make further contacts with community services more meaningful. *Complaints about resources can be entirely justified.* However, it will be found that some clients were not ready to make changes when they used a community service the first time; hence, they have a negative view of the service because their problems were not resolved. This is frequently the case when clients have psychosocial difficulties.

Lack of Knowledge about Available Resources

Clients need to know about resources before they will use them. A key role of the community health nurse is to help clients learn about health care services in the community. Lack of knowledge about resources is a major barrier to the utilization of health care services.

Lack of Understanding of the Need for a Referral

Clients who do not understand the need for a referral frequently do not take action to obtain referral services. This is often true of families who neglect to immunize their children. Many people know that children need "baby shots" but do not understand why. These people will be more likely to follow through on a consistent basis in obtaining immunizations if they know the purpose for receiving immunizations and the consequences of not obtaining adequate protection against communicable diseases.

Client Self-Image

If clients do not have a positive self-image, they may be hesitant to seek care, and they may view themselves as unworthy of such care. The nurse should acknowledge these feelings and develop intervention strategies which will help clients to increase self-esteem.

Cultural Factors

Every culture has definite beliefs regarding health care practices. Resources may not be used if they violate these practices and beliefs. In Arab cultures, for example, women are generally not allowed to leave their homes or immediate neighborhoods without a male escort. Thus, health care services are better utilized by these women if they are located in a neighborhood facility. Within any culture, it will also be found that there is individual variation in how persons respond to the utilization of health care services. That is why it is so important to comprehensively assess strengths, needs, and concerns of each family unit. Lindstrom (1975), studying 30 Mexican-American families, demonstrated that even though the families in her study had a number of shared characteristics, there were also differences which influenced use or nonuse of child health services. Characteristics in common centered on family relationships; these relationships were strong, male-dominated, and extended, with an emphasis on maintaining privacy. In addition, all the families in her study had a minimal income, lived in poor neigborhoods, and many had had little formal education (Lindstrom, 1975, p. 757). Mothers who kept appointments, however, did differ from those who did not. These mothers had to assume more responsibility and independence than mothers who were poor users of child health services. They were likely to be or to have been the head of the household and have been socialized outside the state of Texas. These mothers also reported that they had transportation available and that they utilized either prenatal or child health services because they wanted to be sure that everything was all right. Nonuser mothers tended to live in a nuclear family, to have been socialized in Texas, and to see a doctor only when their children were ill (Lindstrom, 1975, p. 759).

Financial

Many clients do not use community resources because they cannot afford the services offered by these resources. The near-poor client—one who does not qualify for welfare assistance—especially has difficulty paying for the high cost of health care (Skinner, German, Shapiro, Chase, and Zauber, 1978). It is a real challenge for the community health nurse not only to find resources that will assist these clients but also to locate these at-risk individuals. Often, they are unknown to the health care delivery system and only receive needed health care when services are brought to them.

Transportation

Lack of transportation is a major barrier to the utilization of health care services. Increasingly, it is being documented that clients often do not seek assistance from health care professionals because they have problems getting to health care facilities (Lindstrom, 1975; Rossman and Burnside, 1975; and Keith, 1976). If low-cost transportation is not available in the community you are serving, car pooling or establishing clinic services in the neighborhood may reduce transportation barriers.

LEVELS OF NURSING INTERVENTION

The referral process involves different levels of professional intervention by the community health nurse because clients are at varying stages of ability to assume independent functioning when utilizing health care resources. These levels of nursing intervention are discussed below:

LEVEL I: Some clients need assistance with all aspects of the referral process because their life experiences have not prepared them to deal effectively with systems external to their family unit or because their energies are depleted by crises. These clients need considerable support and encouragement and, often, concrete help from the community health nurse before they can follow through on a needed referral. Frequently they assume a passive-recipient role. They may sincerely want assistance from others but fail to take action because they lack the energy to do so, they do not know what it is they need, or they feel inadequate to handle the referral by themselves. Community health nursing intervention with these clients involves health teaching and counseling so that they can identify health needs that necessitate referral. In addition, supportive assistance is necessary while they are learning how to use health care resources. A major goal when working with these clients is to help them to become more actively involved in taking responsibility for meeting their own health needs. At first, the community health nurse may have to assist these clients with making all the arrangements for warranted health care; just keeping an appointment can be a major accomplishment for them. Sometimes it is easier to do for the client than to work with him or her, especially if the client follows through when the nurse makes all the necessary arrangements and decisions. It is important, however, for the community health nurse to always keep in mind the ultimate goal: to help clients to utilize health resources independently.

LEVEL II: At this level, mutual participation is evident. The client does not wait for the community health nurse to initiate discussion about health care needs. Rather, the client actively seeks information to determine what health actions are needed to resolve current health problems or to enhance wellness in the future. Clients at this level may need health teaching to understand the value of preventive health practices, to locate

community resources that they can afford, or to learn about community services such as low-cost or free transportation, which will help them to use needed resources. They are more likely, however, to raise challenging questions and to identify when health care resources are inappropriate to meet their needs. At times, it may be difficult to recognize when these clients need assistance because they are functioning so well in most aspects of their lives.

LEVEL III: At this level, the client can utilize the referral process independently. The nurse may be used as a resource person, but otherwise, she or he assumes a passive participant role.

THE COMMUNITY HEALTH NURSE AS A HOME CARE COORDINATOR: DISCHARGE PLANNING AND THE REFERRAL PROCESS IN ACTION

Home care coordinators are known by many titles, including discharge planner, home care facilitator, and community hospital liaison nurse. Home care coordinators are generally employed by hospitals and community health agencies. Those employed by community health agencies are usually experienced community health nurses who serve one or more area hospitals or health care facilities. Those hired by hospitals have a variety of nursing backgrounds and are usually responsible only to one hospital for coordinating the home care needs of clients. The objectives of the home care coordinator are the following (Gonnerman, 1968, p. 4):

1. To facilitate quality continuous care between health care settings

2. To make optimum use of health care services

3. To help health care and other professionals

recognize and plan for the discharge needs of clients

4. To alleviate client anxiety regarding discharge needs

In assessing client discharge needs, the home care coordinator must be aware that clients with illnesses that are not self-limiting and that involve a residual disability are most apt to need home care services (Gonnerman, 1968, p. 4). These clients may need such things as homemaker services; home health care; assistance with transportation; health teaching in relation to disease processes; medical regimens and environmental modifications which can increase one's self-care capabilities; and counseling relative to career planning, financial management, and structural and process changes needed within the family system as a result of the client's illness. A major role of the home care coordinator is to increase staff awareness about these client needs and about community resources that will assist clients in their home environment. In order for the home care coordinator to keep staff effectively informed about community resources, she or he must maintain open channels of communication with these resources. This is a key role, because without the support and assistance of community agencies, it would be impossible for the coordinator to plan for home care services such as those described above.

Early identification of clients who need home care is essential to ensure sufficient time to make arrangements for care before the client is discharged. Discharge planning can and should begin as early as the day of admission. The home care coordinator should not wait for referrals, but should seek out prospective home care clients. Planning regular visits to the different units within the institution, reviewing client records, and conducting in-service sessions for staff are examples of strategies used by home care coordinators to increase referrals. Staff are more likely to make referrals if they understand how to do so and if administration stresses the importance of continuity of care. It is critical to work with administrative as well as staff level personnel when implementing the home care coordinator role. Administrative personnel can help staff to gain an appreciation for discharge planning and can assist the home care coor-

dinator in obtaining acceptance of her or his role.

The home care coordinator needs to familiarize the staff and others with her or his role, especially if there has never been this type of service provision before. The job description for this position should be circulated to all the staff members, with follow-up meetings to discuss the staff's questions about role responsibilities. The coordinator's office should be easily accessible to staff, clients, and family to promote utilization (Mitch and Kaczala, 1968, p. 35). In addition to accessibility, demonstration of what one can do is one of the best ways to enhance utilization of services.

The home care coordinator needs freedom to develop a role without restrictive rules. She or he must have free access to clients, records, departments, and meetings, be on an equal level with other health team members and have their cooperation, and strive to make discharge planning a multidisciplinary team effort. The home care coordinator must realize that assessment of clients' home care needs in relation to discharge planning is ongoing and done in collaboration with the client, the family, the health care staff, and health care resources. The coordinator is a vital component in any program designed to ensure continuity of care and is increasingly becoming an essential staff member in many health care facilities.

SUMMARY

Community health nurses provide general, comprehensive, and continuous care to clients in the community setting. Through the use of the referral process, they ensure continuity of care by coordinating services with other health care providers and by linking clients to health care resources. Several key concepts are inherent in this process: (1) clients have the basic responsibility for maintaining their health; (2) clients have the right to accept or refuse health care services; (3) planned intervention by

professionals can promote full usage of resources by community citizens; (4) interdisciplinary collaboration and coordination is essential to ensure continuity of care; and (5) clients can learn to independently utilize health care services. Effective utilization of the referral process not only helps clients to resolve their current health needs, but also prepares them to make decisions about how to handle health needs in the future.

REFERENCES

Atwood, J. Principles of the nursing referral process. Ann Arbor, Mich.: University of Michigan, unpublished research project, 1971.

Coombs, P. A. A study of the effectiveness of nursing referrals. *Public Health Reports*, March–April 1976, *91*, 122–126.

Gonnerman, A. M. Introduction of planned discharge coordinators. *Hospital Forum*, January 1968, *10*, 4–6.

Keith, P. M. A preliminary investigation of the role of the public health nurse in evaluation of services of the aged. *Amercian Journal of Public Health*, April 1976, *66*, 379–381.

Lindstrom, C. J. No shows: A problem in health care. *Nursing Outlook*, December 1975, *23*, 755–759.

McCarthy, E. Comprehensive home care for early hospital discharge. *Nursing Outlook*, September 1976, *24*, 625–630.

Mitch, A. D., & Kaczala, S. The public health nurse coordinator in a general hospital. *Nursing Outlook*, February 1968, *16*, 34–36.

Oakland County Health Department (Nursing Division). *Referral form*. Pontiac, Mich.: Oakland County Health Department.

Quinn, J. L. Triage: Coordinated home care for the elderly. *Nursing Outlook*, September 1975, *23*, 570–573.

Rossman, I., & Burnside, I. M. The United States of America. In J. C. Brocklehurst (Ed.), *Geriatric care in advanced societies*. Baltimore: University Park Press, 1975.

Skinner, E. A., German, P. S., Shapiro, S., Chase, G. A., & Zauber, A. G. Use of ambulatory health services by the near poor. *American Journal of Public Health*, December 1978, *68*, 1195–1201.

Stone, M. Dischage planning guide. *American Journal of Nursing*, August 1979, *79*, 1446–1447.

University of Michigan School of Nursing (Family and Community Health Nursing). *Referral guide*. Ann Arbor, Mich.: University of Michigan, 1979.

Wolff, I. Referral—A process and a skill. *Nursing Outlook*, April 1962, *10*, 253–256.

SELECTED BIBLIOGRAPHY

Anderson, J. D. What will social workers "will"? *Social Casework*, January 1979, *60*, 11–18.

Arafeh, M. K., Fumiatt, E. K., Gregory, M. E., Reilly, M., & Wolff, I. S. Linking hospital and community care for psychiatric patients. In *The nurse in community mental health*. New York: American Journal of Nursing Company, 1972.

Bauman, K. E., & Coulter, M. Design and test of a system for tracking referrals. *Public Health Reports*. November–December 1976, *91*, 521–525.

Brill, N. I. *Working with people: The helping process.* Philadelphia: Lippincott, 1973, 140–143.

Elkind, J. S., Berson, A., & Edwin, D. Current realities haunting advocates of abused children. *Social Casework*, November 1977, *58*, 527–531.

Fanslow, C., & Masset, E. Building staff rapport between institutions. *American Journal of Nursing*, August 1979, *79*, 1441–1442.

Habeeb, M. C., & McLaughlin, F. E. Including the hospital staff nurse. *American Journal of Nursing*, August 1979, *79*, 1443–1445.

Hertz, P., & Stamps, P. L. Appointment-keeping behavior re-evaluated. *American Journal of Public Health*, November 1977, *67*, 1033–1036.

Huey, K. Developing effective links between human-service providers and the self-help system. *Hospital Community Psychiatry*, October 1977, *28*, 767–770.

Jacobson, A. M., Regier, D. A., & Burns, B. J. Factors relating to the use of mental health services in a neighborhood health center. *Public Health Reports*, May–June 1978, *93*, 232–239.

Lan, S-P. M., Loewenstein, R., Sinnette, C., Rogers, C., & Novick, L. Screening and referral outcomes of school-based health services in a low-income neighborhood. *Public Health Reports*, November–December 1976, *91*, 514–520.

Lunt, J. Bridging the gap in continuity of care. *Nursing Times*, March 1970, *66*, 372.

Moreland, H., & Schmitt, V. C. Making referrals is everybody's business. *American Journal of Nursing*, January 1974, *74*, 96–97.

Perkins, Sister M. R. Does availability of health services ensure their use? *Nursing Outlook*, August 1974, *22*, 496–498.

Seiler, H. C. Patient discharge planning for continuity of care. *Occupational Health*, March 1978, *22*, 18–19.

Smith, J. A., Buckalew, J., and Rosales, S. M. Coordinating a workable system. *American Journal of Nursing*, August 1979, *79*, 1439–1440.

Wahlstrom, E. D. Initiating referrals—A hospital based system. *American Journal of Nursing*, February 1967, *67*, 332–335.

Will, M. Referral: A process not a form. *Nursing 77*, December 1977, *77*, 44–45.

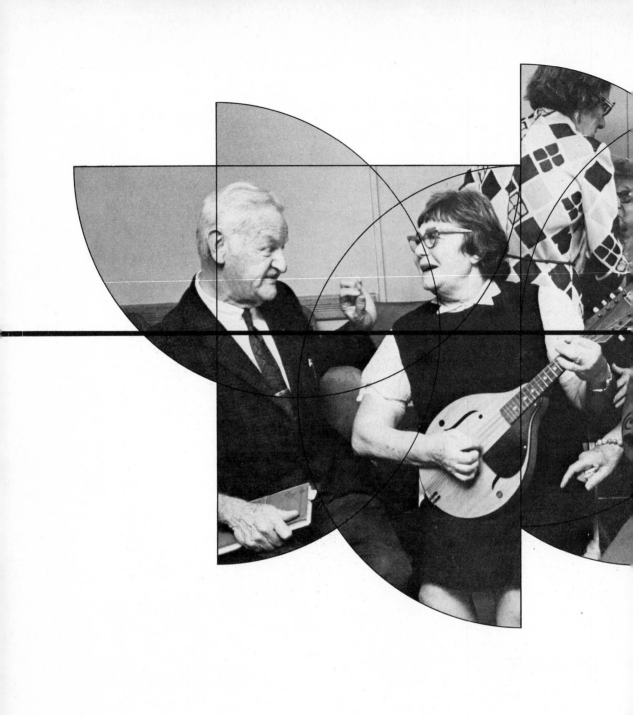

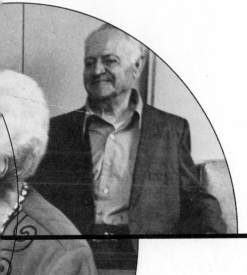

part three

planning health services for population groups

The uniqueness of community health nursing practice lies in the nurse's ability to assess the health needs of a community, to identify populations at risk, and to plan, implement, and evaluate intervention strategies that promote community wellness. A variety of approaches can be used to analyze the state of wellness in a community. Since community health nurses work with individuals, families, and populations across the life-span, a developmental, age-correlated approach to determining populations at risk can be extremely useful.

Community health nurses utilize knowledge from public health practice and nursing practice in order to fulfill their responsibility to the "population as a whole" (American Nurses' Association, 1973). Part 3 explores how knowledge from these two fields of practice is synthesized by nurses in the community when they plan health programs for groups across the life-span. Emphasis is placed on analyzing how nurses utilize epidemiology, community diagnoses, health planning, management, quality assurance, and nursing principles to deliver high-quality services in various community settings.

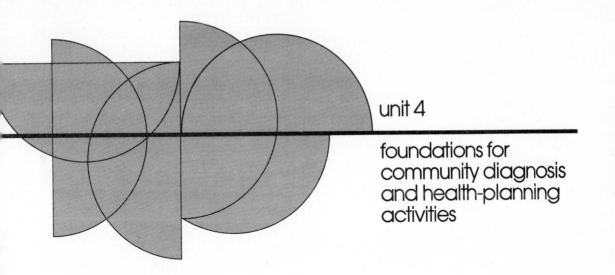

unit 4

foundations for
community diagnosis
and health-planning
activities

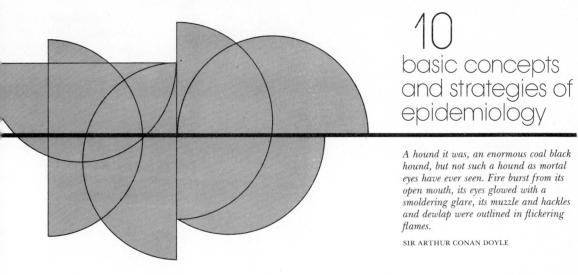

basic concepts and strategies of epidemiology

A hound it was, an enormous coal black hound, but not such a hound as mortal eyes have ever seen. Fire burst from its open mouth, its eyes glowed with a smoldering glare, its muzzle and hackles and dewlap were outlined in flickering flames.

SIR ARTHUR CONAN DOYLE

Thus went the description of the Hound of the Baskervilles, the object of Sir Arthur Conan Doyle's story which was based on an actual Devonshire legend and which was considered to be the greatest of all Holmesian tales. Sherlock Holmes used his brilliant powers of deduction and keen insight to find out why the demonic howl of this hound had brought fear to the Baskerville family. He was able, with his unique problem-solving abilities, to deduce that the howling of the hound was calculated to cause the death of the rightful heirs of the Baskerville fortune. The inheritance would thus fall into the hand of the bastard son of the villainous Hugo Baskerville.

Professionals in community health function very much like the great detective Sherlock Holmes to promote and protect the health of the community. They use an investigative problem-solving process to study the determinants of health and disease frequencies in populations and to plan and implement promotion and disease control programs. These persons use knowledge, concepts, and methods of epidemiology to relate causative events (howl of the hound) to given occurrences (death) in order to identify high-risk populations (Baskerville heirs).

EPIDEMIOLOGY DEFINED

The word *epidemiology* derives from the Greek word *epidemic*. Literally translated this means

The authors are indebted to Associate Professor Elizabeth Keller Beech and to Edna Jennings, friends and colleagues who helped both faculty and students to increase their understanding of the basic concepts of epidemiology and to recognize the value of applying these concepts in the clinical setting. Their support, assistance, and encouragement facilitated learning. Content and illustrations in this chapter reflect many of the ideas shared by them.

epi, "upon," *demos,* "people" (collectively). Historically, the major focus of the epidemiologist was on analyzing major disease outbreaks (epidemics) so that ways to control and prevent *disease* occurrence in populations (people, collectively) could be determined. Today, the definition of epidemiology has been expanded to include the study of variables that affect *health,* as well as those that influence disease occurrence.

There are many variations in the definition

of the term *epidemiology*, but the meanings are essentially the same. In order to have a consistent theme throughout this chapter, the following definition adapted from MacMahon and Pugh (1970, p. 1) will be used:

Epidemiology is the systematic, scientific study of the distribution patterns and determinants of health and disease frequencies in populations, for the purpose of promoting wellness and preventing disease.

Implicit in this definition are two basic assumptions. The first is that patterns and frequencies of health and disease in populations can be identified. The second is that factors which either determine or contribute to the occurrence of wellness or disease can be discovered through systematic investigation.

Community health nurses use the epidemiological process to carry out their systematic investigation of wellness and disease in populations. This process is graphically depicted in Figure 10-1 and will be discussed in detail later in this chapter. When studying Figure 10-1, note that the epidemiological process is similar to the nursing process. The steps are labeled differently but, in essence, they both involve a series of circular, dynamic problem-solving actions. Table 10-1 illustrates this point.

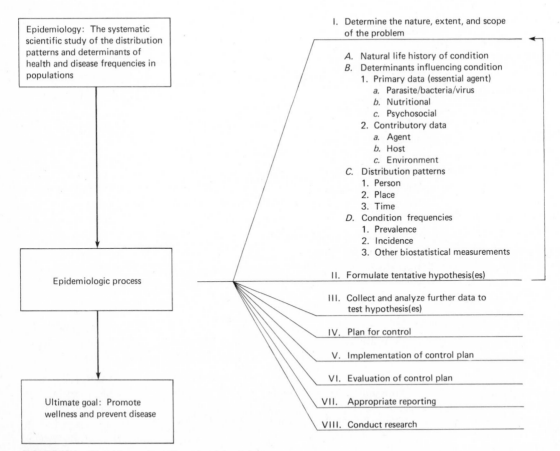

FIGURE 10-1 Graphic explanation of epidemiology.

Learning the language of epidemiology gives one a distinct advantage, however, because the terminology of epidemiology is used by all community health professionals; the terminology of the nursing process is not.

Scope of Epidemiology

Originally, the major focus of epidemiology was the investigation of epidemics caused by communicable diseases such as smallpox, cholera, or scarlet fever. The primary goal was to limit the spread of disease and to prevent its recurrence. Over the years, the scope of epidemiology has changed dramatically. Today, epidemiologists examine variables that keep people healthy, as well as factors that cause the spread and recurrence of disease. In addition to studying causes of communicable disease, epidemiologists analyze the etiology of chronic conditions, accidents, and other health-related phenomena such as child abuse, abortion, and domestic violence.

The reasons for the shift of emphasis in epidemiological study are multiple and relate to changes in diagnostic practices, implementation of effective control measures for communicable disease, changes in the demographic characteristics of the population, scientific advances in medical treatment, and the decline in mortality from communicable diseases. The decline in mortality, however, was probably the major factor. As a result of this decline, life expectancy has risen and the incidence and prevalence of chronic degenerative conditions have increased. As a result

TABLE 10-1 Comparison of the Nursing Process and the Epidemiological Process

Nursing process	*Epidemiological process*

Assessing
    Data collection to determine nature of client problems
	I. Determine the nature, extent, and scope of the problem
	    A. Natural life history of condition
	    B. Determinants influencing condition
	        1. Primary data (essential agent)
	            a. Parasite/bacterium/virus
	            b. Nutrition
	            c. Psychosocial factors
	        2. Contributory data
	            a. Agent
	            b. Host
	            c. Environment
	    C. Distribution patterns
	        1. Person
	        2. Place
	        3. Time
	    D. Condition frequencies
	        1. Prevalence
	        2. Incidence
	        3. Other biostatistical measurements

Analyzing Formulation of nursing diagnosis or hypotheses	II. Formulate tentative hypothesis(es) III. Collect and analyze further data to test hypothesis(es)

Planning
Implementing
Evaluating
Revising or terminating
	IV. Plan for control
	    V. Implement control plan
	    VI. Evaluate control plan
	    VII. Make appropriate report
	VIII. Conduct research

of these changes, it has become imperative that epidemiologists change their focus of study to include noncommunicable entities, as well as communicable ones.

EPIDEMIOLOGY AND THE COMMUNITY HEALTH NURSE

Effective implementation of the epidemiological process requires an interdisciplinary approach. Nurses, environmental engineers, physicians, laboratory technicians, statisticians, health officers, social workers, lay persons, and others all carry out necessary and essential roles in the investigation and control of disease and the promotion of wellness. Any health professional can and should function as a member of the epidemiological team.

Community health nurses participate on the epidemiological team in a variety of ways. Their contacts with families in the home and with groups in various settings (clinics, schools, and industry) put them in a unique position to carry out many epidemiological activities. They regularly become involved in case finding, health teaching, counseling, and follow-up essential to the prevention of communicable diseases, chronic conditions, and other health-related phenomena. Illustrative of this are the actions taken by the community health nurse, in the following case situation, to prevent the spread of a streptococcal infection and the occurrence of chronic complications.

While visiting the Wills family, the community health nurse learned that Bobbie had a severe sore throat. Because Bobbie's symptoms were indicative of a streptococcal infection, the nurse stressed the significance of a proper medical evaluation to rule out or confirm a diagnosis of strep throat. The family followed through immediately. Bobbie's throat culture came back positive for streptococcal disease and he was treated with penicillin. The community health nurse, on a follow-up visit, taught the parents about the necessity of continuing the medication for 10 days even if Bobbie had no symptoms; she knew that a 10-day course of penicillin was needed to eliminate the streptococcal organisms. She also knew from theory and experience that if the organisms were not eliminated Bobbie could have serious chronic complications. By using her epidemiological knowledge, this nurse was able to effectively abort rheumatic fever which can lead to a chronic heart condition or other chronic problems such as kidney disease.

In addition to the activities described above, community health nurses also utilize epidemiological concepts to carry out research in the community setting. A research team may carry out a study to survey major community needs (see Chapter 11) or to identify gaps in knowledge relative to disease causation, prevention, and control. A community health nurse's ongoing, comprehensive contact with the community and its resources allows her or him to make key contributions during these types of studies.

A community health nurse must apply the principles of epidemiology in order to provide preventive health services to *populations* in the community (see Chapter 2). The nurse must understand the significance of expanding epidemiological study to investigate health and disease in populations, as well as with individuals. Only in this way will the community health nurse effectively meet the health needs of the community as a whole.

BASIC CONCEPTS IN EPIDEMIOLOGY

To effectively use the epidemiological process, community health nurses need to have a firm grasp of the basic concepts and tools of epidemiology. Since epidemiology is operationally defined in terms of disease measurements, an understanding of the biostatistical concepts presented in Chapter 11 is essential. Biostatistics help to describe the extent and distribution of health and illness in the community and aid in the identification of specific health problems and community strengths. Biostatistics also facilitate the setting of priorities for program planning.

In addition to biostatistics, there are several basic concepts that guide epidemiological study. These are populations at risk, the natural life history of a disease, levels of prevention, host-agent-environment relationships, multiple causation of disease, and person-place-time relationships. In general, these concepts provide a foundation for explaining how disease develops and how health is maintained, who is most susceptible to disease, and how disease can be prevented and health promoted.

Study of Populations at Risk

A key concept of epidemiology is that the study of disease in populations is more significant than the study of individual cases of disease. Epidemiological research has demonstrated that using large sampling groups is essential for formulating valid conclusions about the distribution patterns and determinants of health and disease frequencies in populations. It is only by observing large groups that commonalities and differences among people who have or do not have a particular disease or condition can be identified.

The identification of commonalities and differences among groups focuses attention on the essential or contributory factors that produce illness or promote health. It has been found through sampling of large groups, for instance, that people who smoke are more likely to develop coronary disease than people who do not smoke (Farquhar, 1977, p. 24). This fact may never have been established if only individual cases had been examined, be-

cause some people who develop coronary disease do not smoke.

A preventive health philosophy has led professionals in community health to emphasize the study of groups. The goal of epidemiological study is to identify *populations at risk*, so that preventive health measures can be used to stop the progression of disease or health-related phenomena. Populations at high risk are those who engage in certain activities or who have certain characteristics that increase their potential for contracting an illness, injury, or a health problem. Parents, for example, who were abused as children are at risk for abusing their own children.

Identifying populations at risk assists community health professionals to utilize more effectively available health resources. Since health resources are not limitless, priorities must be established for the allocation of funds and for the use of health work force time. In Table 20-1, "Priorities in Community Health Nursing," guidelines for determining priorities for community health nursing services are presented. These guidelines are based on the at-risk concept as well as on a philosophy of prevention.

Natural Life History of Disease

In the search for commonalities that may produce disease and health-related phenomena in specific populations, epidemiological study focuses on determining the natural life history of these conditions. Observing the natural life history of disease and health-related phenomena aids in identifying agent-host environmental factors that influence their development, characteristic signs and symptoms during their different periods of progression, and approaches to preventing and controlling their effects on humans.

Leavell and Clark (1965, pp. 17–18) have identified two distinct periods in the natural life history of any disease: *prepathogenesis* and *pathogenesis*. The combination of the processes involved in both of these stages is termed the *natural life history* of a disease or a condition. In the prepathogenesis period, disease has not developed but interactions are occurring between the host, agent, and environment which produce disease stimulus and increase the host's potential for disease. The combination of high serum cholesterol levels and smoking, for example, increases the host's potential for developing coronary heart disease.

The pathogenesis period in the natural life history of disease begins when disease-producing stimuli (smoking or elevated serum cholesterol levels) start to produce changes in the tissues of humans (arteriosclerosis in the coronary vessels). Figure 10-2 shows the interrelationship between the prepathogenesis period and the pathogenesis period and how the latter progresses from the presymptomatic stage to advanced, overt disease. It also shows that disease occurs as a result of processes that happen in the *environment*—prepathogenesis—and processes that happen in *humans*—pathogenesis (Leavell and Clark, 1965, p. 18).

Levels of Prevention

The study of the natural life history of disease facilitates the achievement of the ultimate goal of epidemiology, the development of effective methods for *preventing* and controlling disease or conditions in populations. By identifying significant host-agent-environment relationships which influence the progression of the natural life history of a condition, the epidemiologist can identify populations at risk and develop ways to prevent disease occurrence among them.

A continuum of preventive activities is essential for the promotion of health in any community. As previously discussed in Chapter 2, these activities can be grouped under three levels: *primary* (health promotion and specific protection), *secondary* (early diagnosis, prompt treatment, and disability limitation), and *tertiary* (rehabilitation). Figure 10-3 presents a schema illustrating how to apply these levels of prevention in relation to the natural history

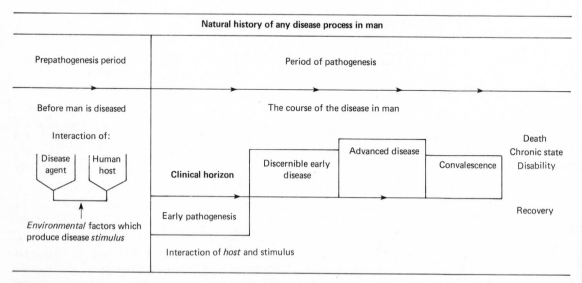

FIGURE 10-2 Prepathogenesis and pathogenesis periods of natural history. *(From H. R. Leavell & E. G. Clark. Preventive medicine for the doctor in his community: An epidemiologic approach. New York: McGraw-Hill, 1965, p. 18.)*

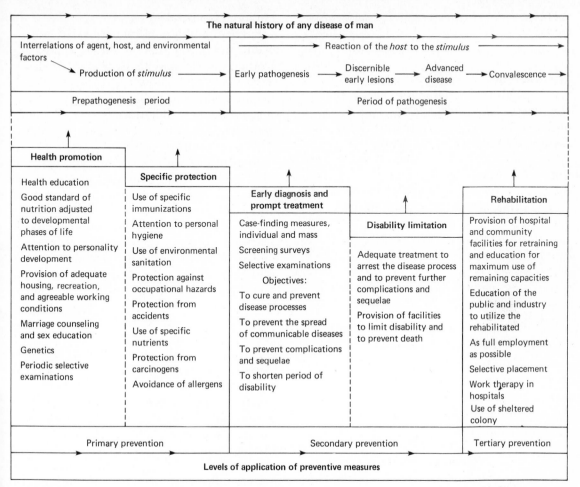

The natural history of any disease of man

Interrelations of agent, host, and environmental factors	Reaction of the *host* to the *stimulus*
Production of *stimulus*	Early pathogenesis → Discernible early lesions → Advanced disease → Convalescence →
Prepathogenesis period	Period of pathogenesis

Health promotion	Specific protection	Early diagnosis and prompt treatment	Disability limitation	Rehabilitation
Health education	Use of specific immunizations	Case-finding measures, individual and mass	Adequate treatment to arrest the disease process and to prevent further complications and sequelae	Provision of hospital and community facilities for retraining and education for maximum use of remaining capacities
Good standard of nutrition adjusted to developmental phases of life	Attention to personal hygiene	Screening surveys		Education of the public and industry to utilize the rehabilitated
Attention to personality development	Use of environmental sanitation	Selective examinations	Provision of facilities to limit disability and to prevent death	
Provision of adequate housing, recreation, and agreeable working conditions	Protection against occupational hazards	Objectives:		As full employment as possible
	Protection from accidents	To cure and prevent disease processes		Selective placement
Marriage counseling and sex education	Use of specific nutrients	To prevent the spread of communicable diseases		Work therapy in hospitals
Genetics	Protection from carcinogens	To prevent complications and sequelae		Use of sheltered colony
Periodic selective examinations	Avoidance of allergens	To shorten period of disability		

Primary prevention	Secondary prevention	Tertiary prevention

Levels of application of preventive measures

FIGURE 10-3 Levels of application of preventive measures in the natural history of disease. (*From H. R. Leavell & E. G. Clark, Preventive medicine for the doctor in his community: An epidemiologic approach. New York: McGraw-Hill, 1965, p. 21.*)

of any disease. It implies that carrying out preventive activities during both the prepathogenesis and pathogenesis periods can alter the progression of a disease. The degree to which preventive activities can be implemented will vary, however, depending on the completeness of knowledge one has about the disease in question (Leavell and Clark, 1965, p. 20).

Host-Agent-Environment Relationships

When analyzing the natural life history of a disease or a condition and how to apply the three levels of prevention, epidemiological study focuses on the relationship of three variables: host, agent, and environment. These variables are defined as follows:

AGENT: An animate or inanimate factor which must be present or lacking for a disease or a condition to occur.

HOST: Living species (humans or other animals) capable of being infected or affected by an agent.

ENVIRONMENT: Everything external to a specific agent and host, including humans and animals.

Various models have been used to study the relationships between the host, agent, and environment. The *epidemiological triangle* is the one most commonly used (Figure 10-4). This model was designed to demonstrate that host-agent-environment factors alone do not produce a disease or a condition. Rather, it is the interactions (depicted by arrows in the model) among these variables that determine whether there is health or disease in a community. Health is maintained when the host-agent-environment variables are in a state of equilibrium. Disease occurs when there is a change in any one of these three variables that disturbs the state of equilibrium between them.

Multiple Causation of Disease

It is only natural to assume that the introduction of a disease agent into a community is enough to cause illness among its citizens. Swine influenza is brought into Ann Arbor, Michigan, and an epidemic takes place!

However, one factor by itself does not cause a disease or a condition. A basic tenet of epidemiology is that more than one factor must be present in order for disease to take place.

This concept is called *multiple causation of disease*. These multiple factors are variables such as the level of immunity in the population, individual susceptibility to disease, availability of vectors, and the amount of contact between members of the population. These variables can disturb the equilibrium between the host, agent, and environment and determine if a disease or condition will result.

The influenza outbreak that occurred in 1978 in the United States demonstrated the concept of multiple causation. The agent introduced into the population at that time was the influenza virus A/USSR. Outbreaks of this disease occurred in groups of young adults and children in environments of close contact: schools, colleges, and military training camps. Attack rates in these areas were high, ranging from 40 to 70 percent in most cases. The disease did not usually appear in adults over 25 years of age.

An analysis of the above situation illustrates that the proper combination of multiple factors is necessary before disease will result. Outbreaks occurred in young adults and children because there were a virulent agent, susceptible hosts who lacked immunity, and crowded environmental conditions that supported the spread of the agent. The disease usually did not occur in those over 25 because they had been exposed to this virus earlier and had developed acquired immunity to the organism. This acquired immunity allowed them to maintain a balance in host-agent-environment factors and to escape the disease. If only one variable, such as a virulent agent, was necessary to cause illness, individuals 25 years and older would also have had high attack rates in 1978.

The concept of multiple causation becomes even more apparent when one studies the natural life history of chronic conditions or health-related phenomena. Friedman's (1976, p. 5) diagram of the web of causation for myocardial infarction (Figure 10-5) clearly demon-

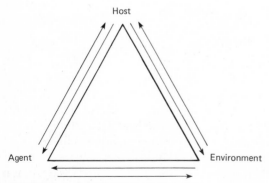

FIGURE 10-4 Epidemiological triangle.

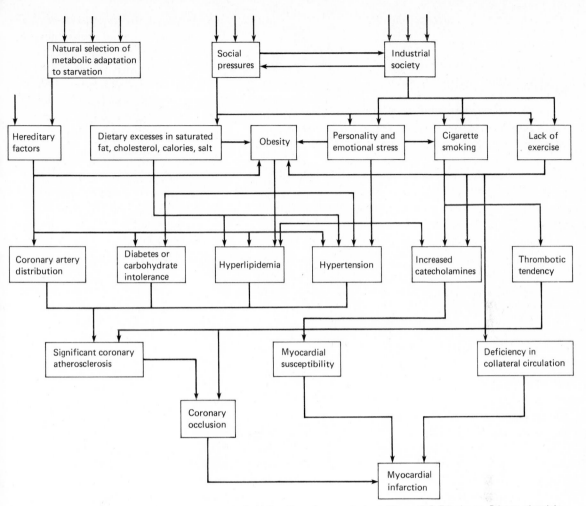

FIGURE 10-5   The web of causation for myocardial infarction: A current view. (*From G.E. Friedman. Primer of epidemiology. New York: McGraw-Hill, 1974, p. 5.*)

strates that it is the interplay between multiple host-agent-environment characteristics that causes a chronic condition.

Person-Place-Time Relationships

It has been emphasized that the study of relationships is necessary for the community health professional to formulate valid hypotheses about disease or condition causation. Identification of measurable variables that can facilitate rapid and efficient data collection is essential to this study. In epidemiological study, the variables that have been found to be most useful are *person* (who is affected), *place* (where affected), and *time* (when affected). Some of the most frequently analyzed characteristics of these variables are the following (MacMahon and Pugh, 1970, pp. 31–32):

1. Person: delineation of group involved

   a. Age, sex, race distribution

   b. Socioeconomic status, occupation, education

   c. Health habits and behaviors

   d. Acquired resistance and susceptibility

   e. Health history—natural resistance, hereditary characteristics

2. Place: geographic distribution in subdivisions of the area affected

   a. Physical environment: weather, climate, geography, radiation, vibration, noise, pressure, animal reservoirs, pollutants, and housing facilities

   b. Social environment: population density and mobility, community groups, occupations and other roles, beliefs and attitudes, technological developments, transportation, educational practices, and health care delivery system

3. Time: chronological distribution of onsets of cases by days, weeks, months

   a. Incubation period: determine life cycle; factors affecting multiplication and virulence of organism

   b. Seasonal trends

   c. Onset of event

   d. Duration of event

Besides the four time factors presented above, immediacy is a primary consideration. Time is a critical factor in disease diagnosis and control. Immediate reporting of a disease outbreak is crucial since the validity of data is often directly proportional to the time lapse incurred in obtaining the information. If a significant amount of time is lost in reporting, the ability to formulate valid hypotheses is decreased.

When monitoring incidence of infectious disease, to note change over time, the terms used to distinguish relative frequency in time and space include the following:

SPORADIC: Presence of occasional cases of the event apparently unrelated in time or space.

ENDEMIC: Constant presence of an event at about the frequency expected from the past history of the community.

EPIDEMIC: Presence of the event at a much higher frequency than expected from the past history of the community; one case of cholera would be labeled epidemic in a United States community. On the other hand, in some foreign countries, several cases of cholera would be considered an endemic occurrence.

PANDEMIC: Presence of an event in epidemic proportions, involving many communities and countries in a relatively short period of time.

When monitoring any disease or condition, it is important to remember that there are wide variations in the degree of symptoms. These variations range from inapparent infection to severe, pronounced symptomatology. It is the inapparent, or subclinical, symptoms that are the most significant in terms of disease transmission or occurrence. If efforts to prevent transmission of infection or efforts to stop the progression of a chronic condition or a health-related phenomenon are limited to people with clinical manifestations, a very large proportion of the problem will be missed.

The iceberg analogy is frequently used to illustrate the importance of identifying individuals with subclinical symptoms during an epidemiological study. Most of the iceberg, as illustrated in Figure 10-6, is submerged. This unseen section is the most insidious and potentially dangerous portion to the seafarer because no action will be taken to avoid it. Individuals with subclinical infections or symptoms, like the submerged portion of the iceberg, present the most danger in a disease-prevention and -control program. Since they do not have obvious symptoms, they are less likely to use preventive measures. An example of this situation is a female client who has asymptomatic gonorrhea. This person frequently transmits gonorrhea for a considerable length of time before it is known, through contact with others, that she has the disease.

Psychosocial phenomena, such as alcoholism, domestic violence, child abuse, and mental illness tend to remain submerged much longer than infectious diseases. Increasingly, it is being recognized that these problems are far more prevalent than statistics reflect. Communities are beginning to conduct epidemiological investigations in order to determine the real magnitude of these problems.

EPIDEMIOLOGICAL INVESTIGATION

In the preceding sections, basic concepts in epidemiology were discussed to lay a foundation for epidemiological investigation of community health problems. These concepts aid in identifying variables to consider when describing the distribution patterns and determinants of health and disease frequencies in populations. They help to analyze causal relationships in disease or condition outbreaks.

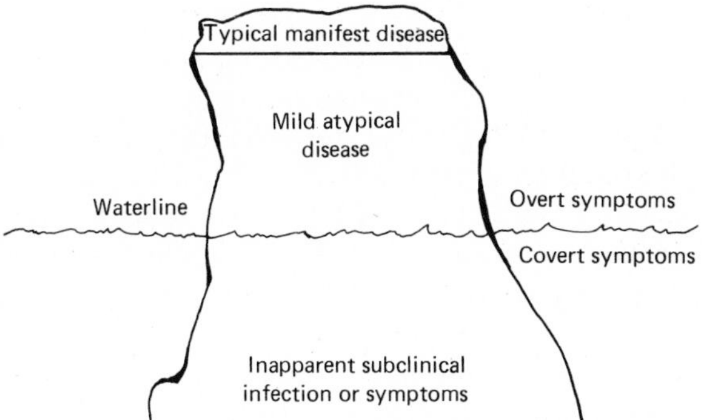

A major goal of epidemiology today is to relate various etiological agents to condition occurrence. Cancer, hypertension, coronary artery disease, accidents, diabetes, and psychosocial phenomena are among the major contemporary problems. Eradication of communicable disease is a continuing and futuristic epidemiological goal. To reach these goals, health professionals have developed and utilized a scientific process known as the epidemiological process.

The epidemiological process is a systematic course of action taken to identify: (1) who is affected (persons); (2) where the affected persons reside (place); (3) when the persons were affected (time); (4) causal factors of health and disease occurrence (host-agent-environment determinants); (5) prevalence and incidence of health and disease (frequencies); and (6) prevention and control measures (levels of prevention) in relation to the natural life history of a disease or a condition.

The epidemiological process has eight basic steps. These steps are graphically illustrated in Figure 10-1. Although each will be discussed separately, it is important to remember that these steps may overlap and do not always follow a sequential pattern. They are interrelated and dependent upon each other. Data, for example, collected in the initial step provide a foundation for all subsequent steps.

FIGURE 10-6 Comparison of inapparent infection to an iceberg. *(Adapted from E. Keller. Environmental health and communicable disease module. Ann Arbor, Mich.: The University of Michigan School of Nursing, 1974, p. 183.)*

Step I: Determine the Nature, Extent, and Possible Significance of the Problem

The primary responsibilities during this initial step are twofold: (1) to verify the diagnosis by data collection from multiple sources; and (2) to determine the extent and possible significance of the verified problem. Data gathering begins when an index case is reported or when there is a noticeable change in the incidence rate for a particular disease or condition. The *index case* is the case which brings a household or other group to the attention of community health personnel. Once this case is known to health professionals, data are collected from a variety of sources in order to determine if a problem really exists. Clinical observations, laboratory studies, and lay reporting assist the epidemiological team in confirming the homogeneity of the current events. If, for instance, four hospital emergency rooms have reported that several individuals were treated for food poisoning in the last 24 hours, health personnel would want to immediately take the following actions:

1. Interview the affected persons to determine the nature of their symptoms and to identify loci of origin according to person, place, and time.

2. Review laboratory studies to confirm a common causative organism. This process could establish that there are several events occurring at the same time.

3. Interview friends, relatives, and lay acquaintances to discern their description of the events which led up to the reported illness and to determine if other individuals have symptoms.

It is important to remember that *time* and *accurate* and *thorough* data collection are critical factors in step I. Significant data may be destroyed if the data collection process is too slow. In addition, if only the "tip of the iceberg" or the most obvious events are observed, the extent of the problem will not be identified. The health professional needs to be like a detective, starting out with interviewing the affected individual and then branching out into this individual's environment to track down the host-agent-environment factors which influence disease occurrence. As previously discussed, the measurable variables which facilitate rapid and efficient data collection about host-agent-environment factors are person, place, and time.

Analyzing data in terms of person, place, and time helps to establish the magnitude of the problem. It tells the health professional the proportion of the people affected, the seriousness of the effects on the host and the community, the improvement or regression over time, and the geographic distribution of the disease or condition. It also helps in identifying potential sources of infection and causal relationships.

The use of spot maps (see Chapter 11, under "Analyze All Available Data") facilitates pinpointing the exact geographic location of the disease or condition. This type of map vividly and visually portrays an epidemiological problem very rapidly. If it is used on a regular basis, health personnel can compare current prevalence and incidence with the expected rates and can identify significant departures from normal. *Incidence* is the number of *new* cases of a disease in a population over a period of time (cases just starting). *Prevalence* is the number of *old* and *new* cases of a specific disease at a given time (see Chapter 11).

When comparing prevalence and incidence rates, one word of caution is necessary. If there is a distinct departure from normal, it must be ascertained that a problem really exists. It may be found that there is only an improvement in reporting, not an actual increase in disease occurrence.

If there has been an actual increase in the

incidence of a particular disease or condition, the health professional makes an *educated guess* as to the nature of the causative agent, based upon the data collected. This formulation of a tentative diagnosis or hypothesis is done in order to enhance further data collection.

Step II: Formulate Tentative Hypothesis(es)

When dealing with infectious diseases, a rapid preliminary analysis of data is imperative. This is essential because infectious diseases can spread quickly, can affect a large number of people in a short period of time, and can have great ranges in severity. Usually this analysis results in the formulation of several hypotheses. Explanation of the most probable source of infection is made in terms of (1) the agent causing the problem; (2) the source of infection, including the chain of events leading to the outbreak of the problem; and (3) environmental conditions that allowed it to occur. An example of how tentative hypotheses are established is provided in the following situation.

From September 5 through 8, 1974, the "World's Largest American Indian Fair" was held near Gallup, New Mexico (Horwitz, Pollard, Merson, and Martin, 1977, pp. 1071–1076). An estimated 80,000 persons attended the fair. Beginning on September 6, 1974, and during the next few days, several hundred people with gastrointestinal symptoms sought attention at two hospitals near Gallup. Over 130 of them had stool cultures positive for a *Salmonella* group C organism, *Salmonella newport*. The hospitals immediately reported the apparent outbreak to the health department. Preliminary tentative hypotheses indicated that either the community water supply of the area or food served at a free barbeque which attracted thousands on September 5, 1974, was the vehicle of transmission for the agent *Salmonella newport*. Evidence favoring a water source included a broken water pipe at the fair grounds in an area soiled with animal feces.

The barbeque was suspected because food preparation practices were reportedly improper and those who attended the barbeque appeared to have a high attack rate of illness.

Since two possible sources of infection were favored in this situation, health personnel took immediate steps to correct both problem situations and collected and analyzed further data to detemine the exact cause of the *Salmonella* outbreak.

Waiting until all data are collected before instituting control measures only amplifies the magnitude of the problem. A health professional must be willing to take risks while carrying out an epidemiological investigation.

Step III: Collect and Analyze Further Data to Test Hypothesis(es)

A basic starting point in this step is to identify the group selected for attack by the disease or problem under investigation. Individual epidemiological health histories should be done to classify persons according to their exposure to suspected or causative agents and to identify the clinical data and bacteriologic findings needed to substantiate the diagnosis. Significant variation of incidence in contrasted population groups should then be noted. These variations can be identified through study of attack rates.

An *attack rate* is an incidence rate which identifies the number of people at risk who became ill. In studying an outbreak of foodborne disease such as the one at the American Indian Fair, the attack rate for persons who ate certain foods would be compared with the attack rate for persons who did not eat certain foods. This is done in an attempt to identify which food was infected by the causative agent. Generally, the food which shows the greatest difference between the two attack rate percentages is the infected food (Communicable Disease Center, 1964, p. 8).

Attack rates are calculated in the following manner:

$$\frac{\text{No. of persons affected}}{\text{No. of persons eating food item}} \times 100$$

$$\frac{\text{No. of persons affected}}{\text{No. of persons } not \text{ eating food item}} \times 100$$

Table 10-2 illustrates how attack rates are graphically summarized. The attack rates in this table were calculated when people became ill after a banquet. They show that one food item, custard, was probably the infected food (note the differences between the two attack rate percentages).

It is essential to remember that attack rates do not positively confirm an infective food. Maxcy and Rosenau (1965, p. 18) have identified the following five reasons why the association of illness with a particular food is often difficult:

1. Some individuals are resistant to the agent and do not become ill even though exposed.

2. The definition of an ill person employed may include some who have unrelated illnesses, unless there is a specific test; and even then, if the illness is one which is prevalent, the ill subjects may include some cases not due to the ingestion of the common vehicle.

3. Contamination of one food by traces of another may take place during serving or before.

4. Errors in history taking may occur. These may be unbiased errors, due to memory lapses or misunderstanding; or they may be due to biases, either on the part of the questioner or the subject. Several kinds of biases are possible; the questioner may have a preconceived notion of what food was responsible and press his questions more vigorously with respect to that food in the case of ill persons than non-ill persons; or the subject may have preconceived notions, leading to the same result. The subject may have reasons for wishing either to claim or disclaim illness. Biases may affect the accuracy either of food histories or illness histories and produce spurious association.

5. Finally, biased sampling may also lead to spurious results.

All the above factors can affect the validity of an attack rate and thereby the choice of the appropriate infective food. Laboratory studies are necessary to confirm the etiologic agent and its vector. A *vector* is an animate or inanimate vehicle such as food, clothing, or insects

TABLE 10-2 Attack Rate Table

Vulnerable food	Persons who did eat vulnerable food				Persons who did not eat vulnerable food			
	Sick	Well	Total	Attack rate, %	Sick	Well	Total	Attack rate, %
Baked ham	19	56	75	25	30	5	35	86
Custard	45	15	60	75	4	46	50	8
Jello	20	35	55	36	29	26	55	53
Cole slaw	48	58	106	45	1	3	4	25
Baked beans	45	55	100	45	4	6	10	40
Potato salad	25	45	70	36	24	16	40	60

SOURCE: From Communicable Disease Center. *Food-borne disease investigation: Analysis of field data.* Atlanta, Ga.: Public Health Service, 1964, p. 8.

which transports disease from an infected host to a new host.

Since one factor alone never causes a disease or condition, it is not sufficient to identify only a causative agent and the infective food. After the possible agents and the attack group have been identified, the common source(s) to which affected individuals were exposed should be investigated. With foodborne disease, the origin, method, and preparation of suspected foods would be primary factors to examine. Concurrently, environmental conditions should be evaluated. These conditions would include such things as the sanitary status of the restaurant, the area where food was served, and the water and dairy supply. Figure 10-7 depicts the type of data which one state, Michigan, collects when enteric infections such as *Salmonella newport* are suspected. Community health nurses are frequently responsible for completing this form during an epidemiological investigation. In some health departments, they are also responsible for collecting specimens for laboratory analysis. Precedures for how to collect these specimens are usually available in the health department. If they are not, the epidemiological division of the state health department will provide information on how to properly collect and preseve specimens for epidemiological analysis.

When completing a case history form during an epidemiological investigation, it is important for the community health nurse to recognize that this task provides an opportunity for health teaching and case finding. Often, the community health nurse identifies new cases during this process and helps clients to learn about the nature of the disease and how to prevent its spread.

It is important to use a variety of data-collection methods in determining the extent and source of an epidemiological problem because individuals who have only minor symptoms of illness often do not seek treatment. In the Gallup, New Mexico, outbreak, the extent of the problem was determined by a large questionnaire survey conducted from September 19 to 25, 1974. Using recently made maps of dwellings in the area, 500 dwellings, housing 2000 persons, were randomly selected for a visit by an interviewer who completed a questionnaire. The interviewer inquired about the occurrence and characteristics of diarrheal illnesses, the types and location of the household water supply, the amount of water consumed at the fair, the time of eating at the barbeque, and the types of food eaten. This survey revealed that attendance at the barbeque was highly associated with illness and confirmed laboratory studies which eliminated water as a vehicle of transmission. It also showed that eating potato salad at the barbeque was strongly associated with illness (Horwitz, Pollard, Merson, and Martin, 1977, pp. 1072 and 1074).

Tentative hypothesis(es) must be tested. The survey conducted at Gallup, New Mexico, helped to confirm one of the original hypotheses on the source of contamination, the food served at the barbeque, and eliminated another, the contaminated water. At times, however, it will be found that none of the original hypotheses is appropriate. That is why it is so important to confirm through laboratory tests and interviews the multiple causes for an outbreak. Identifying only the causative agent does not prevent the further spread of disease. Identifying the agent only helps to treat infected individuals who seek medical care. It does not tell one how the disease is being transmitted. If the chain of transmission is not broken, disease will continue to occur. Benton Roueche's (1968) book, *Eleven Blue Men*, vividly demonstrates how important it is to break the chain of transmission when dealing with both communicable and noncommunicable diseases.

Testing hypothesis(es) helps to determine if the initial control measures were sufficient

ENTERIC INFECTIONS _____ CASE HISTORY
(Insert type)

DIVISION OF EPIDEMIOLOGY
Michigan Department of Public Health   No. _____

Name _____ Birth date _____ Birthplace _____

Address _____

Occupational address _____

Physician _____ Address _____

Health officer _____ Address _____

CLINICAL HISTORY: Date of onset _____ Diarrhea _____

Vomiting _____ Temp. _____ Weight loss _____ Other symptoms _____

_____ Duration of symptoms _____

Present condition _____

Previous pertinent history, if any _____

Source of water: ___ Well   ___ Municipal   ___ Other (specify) _____

Source of milk: ___ Pasteurized (name dairy) _____

                      ___ Unpasteurized (source) _____

Source of food: ___ Restaurant (name) _____

                      ___ Private home, other then given _____

                      ___ Other (specify) _____

Sewage disposal   ___ Privy   ___ Septic tank   ___ Municipal

Additional epidemiological data pertaining to this case:

FIGURE 10-7 Enteric infections case history. *(From Division of Epidemiology, Michigan Department of Public Health, Lansing, Michigan.)*

All other persons in household

	Name	Age	Relation	History of recent illness	Laboratory data
1.					
2.					
3.					
4.					
5.					
6.					
7.					
8.					
9.					
10.					

Visitors to household during past month

	Name	Age	Relation	Address	Laboratory data
1.					
2.					
3.					
4.					
5.					
6.					

Case laboratory data

Specimens					Date	Positive	Negative	Laboratory
Blood	Widal	Feces	Urine	Bile				

Informant _____

Investigation by _____

Health Dept. _____

Date _____

Please use ink in making out histories

to resolve the current outbreak. It also aids in identifying the natural life history of the disease and where further action is needed.

Step IV: Plan for Control

When planning for control, it is essential to identify preventive activities, based on the knowledge of the natural history of the disease in question, which can be used to control the further spread of disease occurrence. Host-agent-environment factors should be analyzed to determine the following:

1. Populations at risk

2. Primary, secondary, and tertiary preventive measures available which would

   a. Alter the behavior or susceptibility of the host (health education, case finding, immunization, treatment, or rehabilitation)

   b. Destroy the agent (heat, drug treatment, or spraying with insecticides)

   c. Eliminate the transmission of the agent (changes in host's health habits or environmental conditions)

3. Feasibility of implementing the control plan, considering such factors as available community resources, time required, cost of control vs. partial or no control, facilities, supplies, and personnel needed

4. Priorities in relation to legal mandates, significance of the problem relative to other community needs, and the feasibility of implementing the control plan

Public opinion can have a significant impact on the effectiveness of any control plan. In the Gallup outbreak of salmonellosis, one control measure could have been to ban future food preparation and consumption for groups of persons numbering over 100 so that careful attention could be given to details. It is highly unlikely that this plan would be well received,

since fairs are a major form of recreation on the Navajo Nation Indian Reservation and the Indians travel considerable distances to attend them. Clearly stating regulations for food preparation, with the mandatory attendance of one environmentalist per 1000 persons to oversee food preparation, would probably be a more realistic control measure for this situation.

Control measures are generally directed toward breaking the chain of transmission. This includes destroying or treating the reservoir of infection, interrupting the transmission of the agent from the reservoir to the new host, and decreasing the ability of the agent to adapt and multiply within the host. A *reservoir* is a living species or an inanimate object such as soil in which an infectious agent lives and multiplies and upon which it depends for survival and reproduction.

Referring again to the Gallup outbreak, the major cause of the disease was error in food preparation. There was prolonged storage of precooked ingredients for potato salad, within the 44 to 114°F range in which *Salmonella* have been demonstrated to multiply. The initial source of the *Salmonella* is unknown (Horwitz, Pollard, Merson, and Martin 1977, p. 1074). As is often the case, the food handlers at this large gathering were lay persons, and their work was unsupervised. Large gatherings of people where food is served should be considered high-risk settings for foodborne disease outbreak. It is advisable to have an epidemiologically trained person monitoring food preparation, storage, and serving at such occasions.

When one is dealing with infectious diseases, the concept of *herd immunity* is also important to consider while establishing a control plan. Herd immunity is the immunity level of a specific group. If, in a given group, 100 percent of the group had received measles vaccine, the herd immunity would be 100 percent. If 80 percent had received measles vaccine, the herd immunity would be at least 80 percent.

Some people in the group have acquired immunity, raising the percentage higher.

Herd immunity does not have to be 100 percent to prevent an epidemic or to control a disease, but it is not known just what percentage is safe. Communities usually strive to achieve an 85 percent herd immunity level. It is important to realize that as herd immunity decreases, the chances for epidemics rise. In the United States today, a major concern is that many school-age children are not receiving immunizations for communicable disease. This greatly decreases the level of herd immunity and is a major barrier to maintaining community health.

Community health nurses are instrumental in helping the public to see the need for effective control of disease by active immunization. This will continue to be a major function of the community health nurse, because immunizing populations at risk is the most effective way to control many of our childhood communicable diseases (see Appendix 13-1 for immunization schedules).

Step V: Implement Control Plan

An active effort should be made to elicit and coordinate the cooperation of the lay public, as well as private and official agencies, when putting control measures into operation. A control program that takes into consideration the beliefs, attitudes, and customs of the community is more likely to be accepted by the public than one that ignores community norms. Health education programs can help to sell a control program in the community, especially if they deal with current community attitudes and beliefs.

In order to evaluate the effectiveness of a control program, broad goals and specific objectives for the program must be identified before the program begins. Defining broad goals and specific outcome objectives such as the ones below makes it easier to determine if control efforts are successful.

BROAD GOAL: To increase the herd immunity level for DPT to 85 percent in Centerville.

OBJECTIVES: To increase the herd immunity level for DPT in census tracts 4 and 5 by 25 percent in 4 months by immunizing kindergarten and first-, fifth-, and tenth-grade students.

To increase the herd immunity level for DPT in census tracts 8 and 9 by 17 percent in 4 months, by immunizing kindergarten and first-, fifth-, and tenth-grade students.

There are many barriers to the successful implementation of a control program for both infectious disease and noncommunicable conditions. Some of the primary ones will be briefly summarized.

Low levels of immunity in an exposed population group increase the likelihood of disease occurrence. Mass and individual immunization programs are effective in raising immunity levels for some diseases. For many diseases, however, there are no specific prophylactic immunizations. An example of one such disease is chickenpox.

Individuals without overt disease symptoms, but who harbor the disease organism, can be a major vehicle in disease transmission. These individuals are known as *carriers*. Typhoid and salmonellosis are examples of diseases that are often transmitted by carriers. Through mass testing of individuals for the suspected agent, carriers can be found and treated. This type of case-finding activity may be the primary factor that stops the spread of a disease. Case finding is a major function of anyone who does an epidemiological investigation.

With any disease and for a variety of reasons, some individuals will delay or not seek treatment. Whatever the reason, a delay in confirmation and treatment of the disease can enhance its spread and continuation.

Individuals for whom the diagnosis is not suspected or confirmed are also barriers to the control of disease. Disease may not be confirmed for several reasons. Some people will evidence atypical symptoms of the disease in question. If clinical symptoms do not fit a disease model, the disease may be missed completely or misdiagnosed. Other individuals are seen too early or too late in the course of the disease process to either suspect or confirm the disease. In these situations, laboratory tests may be falsely negative or they may not be done at all because the clinical symptoms do not reflect a need. There are other times when a diagnosis cannot be confirmed because specimens (stools, emesis, or sputum) have inadvertently been destroyed or handled improperly. When working in the home or in other health care settings, it is vitally important to recognize that laboratory tests are needed to confirm most infectious diseases.

Lack of reporting, often involving nonacceptance of a diagnosis, is one of the key barriers in a control program. This can result from clerical error, indifference, fear, shame, or any of a number of variables. In some instances, professionals may not want to get involved or do not feel it appropriate to become involved. This is especially true when social problems such as gonorrhea or child abuse are the disease or condition in question.

The community health nurse needs to be acutely aware of these barriers because she or he is frequently in a position to help individuals, families, or health care professionals overcome them. Through the use of the referral process, knowledge of community resources, interviewing skills, and the ability to understand both health and disease processes, the community health nurse is uniquely able to assist in resolving these barriers.

Step VI: Evaluate Control Plan

An important part of the epidemiological process is evaluation. This ensures that the next time the process is repeated, it can be improved. It also ensures, through the problem-solving approach, that all elements of a problem have been reviewed. The first step in evaluation is to determine how well the objectives of the process were met. This implies that prior to carrying out the process, objectives were clearly and behaviorally written. The next question to be answered is how the current situation compares to the situation prior to the investigation. Finally, the practicality of the control measures should be determined. Feasibility and cost in terms of money, time, staff, facilities, and community support should be analyzed.

Step VII: Make Appropriate Report

Prompt, accurate, and concise reporting of the outcome of the epidemiological process will provide a basis for future investigations and control measures. Appropriate reporting will also demonstrate accountability to the community of health personnel. It cannot help but clarify the epidemiological situation to both the public and health professionals. Reporting should include what was involved in the epidemiological process: diagnosis, factors leading to the epidemic, control measures, process evaluation, and recommendations for preventing similar epidemic situations.

In actual practice, underreporting of many epidemiological investigations occurs. This happens for many reasons. Completion of necessary forms can be tedious and time-consuming and, therefore, neglected. Frequently there is no one person assigned the responsibility for seeing that reports are completed and the responsibility is overlooked. Usually more effective reporting occurs when one person is designated to coordinate the reporting activities of others.

Societal and individual values and attitudes also contribute to underreporting. At times, conditions such as venereal disease, alcoholism, or mental illness are not discussed because health care professionals are afraid to disturb the status quo in the community.

Accurate reporting is essential for the identification of major community health problems and preventive health action which would correct these problems. Treating only individuals with overt symptoms, rather than collecting and reporting data on populations at risk, does very little to prevent future health problems.

Step VIII: Conduct Research

The ultimate goal of epidemiology, the prevention and control of infectious diseases, chronic conditions, and other health-related phenomena in populations, is far from being realized. Infectious diseases such as gonorrhea, syphilis, hepatitis, enteric disorders, and tuberculosis are still major health problems. Despite scientific advances in the development of immunizations that prevent communicable diseases, epidemic outbreaks of childhood conditions, especially measles and diphtheria, continue to occur. Chronic conditions such as cancer and heart disease are fast-growing problems. Due to their complex nature, very little is known regarding their etiology or ways to prevent and control them. If health services to populations are to be improved, epidemiological research is essential. Health professionals must be prepared to systematically collect and analyze data so that the gaps in knowledge relative to disease causation, prevention, and control are eliminated.

If community health practice is going to be prevention-oriented, all steps in the epidemiological process must be completed. Currently, research in the practice setting is frequently lacking. This is unfortunate because the practitioner is in the best position to identify problems that need further investigation. Research can be exciting and challenging, especially when one discovers significant data that will aid a community to better its health status.

The speed with which one moves through the eight steps of the epidemiological process varies greatly, depending upon the complexity of the given situation, the time it takes for clinical symptoms to develop, and the effectiveness of professionals in obtaining accurate information. Regardless of the rate at which one moves through the steps, the nurse will surely find his or her detective abilities challenged when doing an epidemiological investigation.

EXPANDING EPIDEMIOLOGY TO THE STUDY OF CHRONIC DISEASES AND CONDITIONS

Although communicable diseases are often used to illustrate the application of the epidemiological process, this process is also used to investigate chronic diseases and conditions. In order to do so, one needs to understand the nature of these conditions, approaches used to study them, and inherent problems in identifying their causes and preventing their occurrence. These are discussed below.

Defining Chronic Disease and Conditions

The Commission on Chronic Illness was a national voluntary group that extensively studied chronic disease and illness in the United States from 1949 to 1956. This commission defined chronic diseases as impairments or deviations from normal that have at least one of the following characteristics: permanency, residual disability, irreversible pathological causation and alteration, need for special rehabilitation training, and need for a long period of supervision, observation, or care (Commission on Chronic Illness, 1957, p. 4). People of any age can evidence chronic conditions; these conditions are not synonymous with old age. It should be remembered that aging is the normal process of biological, psychological, and sociological change over time. However, because aging involves a gradual lessening in levels of efficiency and functioning in the different body systems, elderly people are more likely than young people to have chronic conditions. They also are likely to have more of them.

The Scope of Chronic Disease

To show that chronic conditions are evidenced across the age spectrum, Figure 10-8 is presented. This figure illustrates that people of all ages are affected by chronic disease. It should be noted, however, that the predominance of chronic conditions is in the later years, from age 45 and on.

Chronic illness is the major health problem in the American population. This was confirmed by a study carried out during a 2-year period, from July 1965 to June 1967, by the United States Public Health Service. The study showed that approximately 50 percent of the American civilian population had one or more chronic conditions. Of the 95 million Americans affected, approximately 22 million had some degree of activity limitation, and approximately 6.3 million had some degree of activity limitation that was a result of chronic conditions (Mental Health Administration, 1971, pp. 1–4, 8, 11).

Why so much chronic disease? Strauss states that without question the major reason for the high rate of chronic disease in the United States is the elimination or control of infec-

tious and parasitic diseases (Strauss, 1975, p. 3).[1] The industrialized nations of the world are no longer greatly affected by preventable and controllable conditions. Instead, persons in these countries die from cancer, heart disease, stroke, and other long-term conditions such as diabetes.

The relatively low social value given to older people by our culture, as well as the acute care and cure orientation of health personnel, helps to explain why so little attention has been given to the care of persons with chronic conditions. This is unfortunate since there are many physical, social, and psychological components of long-term disease which require organized health care services.

Levels of Prevention for Chronic Disease

The first of a four-volume series, based on the work of the Commission on Chronic Illness, was appropriately titled *Prevention of Chronic Illness*. Prevention must be the underlying approach to chronic conditions or these problems will only increase with time.

Early in its history the commission defined prevention as the means of averting the development of a pathological state, which included all the measures necessary to halt the progression of the condition, especially disability and eventual death (Commission on Chronic Illness, 1957, p. 4). The commission further stated that prevention on all three levels—primary, secondary, and tertiary—is essential for effective management and control of chronic conditions.

Primary prevention of many serious chronic illnesses is frequently impossible because health professionals are unable to determine the exact point in time when a condition begins. When, for example, does schizophrenia, asbestosis, or diabetes begin? Each of these dis-

[1] Anselm L. Strauss. *Chronic illness and the quality of life*. St. Louis: Mosby, 1975.

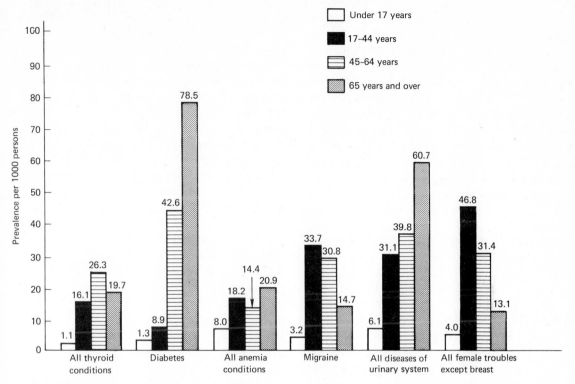

FIGURE 10-8 Prevalence of chronic conditions reported in health interviews per 1000 persons, by age, in the United States, 1973. (*From U. S. Department of Health, Education, and Welfare, Public Health Service, Health Resources Administration. Prevalence of chronic conditions of the genitourinary, nervous, endocrine, metabolic, and blood and blood-forming systems and of other selected chronic conditions, United States—1973. Rockville, Md.: Health Resources Administration, National Center for Health Statistics, March 1977, p. 14.*)

eases goes through a long latent period before symptoms are seen. They may stem from such variables as hereditary characteristics, occupational conditions, environmental stresses, or nutritional factors. There are, however, some chronic conditions that can be prevented. Primary preventive efforts that control communicable disease, reduce accidents, and emphasize adequate care during pregnancy and ways to cope with emotional stress all contribute to the prevention of certain chronic conditions. Primary prevention is an important task of the community health nurse.

Detection and treatment of chronic conditions (secondary prevention) are often possi-

ble. For many conditions such as diabetes, hypertension, breast cancer, and glaucoma, large-scale national programs for early detection represent a profitable and economical approach to secondary prevention.

A major secondary prevention effort relative to chronic illness occurred in the United States when the National Health Survey was authorized and conducted in 1956 to secure information about health conditions in the general population. This survey was enacted under the National Health Survey Act, which was proposed in 1955 by the Department of Health, Education, and Welfare (HEW). Under this act, the Surgeon General of the Public

Health Service was authorized to conduct a survey in order to produce uniform, national statistics on disease, injury, impairment, disability, and related topics.

In 1972, a new survey mechanism initiated by HEW and called HANES, the Health and Nutrition Examination Survey, began. Persons 1 to 74 years of age were examined, with emphasis on their nutritional status. Statistical data were collected on health records, fertility patterns, morbidity, and mortality. HANES is, today, the primary source of nationwide data on illnesses, disabilities, and physiological measurements.

Tertiary prevention activities, as well as primary and secondary ones, should be planned when working with people who have chronic conditions. Tertiary prevention involves rehabilitation, with the ultimate goal being cure or full restoration of the client's level of functioning. For some chronic conditions, this may be impossible; hence, the ideal goal must be replaced by more limited objectives, such as maximizing remaining functional potential or minimizing further deterioration. Another option would be to learn to live within the limitations that the chronic disease has imposed. A more detailed discussion of the concept of rehabilitation is presented in Chapter 17.

Approaches to the Study of Chronic Conditions

Two basic approaches to the study of chronic conditions and other diseases are retrospective and prospective studies. Retrospective and prospective studies are designed to determine if there is a relationship between a factor and a disease, as well as the intensity of that relationship. Mausner and Bahn (1974, pp. 312–325) discuss extensively the principles involved in these types of studies. Since only a brief summary of their thoughts is presented below, the reader should refer to Mausner and Bahn's text to obtain a more in-depth understanding of these approaches.

Retrospective studies look at people who are diagnosed as having a disease, comparing them with those who do not have the disease. The persons who do not have the disease are called *controls*. The controls come from the same general population segment as the individuals who have the condition and have the same characteristics as the study group except for the disease condition. A retrospective study examines factors in the person's past experience. One of the disadvantages of retrospective studies is that detailed information may not be available or accurate. The greatest problem, however, is finding a control group that is alike in all respects except for the condition under study. The advantages of this type of study are cost and the number of subjects needed. Retrospective studies are relatively inexpensive and require a small sampling size, since cases are identified at the onset.

Prospective studies start with a group of people (a cohort), all presumed to be free from a condition but who differ in their exposure to a supposedly harmful factor. This cohort is followed over a period of time to discover differences in the rate at which disease develops in relation to exposure to the harmful factor. A major advantage of this type of study is that the cohort is chosen for study before the disease develops. The cohort is, therefore, not influenced by knowledge that disease exists, as in retrospective studies.

Prospective studies allow calculation of incidence rates among those exposed and those not exposed. Thus, absolute difference in incidence rates and the true relative risk can be measured. The major disadvantage is that a prospective study is a long, expensive project. A large cohort must be used, especially if the disease has low incidence. Also, the larger the number of factors to be studied, the larger the cohort must be. The loss of people from the cohort due to death, lack of interest, or job mobility is a major problem when a study lasts over an extended period of time. Changes in diagnostic criteria, administrative problems, loss of staff or funding, and the high cost of record keeping can all contribute to make this a study that should not be undertaken without careful planning.

Retrospective and prospective studies assist in identifying causes of disease as well as effective disease control mechanisms. It is not intended that this brief description of retrospective and prospective studies will prepare community health nurses to do them. The purpose is to familiarize readers with the basic concepts involved in the study of chronic conditions.

The community health nurse does, however, play an active role in the control of chronic conditions. Case finding through screening programs is a significant aspect of this part of the community health nurse's role.

Screening as a Method for Detection and Control of Chronic Conditions

Screening programs can be an efficient way to identify individuals in a community who may unknowingly have a chronic condition, as well as an infectious disease.

There are two types of screening programs whereby chronic and infectious disease is sought in apparently healthy individuals: the *single screening test* where only one condition is being identified, such as giving a group of teachers a TB tine test, and the *multiphasic screening test* where a battery of tests is used at one time to detect several disease conditions. Doing height and weight measurements, audiometry, and vision screening of all persons at a county fair is an example of multiphasic screening.

Screening tests do not provide a conclusive diagnosis of a disease, but rather are used to identify asymptomatic individuals who may

unknowingly have a problem. Anyone who evidences symptoms of a disease through a screening program should have further medical diagnostic testing. This is essential since early diagnosis and treatment are the primary goals of a screening program. Early diagnosis and treatment are particularly beneficial for conditions such as hypertension and cancer, for which there are treatment measures available to prevent progression of the condition.

Advantages of screening programs are that often they are relatively inexpensive; take little time; need few professionals to administer them; provide opportunity for prevention, early diagnosis, and treatment; and present statistics on the prevalence of disease when there is adequate follow-up. A major disadvantage of screening programs is that people tend to substitute them for medical examination. The findings of screening programs are presumptive and further testing should be done to confirm a diagnosis. In addition, screening programs often do not reach vulnerable groups of people, particularly populations who utilize emergency rooms in a fragmented way for health care. Also, conditions may be missed during screening and persons may be given a false impression of their health status.

Not all chronic conditions lend themselves to screening. Mausner and Bahn (1974, pp. 252–253) have elucidated the following principles that should be the basis of any screening program:

1. The condition sought should be an important health problem [affect a significant percentage of people].

2. There should be an accepted treatment for clients with recognized disease.

3. Facilities for diagnosis and treatment should be available.

4. There should be a recognizable latent or early symptomatic stage.

5. There should be a suitable test or examination [to detect the disease].

6. The test should be acceptable to the population.

7. The natural history of the condition, including development from latent to declared disease, should be adequately understood.

8. There should be an agreed policy about whom to treat as patients [clients].

9. The cost of case-finding (including diagnosis and treatment) should be economically balanced in relation to possible expenditure for medical care as a whole.

10. Case-finding should be thought of as a continuing process and not a "once and for all" project.

It should be clear from reviewing these principles that although screening can be one method for early discovery of asymptomatic disease, it should be used judiciously and discriminately. Screening results need to be thoroughly evaluated and the conditions found must be treated.

In addition to screening for disease and chronic conditions, the community health nurse has a continuing responsibility for case finding through other activities. She or he has the unique opportunity to interact regularly with people in the community through home visits, clinic nursing, school visits, and prenatal classes, to name only a few. A nurse who is able to communicate a sense of caring will hear requests such as, "Say, nurse, my neighbor across the street has a sick baby and she was wondering if you could come and visit her." The nurse in a clinic setting will pick up clues such as a tired young mother who seems unable to handle her four preschool children or possible scoliosis in a preadolescent girl.

A nurse who is open to clues such as those described above will find many situations in which to use nursing skills to prevent disease and promote health.

SUMMARY

Use of the epidemiological process helps community health nurses to identify the health status of the community in which they are working, and to prevent disease, chronic conditions, and other health-related phenomena such as child abuse, mental illness, and domestic violence. This process places emphasis on analyzing the needs of populations rather than the needs of individual clients. Like the nursing process, it is a scientific, systematic problem-solving approach to the study of health needs.

There are several key concepts inherent in the understanding and utilization of the epidemiological process. These are study of populations at risk, natural life history of disease, levels of prevention, host-agent-environment relationships, multiple causation of disease, and person-place-time relationships. In addition to these concepts, a community health nurse must understand biostatistics in order to effectively use the epidemiological process.

By applying the concepts and methods of epidemiology, community health nurses play a vital role in the prevention of disease and conditions in a community. Through their contacts in a variety of settings, they are in a key position to do case finding, to eliminate barriers to the control of disease, and to promote health through teaching and counseling.

REFERENCES

Commission on Chronic Illness. *Chronic illness in the United States. Volume I: Prevention of chronic illness.* Cambridge, Mass.: Harvard University Press, 1957.

Communicable Disease Center. *Food-borne disease investigation: Analysis of field data.* Atlanta, Ga.: Public Health Service, 1964.

Division of Epidemiology. *Enteric infections case history.* Lansing, Mich.: Michigan Department of Public Health.

Doyle, A. C. *The hound of the Baskervilles.* New York: Berkley Publishing Corporation, November 1971 ed., p. 157.

Farquhar, J. W. You can cut the odds on coronary risk. *RN Magazine,* February 1977, *40,* 23–26.

Friedman, G. E. *Primer of epidemiology.* New York: McGraw-Hill, 1974.

Horwitz, M., Pollard, R., Merson, M., & Martin, S. A large outbreak of foodborne salmonellosis on the Navajo Nation Indian Reservation: Epidemiology and transmission. *American Journal of Public Health,* November 1977, *67,* 1071–1076.

Leavell, H., & Clark, G. *Preventive medicine for the doctor in the community: An epidemiologic approach.* New York: McGraw-Hill, 1965.

MacMahon, B., & Pugh, T. *Epidemiology principles and methods.* Boston: Little, Brown, 1970.

Mausner, J., & Bahn, A. *Epidemiology: An introductory text.* Philadelphia: Saunders, 1974.

Maxcy, R. F., & Rosenau, M. J. *Preventive medicine and public health.* New York: Appleton-Century-Crofts, 1965.

Roueche, B. *Eleven blue men.* New York: Berkley Publishing Corporation, 1968.

Strauss, A. *Chronic illness and the quality of life.* St. Louis: Mosby, 1975.

U.S. Department of Health, Education, and Welfare, Public Welfare, Public Health Service, Mental Health Administration. *Chronic conditions and limitations of activity and mobility, U.S., July 1965–June 1967.* Publication No. 1000, series 10-61, Rockville, Md.: Mental Health Administration, January 1971.

U.S. Department of Health, Education, and Welfare, Public Health Service, Health Resources Administration. *Prevalence of chronic conditions of the genitourinary, nervous, endocrine, metabolic, and blood and blood-forming systems and of other selected chronic conditions, United States—1973.* Rockville, Md.: Health Resouces Administration, National Center for Health Statistics, March 1977.

SELECTED BIBLIOGRAPHY

Breslow, L. Risk factor intervention for health maintenance. *Science,* May 1978, *200,* 908–912.

Cassell, M. Potentialities and limitations of epidemiology. In A. Katz & J. Felton (Eds.), *Health and community.* New York: The Free Press, 1965.

Chavigny, C. Self-esteem for the alcoholic: An epidemiological approach. *Nursing Outlook,* October 1976, *24,* 636–639.

Christiansen, E. E. Family epidemiology: An approach to assessment and intervention. In D. P. Hymorich & M. U. Barnard (Eds.), *Family health care. Volume 1: General perspectives.* New York: McGraw-Hill, 1979.

Coulehan, J. L. Screening yield in an urban low income practice. *American Journal of Public Health,* May 1975, *65,* 474–479.

Dean, A. G. Population-based spot maps: An epidemiologic technique. *American Journal of Public Health,* October 1976, *66,* 988–989.

Donabedian, D. Computer-taught epidemiology. *Nursing Outlook,* December 1976, *24,* 749–751.

Greene, M. H. An epidemiologic assessment of heroin use. *American Journal of Public Health,* December 1974, *64* (supplement), 1–8.

Hilbert, M. Prevention. *American Journal of Public Health,* April 1977, *67,* 353–356.

Hingson, R. Obtaining optimal attendance at mass immunization programs. *Public Health Services Reports,* January–February 1974, *89,* 53–64.

International Union of Nutritional Sciences Report. Guidelines on the at-risk concept and the health and nutrition of young children. *American Journal of Clinical Nutrition,* February 1977, *30,* 242–254.

Kessler, I., & Levin, M. L., (Eds.). *The community as an epidemiologic laboratory—A casebook of community studies.* Baltimore: John Hopkins, 1970.

Lenz, P. Women, the unwitting carriers of gonorrhea. *American Journal of Nursing*, April 1971, *71*, 716–719.

Lester, M. R. Every nurse an epidemiologist. *American Journal of Nursing*, November 1957, *57*, 1434–1435.

Morris, J. N. *Uses of epidemiology* (3d ed.). New York: Churchill Livingstone, 1975.

James, S. A., & Kleinbaum, P. G. Socioecologic stress and hypertension related mortality rates in North Carolina. *American Journal of Public Health*, April 1976, *66*, 354–358.

Riessman, C. K. Interviewer effects in psychiatric epidemiology: A study of medical and lay interviews and their impact on reported symptoms. *American Journal of Public Health*, May 1979, *69*, 485–491.

Rosen, F. *Preventive medicine in the United States 1900–1975: Trends and interpretations.* New York: Prodist, 1977.

Ruben, F., Streiff, E., Neal, M., & Michaels, R. Epidemiologic studies of Reye's syndrome: Cases seen in Pittsburgh, October 1973–April 1975. *American Journal of Public Health*, November 1976, *66*, 1096–1098.

Tervis, M. Approaches to an epidemiology of health. *American Journal of Public Health*, October 1975, *65*, 1037–1045.

Venters, M., Schacht, L., & Bensel, R. Report of Down's syndrome from birth certificate data in the state of Minnesota. *American Journal of Public Health*, November 1976, *66*, 1099–1100.

White, K. L., & Henderson, M. M. *Epidemiology as a fundamental science: Its uses in health services planning, administration, and evaluation.* New York: Oxford University Press, 1976.

Wigley, R., & Cook, J. *Community health: Concepts and issues.* New York: D. Van Nostrand, 1975.

Winslow, C. E. A., Smillie, W. G., Doull, J. A., & Gordon, J. E. *The history of American epidemiology.* St. Louis: Mosby, 1952.

Wrona, R. M. A clinical epidemiologic study of hyperphenylalaninemia. *American Journal of Public Health*, July 1979, *69*, 673–679.

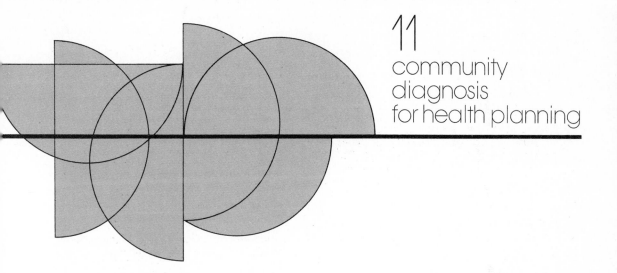

Chapter 2 explored the American Nurses' Association's definition of community health nursing practice which states that the dominant responsibility of nurses in community health is to the population as a whole (ANA, 1973). In order to fulfill this responsibility, community health nurses must "see," "smell," and "hear" the community and describe its people, its environment, its health status, and its health resources. Further, they must systematically analyze all facets of community dynamics (described in Chapter 3) so that populations at risk are determined and ways to meet their needs are identified.

Community health nurses at both administrative and staff levels must become involved in community organizational activities if health

The authors are indebted to A. Josephine Brown, friend and colleague, who encouraged both faculty and students to expand their thinking beyond individual client casework to the community as a whole. Through her efforts, community health nurses have learned how to use the nursing process to plan, implement, and evaluate community health programming. Content and case illustrations in this chapter reflect many of the concepts shared by her.

services are to be available for all citizens. Nursing directors and supervisors should assume leadership in establishing mechanisms for the ongoing survey of community needs and for maintaining collaborative relationships with consumers and other health care resources. They should encourage staff nurses to assess the characteristics of their work community (neighborhood, census tract, or district), so that staff understand how to effect change when resources are lacking as well as how to mobilize resources when they exist. Nursing administrators must provide an atmosphere within their agency which supports staff involvement in community activities; otherwise staff efforts will be focused on individual client casework.

Staff nurses must also take the initiative to expand their thinking to the community as a whole. When handling a family caseload and managing other professional responsibilities, such as clinic and school activities, it is easy for community health nurses to become narrow in their scope of practice. These activities are time-consuming and very important. Thus, the value of taking time to study the community in which the nurse practices is not always readily evident, especially when work demands are heavy.

WHY STUDY THE COMMUNITY?

It is essential for the community health nurse to have an understanding of community dynamics because health action occurs in the community. Every community has *patterns* of functioning or community dynamics, which either contribute to or detract from its state of health. The community health nurse must have a knowledge of these patterns in order to anticipate community responses to health action and to influence the direction of health programming. Without this knowledge, it is difficult to effect change.

Knowledge of community dynamics is obtained through systematic community study. Community study helps the nurse and other health care professionals to identify cultural differences in relation to consumer interests, strengths, concerns, and motivations. This study also assists health care professionals in analyzing processes through which community beliefs, values, and attitudes are transmitted. Having this information allows health professionals to individualize health planning activities for their community.

It is important for the community health nurse to recognize that the traditions in each community vary; hence, the type of programs designed to meet consumer needs should also vary. Programs appropriate for one community or for a group within a community may be ineffective in meeting the needs of other community populations. Walker (1979, pp. 667–671) substantiated this statement when he studied the utilization of health care services by migrant labor families in Laredo, Texas. The purpose of his study was to determine the relationship between economic barriers and the utilization of ambulatory health care services by migrant workers in Laredo. A system of prepaid health insurance was established for families enrolled in a special demonstration project. Three years of study demonstrated that even when economic barriers were removed, the migrant workers in Laredo used ambulatory health care services less often than other impoverished groups in the United States. In addition, the Laredo migrant workers showed lower usage rates than those of other migrant workers in Texas who were covered by the prepaid health insurance project. The conclusion was that further research or community study was needed to determine what unique characteristics of this migrant community influenced use or lack of use of health care services.

Studies such as those conducted by Walker serve to reinforce the need to study the characteristics of the community in which one is working. They demonstrated that assumptions cannot be made about community response to health care delivery efforts, and they point out the relevancy of identifying factors that facilitate or inhibit health action. Such studies also provide data that support the need for collaborative relationships between the consumer and the health care provider to enhance the delivery of health care services.

Study of the community is essential if the community health nurse is truly going to meet the needs of all populations in a given community. Experiences from one community setting cannot always be generalized to another, because health needs and resources are not consistent from one community to another. Data about a specific community are needed if the nature and origin of health problems and the responses to health matters are to be identified.

With the curtailment of federal monies for health care programs, it is even more imperative that community needs and priorities be documented. The Special Health Revenue Sharing Act of 1975 (Public Law 94-63) mandates that dialogue between consumers and health planners occur so that community needs are met. Funds are appropriated on the basis of documented evidence that a planned health program actually reflects a need within the community. Health programs will no longer be federally funded without data that support their need.

Purpose of Community Study for the Community Health Nurse

Within any community setting, there will be professionals from many disciplines and concerned citizens interested in community organizational activities. Since it would be impossible for any one group to handle all the health care needs of a community, efforts by many should be encouraged and supported. Equally important is the need for each discipline to define its responsibilities in relation to community organizational activities so that overlapping and uncoordinated efforts will be avoided. Unfortunately, it is not uncommon to find that the linkages between various community agencies are weak and that health services are planned without taking into consideration the contributions that other health care professionals are making (see Chapter 5). At times, cooperative efforts are not fostered because community agencies are more interested in supporting their own self-interests than in determining how consumer needs can best be met. This practice will not be altered until health disciplines subscribe to the belief that the community is their "client" and that interdisciplinary efforts are needed to achieve wellness for the population as a whole.

When studying the community, the community health nurse must recognize that she or he is a member of an interdisciplinary team whose activities should not be carried out in isolation. Implicit in the concept of interdisciplinary functioning are several major premises: (1) there is a common endeavor that all professionals are working toward; (2) interdisciplinary teams are established to meet client needs and, thus, the client is the key member on the team; (3) professionals will share knowledge and information across disciplinary boundaries so that team goals can be reached; and (4) all disciplines will delineate and share the unique talents they have, so that the team can delegate responsibilities to appropriate team members.

The unique perspective that the community health nurse brings to an interdisciplinary community team is a holistic philosophy derived from a synthesis of nursing and public health knowledge. The community health nurse's professional experience, educational preparation, value system, and relationships with consumers, provide the skills that allow her or him to integrate biopsychosocial data into a meaningful whole. Since it is known that all parameters of human functioning and all aspects of community dynamics have an impact on the client's (community) health status, the whole must be analyzed. Only when this is done will health programs truly reflect the needs of the consumer.

Prevention is often the one aspect of wholeness that is overlooked when community problems are analyzed and health services developed. This happens because many health care professionals have a curative rather than a preventive health philosophy. Because community health nurses, as well as other health department personnel, have educational preparation which enhances their ability to examine the preventive aspects of health behavior, they are delegated the major responsibility for monitoring preventive health practices in the community.

The community health nurse's primary

purpose when studying the community is to identify strengths and deficiencies in relation to preventive health practices. She or he places emphasis on examining the health care delivery system to determine if there are structural or process characteristics within this system that impede preventive health programming. In addition, the community health nurse works with consumers and other health care professionals to improve the quality of preventive health activities when deficiencies are identified.

DIAGNOSING PREVENTIVE HEALTH NEEDS IN THE COMMUNITY

When participating in community diagnostic activities, the community health nurse uses the nursing process as described in Chapter 8, but shifts emphasis from the family to the community as a whole. Data are collected from multiple sources (assessing) in order to formulate nursing diagnoses (analyzing) about community health problems. Nursing diagnoses about health needs that exist, about health needs that are and are not being met, about community dynamics which either positively or negatively influence health action, and about deficiencies in the existing health care delivery system are generated for the purpose of facilitating health planning. In addition, nursing diagnoses about community strengths are made, because it is through its strengths that a community is able to resolve its health problems. Some examples of nursing diagnoses that might be made after the community health nurse has assessed the community are listed below:

· Children in census tracts 10 and 11 are at risk for lead poisoning because of the inadequate enforcement of housing regulations in these areas.

· Thirty-five percent of the aging persons in the community are experiencing social isolation because recreational activities and transportation for these persons are lacking.

· Teenagers are at risk for unwanted pregnancies because health care resources in the community refuse to provide birth control information for teenagers without parental consent.

· Community health nursing services need to be increased in census tract 5, because the number of new referrals from this area exceeds the time the current nurse has available for home visiting.

· Local churches within the community readily support health education efforts.

· Service clubs within the community respond very favorably when health care professionals request financial assistance for meeting unresolved health problems.

Once nursing diagnoses are established, the community health nurse uses the principles of planning (see Chapter 12) to prioritize health needs, to determine alternative ways to resolve these needs, to develop specific objectives for health programming, and to identify ways to accomplish the stated objectives (planning). The following are a few examples of objectives that might be developed when planning a health program to meet the social needs of aging citizens in the community:

· The county commissioners will appropriate funds for a senior citizens project in census tract 2.

· St. Francis Catholic Church will donate space in their facilities once a week for recreational activities for the aging.

· Community volunteers will plan and implement recreational activities for the aging at St. Francis Church.

· The local chapter of the American Red Cross will provide transportation for aging citizens once a week, so that these persons can participate in the social activities planned at St. Francis Church.

The above objectives can be met in several ways. For example, the community health nurse might make all the necessary contacts personally or delegate responsibilities to others, perhaps by obtaining volunteers. Church groups, service clubs, and social workers from community agencies, for instance, often know of individuals who are interested in volunteering their time and energies for worthy community projects. Community health nurses usually seek help from others when planning a health program because they know that active participation by consumers and other professionals promotes long-term support and involvement.

Planning must result in action (implement-

ing), and action must be evaluated; otherwise time and effort are wasted and community needs go unresolved. When one is evaluating action, it may be found that new problems emerge because insufficient data or data that are no longer valid, were collected during the assessment phase (evaluating). If this is the case, objectives and intervention strategies should be altered so that they reflect ways to resolve existing needs.

Diagnosing community health problems and planning action to correct these problems are far more difficult than was just indicated. The point being made above is that the community health nurse uses the nursing process—assessing, analyzing, planning, implementing, and evaluating—when intervening with the population as a whole, as well as when working with individual families. How community health nurses assess the health status of populations and how they analyze community data is further elaborated on in this chapter. An overview of health planning is presented in Chapter 12.

METHODS FOR ASSESSING A COMMUNITY'S STATUS

There are a variety of strategies a community health nurse can use to obtain data about community needs. Before selecting any method for data collection, the community health nurse must first define what needs to be assessed. Establishing guidelines for assessment helps the nurse to organize the data-collection process and to identify significant factors that have an influence on a community's state of wellness.

Figure 11-1 summarizes the various parameters the community health nurse should examine when analyzing the health status of any community. It points out that the physical, social, and mental aspects of wellness are interrelated and that people, environmental, and health resource characteristics make an impact

on a community's state of wellness. If there are changes in any one of these components, the balance of health is altered in the community setting. When diagnosing community needs, it is important to examine all components of wellness and to identify community dynamics that detract from or enhance community growth. Chapter 3 presents the knowledge needed to analyze community dynamics.

After determining the information needed to establish appropriate nursing diagnoses about community problems, the community health nurse uses both subjective and objective data-collection methods to obtain this information. These methods are discussed below. It is important to keep in mind that no one method is sufficient for obtaining a compre-

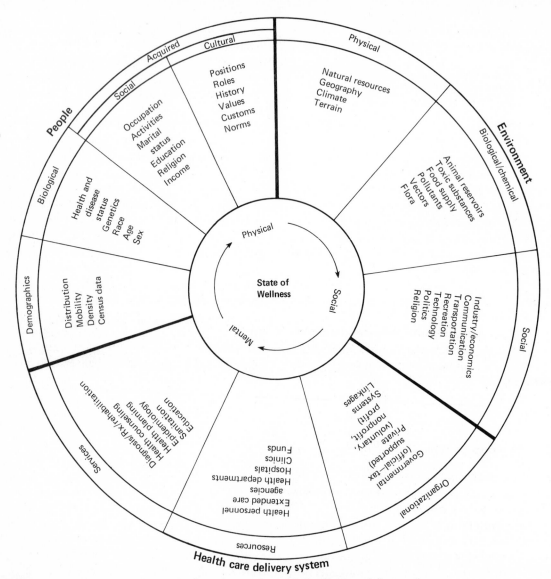

FIGURE 11-1 The community: its people, its environment, and its health care delivery system.

hensive view of how a community is functioning.

Analyze Available Statistics

Many people immediately associate the term *statistics* with a long list of numbers, boring to read and difficult to use. If used effectively, however, statistical data can be exciting and intriguing. It can quickly reveal facts about a community, including clues about why citizens do or do not become involved in health projects, as well as concrete information about the characteristics of the population being served. For example, one community health nurse was concerned because parents in one of the schools she serviced were not participating in health activities designed to promote child safety.

When this nurse looked at census tract data, she found that 64 percent of the households in her district were headed by single-parent, working mothers who had a marginal income. This information suggested to the nurse that in order to reach these women, she would have to plan activities outside the traditional 8 to 5 working hours. It also pointed out to her that she was dealing with families who were at risk for financial, social, and psychological crises. This data stimulated the nurse to design health programs that were relevant to mothers' as well as children's needs. One program, How to Meet Your Social Needs While Caring for Small Children, was particularly well-received. This program was planned because the nurse on several home visits heard mothers complain about the lack of time for leisure activities. The expressed concerns of these mothers, coupled with knowledge obtained from census tract data, led the nurse to believe that there were other mothers in the area who had the same concern. Her nursing diagnosis was valid and resulted in a meaningful health program that was well attended. Because this one program was so well received, an ongoing activity and discussion group for these mothers was established, with equally positive results. The processes this nurse used to develop her mother's group and to maintain it are presented in Chapter 19.

Use of statistical data can be very beneficial in community health nursing practice. The nurse in the above illustration found that statistical data provided her with clues about why families were not responding to school health activities. Statistical data also helped this nurse to identify some of the possible concerns of the population she was serving and, thus, she was able to predict health interests and plan health programs accordingly.

Statistical data often provide the basis for decision making in the face of uncertainty. The community health nurse frequently finds that there are several requests for nursing service and it is necessary to plan time to ben-

efit the greatest number of people. Using census tract data, vital statistics, and health statistics can help community health nurses to determine where to focus their efforts. Take, for instance, the community health nurse who has several requests for the establishment of a well-baby clinic in various locations. If only one clinic can be funded, this nurse may use statistical data to document a need for a clinic in one location rather than another. The concentration of preschool children in a given area, the illness and death rates of these children, and the level of immunization protection can all be obtained from statistical data. These data provide information about where the greatest need exists and can be used to substantiate a decision a nurse might make about clinic location.

The importance of understanding and using statistical data becomes increasingly apparent to the community health nurse when decisions such as those described above must be made. Statistical data help the community health nurse to more effectively carry out many daily responsibilities. These data help the nurse to:

· Predict health needs of individuals, families, and populations

· Identify groups at risk

· Determine priorities when needs are greater than staff time available

· Evaluate the outcomes of nursing services

· Document accountability

· Support the need for increased funding for nursing services

Statistics Defined

The term *statistics* is generally used to describe two different phenomena: (1) numerical data which reveal actual counts of a given occurrence, such as the number of cases (325) of reported hepatitis in a given community; and (2) methods or procedures developed to analyze and interpret numerical data. These methods are labeled either *descriptive* or *inferential*. The descriptive methods will be emphasized in this chapter because they are used more frequently by the practitioner than are the inferential methods.

Descriptive methods involve relatively simple mathematical procedures, including such things as the construction of tables, graphs, or frequency distributions and the calculation of rates, percentages, or averages. These methods are used to organize and synthesize a mass of data. They help to describe and communicate to others, such facts about a given population as age, height, weight, or causes of disease and death. *Inferential* methods are more sophisticated, mathematical tools (analysis of variance or t-tests) used by researchers and statisticians to draw generalizations from data obtained from a sample population. The term *population*, as it is used here, does not necessarily imply individuals living in the same geographic area. Rather, it means a set of individuals who have some characteristics in common. Sample populations are studied in order to make inferences about individuals who are at risk for developing health or health-related problems.

In community health, several terms are used to describe health or health-related data. These are *biostatistics, vital statistics, demographic statistics,* and *morbidity and mortality statistics*. *Biostatistics* is the overall broad term used to identify any data that delineate health or health-related events. Health statistics that describe birth, adoption, death, marriage, divorce, separation, and annulment patterns are labeled *vital statistics*. Because these events must be registered in each state, trends can be ascertained within each state and the country as a whole. Usually at least 5 years' data should be examined to see if significant patterns are occurring over time. Monitoring these signif-

icant changes helps the community health nurse to identify health promotion activities needed across the life-span. For example, major causes of death for each developmental age group (see Chapters 13 through 18) are calculated from death registries each year. These death rates assist the health professional in determining key community health problems and in substantiating a need for specific health programs. The development of programs to prevent accidents and the establishment of screening clinics to identify at-risk persons for hypertension are examples of health activities that have been initiated to reduce the number of unnecessary deaths in the United States. Data related to the analysis of death trends are classified as *mortality statistics*.

Infant and maternal death rates or mortality statistics have traditionally been used in community health to make judgments about the health status of a community. Deaths in these two population groups are considered to be unnecessary and often associated with poor environmental conditions and inadequate health care. Thus, they may reflect not only unmet health needs but also deficiencies in the health care delivery system which need to be corrected.

Demographic statistics also aid the practitioner in identifying significant characteristics of a population, such as socioeconomic status, which influence the delivery of health care services in a community. Demographic data describe the size, distribution, structure, and change in populations over time (Shryock, Siegel, and Associates, 1971, p. 1). These data are collected by census and special surveys.

Census data provide a wealth of information about a community's population characteristics. Census tracts have been established and maintained in large cities throughout the country, so that social and economic changes can be easily identified from one census to another. Census tracts are "small areas in large cities, having a population between 3,000 and

6,000 with fairly homogeneous characteristics with respect to ethnic origin, economic status, and living conditions" (Shryock, Siegel, and Associates, 1971, p. 39). Census tract boundaries are preserved from one national census to another so that variations in population characteristics can be studied over time.

Presented below is an outline of the data available on census tracts in the United States, from the 1970 census (Shryock, Siegel, and Associates, 1971, appendix B). Similar information will be available from the 1980 census. Health professionals analyze census data because it has been documented that there is a significant relationship between educational background, economic status, and living conditions and the number of health needs in specified populations (Miller, 1975, p. 355). This information can be obtained at a nominal cost from the United States Bureau of the Census, Washington, D.C.

I. General characteristics of the population: 1970

  A. Race

  B. Age by sex

  C. Relationship to head of household

  D. Type of family and number of own children

  E. Marital status

II. Social characteristics of the population: 1970

  A. Nativity, parentage, and country of origin

  B. School enrollment

  C. Years of school completed

  D. Children ever born

  E. Means of transportation and place of work

III. Labor force characteristics of the population: 1970

  A. Employment status

  B. Occupation

  C. Industry

  D. Class of worker

IV. Income characteristics of the population: 1970

  A. Income in 1969 of families and unrelated individuals

  B. Type of income in 1969 of families

  C. Ratio of family income to poverty level

  D. Income below poverty level: families, family heads, unrelated individuals, persons and households

V. Occupancy, utilization, and financial characteristics of housing units: 1970

  A. Tenure, race, and vacancy status

  B. Lacking some or all plumbing facilities

  C. Complete kitchen facilities and access

  D. Rooms

  E. Persons

  F. Persons per room

  G. Value

  H. Contract rent

VI. Structural equipment and financial characteristics of housing units: 1970

  A. Year moved into unit

  B. Automobiles available

  C. Gross rent

  D. Gross rent as percentage of income by income

  E. Units in structure

  F. Year structure built

  G. Heating equipment

  H. Basement

  I. Selected equipment (air conditioning, public sewer, water supply, more than one bathroom)

In addition to vital and demographic statistics, the community health nurse uses morbidity statistics to assess the health status of the community. *Morbidity data* describe the extent and distribution of illness in a community.

These data assist the nurse in identifying specific health problems and in setting priorities for program planning. One Midwestern community, for example, used morbidity statistics to support the need for a neighborhood health clinic in one of their inner-city districts. A comprehensive analysis of these statistics revealed that 52 percent of all new tuberculosis cases, 61 percent of all new syphilis cases, 72 percent of all new gonorrhea cases, and 37 percent of all accidental poisoning cases occurred in one particular section of the city in a given time period. It was evident from this information that the health needs in this district were much greater than in other sections of the city. Special funds were allocated to determine if a new approach for delivering health services could alter the disease trends in this area; significant positive changes were noted within a 3-year time frame. Because morbidity statistics were collected prior to and during the time the clinic was in existence, state legislators responded favorably to a request for additional funds to keep the clinic open. Health professionals in this situation had documented the need for and the effectiveness of their pilot health clinic. The use of statistics helped these health professionals to establish a neighborhood health center, as well as to keep the center functioning after the trial period.

How to Use Statistical Data[1]

Usually community health professionals express absolute numbers or actual counts in terms of relative numbers. This is done because relative numbers make it easier to compare results in populations of differing sizes or to visualize what proportion of a given population is affected by a given phenomenon. A *relative number* is one which shows a relationship between two absolute numbers; this relationship is expressed in terms of a round

[1]Handout materials distributed in 1968 by the community health nursing faculty at Michigan State University, East Lansing, Michigan, provided the framework for this section.

number. A *percentage* is an example of a relative number; 100 is the round number used to show relationships when percentages are calculated.

The value of using relative numbers becomes clearer when the nurse actually works with raw data. For example, stating that 45 teenagers in a mental health institution need foster home placement has very little meaning until this number is related to the total number of teenagers in the institution. If there are only 100 teenagers in this setting, then 45 is a significant proportion (45 percent) of this given population. If, on the other hand, there are 1000 teenagers in this environment, 45 is a relatively small proportion (4.5 percent) of the total population. The percentages are identified by relating 45 (absolute number) to 100 or 1000 (absolute numbers) and then multiplying the results by 100 (round number).

Raw data from populations of differing sizes cannot be compared unless absolute numbers are converted to relative numbers. For instance, knowing the number of students who received free lunches in 1980 in each school in the county only becomes relevant when one summarizes the percentage of children in each school who received free lunches. The following figures illustrate how deceptive absolute numbers can be when making comparisons from one population to another; even though the number of children (250 vs. 75) receiving free lunches is much higher in the Burns Park High School, the proportion of childern needing free lunches in Kent Elementary School is five times greater than the proportion of children needing free lunches in Burns Park High School:

$$\frac{75}{150} \times 100 = 50\%$$ of the children in Kent Elementary School received free lunches in 1980

$$\frac{250}{1000} \times 100 = 10\%$$ of the children in Burns Park High School received free lunches in 1980

Besides percentages, two other relative numbers, ratios and rates, are commonly used to analyze health or health-related events. A *ratio* expresses the size of one number in relation to the size of another number. The number of females to males (sex ratio) or per capita expenditure for health care in a given state are examples of ratios. Per capita ratios are obtained by dividing the amount of money spent for health care (event) by the population in a given state (population).

A *rate* is actually a ratio but with the additional features of expressing what has happened in terms of a certain unit of *time* and the *population at risk* for a given event. It delineates the relationship between the number of times an event has occurred to the size of the population at risk. In demographic study, the unit of time for a rate is usually a year unless otherwise stated.

The formula for a rate is given as follows:

$$\frac{\text{Event in a given time}}{\text{Pop. at risk in same time period}} \times \text{round no.}$$

The *event* in this formula is the number of times a phenomenon (births, deaths, or disease) has occurred. The *population* is usually the number of persons at risk for a given event. The round number is one which makes the rate above the value of 1. If, for instance, an event such as polio occurs infrequently within a large population at risk, the round number used would be 100,000. On the other hand, when an event such as death occurs frequently within a population at risk, the round number used would be 1000.

Following are examples of how to apply the rate formula. Note particularly the population at risk, which varies depending on the nature of the event. When morbidity rates (incidence and prevalence) are calculated, the total population of the community may be at risk. In determining infant mortality rates, only infants born within a certain time period are at risk.

Incidence rate. This is the number of new cases of a disease in a population over a period of time.

Incidence rate = number of "new" cases of a specified disease or condition occurring during a given time period (as during a year) ÷ population at risk during a given time period × 100,000

Bay City, January through December 1980, 50 new cases of diabetes in a population of 75,000.

$$\text{Incidence rate} = \frac{50}{75,000} \times 100,000 = 66.3$$

Incidence rate for diabetes in Bay City 1980: 66.3 new cases of diabetes per 100,000 population.

Prevalence rate. This is the number of old and new cases of a specified disease existing at a given time.

Prevalence rate = number of "old" and "new" cases of a specified disease or condition existing at a "point" in time ÷ total population at a point in time × 100,000

Bay City, December 1980, 1200 cases of diabetes in a population of 75,000.

$$\text{Prevalence rate} = \frac{1200}{75,000} \times 100,000 = 1600$$

Prevalence rate for diabetes in Bay City, December 1980: 1600 cases of diabetes per 100,000 population.

Infant mortality rate. This is the number of deaths of infants under 1 year of age per 1000 live births during a given year.

Infant mortality rate = number of deaths under 1 year of age during a given year ÷ number of live births during a given year $\times$ 1000 live births

Bay City, 1980: 25 infant deaths.

Infant mortality rate $= \dfrac{25}{1275} \times 1000 = 19.6$

Infant mortality rate Bay City 1980: 19.6 infant deaths per 1000 live births.

Frequently Calculated Rates and Ratios

In addition to the above examples, there are several other rates and ratios that are used to measure the state of health in a community.

The formulas for calculating these are presented in Table 11-1. Besides helping to identify the major health problems in a community, these statistics aid in projecting future health service and personnel needs. For example, examining the crude birth rate assists health care professionals in determining the demand for childhood health services over the next 20 years.

Rates, ratios, or percentages are the types of descriptive statistics most commonly used in community health nursing practice. At times, however, there is a need to use other descriptive measures, such as averages, in order to organize and characterize data. This is so when a series of measurements or quantitative

TABLE 11-1 Formulas for Rates and Ratios Frequently Calculated in Community Health Nursing Practice

Rate or ratio	Formula	Commonly used round number
MORTALITY STATISTICS		
Crude death rate	Number of deaths from all causes during a given year ÷ population estimated at midyear	× 1000 population
Age-specific death rate	Number of deaths for a specified age group during a given year ÷ population estimated at midyear for the specified age group	× 1000 population
Specific-cause-of-death rate	Number of deaths from a specific condition during a given year ÷ population estimated at midyear	× 100,000 population
Maternal mortality rate	Number of deaths from puerperal complications during a given year ÷ number of live births during the same year	× 100,000 population
Infant mortality rate	Number of deaths under 1 year of age during a given year ÷ number of live births during the same year	× 1000 live births
Neonatal mortality rate	Number of deaths under 28 days of age during a given year ÷ number of live births during the same year	× 1000 live births
Fetal mortality rate	Number of fetal deaths 20 weeks gestation or more during a given year ÷ number of live births and fetal deaths during the same year	× 1000 live births and fetal deaths
Birth-death ratio	Number of live births in a specified population ÷ number of deaths in a specified population	× 100

data is being analyzed. Generally, in any series of data, characteristic values tend to cluster near the center of the distribution. Thus, averages are often labeled measures of central tendency.

Measures of Central Tendency

Averages help to identify a value which is most characteristic of a set of raw data. There are several kinds of averages used to summarize quantitative measurements; the most frequently used ones in community health nursing practice are the arithmetic mean, the median, and the mode.

The *mean* is the arithmetic average of a set

of observations. It is the value in a series of data equivalent to the sum of the measurements divided by the number of measurements. The formula for calculating the mean is:

$$\text{Arithmetic mean} = \frac{\text{sum of measurements}}{\text{no. of measurements}}$$

A community health nurse who wanted to determine the average weight of children in a second-grade classroom would compute the average or mean as follows:

Weight of children in pounds: 51.2, 53.1, 55.1, 54.1, 53.0, 47.5, 48.8, 52.9, 50.5, 51.5, 53.1, 49.5, 53, 55.1, 49.9

TABLE 11-1 Formulas for Rates and Ratios Frequently Calculated in Community Health Nursing Practice (*Continued*)

Rate or ratio	Formula	Commonly used round number
Case fatality ratio	Number of deaths from specified disease or condition ÷ number of reported cases of the specified disease or condition	× 100
MORBIDITY STATISTICS		
Incidence rate	Number of "new" cases of a specified disease or condition occurring during a given time period ÷ population at risk during the same time period	× 100,000 population
Prevalence rate	Number of "old" and "new" cases of specified disease or condition existing at a "point" in time ÷ total population at a point in time	× 100,000 population
VITAL AND DEMOGRAPHIC STATISTICS OTHER THAN MORTALITY		
Crude birth rate	Number of live births during a given year ÷ population estimated at midyear	× 1000 population
General fertility rate	Number of live births during a given year ÷ population estimated at mid-year for females ages 15–44 during the same year	× 1000 female population (15–44 years old)
General marriage rate	Number of marriages during a given year ÷ number of persons 15 years of age and over in the population in the same year	× 1000 persons 15 years of age and over
General divorce rate	Number of divorces during a given year ÷ persons 15 years of age and over in the population in the same year	× 1000 persons 15 years of age and over
Dependency ratio	Persons under 20 years of age and persons 65 years and over ÷ total population ages 20–64	× 100

Sum of measurement $= 778$

Number of measurements $= 15$

Mean weight $= 51.9$

Arithmetic mean $= \dfrac{778}{15} = 51.86$ or 51.9

Knowing the mean or "average" value of a series of measurements helps the community health nurse to identify quickly persons who may have health needs or who are at risk for health problems in the future. Persons who fall far below or far above the average should be comprehensively assessed to determine why this is happening.

The *median* is the "middle" value in a series of quantitative data which divides the measurements into two equal parts. That is, 50 percent of the measurements are less than and 50 percent are greater than the median value. To calculate the median, the measurements in the distribution must be arranged in order of size. Referring again to the children in the second-grade classroom, the median weight of these children would be determined by putting all of their weights in numerical order so that the middle value can be identified. This is illustrated below:

47.5, 48.8, 49.5, 49.9, 50.5, 51.2, **52.9** (median) 53, 53, 53 (mode), 53.1, 54, 55, 55.1

The median is *52.9*, or the eighth measurement because 50 percent of the measurements are less than this value and 50 percent are greater than this value. If there had been an even number of measurements, the median would be found by dividing the sum of the two middle measurements by two.

48.8, 49.5, 49.9, 50.5, 51.2, 51.5, **52.9, 53**, 53, 53, 53.1, 54, 55, 55.1

Middle measurements $= (52.9 + 53.0) \div 2 = 52.95$ (median)

The median is usually computed when there are very high or very low extremes in a series of measurements because the mean is distorted by very high or low values but the median is not. When census tract data are reported, for instance, median income is usually given because there is such a great variation in family income, ranging from below poverty level to over $50,000. Generally, however, the mean is the most frequently used measure of central tendency in community health practice because it takes into account all measurements in a series and is the most stable.

The *mode* is the measurement that appears most frequently in a series of quantitative data. It is identified by counting the number of times a particular value appears. The measurements do not have to be ordered. Fifty-three points is the mode or typical value of the weights of our second-grade classroom children because it occurred more frequently than any other weight. The mode is helpful when one wants to identify an average value very quickly. It is only an estimate, however, and not too reliable; other measurements of central tendencies should be used when refining data analysis.

Relative numbers, including rates, ratios, percentages, and measures of central tendency are computed so that comparisons between sets of absolute numbers can be made. When a series of relative numbers is being studied, it is helpful to present the data graphically.

Graphic Presentation of Data

Graphic presentation of data is an efficient way to show large numbers of observations at one time. Numerical figures are more easily remembered when presented graphically because data are organized and relationships are demonstrated. Tables, graphs, and charts are some of the instruments used to present statistical information symbolically. Guidelines for presenting data in this form include the following:

- Illustrate only the amount of data which are appealing to the sight.

- Number a table, graph, or chart if more than one is used (Table 11-1, Table 11-2, or Table 11-3).

- Title each table, graph, or chart, including in the title information identifying what, where, and when.

- Label both the horizontal and vertical axes of the graphic presentation.

- Identify the source of the data at the bottom of the chart, including author, title of publication, publisher, date of publication, and reference page number.

When these guidelines are used, a table would look like the example that is presented in Table 11-2.

Graphic presentation of data has popular appeal and is frequently used to portray quickly a large number of facts. Graphs, charts, and tables can be misused or misunderstood, however, especially if one attempts to relate data which are unrelated. Also, attempting to present too many facts on one table defeats the purpose for using visual presentations of data; when this is done, it confuses rather than clarifies the events being illustrated.

Available data on a community should be used in the most effective way possible to get across the significance of a community's health problems. These data should not, however, be misrepresented on tables, graphs, and charts. If available data are not sufficient to reach decisions about a community's state of health, do not try to make them be so by graphically presenting incomplete findings. Rather, use other methods to collect the data needed to analyze what is happening in the community.

Carry Out Surveys

Surveys are commonly conducted in community health nursing practice because existing data from census, vital statistics, and morbidity

Table number and title:

TABLE 11-2   Leading Causes of Death and Cause-Specific Rates, Michigan and United States Residents, 1976

Horizontal axes:

Vertical axes:

Rank	Cause of death	Number of deaths Michigan	Number of deaths U.S.	Rate Michigan	Rate U.S.
1	Diseases of the heart	29,233	723,878	321.1	337.2
2	Malignant neoplasms	14,880	377,312	163.4	175.8
3	Cerebrovascular diseases	7,354	188,623	80.8	87.9
4	Accidents	3,912	100,761	43.0	46.9
5	Influenza and pneumonia	2,106	61,866	23.1	28.8
6	Diabetes mellitus	1,719	34,508	18.9	16.1
7	Cirrhosis of the liver	1,486	31,453	16.3	14.7
8	Arteriosclerosis	1,207	29,366	13.3	13.7
9	Suicide	1,182	26,832	13.0	12.5
10	Homicide	1,092	19,554	12.0	9.1
	Subtotal	64,171	1,593,153	704.9	742.7
	All other causes	11,630	316,287	127.7	146.9
	Total	75,801	1,909,440	832.6	889.6

Source note:

SOURCE: From Office of Vital and Health Statistics. *1976 Michigan Health Statistics*, Lansing, Mich.: Michigan Department of Public Health, 1976, p. 35.

records are inadequate to substantiate a need for the development of a particular health program. Standard sources of data, such as those mentioned above, may show that suicide is one of the leading causes of death for older adolescents. This information is significant in that it focuses attention on a major health problem of this developmental age group. It is not sufficient, however, to identify health action needed in a particular community for reducing adolescent mortality due to suicide. Other types of information must be collected before a health project is initiated in a local community. Data about such things as the usage of available mental health resources by teenagers, attitudes of professionals and consumers in relation to the needs of the adolescent, and reasons for teenage suicidal actions must be ascertained before health planning can be effective. A survey is frequently conducted to obtain this type of information.

A community survey is a systematic study designed to collect data about a community's functioning. Data about a specific segment of the population, about a particular component of the health care delivery system, or about health needs of the entire community may be collected when conducting a survey. The scope varies depending on the purpose and the financial and work force resources available. It is important to define specifically the reason for doing a survey because this process can be costly and time-consuming. On the other hand, this process can provide essential data for health programming and may save time and monies if it is planned carefully.

Sometimes health care professionals become enthusiastic and attempt to speed up the survey process by decreasing planning time. This practice is not wise because planning can actually decrease the time it takes to effectively implement a survey. For example, conducting a pilot study or a small-scale survey during the planning phase can help to eliminate major problems in the survey process before an extensive study is initiated. This, in turn, could significantly reduce the amount of time needed to obtain appropriate data.

There are a variety of ways in which a community can survey its needs. Personal interviews, telephone interviews, or written questionnaires are a few examples of the methods that can be used to collect data about community health problems and strengths. It is important to select carefully survey methods and tools because resources and needs vary from one community to another. Reviewing the literature about what other professionals are discovering in their work is useful.

Siemiatycki (1979, p. 238), examined the cost and quality of data collection when utilizing three different survey strategies: mail, telephone, and home interview. It was found "that telephone and mail strategies with intensive follow-up achieved response rates comparable to these achieved by the home interview strategy and for between 45 and 56 percent of the cost." It was also discovered in this study that home interviews did not improve the quality of data collected. In fact, respondents answered questions about sensitive topics more readily by mail than during a home interview (Siemiatycki, 1979, pp. 243–244).

Studies like the one conducted by Siemiatycki can provide data that help a community to make a more knowledgeable decision about fact-finding methods. They support the value of investigating the literature before initiating a costly project to determine community needs. If a community can obtain information at less cost and still preserve the quality of data that are collected, considering the use of the less costly method is warranted. If time is not taken to review what others have done, a less costly method may never be considered. It must be remembered, though, that research studies do not provide all of the answers for a particular community. A more costly method might be selected if that is the only way to obtain certain types of data. Home interviews should be used, for instance, if environmental conditions need to be observed.

Surveys should be used to obtain data that are not available from other sources. Generally, accurate data can be obtained about vital events (births, deaths, or marriages), but morbidity data are often incomplete. Disease rates and data about health-related phenomena (alcoholism, mental disorders, or child abuse) are usually only estimates, due to the lack of adequate reporting. It is frequently unknown how many individuals are affected by these conditions or how many who are affected are receiving adequate care. Surveys may be able to elicit this type of data. In addition, a survey can help to determine comprehensive needs of a particular segment of a population. Census information provides data about a census tract in relation to income, housing, education, and transportation. It does not provide data about specific health problems, social needs, or health care resources.

Data obtained from a survey provide the foundation for more extensive investigation of health needs in a community. Research is frequently conducted after surveys are completed to explore the potential cause-and-effect relationships between differing community phenomena. Surveys do not provide sufficient evidence to substantiate cause-and-effect conclusions because generally there are very few controls built into a survey design (Polit and Hungler, 1978, p. 207).

Conduct Research

Research to document the effectiveness of nursing services and to identify cause-and-effect relationships is critically needed in the community health nursing setting. Funders of health care services are demanding concrete data that support the need for nursing personnel, the need for certain health programs, and the value of using one intervention strategy rather than another. If qualitative data are not available, funders evaluate effectiveness only on the basis of quantitative counts, such as the numbers of home, school, or clinic visits. When this happens, the quality of nursing care suffers.

Research can help the health care professional to document effectiveness of quality, as well as to identify community needs and to propose intervention strategies that best meet these needs. Illustrative of this statement is the study conducted by Skinner, German, Shapiro, Chase, and Zauber (1978, pp. 1195, 1201), which demonstrated that the near-poor population—those families who did not qualify for Medicaid benefits but who had inadequate financial resources to meet health care costs—were a special population at risk within a community. This study showed that the near-poor in East Baltimore were using fewer health care services than were Medicaid recipients. When financial barriers were removed by enrolling the East Baltimore near-poor in a prepaid health plan, this difference in usage was minimized.

Time must be provided so that practitioners can investigate clinical practice issues and concerns. It is only in this way that a profession can remain viable. Collaborative relationships established between service settings and academic environments can facilitate practitioners' involvement in research. Research can be stimulating and challenging to practitioners, especially if they have support and encouragement from individuals who are involved in clinical research on a regular basis.

Lindeman (1975, p. 697) conducted a nationwide survey among nurses to determine priorities for clinical nursing research. Among the top 15 priorities identified were items related to the improved use of the nursing process, evaluation of quality care, and the role of nursing in the provision of preventive health services. These priorities reflect concerns experienced daily by the community health nurse.

Contact Consumers and Community Leaders

Research and surveys tend to focus on the present. Since a community's current characteristics are an outgrowth of its historical development, it is beneficial to interview consumers and community leaders to identify what has gone on in the past and how the past is affecting the present. The values, attitudes, and interests of previous community leaders often subtly influence the current direction of health planning. Contact with key community persons can help community health nurses to understand why there is resistance to certain health programs, how to reduce resistance to change, and who nurses might work with to enhance their productivity in the community setting.

Directors of housing projects, clergy, professionals in other health care agencies, local politicians, owners of long-established businesses, and unofficial community spokespersons are some of the individuals a nurse might contact to attain information about community dynamics. These individuals can help the nurse to gain knowledge about the power relationships within a local area, community values and attitudes, and environmental factors which enhance or detract from a community's state of health. Unofficial spokespersons often provide the most candid opinion of how the consumer views health and the health care delivery system. Clergy, agency clients, and cultural organizations, such as International Neighbors or the Polish club, can frequently assist a community health nurse in identifying these spokespersons.

A community health nurse should use every opportunity available to relate to community people outside and within the agency. The opportunities are limitless and only require motivation on the part of the nurse and supervisory support to take advantage of them. A visit to the local library can provide very valuable information about a community's history. On the other hand, talking with people the nurse meets while carrying out regular caseload responsibilities can be just as valuable. Spontaneous interchange often provides an atmosphere for free, honest communication. This type of dialogue also helps to create a positive image in relation to what health care professionals are doing to improve the health of people. The ability to relate to others in the community, such as school principals, physicians, administrators in mental health agencies, secretaries, and clergy, is essential if one wants to diagnose community needs accurately.

Observe, Listen, and Analyze

Data about a community can be obtained daily by observing, listening, and analyzing. What the environment looks like when the nurse drives in the district, how families are dressed when they are seen in the clinic setting, and who relates to whom during community meetings all provide the community health nurse with clues about a community's state of health. Community health nurses who are really interested in the welfare of their community will take time to analyze what has been observed and heard. They will be alert to environmental conditions that adversely affect the state of a community's health. If, when driving through the district, a nurse finds older homes in poor repair, he or she can raise questions about the potential for lead poisoning and the need for enforcement of housing legislation. An astute nurse will not ignore observations or accept them as a matter of fact without trying to effect change.

Analysis of community observations must focus on strengths as well as needs, because it is through a community's strengths that health problems are resolved. One community health nurse, for example, was able to effect environmental changes in her district because she had identified that the parents in the area were genuinely concerned about the welfare of their children. Rat-infested vacant lots in the neighborhood provided a serious threat to the children who played in them. This nurse, with the assistance of a minister, was able to mobilize parents' energies so that the garbage from these lots was removed and rats were killed. Maintaining the lots as suitable play areas became a major community project.

A community health nurse who views the community as the unit of service is more likely to meet the needs of individual families than the nurse who only focuses on family health care needs. Family problems are interrelated with community problems and often cannot be resolved until changes occur within the community system. A nurse needs to collect data on the community in order to determine the extent to which family health problems are influenced by community values, attitudes, and beliefs. Frequently, families from differing ethnic backgrounds are labeled social problems because they do not relate to social systems as do middle-class white Americans. When this is the case, change will not occur if the community health nurse only works with individual families. In these situations, the community health nurse needs to help social systems gain an appreciation of different cultural values and attitudes and must help families learn how to interact with social systems unfamiliar to them.

SOURCES OF COMMUNITY DATA

There are numerous federal, state, and local agencies and individuals that a community health nurse can contact in order to obtain data about the community. Some have been mentioned previously in this chapter but will be summarized here to give a composite picture of the multiple sources of data one can use when diagnosing community needs.

The only federal agency specifically established for the collection and dissemination of health data is the National Center for Health Statistics. This agency conducts the National Health Survey, which provides valuable information on the health and illness status of United States residents (see Chapter 10). In addition, this agency provides official information on vital statistics and data about the supply and use of health resources (Office of the Federal Register, 1978, p. 265).

Several other federal agencies will supply health data on request. The National Institutes of Health, the Center for Disease Control, and the Health Resources Administration are a few examples of such agencies. The *United States Government Manual*, which can be purchased from the Superintendent of Documents, U.S. Government Printing Office, Washington, D.C., is a valuable reference for identifying other governmental agencies that disseminate health data. This manual describes the purposes and programs of most federal agencies.

The importance of obtaining data from the Bureau of the Census on the size, distribution, structure, and change of populations in the United States cannot be overemphasized. These data demonstrate patterns over time and provide general characteristics of a community's total population. Knowing that there is a high concentration of individuals 65 years and over, or of children ages 1 through 5 in a community, assists health care professionals in predicting the type of health problems and health care services needed in a particular community. For example, a community health nurse who knows from census tract data that 30 percent of the people in his or her census tract are 65 years or older should become concerned if no geriatric families are in the caseload and then investigate why referrals for this age group are not being received.

In addition to helping individual staff nurses, census tract data help nursing administrators to determine where nursing services are most needed. Knowledge about the concentration of people, the economic status, and housing conditions in an area assists administrators in predicting populations at risk in segments of their community. Often, state health departments will help local health departments to use census tract data to identify at-risk groups. State health departments have statistical divisions that provide consultation in relation to data collection and analysis.

State health departments are a major source of data for identifying the health status of citizens in a particular state. Vital statistics, morbidity data, health work force, and resource information are usually collected and disseminated by this agency. The department of education, the bureau of mental health, and health service agencies (HSAs) are some other state agencies that supply health and health-related information. Obtaining a state directory of social agencies will help each reader to determine which agencies in her or his state furnish information about specific health needs in local communities. The number of state agencies that supply health and health-related data are too numerous to list here.

On the local level, some key sources for obtaining community data are the chamber of commerce, city planner's office, health department, county extension office, intermediate school districts, libraries, health and welfare professionals, hospital records, clergy, community leaders, and consumers. Again, sources are too numerous for all of them to be listed here. Most cities and counties have social services directories which provide information on the major health and welfare resources in their community. Experienced practitioners can also help new community health nurses to identify the most appropriate source for obtaining specific data about the area in which they are functioning.

Legislators and public officials on all three levels of government are usually more than willing to assist the health care professional in analyzing social and health care legislation. Laws and ordinances related to community health reflect the values and priorities of a community, the state, and the federal government. Every health care professional should be familiar with legislation that influences the health of his or her community. Specific laws and ordinances are discussed throughout this text. Here it is sufficient to emphasize the importance of studying legislative trends in order to gain an understanding of a community's priorities in relation to health care issues.

ANALYSIS OF ALL AVAILABLE DATA

Data should not be collected for the sake of having data. Unfortunately, this is often the case. Daily activity reports, vital statistics, and census data are frequently collected, but just as frequently filed in a drawer without being used. This benefits no one. Once community data are assembled, they should be organized in a meaningful way so that patterns of functioning and trends can be ascertained. Many techniques can be used to synthesize community data. Charts, figures, and tables are often used for this purpose. Graphic presentation of such things as population distributions, morbidity data, or vital statistics for several decades can be very effective in pinpointing significant community problems. Growth or lack of growth in a community, for instance, can be identified when population distributions are graphically visualized. Lack of growth in a community can be a very serious problem, because many federal and state health funds are allocated on a per capita basis, that is a given amount of money is allocated for each person residing in the area.

Mapping is another technique that facilitates data analysis. Dotted scatter maps can be used to determine at a glance such things as high-risk populations, poor environmental conditions, the distribution of illness, disease, and health, and the accessibility of health care services. When this technique is used, school districts or political jurisdictions are usually outlined on a county map. Point symbols or spots are then distributed within these divisions as specified events happen (disease, death, health-related phenomena, or condemned housing), at the exact locations where the events occurred. Figure 11-2, Reported Cases of Hepatitis in Howard County, illustrates the mapping technique. The clustering of hepatitis cases in census tracts 12, 13, and 9 was related to an outbreak of hepatitis that occurred in a trailer camp in census tract 12. Relatives and friends from census tracts 9 and 13 had contact with family and friends in census tract 12 while they were in a communicable state. An epidemiological investigation provided evidence which supported that a major outbreak of hepatitis had occurred in a very short time period. The clustering of hepatitis cases in census tract 6 was a result of drug problems.

Dotted scatter maps can be very impressive and useful, but they can also be misleading if the population base is not analyzed. A geographic area may have far fewer cases than another because there are far fewer people in that area. Calculating rates, ratios, and percentages aids in making comparisons from one census tract to another. These descriptive statistics also help to compare the occurrence of significant events with other communities and with state and national rates.

Comparing community rates with state and national rates is very beneficial. It can highlight specific health problems as well as community strengths. It helps a community to determine priorities for program planning. If a community's infant and maternal mortality rates, for instance, are much higher than state and national rates, a community would want to examine carefully its maternal-child health programming. On the other hand, a community may find, when making these comparisons, that its maternal-child health statistics are far superior to those of other areas. This, in turn, could demonstrate to the community the value of maintaining adequate health programs for these two age groups in the population.

Analysis of data often supports the need for further data collection. This is illustrated in the following case situation:

In one census tract of a large urban area, the health department became aware of a maternal infant health problem. This census tract was a residential rental area with basement efficiency apartments renting for $240.00 or higher per month. The population was 75 percent students and young working people, referred to as the "swinging singles." Of the remaining 25 percent, 20 percent were elderly first-generation Jewish merchants, and 5 percent were young black families living in the city housing project. The area had a high reported incidence of mugging, purse snatching, and apartment thefts, with rumors of drug manufacturing, pushing, and usage.

Few referrals were made to the health agencies in the area; case finding was negligible; records of nursing services showed few home visits to individuals in this district. The explanation given for this situation was that the majority of the population in this census tract was either at school or working and, therefore, inaccessible to agency personnel during the working day. Evening office hours were scheduled by private physicians as well as by several health clinics in the area. The health department became particularly concerned about the lack of referrals from this census tract when they analyzed the infant and maternal death rates for the entire county. It was discovered that only in this census tract did these rates significantly vary from national statistics.

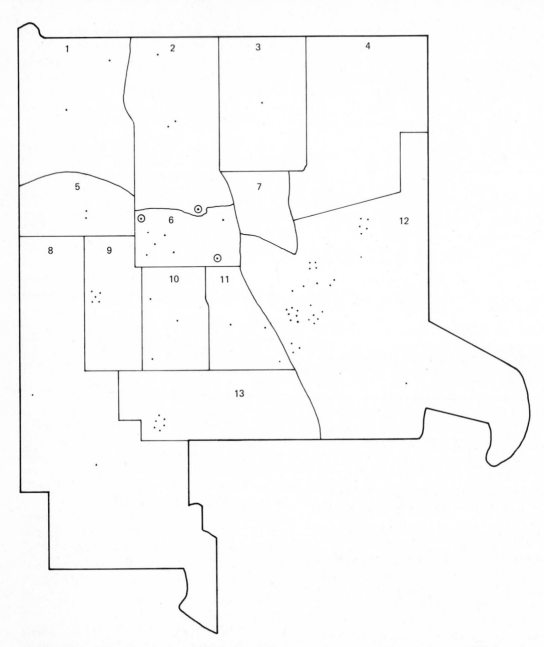

FIGURE 11-2   The mapping technique: reported cases of hepatitis in Howard County, January 1979 through June 1979. Key: • = cases of hepatitis; ⊙ = drug suppliers.

Infant and maternal mortality rates for the specified census tract:

27.4 infant deaths per 1000 live births

8.4 maternal deaths per 1000 live births

Infant and maternal mortality rates in the United States during the same time period:

16.1 infant deaths per 1000 live births

3.1 maternal deaths per 1000 live births

It was obvious from the vital statistics that something had to be done to improve the health status of mothers and children in this area. However, more specific data were needed to determine causes of death, health status of area residents, and usage of health care services, as well as related health problems, including socioeconomic difficulties, drug usage, and attitudes about the "establishment." Personnel from a drug clinic and the student organization at a local college assisted the health department in collecting the data they needed. Lack of transportation, extremely limited incomes, lack of knowledge, inadequate nutrition, and resistance to normal channels of health care were some of the major problems identified. The establishment of a neighborhood health clinic, staffed mostly by college students and area residents, produced positive results. Data analysis at the end of 2 years reflected a significant decrease in the infant and maternal mortality rates for this area.

The above situation dramatically illustrates the importance of analyzing data once they are compiled. Community diagnostic activities are carried out so that appropriate decisions about health planning can be made. If data are not analyzed, health action will probably not occur.

PRACTICAL TIPS FOR IMPLEMENTING COMMUNITY DIAGNOSTIC ACTIVITIES

Community diagnostic activities are exciting and challenging. It should be apparent, however, that they cannot be left to chance. If these activities are to be implemented effectively, time for planning, assessment, and analysis must be set aside and administrative support must be available. Equally important is the need to always keep the framework of the "community" in clear perspective when providing nursing care. Community dynamics that adversely affect the health status of individuals, families, and populations at risk should not be ignored. Nursing intervention strategies should be planned to resolve community problems as well as to resolve needs of individual clients.

New practitioners often experience feelings of frustration and disillusionment when first entering into the practice setting because there are tremendous gaps between reality and the ideal. Presented below are some suggestions for bridging some of these gaps in relation to community organizational activities.

Do Preliminary Community Study during Orientation Period

It is only natural for newly employed nurses to want immediate involvement in client casework. Reading policy and procedure manuals and attending orientation meetings can be tiring and less than rewarding. It is important, however, to remind oneself that orientation periods are designed to facilitate functioning in relation to all aspects of one's job responsibilities. Do not overplan family visits during this time period. Rather, balance family and community activities so that time is available to learn about community dynamics and population characteristics. Allowing time in your schedule to engage in the following activities during the orientation period will help you to function more effectively in the community health setting.

· Analyze census tract and vital statistics data to learn about population characteristics in your district.

- Attend case conferences and community meetings (PTA, social service council, citizen group activities) with an experienced employee.

- Attend a board of health meeting to identify the values and attitudes of those responsible for policy making in the health department.

- Drive through your district, observing environmental conditions, interactions between people, and the location of health care and welfare resources, recreational facilities, local churches, school systems, and shopping areas.

- Shop in your district to determine cost of essentials, such as food and clothing.

- Make field visits with personnel from other departments in your agency (environmental health, mental health, or nutrition).

- Observe in clinic settings (well-baby, venereal disease, adult screening, or prenatal).

- *Ask questions.*

Most agencies allow new employees to help design their orientation. The above activities should be planned for, even if similar experiences were available during your course of study in the academic environment. In the educational setting, these types of experiences are planned so that students have the opportunity to apply theoretical concepts in the practice setting. Educational experiences cannot, however, provide the practitioner with the specific information needed to understand the unique characteristics of the population being served.

Discuss Community Problems during Supervisory Conferences

In community health nursing practice, the practitioner is frequently unable to meet client needs because of deficiencies in the health and welfare systems. The nurse may also find that there is insufficient time to work comprehensively with all the families referred to him or her. These difficulties should be discussed with the nursing supervisor because the supervisor is in a favorable position for initiating major change in community systems. In addition, the supervisor can provide support and assistance in relation to caseload management activities as well as give suggestions about innovative intervention strategies for dealing with community problems. For example, it is not uncommon for the nursing supervisor to help the staff develop a new well-baby clinic when child health services are lacking. It is also not uncommon for the nursing supervisor to provide support and assistance when a staff member wants to establish group activities in order to expand her or his services to a larger number of clients.

Include Community Organizational Activities on Evaluation Tools

Staff-level community organizational activities are seldom evaluated or rewarded. As a result, very little priority is placed on these types of activities and the focus of service shifts from the community as a whole to individual clients. To alter this practice, the practitioner must take time to revise evaluation tools and procedures so that community activities are assessed during the evaluation process. Only if this is done will time be allocated for community work. Listed below are a few examples of items one might want to include under a community service category on a staff evaluation tool:

- Assesses health needs and strengths of specific populations (school, clinic, industry) in assigned district

- Works with nursing supervisor to discern health action needed for at-risk populations in assigned district

- Works with the nursing supervisor to develop

intervention strategies (group work, clinic services) for populations at risk in assigned district

· Collaborates with other professionals on health-planning projects for populations at risk in the community

SUMMARY

Meeting the health needs of high-risk populations is a major function of the community health nurse. A nurse must know the community before this responsibility can be effectively carried out. A variety of strategies must be used to assess the health status, the health capability, and the health action potential of the nurse's community. Data must be analyzed as well as collected so that target groups for nursing service can be identified. Use of the nursing process facilitates implementation of these activities.

There are numerous professionals and consumers who will assist the community health nurse in identifying community health problems and strengths. Interdisciplinary collaboration and consumer participation must be fostered during the community diagnostic process, because no one person alone can appropriately diagnose community needs.

Exploring the community, its organization, and its activities is extremely rewarding because it gives one a clearer picture of community health action. It provides the foundation for health-planning activities which are designed to improve the health status of high-risk groups. It further helps the community health nurse to intervene more effectively with individual families, because often family health problems cannot be resolved until changes occur in the health care delivery system. It may be difficult for the community health nurse to integrate community organizational activities into an already busy schedule, but it is essential to do so in order to meet the needs of individuals, families, and populations at risk.

REFERENCES

American Nurses' Association. *Standards of community health nursing practices.* (CH-25M) Kansas City: ANA Publications, 1973.

Community health nursing faculty. *Public Health Statistics Notes.* East Lansing, Mich.: Michigan State University, 1968.

Lindeman, C. A. Priorities in clinical nursing research. *Nursing Outlook,* November 1975, *23,* 693–698.

Miller, C. A. Health care of children and youth in America. *American Journal of Public Health,* April 1975, 165, 353–358.

Office of the Federal Register. *1977/78 United States government manual.* Washington, D.C.: Office of the Federal Register, 1978.

Office of Vital and Health Statistics. *1976 Michigan health statistics.* Lansing, Mich.: Michigan Department of Public Health, 1976.

Polit, D. F., & Hungler, B. P. *Nursing research: Principles and methods.* New York: Lippincott, 1978.

Shryock, H. S., Siegel, J.S., & Associates. *The methods and materials of demography.* Washington, D.C.: U.S. Department of Commerce, 1971.

Siemiatycki, J. A Comparison of mail, telephone and home interview strategies for household health surveys. *American Journal of Public Health,* March 1979, *69,* 238–245.

Skinner, E. A., German, P. S., Shapiro, S., Chase, G. A., and Zauber, A. G. Use of ambulatory health services by the near poor. *American Journal of Public Health,* December 1978, *68,* 1195–1201.

Walker, G. M. Utilization of health care: The Laredo migrant experience. *American Journal of Public Health,* July 1979, *60,* 667–671.

SELECTED BIBLIOGRAPHY

Balinsky, W., & Berger, R. A review of the research on general health status indexes. *Medical Care*, April 1975, *13*, 283–292.

Breslow, L., & Somers, A. R. The lifetime health-monitoring program. *New England Journal of Medicine*, March 17, 1977, *296*, 601–608.

Bruhn, J. G. Planning for social change: Dilemmas for health planning. *American Journal of Public Health*, July 1973, *63*, 602–605.

Bureau of the Census. *Statistical abstract of the United States*. Washington, D.C.: U.S. Department of Commerce, 1979.

Burgess, A. W., & Lazore, A. *Community mental health: Target populations*. Englewood Cliffs, N.J.: Prentice-Hall, 1976.

Connor, D. M. *Diagnosing community problems*. Antigonish, Nova Scotia: Demond M. Connor, 1966.

Cordes, S. M. Assessing health care needs: Elements and processes. *Family and Community Health*, July 1978, *1*, 1–16.

Cox, F. M., Erlich, J. L., Rothman, J., & Tropman, J. E. (Eds.). *Strategies of community organization: A book of readings*. Itasca, Ill.: F. E. Peacock Publishers, 1974.

Crawford, C. O., & Leadley, S. M. Interagency collaboration for planning and delivery of health care. *Family and Community Health*, July 1978, *1*, 35–46.

Gilson, B. S., Gilson J. S., Bergner, M., Bobbitt, R. A., Kressel, S., Pollard, W. E., & Vesselago, M. The sickness impact profile: Development of an outcome measure of health care. *American Journal of Public Health*, December 1975, *65*, 1304–1310.

Hanchett, E. *Community health assessment: A conceptual tool kit*. New York: Wiley, 1979.

International Union of Nutritional Sciences Report. Guidelines on the at-risk concept and the health and nutrition of young children. *American Journal of Clinical Nutrition*, February 1977, *30*, 242–254.

Klein, D. C. Assessing community characteristics. In B. W. Spradley (Ed.), *Contemporary Community Nursing*. Boston: Little, Brown, 1975, pp. 415–424.

Kosa, J., & Zola, I. K. *Poverty and health*. Cambridge, Mass.: Harvard University Press, 1975.

MacStravie, R. E. *Determining health needs*. Ann Arbor, Mich.: Health Administration Press, 1978.

Meltzer, J., & Hochstim, J. Reliability and validity of survey data on physical health. *Public Health Reports*, December 1970, *85*, 1075–1086.

Montoye, H. S. *Physical activity and health: An epidemiologic study of an entire community*. Englewood Cliffs, N.J.: Prentice-Hall, 1975.

Murphy, M. J. The development of a community health orientation scale. *American Journal of Public Health*, December 1975, *65*, 1293–1297.

Reinhardt, A. M., & Chatlin, E. D. Assessment of health needs in a community: The basis for program planning. In A. M. Reinhardt & M. D. Quinn (Eds.), *Current practice in family-centered community nursing*. Saint Louis: Mosby, 1977, pp. 138–185.

Roemer, M. I. *Rural health care*. Saint Louis: Mosby, 1976.

Rosen, G. Preventive medicine in the United States 1900–1975: Trends and interpretation. In *Preventive Medicine USA*. New York: Prodist, Division of Neale Watson Academic Publishing Co., 1976, pp. 716–791.

Sandahl, B. A paradigm for progressive health promotion problem identification and resolution of health status. *Nurse Practitioner*, September–October 1977, *2*, 20–21.

White, E. H. Health and the black person: An annotated bibliography. *American Journal of Nursing*, October 1974, *74*, 1839–1841.

Wing, K. R. *The law and the public's health*. Saint Louis: Mosby, 1976.

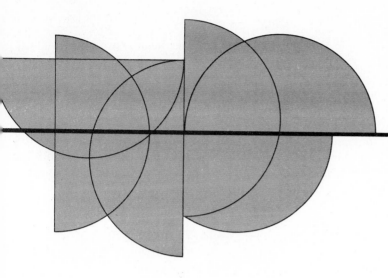

12
community health planning for population groups

There was a little girl who had a little curl
Right in the middle of her forehead;
When she was good she was very very good
And when she was bad she was horrid.

This nursery rhyme describes the state of health care services in the United States: some of them are very very good and some of them are appalling. One can say with certainty that the overall picture of health care services is not orderly, equitable, or logical. Failure to reach certain segments of the population, notably low-income and rural people, is a reflection on health planning activities.

Nursing has often not been assertive in health-planning activities for population groups. This has historical roots in nursing practice. In 1903 Lavinia Dock, a nurse, wrote that "nursing has not made itself a moral force; is not a public conscience, takes no position in large public questions, is not feared by those of low standards; allows all manner of new conditions and developments in nursing affairs to arise, flourish, succeed, or fail" (Ashley, 1975, p. 1466). Nursing has come a long way from those nonassertive days but still has significant strides to make.

Today the professional nurse is beginning to assume assertive leadership roles in meeting the health needs of consumers. She or he is becoming increasingly involved in health planning and political activities and is realizing the importance of understanding health legislation and financing. Unfortunately, nurses have often thought that the subjects of health planning, politics, legislation, and financing were dull or "not nursing." Yet, nursing involves all these things.

Health planning is one of the primary functions of a community health nurse. The American Nurses' Association states that the dominant responsibility of nurses in community health is to the population as a whole and that the nurse must acknowledge the need for comprehensive health planning to implement this responsibility (ANA, 1973). This chapter will emphasize the role of the community health nurse in health planning for population groups.

DEFINING HEALTH PLANNING

Health planning is an ongoing process whereby information about a community is systematically collected and used to structure a usable community health plan (Ruybal, 1978). It is a process based upon scientific principles and methods.

Health planning is a problem-solving approach which helps a community to evaluate and bring about specific changes in its health care delivery system. The problem-solving approach is the basis for planning nursing care with individuals and families, and it can be expanded to population groups. The health planning process for population groups involves the same steps used in the nursing process: assessing, analyzing, planning, implementing, and evaluating. Basic concepts of epidemiology (Chapter 10), biostatistics (Chapter 11), and management (Chapter 20) are used to refine decision-making and diagnostic skills and to expand intervention options during the health planning process.

The assessment phase of health planning begins with data collection. Data is collected when a nursing or health policy problem is recognized or a community desires to evaluate its current health status. Methods used by the community health nurse to collect information about a community and to analyze and prioritize community needs are presented in Chapter 11.

Data collection and analysis, the first two steps of the planning process, identify conditions which warrant health planning action. When the need for health planning action is diagnosed, the planning phase starts. This stage involves looking at various alternative solutions, selecting a solution to implement, developing measurable objectives, determining the cost of implementing various options, and choosing the appropriate time to implement the selected solution.

The implementation phase occurs when the solution is carried out through specific actions.

These actions may be carried out by the nurse, consumers, or other health care professionals.

Evaluation looks at what actions were successful or unsuccessful as well as why. It also compares predicted outcomes with unpredicted ones and helps to identify new problems.

For the community health nurse, the emphasis in health planning is on the health of population groups within the community, and problems, solutions, and actions are defined on this level. By comparison, in clinical nursing, the emphasis is on the individual as the unit of service (Williams, 1977, p. 251). In community health nursing, the family is the unit of service and the client is the community.

The Community Health Nurse and Health Planning

The community health nurse is particularly well qualified to carry out health planning. Each day the nurse sees the needs of population groups within the community through home visits, clinics, classes, schools, and other nursing activities. She or he is able to obtain a composite picture of the health needs of a population group such as lack of prenatal care, family-planning services, or public transportation. The nurse's continual, comprehensive contact with the community makes her or him knowledgeable about available resources and gaps in service provision. The staff nurse should share these assessed health needs with supervisory personnel, and together they can discuss the alternatives to the situation. The agency's philosophy of service, policies, priorities, and staff variables will affect the alternatives offered. By sharing assessed needs with people in an agency who are in the position to assist in implementing change, the nurse is taking a beginning step in health planning for the needs of the community.

Nurses usually see only the "tip of the iceberg" when diagnosing problems common to families in the caseload they carry. What has been assessed, however, can become the basis for an epidemiological investigation of community needs, because the family is the smallest epidemiological group (Taylor and Knowelden, 1964, p. 303). Epidemiological studies examine groups larger than the family. They frequently involve investigation of needs in census tracts or specific political boundaries such as cities, towns, or counties.

Health needs of population groups can also be dealt with by building upon research studies and known problems and solutions. How this is done was illustrated by community health nurses in a southern city who served schools as well as provided general nursing service to the community. The school intervention program included only hearing and vision screening and episodic encounters with children who were referred by others or themselves. The community health nurses were aware that such a program did not involve continuous problem solving or comprehensive services. A decision was made to continue the usual nursing services to the school and to begin a pilot program that was preventive and directed to a defined group.

The pilot program was based upon research that demonstrated that (1) a small proportion of persons have the greatest number of illnesses in a group, (2) a good predictor of a student's absence is the past attendance record, and (3) at least 80 percent of school absences are for health reasons. Using this data, personnel decided that children with a record of many absences and their families could benefit from nursing service. The major objectives for the study were "1) to consider the utility of directing nursing services to a defined risk group and 2) to document the results of the experience in terms of patient outcomes, specifically, change in absence experience" (Long, Whitman, Johansson, Williams, and Tuthill, 1975, p. 389). The study validated that "it is possible to incorporate a prevention-oriented service directed to a defined risk group into an on-going school health program" (p. 392).

The primary goal of health planning activities such as those described above is to develop comprehensive health care options for all citizens in the community. Working with one community subgroup, school-age children, helps health planners to begin to develop comprehensive services for all.

FRAMEWORK FOR HEALTH PLANNING WITH POPULATION GROUPS: THE DEVELOPMENTAL APPROACH

A variety of approaches have been used to identify and act upon health problems of population groups. Groups are defined as aggregates of persons who have one or more personal or environmental characteristic that is similar. Often select groups have been identified on the basis of a shared health condition such as drug abuse or diabetes. Other groups have been identified according to the characteristic they share by living in a particular geographic area. Students in married housing (Figure 12-1), for example, share stresses re-

lated to obtaining an educational degree and to living in crowded conditions. Since this text emphasizes planning preventive services for groups across the life span, a developmental, age-correlated approach to grouping is used. By using this approach, the community health nurse can assess the health needs of all individuals and groups within the community and can identify health promotion activities needed to enhance the health status of all developmental age groups.

The developmental approach views human

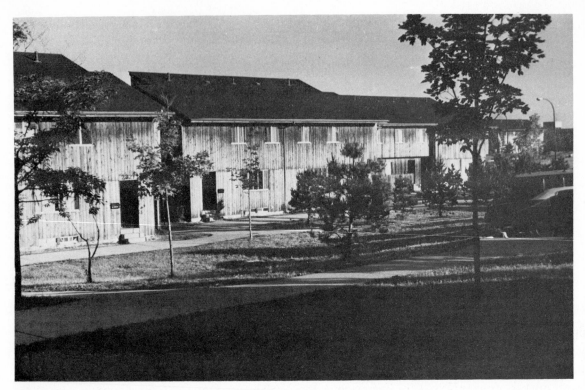

FIGURE 12-1 A university married student housing community.

life as a process of continued development. Erikson (1950), Havighurst (1952), Freud (1965), and Piaget (1969), along with others, have written about the process of human development throughout the life span and have outlined critical stages of human development. Erikson's eight stages of the life cycle (infancy, early childhood, play age, school age, adolescence, young adulthood, adulthood, and senescence) have been used widely in nursing (Erikson, 1950). Duvall (1977) continues to be a source for the study of developmental tasks to be accomplished by individuals and families. Reviewing the writings of the above authors will give the reader an in-depth perspective on individual development throughout the life-span and family development across the family life cycle.

The developmental approach is based on the theory that individuals develop in their own way, yet in conformity with a common developmental pattern. It postulates that failure to accomplish developmental tasks at the appropriate time makes subsequent development more difficult. Community health nurses can use the developmental framework as a foundation for identifying problems that exist or have the potential to exist and for determining health programs needed in a community for a particular developmental age group. For example, a major developmental task of aging is to make an adjustment to changing sensory perceptions and strengths. These changes may increase the aging person's need for medical care and decrease the aging person's ability to handle activities of daily living.

If vital statistics indicate an increasing number of aging citizens living in the county, the nurse may want to look at the supportive services such as Meals-on-Wheels, transportation, and medical care that are accessible to them.

KEY PRINCIPLES INVOLVED IN HEALTH PLANNING

When studying the subject of comprehensive health planning for developmental population groups, a number of principles emerge.

Community Diagnosis

Understanding the concepts presented in Chapter 11 relative to community diagnosis, along with the epidemiological variables of person, place, and time is essential to answer the key questions that health planners must ask as they assess health planning needs. *People* involve the "who" of community diagnosis. The cultural, ethnic, psychological, and biological characteristics of the person variable must be considered when planning health services. These characteristics influence how persons define health and illness. Since these terms do not have a common meaning to all people, it is crucial to identify how the population being served views these concepts. If, for instance, a population narrowly defines health as the absence of disease, this population would probably respond more favorably to the provision of curative care than to the provision of preventive care.

Place describes the setting where services are planned. It may be rural or urban, the inner city or suburbia. When examining the characteristics of place, the availability, accessibility, and cost of present services should be analyzed. Size is also a factor to consider when looking at place. A community with 1000 residents will have different needs from a community which has a population of 1 million. The cost to deliver health services, the kinds of personnel and financial resources that are available, and the complexity involved in planning and implementing services are some factors that vary among populations of different sizes.

The basic unit of service in health planning is the population to be served and their distribution. Any planning that is done should take into consideration population size and distribution and needs as reflected by health statistics. Population size and mortality and morbidity rates for the future should be estimated. Future demands on the health care delivery system are determined in this way.

Time in relation to urgency needs to be considered when doing health planning. If the problem under consideration, for example, is an emergency such as influenza among aging citizens, immediate action must be taken. Other health problems such as accident prevention may not require immediate action but can necessitate action over time.

Long-term action presents more complex demands on the health planner. When long-term intervention is needed, mechanisms must be established to ensure that evaluation occurs periodically during the intervention phase, that coordination of all persons involved in the process is supported, and that public awareness of the problem and the health program is maintained.

It is extremely important to determine when the time is appropriate to initiate the health program under consideration. Analyzing such things as community values and attitudes, availability of resources, and cost-benefit factors helps the health planner to determine the appropriate time to begin health-planning intervention.

Examining a community's developmental

history is another significant factor to consider when looking at the time variable. An older, inner-city ethnic community would probably have more set values and attitudes about health and illness than would a newer community, such as a prospering subdivision. Analyzing how values and attitudes have evolved over time in an older community assists the health planner in identifying key community leaders who can influence value and attitude changes and intervention strategies which have facilitated health behavior change in the past.

Planning for Comprehensive Care

A comprehensive health care system should plan for preventive, episodic, and catastrophic health care services for the entire population. Preventive services focus on the prevention of condition occurrence. Episodic services are diagnostic, curative, and restorative. Catastrophic services are designed to handle emergency and disaster situations and to help families who incur health situations beyond the scope of their financial resources.

Within the health care system there are various patterns for providing comprehensive services to populations. Generalized and specialized school health services, as well as generalized and specialized medical care offices, are examples of the types of patterns used to deliver health care. However, within each of these patterns, comprehensive care needs to be built into the program. How the nurse in the school setting plans for the delivery of comprehensive services to the school-age population is discussed in depth in Chapter 14. Planning preventive focused immunization programs against measles, rubella, and diphtheria, developing protocols for the handling of episodic health care needs, such as outbreaks of nuisance diseases, and establishing guidelines for handling emergency or catastrophic incidents are examples of some of the activities a nurse in the school setting

would carry out to ensure that comprehensive care is available for the entire school-age population.

Communication

To function in a health-planning group, the nurse must be able to communicate well, openly, and assertively. The nurse must understand the contributions nursing can bring to the health of people and be able to explain these contributions to others. This skill develops with time and experience. Because functioning in a health-planning group with other professionals is an expected activity of every nurse working in community health, supervision must be available until the nurse learns the process and becomes more confident about his or her skills.

Communicating effectively in a health-planning group requires a firm understanding of group dynamics and a knowledge about population needs. A change in mindset is frequently necessary when beginning to plan for groups because nurses are often only prepared to work with individual clients. A concern for the problems of a community and planning for a group of people with similar characteristics means that the nurse must deal with problem-defining and -solving on a group level, involving health care professionals. Nurses cannot, by themselves, resolve all the health care needs of a community.

Integration of Health Care Services

The integration of health care services to clients should be a high priority. In our present health care system, clients are seen by numerous care givers and gaps in services and duplication of services are evident. Settings such as well-child clinics and school health services have often fostered the inefficient separation of routine physical examinations from diagnostic and treatment services. It is possible to establish protocols or standards of care within health care settings so that one health professional is able to take care of most client needs. At this time, a concentrated effort to integrate health care services and to develop standards for care is needed.

Total Health Care Programs

The concept of a total health program is basic to comprehensive health care. Rather than thinking of a nursing program offering health services, planners should identify the role of nursing in a health care program as well as the role of other disciplines, such as physicians, occupational therapists, nutritionists, and social workers.

No one single discipline has all the answers in health planning. Team members need to acknowledge and respect each other's contributions. Team members may include ministers, priests, rabbis, pharmacists, health educators, school personnel, architects, physicians, psychiatrists, social workers, and environmentalists. Each of these professions brings a skill that aids clients with specific problems: the rabbi deals with spiritual affairs, the pharmacist deals with medicine regimens, and the nutritionist deals with nutritional concerns. The nurse's unique role is to be able to collate all of the information gathered by other professionals and to synthesize it when analyzing health care situations (Kinlein, 1977, p. 10). In addition, the nurse is in a key position to collect data that provide a foundation for understanding the health care needs of groups. For example, as the nurse visits homes, where and how families obtain food, prepare it, and eat it becomes known. The nurse may also learn where and how people buy medications, how well they do or do not follow prescribed therapy, and where health care services are or are not available.

The community health nurse is skilled in forming health care plans based on clients'

life-styles and the cultural and socioeconomic factors of the community. This knowledge, as well as data collected during home visiting, should be transmitted to other members of the health team when health planning for groups within the community takes place.

Consumer Participation

Consumer participation during the health-planning process is an absolute necessity for several reasons. The consumer is the recipient of care and can help to ensure that the provided services will be of high quality and at a reasonable cost. Consumers can also ascertain whether or not the services are responsive to the needs of those for whom they are intended. In addition, they can help to evaluate whether or not health-planning action has been effective. Finally, involving the consumer in the planning process helps to raise the consciousness of those participating about what constitutes good health and how to reach optimal health.

Lip service is more often given to the concept of consumer input than effort to effect actual consumer involvement. Consumers need to feel wanted and their efforts utilized. They need to be well informed about the health needs of the community and reasons for various health programs. They need the opportunity to share their concerns and needs and to influence community health action.

There is much literature available about how to involve consumers in health planning (Pecarchik, Ricci, and Nelson, 1976; Geer, 1976). It is significant to note when reviewing the literature how values influence the decisions made by consumers and health care professionals. Nurses need to be aware that values determine which goals are formulated and how decisions are made by consumers and providers. Facts will be used to predict choices, but values will decide what alternative is selected out of a range of alternatives.

SIGNIFICANT HEALTH LEGISLATION

For a long period of time, health planning was primarily reactive. Only after a health problem that affected a large number of people had been found was there an attempt to solve it. Beginning with some of President Johnson's Great Society programs in the 1960s, however, health planning was emphasized at the federal level. As described in Chapter 4, Public law 89-239, the Heart Disease, Cancer, and Stroke Amendment, known as the Regional Medical Program, actively involved professionals in health planning. In 1966, Public Law 89-749, the Comprehensive Health Planning and Public Health Service Amendment, was passed. This was a significant document written to enable states and communities to plan for better usage of health resources. There were many problems with this law, one being that no new plans could interfere with existing patterns of private practice of medicine and dentistry. The law was also inadequately funded. Because of these problems, other legislative action was taken in the midseventies.

The National Health Planning and Resources Development Act of 1974 (Public Law 93-641) was signed by President Gerald Ford on January 4, 1975. Its purpose was to provide funding for program development activities and services which would improve the delivery of health care in local communities. It is hoped that this legislation will improve accessibility of health care services, curtail rising costs, and monitor the quality of care being provided.

The goals of the National Health Planning and Resources Development Act were clearly delineated in the preamble to this act. The preamble of Public Law 93-641 stated that this law was passed "to facilitate the development of recommendations for a national health planning policy, to augment area wide and state planning for health services, manpower and facilities, and to authorize financial assistance for the development of resources to further that policy" (Rubel, 1976, p. 3).

The terms of Public Law 93-641 ended the existing Hill-Burton Act (1947–1974), Regional Medical Programs (1966–1974), and the Comprehensive Health Planning Programs (1966–1974). All of these were programs to correct health care delivery problems but none had power to be comprehensive.

There are two new titles in Public Law 93-641: title XV and title XVI. Title XVI provides federal financial assistance for construction and modernization of health care facilities. Title XV creates a national network of local health systems agencies (HSAs), state health planning and development agencies (SHPDAs), and statewide health coordinating councils (SHCCs). These agencies are regulatory and are responsible for health planning and the development of resources under the law. The HSAs are very important elements of Public Law 93-641. They are geographically located in designated regions where effective planning and development of resources can be implemented at the community level. Their purpose is to improve the health of residents in the area by increasing the availability, continuity, and quality of health services while simultaneously limiting the costs of health care. Decreasing duplication of services is also a major goal of these HSAs. Specifications for an HSA are as follows (Rubel, 1976):

1. The HSA area must be geographically appropriate for planning and development. The resources should provide all the necessary health services for the residents.

2. The HSA should have a population of 500,000 to 3 million.

3. The HSA should include one center for the provision of highly specialized services.

4. The HSA planning boards must have at least 51 percent of its membership made up of consumers who are representative of the areas' groups, minorities, and geographical regions. One-third of the board must be direct providers of care, including physicians and nurses. The remaining percentage may be indirect providers such as drug suppliers and insurance personnel.

Public Law 93-641 has also created a new National Council for Health Policy (NCHP). This council is located within the Department of Human Resources and Development, formerly the Department of Health, Education, and Welfare, and will make recommendations to the secretary of HRD on national health policy planning.

There are several major elements in the law that represent a new approach to planning for health services (Rubel, 1976, p. 4). First, there is an emphasis on strong local planning as well as local control over the development of services. All segments of the health care system, including providers of care, consumers, and third-party payers, must be part of health-planning boards. Second, the certificate of need (CON) program will ensure that states do not develop health services that are not needed. Last, there are incentives to states to hold the cost of health care down.

National Health Priorities

The following 10 national health priorities are listed in Section 1502 of Public Law 93-641 (Chopoorian and Craig, 1976, p. 1989):

1. The provision of primary care services for medically underserved populations, especially those which are located in rural or economically depressed areas;

2. The development of multi-institutional systems for coordination or consolidation of institutional health services (including obstetric, pediatric, emergency medical, intensive and coronary care, and radiation therapy services);

3. The development of medical group practices (especially those whose services are appropriately coordinated or integrated with institutional health services), health maintenance organizations, and other organized systems for the provision of health care;

4. The training and increased utilization of physician assistants, especially nurse clinicians;

5. The development of multi-institutional arrangements for the sharing of support services necessary to all health service institutions;

6. The promotion of activities to achieve needed improvements in the quality of health services, including needs identified by the review activities of Professional Standards Review Organizations under Part B of Title XI of the Social Security Act;

7. The development of health service institutions of the capacity to provide various levels of care (including intensive care, acute general care, and extended care) on a geographically integrated basis;

8. The promotion of activities for the prevention of disease, including studies of nutritional and environmental factors affecting health and the provision of preventive health care services;

9. The adoption of uniform cost accounting, simplified reimbursement, and utilization reporting systems and improved management procedures for health service institutions;

10. The development of effective methods of educating the general public concerning proper personal (including preventive) health care and methods for effective use of available health services.

How does Public Law 93-641 affect nursing? The answer is, greatly, if the profession wants to have a role in the planning of health services for the 1980s. The first question that should arise is how can nurses influence the planning that Public Law 93-641 offers at the local level? On a volunteer basis, nurses can attend public hearings and serve on HSA and SHCC committees and boards. They must, however, become involved on a professional level also. State and district nursing organizations should use their collective power to ask for positions on HSA boards and committees. The number of nurses currently serving on HSA boards is very limited.

In an August 1977 study of HSAs, the Department of Health, Education, and Welfare found the following data about the make-up of the governing boards of HSAs. During the time of this particular study, the boards of 204 HSAs totaled 5931 people, 2820 of whom were provider members. Nurses comprised only 6 percent of these provider members (National League for Nursing, July 1979, p. 3):

Members	Number	Percent
Physicians	637	22
Dentists	135	5
Nurses	164	6
Health care institutions	882	31
Health care insurers	142	5
Health professional schools	157	6
Allied health professionals	233	8
Not classified	490	17

Nurses can help decide the directions health care will take, or they can sit back and let others decide their role for them. Nurses must become more visible in health policy making. Nursing is the largest of the health care professions but constitutes only 6 percent of the health care providers on HSA boards. The need for nurses to get involved is obvious.

INTERDISCIPLINARY FUNCTIONING

Nursing's role in the formulation of health policy remains to be developed almost from the ground floor. Collaboration with other members of the health team in this formulation is an exciting, evolving responsibility of nurses in all settings. It is a responsibility that provides challenging opportunities for expanding one's awareness of community needs and for influencing community health action.

A team is a group of persons who have a set of tasks that need to be accomplished. A cooperative and collaborative effort is essential if tasks are going to be completed. To be truly effective, the energy of the group should be spent on accomplishing the tasks of the group as well as developing team cohesiveness and satisfaction. Defining team tasks is not an easy process, but if it is not done, confusion and lack of direction and decision making results.

Defining tasks for an interdisciplinary team in the community setting presents special planning challenges for the community health nurse and other health care professionals. This is so because professionals in the community setting have a much broader health focus than do professionals in other settings. Identifying specific tasks to be accomplished when one has a broad focus can be difficult and more time-consuming. Beckhard (1972) substantiated this fact when he compared the effectiveness of a surgical team and a community primary care team. Both were defined as teams, and yet the amount of time to maintain the community care team was lengthy compared with the surgical team. Table 12-1 presents some of the reasons why the community team was less effective in this particular study. Beckhard's findings are not atypical, however. Handling role ambiguity concerns, resolving priority issues, defining specific tasks when goals are very broad, and facilitating group decision making are common activities that all interdisciplinary community health teams need to address.

Every interdisciplinary team needs to openly discuss, very early in the planning phase, the problems identified by Beckhard. Group members need to state what contributions they can make during the health-planning process and the role of their discipline in the community setting. The group's end goals must be defined so that each team member is working toward the same goal. Mechanisms for enhancing decision making must be established, otherwise goals will never be reached. Communication should be open so that differences of opinion can be questioned and ambiguities can be addressed.

Communicating effectively takes time, is never perfect, and requires the leadership of a person who is skilled in helping each person to contribute. Individuals on the health-planning team will communicate in a group as they communicate in other settings: some are aggressive and others will withdraw. The seasoned leader can aid the group in functioning effectively. This leader may be part of the administration of the agency or may be a state-level or university consultant.

There is a wealth of information written for those who are interested in perfecting the state of working collaboratively with other disciplines (Wise, Beckhard, Rubin, and Kyte, 1974). The reader may wish to refer to these writings to obtain a more in-depth view of interdisciplinary team functioning.

Guidelines for Group Functioning

Rubin and Beckhard (1972, pp. 332–333) have developed general guidelines that help members of health teams to develop effective working relationships. These guidelines are as follows:

1. No health-planning team automatically becomes a team just by sitting together and calling itself a team. Members have to consciously examine their goals, tasks, relationships, decision making, backgrounds, norms, and values. This is basic to the effective functioning of the team.

2. The team must be able to evaluate period-

TABLE 12-1 Comparison of Effectiveness of Two Different Teams

Condition	Surgical team	Community primary care team
Purpose	Specific: to operate and heal	General: comprehensive care
Task	Very clear	Somewhat unclear: probably many tasks
Who does what?	Roles and functions very clear	Roles ambiguous: several members may perform same functions for different patients
Where work is performed	In one location	In a number of locations
Decision making	Clear hierarchy: surgeon, first assistant, scrub nurse	Unclear: group of colleagues with different information and skills; group decisions sometimes required
Communication	One-way command system	May be discussion and problem solving
Goal priorities	Same for all members	May vary among members

SOURCE: From R. Beckhard. Organizational issues in the team delivery of health care. *Milbank Memorial Fund Quarterly*, July 1972, *1*, 293.

ically what it is doing, perhaps using methodology developed in nonmedical settings. The team can view itself as a "patient" and assess, diagnose, and treat itself. It will renew itself in this way.

3. The agencies in which teams work need to support them so that continuity, follow-up, and reinforcement of activities takes place.

4. Ideally, every team member should participate in each group task. Each member can be both a leader and an observer of the group process. Leaders need to be trained to help groups look at this method of functioning.

5. Cultural differences and expectations can be the basis for many problems between health team members as well as between the team and the population being served. The team needs to be aware that this is happening and to focus on the problem of how to cope with cultural differences.

6. Each team member needs to learn to listen.

7. If a team member does not know how to be a leader, training opportunities should be supplied.

8. Some concepts that are basic to health planning for population groups may need to be taught to both individuals on the team and the team as a whole. Working with population groups, for instance, rather than individual clients may be an important new concept to some members.

9. New team members need to be socialized and oriented to the group. Consumers or inexperienced professionals may feel very uncomfortable until this is taken care of.

10. Health planning teams need to remember that they have two functions: planning health care and maintaining themselves as well-functioning teams.

BARRIERS TO HEALTH PLANNING

Each step in the process of health planning goes down neatly on paper. Carrying out the process in "real life" is a different and challenging activity. There are several barriers to health planning that need to be acknowledged. Some of these, such as unavailability and inaccessibility of resources, inadequate knowledge, and lack of commitment to health planning, were addressed previously. Others are presented below.

A major barrier to effective health planning is a lack of understanding of the term *health*. Health is an elusive state that is difficult to define. What causes health is not easy to enumerate. It is possible to list healthy behaviors, but no one can guarantee health because both health and disease are affected by multiple, interrelated variables (multiple causation prin-

ciple). Epidemiological research has not yet been sufficient to document what these multiple causes are for many conditions or what health actions most effectively promote health and prevent disease. Thus, it is difficult for health planners to develop health action strategies for many situations. As more epidemiological research is conducted, this barrier should become less acute.

The hospital-based, disease-oriented focus in our present health care delivery system presents another key barrier to health planning. Health promotion and prevention concepts are very often not grasped by lay and professional people alike in this system. Skyrocketing hospital costs have severely disrupted the health care system of the country and, thus, community health prevention programs have been badly neglected. Basically what has happened is that persons spend so much money curing illness that there is no money left for preventive health care.

Lack of sufficient money and personnel is a constant barrier. Health may not be a priority for communities so that energy and money are spent in other directions. Health planning is often a political rather than a technical or analytical exercise, and it is possible to see an ongoing contest between local, state, and federal governments for control of planning agencies and money.

Noncompliance with health-planning activities is also a barrier. In the United States, freedom of choice is a highly prized right. Safety belts save lives, but one may choose whether or not to use them. Healthy behaviors can be presented as options but that is all. Differing values promote different priorities. If an individual is not motivated to seek preventive care, preventive health-planning action will be ineffective.

The health care system in the United States is an enormous industry that has unbelievable growth each year. Health care is a basic part of the American economy; it is inevitable that is should not function perfectly. Efforts are being made, however, to improve the quality of health care in our country.

SUMMARY

Health planning for population groups is a major function of the community health nurse. In any community setting, there are groups at risk for specific health problems. The developmental framework helps the community health nurse to identify groups at risk across the life span.

Community health nurses provide unique contributions during the health planning process. Educational experiences prepare the nurses to comprehensively analyze needs of families as well as populations. Clinical practice brings them in touch daily with consumer concerns and helps in identifying gaps or duplication in the health care delivery system.

Currently, there are obvious deficiencies in the health care delivery system which warrant health planning action. Health care services are frequently fragmented, extremely costly, and often lacking for specific segments of the population. However, there has been a positive trend evolving which places emphasis on developing new ways to meet the health care needs of all citizens. In 1975, the National Health Planning and Resources Development Act was passed. This act provides funding for program development activities and health sevices that will improve the delivery of health care in local communities.

Involvement in health-planning activities can be exciting and rewarding. Nurses are increasingly recognizing the importance of actively participating on health-planning teams and engaging in political activities aimed at changing health policy.

REFERENCES

American Nurses' Association. *Standards of community health nursing practice.* (CH-2SM) Kansas City: ANA Publications, 1973.

Ashley, J. A. Nursing and early feminism. *American Journal of Nursing,* September 1975, *75,* 1465–1467. Reprinted with the permission of the American Journal of Nursing Company. Copyright by the American Journal of Nursing Company.

Beckhard, R. Organizational issues in the team delivery of comprehensive health care. *Milbank Memorial Fund Quarterly*, July 1972, *1*, 287–316.

Chopoorian, T., & Craig, M. M. PL 93-641, nursing and health care delivery. *American Journal of Nursing*, 1976, *76*, 1988–1991.

Duvall, E. M. *Marriage and family development* (5th ed.). Philadelphia: Lippincott, 1977.

Erikson, E. H. *Childhood and society*. New York: Norton, 1950.

Freud, S. *New introductory lectures on psychoanalysis*. J. Strachey (Ed. and Trans.). New York: Norton, 1965 (originally published 1933).

Greer, A. Training board members for health planning agencies. A review of the literature. *Public Health Reports*, January 1976, *91*, 56–61.

Havighurst, R. J. *Developmental tasks and education*. New York: McKay, 1952.

Kinlein, M. L. *Independent nursing practice with clients*. Philadelphia: Lippincott, 1977.

Long, G. V., Whitman, C., Johansson, M., Williams, C., & Tuthill, R. W. Evaluation of a school health program directed to children with a history of high absence. *American Journal of Public Health*, April 1975, *65*, 388–393.

National League for Nursing, Public Affairs Advisory. *The purposes and politics of HSA's*. July 1979, pp. 1–4.

Pecarchik, R., Ricci, E., & Nelson, B. Potential contribution of consumers to an integrated health care system. *Public Health Reports*, January 1976, *91*, 72–76.

Piaget, J., & Inhelder, B. *The psychology of the child*. New York: Basic Books, 1969.

Rubel, E. J. Implementing the national health planning and resources development act of 1974. *Public Health Reports*, January 1976, *91*, 3–8.

Rubin, I. M., & Beckhard, R. Factors influencing the effectiveness of health teams. *Milbank Memorial Fund Quarterly*, July 1972, *1*, 317–335.

Ruybal, S. E. Community health planning. *Family and Community Health*, April 1978, *1*, 9–18.

Taylor, I., & Knowelden, J. *Principles of epidemiology* (2d ed.). Boston: Little, Brown, 1964.

Williams, C. A. Community health nursing—What is it? *Nursing Outlook*, April 1977, *25*, 250–254.

Wise, H., Beckhard, R., Rubin, I., & Kyte, A. *Making health teams work*. Cambridge, Mass.: Ballinger, 1974.

SELECTED BIBLIOGRAPHY

Altman, D. The politics of health care regulation: The case of the national health planning and resources development act. *Journal of Health Politics and the Law*, 1978, *2*, 560–580.

Elinson, Jack, Insensitive health statistics and the dilemma of the HSA's. *American Journal of Public Health*, May 1977, *67*, 417–418.

Hyman, H. *Health planning, a systematic approach*. Germantown, Md.: Aspen Systems Corporation, 1975.

Kalisch, P. A., & Kalisch, B. J. *Nursing involvement in the health planning process*. DHEW Publication No. HRA 78-25. Hyattsville, Md.: U.S. Department of Health, Education, and Welfare, September 1977.

Kark, S. *Epidemiology and community medicine*. New York: Appleton-Century-Crofts, 1974.

Lane, D., & Mazzola, G. The community hospital as a focus for health planning. *American Journal of Public Health*, May 1976, *66*, 465–468.

Mott, P., Mott, A., Rudolph, J., Lane, E., & Berg, R. Difficult issues in health planning development and review. *American Journal of Public Health*, August 1976, *66*, 743–746.

Scipien, G. M., Barnard, M. U., Chard, M. A., Howe, J., & Phillips, P. J., *Comprehensive pediatric nursing*. New York: McGraw-Hill, 1975.

Shonick, W. *Elements of planning for area-wide personal health services*. St. Louis: Mosby, 1976.

Spiegel, A. D., & Hyman, H. H. *Basic health planning*

methods. Germantown, Md.: Aspen Systems Corporation, 1978.

Spiegel, C., & Lindaman, F. Children can't fly: A program to prevent childhood morbidity and mortality from window falls. *American Journal of Public Health,* December 1977, *67,* 1143–1146.

White, K. L., & Henderson, M. W. (Eds.). *Epidemiology as a fundamental science. Its uses in health services planning, administration, and evaluation.* New York: Oxford University Press, 1976.

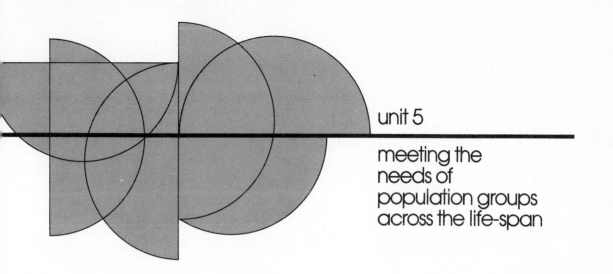

unit 5

meeting the
needs of
population groups
across the life-span

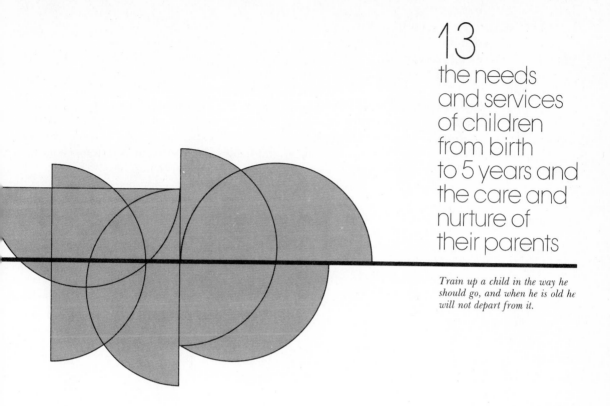

13
the needs and services of children from birth to 5 years and the care and nurture of their parents

Train up a child in the way he should go, and when he is old he will not depart from it.

The wise King Solomon wrote this proverb 3000 years ago. Today, parents are still struggling to find out what it means to "train up a child in the way he should go," although a modern version would certainly translate the end result to be the maximizing of the child's potential and helping him or her maintain balance and direction in the environment (Dunn, 1973, p. 4). Maximizing the potential and maintaining balance is not easy. Children and their parents form an important team in reaching developmental milestones. It is difficult to separate the health of one from the health of the other. Although parents struggle with all of the child's developmental age levels, the first 5 years in a child's life are the most important for the simple reason that they

come first. They are the formative years and their influence upon the years that follow are beyond calculation.

Federal, state, and local health professionals have had concern for maternal-infant health that can be traced to the turn of the century. The concern for maternal-infant health stems from the fact that the health of the infant cannot be separated from the health of the parents, and particularly the mother. In 1900 deaths of mothers and children were major contributors to mortality figures: approximately 60 mothers died for every 10,000 pregnancies that produced live-born infants; out of every 1000 of these infants, 100 did not survive the first year of life (Wilner, Walkley, and Goerke, 1973, p. 365).

These statistics were high and they motivated concerned individuals to develop community maternal-child health programs; nursing assumed a major leadership role in this effort. Lillian Wald, a pioneer community health nurse and feminist, helped establish milk stations in 1903 at the Henry Street Settlement House in New York City to ensure the safety of milk for babies. Diarrhea caused by contaminated milk in the summer months was the cause of many deaths. The city of New York followed this example and in 1911 authorized the establishment of 15 milk stations:

A nurse is attached to each station to follow into the homes and there lay the foundation, through education, for hygienic living. A marked reduction in infant mortality has been brought about and moreover, a realization, on the part of the city, of the immeasurable social and economic value of keeping the babies alive. (Wald, 1915, p. 57)

Traditionally, childbearing women, infants, and children are considered to be the more dependent and vulnerable members in a society. As the society develops, there is a trend toward greater concern for this segment of the population. The health of a society's children ensures that society's future, so this concern for infants and children is justified on economic as well as other grounds.

The mortality rates for mothers and children are frequently used to assess the health of populations. Since the turn of the century, great progress has been made in the United States in reducing maternal and infant mortality. During the 55 years after World War I, maternal mortality decreased 95 percent and infant mortality 90 percent (Hanlon, 1974, p. 320). This progress was due to factors such as improved medical care, better housing, sanitation, and nutrition, as well as the decline of infectious diseases because of immunizing agents and the introduction of antibiotics and other therapeutic medicines.

During the period 1965 to 1970, the infant mortality rate declined from 25 to 20 deaths per 1000 live births. Data through 1975 indicated that it continued to fall at the same rate (Morris, Udry, and Chase, 1975, p. 359). Explanations for this decline include the falling birth rate and the advent of better maternity and infant care services for high-risk mothers and babies. The outcome is that more mothers and babies are surviving.

The increasing complexity and cost to the public of meeting the needs of those 0 to 5 years old, as well as the numbers of deaths and handicapping conditions that are present, make it essential that efforts to fulfill the health needs of this age group and their parents be organized on all levels of society. Everyone, regardless of race or economic level, has the right to health care and health education. They also need assistance in changing unhealthy behavior to healthy behavior. This is not presently the situation. Consider the following statistics presented by the *American Journal of Public Health* in a lead article in 1975 (Miller):

· In New York City, 80 percent of white children had a well-baby checkup in the first 2 months of life, but only 56 percent of the babies of Spanish origin had a well-baby examination in the first 2 months of life. By 1 year of age, only 0.5 percent of white non-Spanish babies had received no checkup at all; 7.6 percent of the Spanish babies had had no checkup.

· Between the ages of 1 and 4, a nonwhite child is three times more likely than a white child to die of influenza or pneumonia and twice as likely to die of accidental death.

· Prematurely born infants present increased medical requirements in the first weeks of life and they are vulnerable to life-long danger.

They are born three times more frequently to poor women than to others.

· Three-fourths of the nation's children who are mentally retarded are found in impoverished rural and urban slums. A child from a low-income family in these areas is 15 times more likely to be diagnosed as retarded than a child from a high-income family.

Figure 13-1, which gives infant mortality rates by color in the United States from 1925 to 1974, graphically illustrates that the color of an infant's skin affects the chances of that infant's survival. Though whites and nonwhites have decreasing mortality rates, the mortality rate for minority infants is two-thirds again as high as the rate for white infants. This is related to the fact that poverty is much more prevalent among minority groups. The death rate for minority preschool children is approximately 50 percent higher than for white children. These children also have high death rates from influenza, pneumonia, and other infectious diseases (*Health*, 1975, p. 341).

Despite the decreasing death rates among infants, the United States still has much work to be done when compared with other countries in the world. Table 13-1, which shows infant mortality rates for selected countries in 1973, illustrates that 14 countries have lower infant mortality rates than the United States.

Morbidity among the 0 to 5-year-old population, as well as mortality, presents a major public health concern. In the process of growing up, children encounter injuries and illnesses that interfere with normal functioning. Jack and Jill's broken crown and Humpty Dumpty's fall off the wall are common experiences known to every child.

There are health problems common to the 0- to 5-year age group that can be prevented as well as problems that necessitate secondary and tertiary prevention. In order to plan

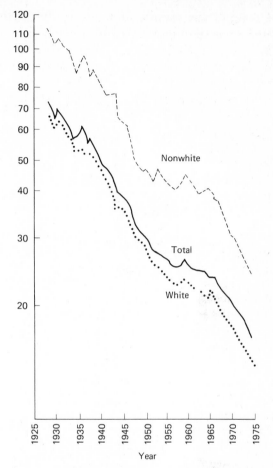

FIGURE 13-1 Infant mortality rates by color: United States, 1926–1974. Rates are the number of deaths under 1 year of age per 1000 live births. 1925–1932, includes birth-registration status only; 1932–1934, Mexicans are included with "nonwhite"; 1962–1963, figures by color exclude data for residents of New Jersey; 1974, provisional. (*From National Center for Health Statistics. Vital Statistics Rates in the United States, 1940–1960. PHS Pub. No. 1477; and Monthly Vital Statistics Report, Provisional Statistics, Annual Summary for the United States, 1974, 23, 13.*)

health services for this group, the community health nurse should be familiar with these problems to facilitate application of the three levels of prevention as well as case finding.

TABLE 13-1   Infant Mortality Rates: Selected Countries, 1973*

Rank	Country	Rate	Rank	Country	Rate
1	Sweden	9.6	21	Austria	23.7†
2	Finland	10.1†	22	Spain (1972)§	25.2†
3	Norway (1972)	11.3	23	Italy	25.7†
4	Netherlands	11.6†	24	Bulgaria	25.9†
5	Japan (1972)‡	11.7	25	Jamaica	26.2
6	Switzerland	12.8†	25	Trinidad and Tobago (1972)	26.2
7	Denmark (1971)	13.5	27	USSR¶	26.3†
8	France (1972)§	16.0†	28	Greece (1972)	27.8†
8	German Democratic Republic	16.0	29	Poland (1972)	28.5
10	New Zealand	16.2	30	Hungary	33.5†
11	Australia (1972)	16.7†	31	Romania	38.2
12	Canada	16.8	32	Uruguay (1971)	40.4
13	Belgium	17.0†	33	Yugoslavia	43.3
14	United Kingdom (1972)	17.5	34	Portugal	44.8†
15	*United States*	*17.7*	35	Sri Lanka (1972)	45.1†
16	Ireland	17.8†	36	El Salvador (1971)	52.5
17	Federal Republic of Germany (1972)	20.4†	37	Costa Rica (1971)	56.5
18	Singapore	20.4†	38	South Africa (1971)	63.2†
19	Czechoslovakia	21.2†	39	Chile (1970)	78.8
20	Israel	22.1	40	Guatemala	79.1

*Rates are deaths under 1 year of age per 1000 live births.

†Provisional.

‡Excludes data for Okinawa.

§The 1973 rates of 12.9 for France and 15.1 for Spain were not used because they exclude live-born infants dying before registration of birth.

¶Data exclude infants born alive of less than 28 weeks' gestation, less than 1000 g in weight and 35 cm in length, who die within 7 days of birth.

NOTE: This table is limited to sovereign countries with estimated populations of 1 million or more and with "complete" counts of live births and infant deaths, as indicated in the 1973 *Demographic Yearbook* of the United Nations.

SOURCE: From National Center for Health Statistics. *Health: United States 1975.* PHS Publication No. HRA76. Rockville, Md., 1975, p. 349.

COMMON HEALTH PROBLEMS

Table 13-2 shows the leading causes of death for all ages and lists separately the causes for children under 1 year as well as children 1 to 4 years. For children under 1 year, complications of pregnancy and birth are important death factors. As children become mobile and walk, after the age of 1, accidents (in cars, fires, drownings, falls, and ingesting substances and other objects) become the major cause of death.

TABLE 13-2   Leading Causes of Death, 1977

	No. of deaths	Death rate*		No. of deaths	Death rate*
All ages	1,899,597	878	Accidents:	1,173	37
Heart disease	718,850	332	Ingestion of food object	275	9
Cancer	386,686	179	Motor-vehicle	253	8
Stroke†	181,934	84	Mechanical suffocation	206	6
Accidents:	103,202	48	Fires, burns	159	5
Motor-vehicle	49,510	23	Other	280	9
Falls	13,773	6	1 to 4 years	8,307	69
Drowning	7,126	3	Accidents:	3,297	27
Fires, burns	6,357	3	Motor-vehicle	1,219	10
Other	26,436	13	Drowning	650	5
Under 1 year	46,975	1,485	Fires, burns	608	5
Anoxia	10,604	335	Ingestion of food object	168	1
Congenital anomalies	8,420	266	Falls	121	1
Complications of pregnancy and childbirth	5,786	183	Other	531	5
			Congenital anomalies	1,066	5
Immaturity	3,714	117	Cancer	631	5
Pneumonia	1,665	53			

*Deaths per 100,000 population in each age group. Rates are averages for age groups, not individual ages.

†Cerebrovascular disease.

SOURCE: From National Center for Health Statistics, Public Health Service, U.S. Department of Health, Education, and Welfare, in National Safety Council. *Accident Facts 1979 Edition.* Chicago, Ill.: National Safety Council, 1979, p. 8.

Problems before Birth

Table 13-3 lists the factors associated with high-risk pregnancies. These factors are important to know because they provide the basis for the high mortality and morbidity rates during the first year of life and contribute to the high maternal mortality rates. They are danger signs, signaling threat to the newborn and the mother. Those caring for the pregnant mother can effectively use this guide to identify high-risk mothers and infants and to implement preventive measures. As is demonstrated by this table, socially and economically deprived persons are more likely than others to have high-risk babies. This is at least par-

tially explained by the lack of adequate prenatal care, which is unavailable in urban and rural slums.

About 70 percent of the women giving birth in 1973 began prenatal care before the end of the first trimester of pregnancy. Married women began care much earlier than unmarried ones; only 40 percent of the latter had any care before the end of the first trimester even though they were predominantly young, when the risks to both mother and child are very high (*Health*, 1975, p. 364). This fact is significant to the community health nurse who may be able to influence the young, unmarried mother to utilize antepartal services.

TABLE 13-3   Factors Associated with High-Risk Pregnancy

1. Demographic factors

   a. Lower socioeconomic status

   b. Disadvantaged ethnic groups

   c. Marital status: unwed mothers

   d. Maternal age

       1. Gravida less than 16 years of age

       2. Primigravida 35 years of age or older

       3. Gravida 40 years of age or older

   e. Maternal weight: nonpregnant weight less than 100 lb or more than 200 lb

   f. Stature: height less than 62 in (1.57 m)

   g. Malnutrition

   h. Poor physical fitness

2. Past pregnancy history

   a. Grand multiparity: six previous pregnancies terminating beyond 20 weeks' gestation

   b. Antepartum bleeding after 12 weeks of gestation

   c. Premature rupture of membranes, premature onset of labor, premature delivery

   d. Previous cesarean section or mid- or high-forceps delivery

   e. Prolonged labor

   f. Infant with cerebral palsy, mental retardation, birth trauma, central nervous system disorder, or congenital anomaly

   g. Reproductive failure: infertility, repetitive abortion, fetal loss, stillbirth, or neonatal death

   h. Delivery of preterm (less than 37 weeks) or postterm (more than 42 weeks) infant

3. Past or present medical history

   a. Hypertension or renal disease or both

   b. Diabetes mellitus (overt or gestational)

Problems after Birth

Once a baby is born, gestational age, birth weight, and environment are significant factors in its chances for survival. The newborn period (birth to 1 month) is particularly important since nearly three-fourths of all infant deaths occur within the first 28 days of life (*Health*, 1975, p. 346). Most of these deaths are associated with prematurity. Premature infants are usually of low birth weight, that is, less than $5\frac{1}{2}$ lb (2500 g). Prematurity also can have an adverse effect on the establishment of maternal-infant bonding. Low-birth-weight infants are not necessarily premature. All low-birth-weight infants, whether premature or not, are highly vulnerable to disease and death. About 5 out of every 100 of these babies, 150,000 babies a year in the United States, are so ill that they require intensive care (Schwartz and Schwartz, 1977, p. 2). The incidence of neurological and psychological ab-

TABLE 13-3   Factors Associated with High-Risk Pregnancy (*Continued*)

   c. Cardiovascular disease (rheumatic, congenital, or peripheral vascular)

   d. Pulmonary disease producing hypoxemia and hypercapnia

   e. Thyroid, parathyroid, and endocrine disorders

   f. Idiopathic thrombocytopenic purpura

   g. Neoplastic disease

   h. Hereditary disorders

   i. Collagen diseases

   j. Epilepsy

4. Additional obstetric and medical conditions

   a. Toxemia

   b. Asymptomatic bacteriuria

   c. Anemia or hemoglobinopathy

   d. Rh sensitization

   e. Habitual smoking

   f. Drug addiction or habituation

   g. Chronic exposure to any pharmacologic or chemical agent

   h. Multiple pregnancy

   i. Rubella or other viral infection

   j. Intercurrent surgery and anesthesia

   k. Placental abnormalities and uterine bleeding

   l. Abnormal fetal lie or presentation, fetal anomalies, oligohydramnios, polyhydramnios

   m. Abnormalities of fetal or uterine growth or both

   n. Maternal trauma during pregnancy

   o. Maternal emotional crisis during pregnancy

SOURCE: Adapted from V. C. Vaughn and R. J. McKay (Eds.) and W. E. Nelson (Con. Ed.). *Textbook of Pediatrics*, 10th ed. Philadelphia: Saunders, 1975.

normalities occurring during the first year of life is four times as high for low-birth-weight infants as others. Low-birth-weight children represent a major public health problem.

Problems developing before the infant reaches 1 month of age are usually related to gestational age and birth weight and in utero problems. Problems after 1 month are more often related to environmental factors. Here the community health nurse plays a significant role in prevention, especially in relation to morbidity.

Parent-Child Bonding

Parent-child bonding can be adversely affected when an infant is separated from its primary care giver for a period of time. This separation can occur when an infant is premature or otherwise at risk and must have long-term health care away from parents. Even with normal hospital deliveries, mothers may not see their infants for 12 to 24 hours following delivery. Studies have shown that this period is crucial for the formation of attachment bonds between mothers and their babies and is important for establishing the mothering behavior of mothers (Klaus and Kennell, 1976). Klaus and Kennell hypothesize that all disorders of mothering, ranging from a persisting concern about a minor abnormality, to abusing and neglecting children, are in part the end result of separation in the early newborn period (Klaus and Kennell, 1976, p. 124).

Another problem associated with high-risk infants—those who are small, or have other physical, familial, and psychological problems—can be failure to thrive on the part of the child. A child who fails to thrive is one in whom no clear organic etiology can be demonstrated for the growth failure. Instead, the problem seems to arise from situations of environmental, sensory, or parental deprivation. Placement of a child in a nurturing atmosphere often brings improvement.

In one study of 39 infants who failed to thrive, 41 percent were below 5 lb 8 oz at birth and 57 percent were the results of complicated pregnancies (Shaheen, Alexander, and Barbero, 1977, pp. 205–206). Other areas of stress that contributed to the child's failure to thrive in this study were the family constellation, socioeconomic status, and disruption in the infant's immediate and extended family. Sixty-two percent of the families had had involvement with community agencies prior to the child's hospitalization.

Harrison (1976) has suggested that nursing care with families that fail to thrive must include support that encourages adaptive mothering behaviors and promotes mother-child attachment. The nursing care should also include teaching specific nurturing techniques, including adequate feeding and interaction with the environment. Assistance to the family with resolving problems that interfere with the family's ability to provide a nurturing environment is another element of nursing care that Harrison suggests. She has also developed three tools which assist the community health nurse to analyze the mothering behaviors, including infant behaviors, and the nursing intervention with these families.

Abuse and Neglect

In general, abuse refers to acts of *commission* such as beating or excessive chastisement. Neglect refers to acts of *omission* such as failure to provide adequate food, clothing, or emotional care. However, the line separating the two is a very thin one. The problem of abuse and neglect is a growing one. In 1975, there were approximately 555,000 reported cases of suspected child abuse and neglect and the Department of Health, Education, and Welfare estimates the actual number to be over a million (Helfer and Kempe, 1976, p. xvii). It is also a cumulative problem since the scars of abuse and neglect have long-term effects. The most damaging aspect of child abuse and neglect is on the developmental process and emotional growth of the child. Abused children do not feel safe and are unable to trust others, Erikson's first stage in development.

Parents tend to follow their own parent's style of child rearing: if it was characterized by abuse and neglect, their own child-rearing style is likely to repeat these characteristics. Children who are abused or neglected have parents who were often themselves neglected and abused as children. This one factor is more significant among parents who maltreat their children than any other factor, including socioeconomic status, living conditions, race, religion, education, emotional status, and cultural and family background (Steele, 1976, p. 14).

Parents of abused children often do not understand the normal growth and development patterns of their children and expect too much of them. As a result, the child is criticized and physically and emotionally punished. A sense of failure, lack of confidence and faith in one's own abilities often results in abused and neglected children.

Many factors in a family contribute to the

abuse and neglect of children by parents (Garbarino, 1977). These include blocks to the role transition of parent as a result of not having been able to develop the role of care giver. The parents may also have had inadequate role models. Such parents have a lack of knowledge about what is involved in parenting, both physically and emotionally, and thus do not know what to expect realistically of themselves or their children. Abusing parents often consider their own needs as more important than their children's needs: they have an inappropriate concept of the legitimacy and value of their own needs when ranked with their children's needs. Expecting children to fulfill parents' needs is another problem. Abusing parents feel that they are unable to have any effect and control over events inside and outside the family. Unfortunately, these same families are often characterized by great demands for adjustment to stresses such as moves, job changes, and illnesses. Difficulties may also arise when children begin demanding independence, pushing away from families, or when they are negativistic.

Garbarino also suggests that abusing families are socially isolated from support systems. This isolation may be a result of mobility patterns, characteristics that alienate others, social stresses that cut families off from potential and actual supports, as well as social service agencies that are unable to identify and care for high-risk families.

Community health nurses need to be alert to situations where abuse and neglect have the possibility of occurring and intervene before this happens. Marital strain, poverty, isolation, and overwhelmed mothers are signals to be heeded. Premature births or having children with developmental disabilities are stressful situations that need to be noted. Parents who expect infants to be responsible for their acts and who respond with physical punishment provide another situation to watch.

Mental retardation, emotional disorders, and learning disorders can be other evidences of a less-than-positive nurturing environment for infants. Organic pathologic factors are contributors to these disorders, but there are also psychosocial and other factors which influence the development of these disorders.

Presently there are no states with enough resources and personnel to deal adequately with the increasing number of reported cases of abuse and neglect, not to mention working with families who have already been identified as needing care.

Sudden Infant Death Syndrome

Another sequel to high-risk pregnancy may be the sudden infant death syndrome (SIDS). In the United States, 1 out of every 300 live-born infants a year dies from SIDS. It is the number-one cause of death in infants after the first week of life. Although SIDS is as old as the New Testament, the cause of this disease is not known (National Foundation for Sudden Infant Death, p. 2). Helping parents handle grief and guilt feelings is the major role of the community health nurse in these situations. The impact of death on siblings is another area where the nurse must intervene.

Increasingly, communities are setting up crisis teams to assist families who have experienced a child's death from SIDS. One health department in a Northern city employs a pediatric nurse practitioner who works full-time with such families. She facilitates family adjustment as they work through the grief process after death has come to a seemingly healthy infant.

Acute Illnesses

Respiratory diseases and other conditions such as diarrhea result in short-term disability and account for many doctor visits among infants. These diseases caused much death in the past. Today, there is less mortality from these conditions but a tremendous amount of professional time is spent in controlling acute illnesses. The nurse in the pediatric clinic or the nurse who makes home visits will see these kinds of problems and will need the expertise to explain their origin and treatment to parents.

Problems among Children Age 1 to 5

Children do change in their capacities. As developmental growth occurs, infants and children's needs and problems become different.

Accidents

As Table 13-2 demonstrates, accidents causing death during a child's first year are not usually major public health problems. After this period, however, accidents become the leading cause of death in children 1 to 14 years of age.

When the accidental death rate for children between 1 and 5 years of age is compared with the other causes of mortality in this age group, accidental injury is by far the most prevalent. Of all accidents, 33 percent of the deaths are from motor vehicles, 22 percent are from fires and explosions, 14 percent are from drowning, 13 percent are from inhalation and ingestions, 12 percent are from falls, and 6 percent are from various other accidents. It is not difficult to see that accidents are a major health problem and that present education and legislation are not as effective as they should be in combating a problem that is preventable.

Respiratory and Gastrointestinal Problems

Upper respiratory infections become a common cause of illness in the 1 to 5 year age group, especially when they begin to play in groups of children. Upper respiratory infections can be minor and cause only minimal interference to living. Others can be life-threatening, especially when no treatment is obtained. Lower respiratory tract infections result generally from infections of the upper respiratory tract.

Minor gastrointestinal problems are almost as common as respiratory infections. The use of epidemiology in examining the numbers of cases in a family and a community helps to determine whether the causative agent is or is not communicable. Epidemiological investigation also helps to identify significant environmental conditions that need changing, especially when a child has repeated infections.

Prompt treatment of acute conditions, ongoing medical care, educating parents regarding good health care practices, and early detection of illness can help to prevent or curtail respiratory and gastrointestinal problems.

Chronic Diseases

Chronic diseases are important because of their long-term effects. During the 1960s, 15 percent of the 18-year-old males were rejected for military service because of long-term medical problems that could have been lessened or prevented by appropriate health care (*Health, 1975*, p. 342).

A death rate of 6 out of every 100,000 of the 1- to 5-year population results from cancer. The types of cancers that are seen in children differ from those seen in adults. Those affecting children are the leukemias, embryonal tumors, and sarcomas. Regular medical follow-up can aid in early diagnosis of such conditions.

Under the category of chronic problems come children with developmental disabilities such as phenylketonuria, Down's syndrome, cerebral palsy, blindness, mental retardation, or deafness. Also included are children with physical health problems such as diabetes, rheumatoid arthritis, and kidney disease. These children present problems to their families that demand special attention, study, and creative problem solving.

Between 100,000 and 200,000 babies born each year in the United States are mentally retarded. The causes of the retardation can be identified in only one-fourth of the cases. In the other three-fourths, inadequacies in prenatal and perinatal care, nutrition, child rearing, and social and environmental opportunities are suspected as causes (White House Conference on Children, 1970). Many of these suspected causes can be dealt with in some manner by the community health nurse.

Communicable and Preventable Diseases

Preventable communicable diseases are still a major community health problem. In 1977, 54,847 cases of measles were reported to the Center for Disease Control in Atlanta, Georgia. This is a 33.4 percent increase over the 1976 rates and the largest number of cases reported since 1971 (Center for Disease Control Feb. 3, 1978, p. 39). The current herd immunity is low. Only 60 percent of American children under 15 years of age are completely immunized (Garner, 1978, p. 132). Community health nurses need to make an effort to increase this level to at least the desired level of 85 percent.

Table 13-4, relating complications from childhood diseases, summarizes the problems that can result from the preventable childhood diseases. The contributing factors that allow children to remain unimmunized include the lack of consumer awareness, understanding, and responsibility; the complicated vaccine schedule which can be easily misunderstood; the increased mobility of families, which can lead to fragmented health care; inadequate funding for immunization research on the federal level; resistance by public school systems to compliance with state immunization requirements; and apathy because the evidences of childhood disease are no longer obvious.

Lead Poisoning

Mental retardation and other neurological handicaps are needless results of lead poisoning in children. Lead poisoning results mainly from ingestion of chips of lead-containing paint from walls and woodwork, often in older, dilapidated housing. Its etiology, pathophysiology, and epidemiology are well known as are methods for its screening, diagnosis, prevention, and treatment. Yet each year it continues to cause death, mental retardation, and other problems in many children. The long-term effects of lead poisoning can be subtle; the neurological defects may not be discovered until a child enters school and the teacher notes a *slight* deficiency in the performance of the child.

With the passage of laws banning the use of lead paint, the problem has greatly decreased. Children living in old housing where peeling exposes old lead paint are still most vulnerable. Pica, the appetite for unusual foreign materials, is also significantly related to this problem. Children between the ages of 1 and 6 years are the main victims; those between 1 and 3 years of age comprise approximately 85 percent of the cases, with the highest incidence coming at 2 years of age. Over 50 percent of all deaths from lead poisoning occur in 2-year-olds (Lin-Fu, 1975, p. 5). This particular statistic is related to the 2-year-old's normal developmental need to explore and sample the environment.

The diagnosis of this problem is made if there is a history of ingestion, a blood lead level of 0.06 mg per 100 mL or higher, and the presence of two or more of the following symptoms: gastrointestinal symptoms of anorexia, nausea, vomiting, abdominal pain, constipation; hematological findings of anemia or pallor; neurological signs of stupor, lethargy, or convulsions; and x-rays showing increased density of the long bones or opacities showing lead flakes in the abdomen (Lin-Fu, 1975, p. 8).

Physicians and other health professionals, as well as the public, are not aware of the existence or magnitude of this problem. One result is a high rate of recurrence of lead poi-

TABLE 13-4 Some Complications from Selected Childhood Diseases for Which Immunizations Are Available

Complications	Mumps	Measles (rubeola)	Rubella	Rubella (in utero)	Polio	Tetanus	Pertussis	Diphtheria
Mental retardation		X	X	X			X	
Brain damage		X	X	X			X	
Meningoencephalitis	X	X	X	X				
Paralysis					X			X
Blindness		X	X	X				
Deafness	X	X	X	X				X
Pancreatitis	X							
Juvenile-type diabetes	X							
Orchitis (postpubertal)	X							
Oophoritis (postpubertal)	X							
Sterility (males)	X							
Pneumonia	X	X				X	X	X
Heart damage, pericarditis	X							X
Polyarthritis			X					
Hepatitis	X							
Nephritis	X							X
Cerebral hemorrhage							X	
Muscle spasm						X		
Death	X	X	X	X	X	X	X	X

SOURCES: Adapted from M. K. Garner. Our values are showing: Inadequate childhood immunization. *Health values: Achieving high level wellness*, May–June 1978, *2*, p. 130; R. A. Hoekelman, Saul Blatman, Philip A. Burnell, S. B. Friedman, & H. M. Seidel. *Principles of pediatrics health care of the young*. New York: McGraw-Hill, 1978; and G. M. Scipien, M. U. Barnard, M. A. Chard, J. Howe, & P. J. Phillips. *Comprehensive pediatric nursing*. New York: McGraw-Hill, 1975.

soning among children because of the lack of an epidemiological follow-up of reported cases of this disease. Children are treated and then sent back into the same environment that produced the poisoning; the cycle then repeats itself.

Another problem is the weak and ineffective housing laws and lack of enforcement. One community health nurse visited a family who rented an older home with lead paint on the outside. They lived in a neighborhood heavily populated with children. Two children ingested peeling paint chips and as a result the nurse had the environmental department check the paint for lead content. The city housing department was contacted; they in turn contacted the landlord who was informed of the need to scrape and repaint the house with nonlead paint. The request was never enforced and the house remains a hazard in the community.

Not all situations are the same, however. One community utilizes community health nurses for epidemiological investigation and follow-up of lead-poisoning referrals. The largest hospital in that city will not release children diagnosed with lead poisoning back into their same environments. Families must make alternative housing arrangements until the source of the lead poisoning is eliminated.

Nutritional Inadequacies and Dental Problems

Another condition seen by the community health nurse when working with children ages 1 to 5 is nutritional inadequacy and anemia. Brain cells reach adult numbers by 18 months of age. Severe early malnutrition during the first year of life will retard cell division rate and result in a brain with fewer cells. This change is irreversible, regardless of the nutritional intake thereafter (Medcom, 1975). Quality and quantity of the diet are also important since early nutrition affects the rate of fat cell proliferation.

Two feeding problems seen by the nurse are overfeeding of infants and young children and too early an introduction of beikost (foods other than milk or formula). Feeding beikost at an early age is viewed by parents as a developmental milestone and thus they push the infant before he or she is ready. There appears to be little evidence to support giving solids before the age of 3 to 4 months, because the result of this practice is the replacement by solids of the milk the infant needs for growth. Another result is that the child may be overfed if the amount of milk given is not decreased when solids are given. Solids are not digested well by young children because of their immature gastrointestinal systems. Spoon feeding begun too early can result in frustration for both parent and child.

There is a high prevalence of iron-deficiency anemia in infants and children of all socioeconomic levels, even among those who supposedly have an adequate diet (Medcom, 1975, p. 36). Infants and children particularly at risk are those who are born prematurely, have perinatal blood loss, have congenital heart disease, are irritable and anorexic, have pica or disturbed sleep patterns, and are fed homogenized cow's milk before the age of 9 months. Cow's milk induces enteric blood loss and contributes to at least 50 percent of the cases of iron-deficiency anemia in the United States.

Another problem, overnutrition, results from the popular notion that to be healthy is to be fat and the equating of rewards for good behavior with food. Obesity is not condoned for adults, but fat children are often considered cute. Unfortunately, childhood fat may not disappear in adulthood. Plotting body weight in comparison with body height helps parents and nurses to determine whether obesity is a problem.

Poor dental hygiene is another problem that can begin with this age group. As early as 1862, one researcher was calling attention to the association of dental caries with the practice of offering milk or sugared water at bedtime (Foman, 1974, p. 345). More recent research supports the idea that milk with an added carbohydrate or a sugared pacifier at bedtime, after teeth have begun to erupt, increases the likelihood of dental caries (Foman, 1974, p. 346). The "nursing bottle" syndrome is promoted by constant bottle sucking. With this syndrome, the maxillary anterior teeth are destroyed and caries develop on the maxillary and mandibular molars. Eating frequent between-meal snacks also contributes to caries because the carbohydrates in the snacks are in frequent contact with the teeth.

Unfortunately, it is often only after children reach school age that parents become concerned with dental hygiene, and by then much damage may have been done to the teeth. The appearance of their mouth contributes to the way people feel physically and emotionally, and the financial cost of dental repair can be very high.

Behavioral Problems

Disturbance of sleep patterns, toilet training, eating, and relationships with strangers and continual whining and crying are some behavioral problems seen by the nurse who works with children. Parents will often have questions about problems in these areas that seem minor but can cause daily discomfort to a family and develop into more major problems.

HEALTH PROMOTION NEEDS

Identifying areas where families and larger groups can increase the state of their health, where they are working toward maximizing their potential, is one of the most exciting and challenging aspects of family and community health nursing.

Health promotion in the 1- to 5-year age group is particularly important because this period provides the foundation of the physical, intellectual, and emotional health for the rest of the child's life.

The nurse needs to remember the concept that behavior changes with age in a patterned, predictable manner. Behavior has form and shape just as physical patterns do. All growth, whether physical or emotional, implies organization.

Norms for various ages can be dangerous if they are used as absolute standards because each child develops with a different rhythm. Making diagnoses from the behavior a child exhibits takes knowledge, skill, and experience. However, norms for various ages can be guides for planning health promotion programs. Brazelton's *Infants and Mothers* (1969) describes the range of differences infants of the same age can have. The Denver Developmental Screening Test and the Washington Guide, which will be discussed later, also give normal ranges.

Health Promotion before Birth

Good health begins before a child is conceived. Children need to be wanted and planned, and people need to learn how to be parents. Becoming pregnant does not confer readiness for children because an individual does not automatically put aside all personal needs to prepare for a child's world, which is in itself not a rational world. Thus, parent education needs to start early. It needs to become a part of school curriculums, community organizations, and church groups. Apprenticeship programs in which young people go into families and work with children in group settings has already begun (Callahan, 1973, p. 193). Parenting programs need to include information regarding the physical aspects of child care; nutrition for the mother and the child; the physical, intellectual, and emotional development of children; and the stresses of role changes for parents. Some schools use the team approach, with the teacher, the school nurse, the social worker, and the nutritionist all working together to present the parenting program.

The nurse in the school setting can help teachers and administrators plan parenting classes at the junior- and senior-high level. Accompanying information on parenting must be courses on responsible sexuality, the physiology of sexual development, the part optional parenthood and contraception play in teenagers' sexuality, and the consequences of poor health practices during adolescent years.

The nutrition of the female throughout her life plays a role in the health of the children she delivers (National Academy of Science, 1975). As girls become responsible for their own nutrition and can make choices about what they eat, they need to know what proper nutrition is. They also need to be aware that their choices are affecting the health of their future children. The school setting is an appropriate place to teach this kind of information. Health professionals must include adolescents' preferences for fast foods (those prepared with minimum time in franchise restaurants) when planning lunch meals and doing nutritional counseling. Fast foods are eaten as meals and as snacks and, for many people, they provide 25 percent of the daily caloric intake (Thomas and Call, 1973). Hanson and Wyse (1979) have developed "nutrient profiles" of fast foods, some of which contain significant quantities of nutrients. The community health nurse can utilize these profiles to make eating of fast foods more positive.

Research is beginning to demonstrate that fathers, as a result of their habits, may cause defects in their children. Work with laboratory animals has shown that male rats who have been given methadone produce offspring with low birth rates and excessive numbers of deaths. The research needs to be confirmed, but fathers may play significant roles in the health of their children (*Time,* July 2, 1979).

Health Promotion during Pregnancy

Pregnancy is a developmental task for both parents. Parents need support throughout pregnancy because this is a time of change and of strong emotions, some positive, some negative, and most ambivalent. How people feel about pregnancy varies widely and depends upon whether the pregnancy was planned, whether or not the parents are married, whether they have other children, whether the mother is working, whether memories of their childhood are positive or negative, and how they feel about their parents. Lack of support can cause the parents to feel stress, can delay preparation for the infant, and can retard

bond formation. Supportive treatment of parents during pregnancy and the few months following the birth may well help to prevent child abuse and neglect (Kennell, Voos, and Klaus, 1976).

Prenatal classes, groups such as La Leche League, and visits by the community health nurse can help with this kind of support. The nuclear family system of the United States as well as the mobility of many Americans often means that the parents do not have other family members, family physicians, close friends, or neighbors who can be helpful in this period.

Concerns that parents have during the time of pregnancy, which should be addressed during prenatal classes, involve preparing for labor and delivery, how to physically prepare the home environment for the new baby, whether or not to breast-feed, whether or not the new mother should work outside the home, and how to prepare other siblings for the additional family member. Moreover the mother needs to know that alcohol, smoking, and other drugs can adversely affect the fetus; she should, of course, begin seeing her obstetrician or family doctor as soon as she suspects she is pregnant.

Parents should know that their genetic backgrounds can play a crucial role in their child's health. Ideally, this concern would occur prior to marriage, but often it does not. Down's syndrome, Tay-Sachs disease, sickle-cell anemia, cystic fibrosis, hemophilia, and Huntington's disease are some diseases which have a genetic origin. When parents know that these diseases are in their family constellations, they have several choices. They may have genetic testing prior to conception, they may adopt, or they may choose not to bear a child. They may also choose to conceive and then have genetic testing to ascertain whether or not the fetus carries the disease. Other alternatives include to have a defective child and to conceive and deliver without having genetic tests. If couples know about genetic problems before they marry, they may also make the decision not to marry. The community health nurse needs to be able to help people look at alternatives and provide sources of genetic counseling. There are an increasing number of genetic counseling centers throughout the country (Henden and Marks, 1978).

Expectant parents need more than knowledge to make the transition to parenthood successfully. They need the chance to look at the various situations that arise in parenting, compare different ways of dealing with them, and develop their own style of parenting. Nurses have used prenatal class settings to provide clarification about the role of the parent, to do actual role modeling by actively discussing problems and exploring alternatives, and to provide opportunities for role rehearsal. Role rehearsal can be done by using case studies and situations with the opportunity for parents to react and respond. Case studies and sharing of personal experiences to stimulate problem solving can be used with parents throughout any of the developmental and maturational crisis periods they may experience with their children.

Health Promotion after the Birth

The community health nurse should be cognizant that sometimes health services are not offered to new parents between the postpartum hospital discharge and the sixth-week checkup. The mother is often not in optimum physical condition after experiencing a loss in blood volume, rapid weight loss, and displacement of internal organs during the birth process. Yet she needs to meet the needs of a dependent infant whose respirations are not well established, who is undergoing massive blood changes, and who may be weak, dehydrated, and irritable. In addition, when the mother goes from the protected hospital environment to the home setting, she needs to adjust to role changes and the responsibility of infant care.

Nurses in the hospital who work with parents postpartum should make selected referrals of those families needing the services that a community health nurse can offer. The nurse, with observation, is able to pick up stresses and provide needed help.

The community health nurse has an important role in the referral process from hospital to home with families who have newborns. The community health nurse can discuss with the hospital nurse the types of families who need referrals. The hospital nurse should assess the entire family situation, assess the parent-child bonding, and make appropriate referrals based upon this information. The referral process is based upon the hospital nurse's assessment, and it is vital that she or he understand what an appropriate referral is and what the community health nurse can do with families who have newborns.

Table 13-5 is a compilation of concerns with which new parents may desire help during the puerperium. The puerperium is a short period of time, but it can be a highly troubled one if needed help is not present. These concerns should be taken into consideration when a nurse is identifying parents for referral or when a community health nurse is making a home visit.

Parenting

Parenting is a developmental stage in the life cycle of persons, and growth and development should continue for the parent as well as for the child. Ideally, this stage would be fairly free of anxiety and guilt, but that is not always the case. Most parents, in fact, experience some stress. The huge numbers of best sellers written for parents on how to do the job well testify to the insecurity that many parents feel (Robertiello, 1975; Salk, 1974; Spock, 1974; Illingsworth and Illingsworth, 1977; Comer and Poussaint, 1975; Biller and Meredith, 1974).

TABLE 13-5   Percentages of Mothers Noting Specific Concerns during the Puerperium

Area of concern	Percent of mothers concerned			Area of concern	Percent of mothers concerned		
	Minor concern	Major concern	Total		Minor concern	Major concern	Total
Return of figure to normal	30	65	95	Discomfort of stitches	33	20	53
Regulating demands of husband, housework, children	42	48	90	Breast care	40	10	50
				Constipation	35	15	50
Emotional tension	48	40	88	Setting limits for visitors	27	23	50
Fatigue	28	55	83	Interpreting infant's behavior	27	23	50
Infant behavior	47	33	80				
Finding time for self	45	33	78	Breast soreness	35	13	48
Sexual relations	53	20	73	Hemorrhoids	25	23	48
Diet	33	40	73	Labor and delivery experience	28	20	48
Feelings of isolation, being tied down	42	28	70	Father's role with baby	22	23	45
Infant's growth and development	45	25	70	Lochia	35	5	40
				Other children jealous of baby	27	13	40
Family planning	25	43	68	Other children's behavior	25	15	40
Exercise	23	45	68	Infant's appearance	18	20	38
Infant feeding	43	25	68	Traveling with baby	27	8	35
Changes in relationship with husband	35	25	60	Clothing for baby	20	10	30
Physical care of infant	45	13	58	Feeling comfortable handling baby	15	8	23
Infant safety	33	25	58				

SOURCE: From Marcia Gruis. Beyond maternity: Post partum concerns of mothers, *American Journal of Maternal Child Health*, May–June 1977, *2*, 185.

Each of the sources listed above proclaims the "right" way to parent. Which one should parents choose? How can parents do the "right" things for their children?

If they are interested in promoting moral and social maturity in later life, the answer is simple: they should love them, enjoy them, and want them around. They should not use their power to maintain a home that is only designed for the self-expression and pleasure of adults. They should not regard their children as disturbances to be controlled at all cost. (McClelland, Constantian, Regalado, and Stone, 1978, p. 53)

In the study cited above, which investigated child rearing, it was the easygoing, loving parents whose children turned out to be the most mature (this is basically common sense) and what counted most among the different methods of child rearing that were studied was the child's feeling that he or she was loved and wanted.

Parenting also involves the father; his important role in the child-rearing process has long been neglected, but this is changing. Fatherhood begins when the woman first finds out that she is pregnant. As she goes through many physical and emotional changes, so does he. Even though his body is not physically altered, he may experience body-image changes, such as gastrointestinal disorders, backaches, toothache, leg ache, and syncope, that can have a profound effect on the pregnancy experience (Fawcett, 1978). The nurse can help reduce the father's anxiety and confusion resulting from these changes by providing information about them and encouraging him to share them with others in group situations. The nurse can help parents to understand that although the changes are a concern, they are normal and learning to adapt to them is part of the process that occurs as the pregnant family takes on the parent role.

Fathers have to learn how to be fathers just as mothers need to learn how to be mothers. Our society has often given males the message that being an involved father is not a major goal for a man. The result has been that fathers and babies are often deprived of a warm relationship. One study showed that middle-class fathers of infants spent only 15 to 20 minutes per day with their babies (*American Baby*, June 1976, p. 38). Fathers can offer different stimulation, handling, and voice qualities from mothers, which enlarges the infant's environment. A positive relationship between baby and father benefits the entire family.

The nurse should realize that an increasing number of children are being parented completely by divorced, widowed, and single fathers and mothers. Health programs need to specifically address the needs of parents and children in these situations.

Single Parents

The adolescent single parent and her infant are at high risk both emotionally and physically. Help with parenting skills for this age group is a high priority for the community health nurse. The adolescent usually has not completed her own physical, mental, and emotional growth, and becoming responsible for another human being presents both a maturational and a situational crisis for her. Pre- and postnatal clinics set up for intensive and personal care for this group, as well as alternative education classes within the school system, have been ways in which this has been accomplished. Chapter 14 discusses adolescent parenthood in depth.

Divorced, single, or separated parents often find themselves fulfilling the roles of individual, father, mother, breadwinner, homemaker, and citizen. This can be an overwhelming situation unless appropriate resources are available and utilized. The community health nurse is able to help single parents look at the reality of their situation and at the options and resources available to them. Community groups, such as Parents Without Partners and local family counseling centers, may be helpful. Many times these parents are functioning quite well in relation to the responsibilities they encounter. The positive aspects and actions evidenced should be reinforced.

The single father can be at a greater disadvantage for receiving societal supports than the single mother. Many programs have been designed and implemented for maternal-child health, since this is considered the natural occurrence. The father, whose involvement with his children has only recently received societal sanction, often finds himself less prepared and with fewer supports in his dual-parent role.

Another dilemma of the single parent is that of the "weekend parent." Many divorced fathers are put in the role of seeing their children on a limited basis. They are unsure of their role with their children and have many concerns about how to facilitate their children's developmental growth. Again, the nurse, with counseling and referral to appropriate resources, can be helpful and can facilitate adjustment to the weekend parent role.

Preventive Health Care

Newborn Assessment

Assessment of the newborn is viewed as a decisive foundation for early case finding and preventive care. The kinds of observations that are made help to determine the nursing and medical care that the infant will receive as well as the kind of parenting that is given.

During the assessment, the nurse should get baseline data about the infant's surface features, movement patterns, and general health for comparisons with future examinations. Since health promotion is the concern, systematic periodic assessment over a period of time is important. The developmental approach, rather than the traditional disease-oriented model, should be the focus. Parental involvement in the assessment process helps the nurse to see how the family interacts. It also provides the opportunity to begin anticipatory guidance and problem solving.

The Neonatal Behavioral Assessment Scale developed by T. Berry Brazelton (Brazelton, 1973) is a valid and useful method for observing, making judgments, and scoring selected reflexes, motor responses, and interactive behavioral responses of newborns. The main focus of the scale is on the observation and rating of the infant's interactive behavior. It measures a total of 27 behavioral responses of the infant organized into the following six categories:

1. Habituation—how soon the infant diminishes responses to specific stimuli.

2. Orientation—when and how often the infant attends to auditory and visual stimuli.

3. Motor maturity—how well the infant coordinates and controls motor activities.

4. Variation—how often the infant coordinates and controls motor activities.

5. Self-quieting abilities—how often, how soon, and how effectively the infant uses personal resources to console himself or herself.

6. Social behaviors—smiling and cuddling behaviors.

Using the Brazelton scale points out vividly that newborns are able to control their responses to external stimuli. Generally, the abilities of newborns have been underestimated by both parents and health professionals. Erickson (1976) has described how child care professionals can best utilize the Neonatal Assessment Scale.

Anticipatory Guidance

Anticipatory guidance in helping parents to know what to expect of their children at different stages is one of the *most basic and significant* health promotion needs of parents. Through anticipatory guidance, parents can gain knowledge about average development and, thus, may not expect too much or too little from their children. They can also learn that, although there are patterns, each child is unique within that pattern. Parents readily acquire literature on growth and development from the hospital or pediatrician. The community health nurse should be familiar with this material and explain to parents that it is to be used a guide.

Parents are able to assess quite accurately their children's problems when they are given adequate information. This is logical because their proximity makes them frequent observers. Parents' assessment is important because how they define health or behavior as a problem influences interaction in the home and the child's further development.

Since an infant's growth and development is so rapid during the first 2 years, it is imperative that periodic and systematic screening be done. An illustration of this is the infant's reflexes which are present during the first weeks and then develop into purposeful movements as the central nervous system develops. Periodic comprehensive assessment and use of the developmental model facilitates the study of an infant's growth, early behavior patterns, and general development. If, for example, the infant's reflexes are questionable in symmetry, equality, or movement, this might be a sign of immaturity or a lack of integration in the central nervous system. These might also be signals of serious impairment of the central nervous system. Periodic screening and evaluation helps parents and professionals to evaluate more carefully the questionable status of the reflexes and to plan stimulation that enhances sensory development.

Baseline information compiled through periodic assessment is the key to planning early intervention. It allows for objectivity in conclusions that can be made about an infant's early development and can aid in planning interventions. The baseline data also serve as a basis for self-comparison of an infant or child over a period of time. It is imperative that the nurse know "normal" expectations for development so that what is unusual, abnormal, or delayed can be quickly recognized.

There are numerous schedules available for preventive child health care. Appendix 13-1 presents a summary of the health care which should be provided at specified intervals. It includes the suggested immunization schedule for children. The schedule can sound complicated, so giving parents a written immunization schedule and method for record keeping might be helpful. Effective anticipatory guidance helps parents to determine when children should have immunizations.

Immunizations are important, but they are not without their problems. If a child has a fever, immunizations are not to be given since they result in increased fever. Usually a child with a chronic illness, especially allergies and a central nervous system disorder, should have a physician's order for an immunization. Open skin lesions of any kind are contraindications for smallpox vaccine. Allergy to the substance any vaccine was grown on is an indication that the immunization should not be given. Another consideration is that at least 1 month should elapse between injections of live vaccine because live organisms can reduce the immunity potential of other live organisms. In general, problems of immunologic deficiency and immunosuppressive therapy, such as the use of corticosteroids, are contraindications for vaccines without a physician's specific order.

Also included in the preventive child health care schedule are the history to be obtained from parents and physical measurements to be done.

The Denver Developmental Screening Test (Erickson, 1976, pp. 173–192) and the Washington Guide (Barnard and Erickson, 1976, pp. 75–95) are valuable tools that assist the nurse in checking for developmental landmarks, giving norms for their attainment. Areas of concern to parents about infants include nutrition, frequency and amounts of feedings, weaning, sleeping patterns, teething, handling of the genitals, and dealing with common illnesses. After the first year of life, the child matures and new behavior patterns develop. Parents thus have additional areas of concern after a child is a year old, such as how to provide adequate nutrition when appetite decreases. This is normal, because the child is also having a decrease in growth. Other concerns during this period include sleep disturbances and nightmares, nocturnal enuresis, bowel and bladder training, thumbsucking, temper tantrums, masturbation, stuttering, negativism, and the increased need for independence and exploration. A thoughtful hearing of questions in relation to these concerns gives the nurse an idea of how the parents perceive the problem. Answers based on the child's development are supportive and help to eliminate some major concerns and problems.

Helping parents to know when a child is ill enough to call a doctor is important. This action can help to prevent minor upper respiratory infections (URIs) and gastrointestinal (GI) upsets from becoming major problems. Fever of 101° or over for 24 hours is a signal to parents to call the doctor.

The possibilities for preventive health care are varied and almost endless when helping parents to learn to handle childhood illness. Questions such as the following help a community health nurse to determine what information parents need in order to prevent serious illness. Do the parents have a thermometer and do they know how to use it? Do they understand the concept of dehydration? Do they know basic first aid and when to call a physician?

Accident Prevention

Since accidents are the major cause of death after the age of 1 year, prevention of them is critical. Appendix 13-2 summarizes typical actions that cause accidents and lists precautions to take at varying age levels to avoid accidents.

Fontana (1973) has listed several factors in the human environment that lead to accidents. Each of these factors can be dealt with to bring about positive change and reduction in accidents:

1. What and how adults learned as children on the subject of safety affects how parents teach children about the subject.

2. Children under stress from elements such as hunger and anger are likely to have more accidents than others.

3. Stress within a family leads to parental preoccupation and faulty supervision.

4. Self-discipline in children as well as common sense and sound judgment stem from loving, consistent parental discipline. Lack of these are factors in accidents.

5. Children who are protected from harm only by "no" do not develop self-reliant behavior. Constant warnings of danger are not conducive to growth.

6. Lack of knowledge about a child's normal growth and development contributes to accidents. Children make first-time movements before parents expect them.

7. Lack of knowledge about the individual child's development contributes to accidents. Some children grow faster or are more aggressive than others in the same family, and parents are not ready for the differences.

8. The early hours of the morning when parents are asleep and preschoolers are awake are prime times for accidents.

9. Accidents tend to cluster in a family around the time of a household move. Changes in the environment and routine as well as tension are precipitating factors.

There are also factors in the physical environment that parents need to be alerted to, such as the following:

1. Products intended for children but not safely designed, such as rattle parts that can be aspirated

2. Products such as drugs, cleaning agents, and power mowers never intended for children

3. Products such as can zip-tops, whose design causes injuries

4. Elements such as steep stairs, scatter rugs, and sharp corners that are a hazard

Parents cannot remove all environmental

hazards and they *cannot* and *should not* control their children 24 hours a day. However, with a combination of child supervision, education of parents, and legislative and environmental changes to get rid of hazards, accidents can be reduced. Families need an understanding of the philosophy of accident prevention. As specified by the National Safety Council, it is not a barrage of dos and don'ts but rather it is doing things the right way in the interest of the welfare of others.

One method the nurse can use to improve the family approach to accident prevention is accident analysis after an accident occurs. What, how, to whom, where, when, and why did the accident happen? Families must understand that the purpose of this is not to fix blame but rather to prevent a recurrence. Often, teaching the parent who is the primary care provider for the child will have an impact on accident prevention. The nurse can help this parent to be alert to hazards in the environment when home visits are made.

Automobiles are also killers of children. Safety belts or safety car seats should always be used by children in the car since children can become flying missles against the dashboard or window. Children can fall from moving cars if they are able to manipulate the locks. Obviously, seatbelts preclude such an accident from happening. Children should never be left alone in parked cars. The cigarette lighter, gear shift, steering wheel, and clutch are all very dangerous playthings.

There are community approaches to the problem of accident prevention as well as individual ones. "Children Can't Fly" was a program developed by the New York City Department of Health to combat the high incidence of child morbidity and mortality due to falls from windows. As a result of the community education approach, including counseling, referral, data collecting, media campaign, community education for prevention, and the provision of free window guards, falls were reduced by 50 percent from 1973 to 1975

(Spiegel and Lindaman, 1977). The program continues as a result of its success.

Prevention of Child Abuse and Neglect

As previously mentioned in this chapter, abuse and neglect are symptoms of stress in a family. The conditions of poverty, undernutrition, unemployment, overcrowding, restricted physical surroundings, and inadequate education support this problem. Knowledge currently available tells us that antenatal poverty and nutritional deficits produce a high-risk infant; at the same time, high-quality medical care is least available to the very people who are at highest risk. The high-risk infant and ill-prepared parents have the fewest resources for achieving the best health possible. Communities can deal with these poverty problems on a local level. However, the nation needs to deal with them on a federal level to make the fullest impact.

To save a child from the serious effects of abuse and neglect, nurses need to be alert when they notice that families are having children very quickly with no relief between pregnancies. The danger signs of marital stress, isolation, and overwhelmed parents need to be seen also. Premature births, where questionable bonding has taken place, indicate a need for priority service, as do families where there are children with developmental disabilities and chronic disease.

Every parent needs to know how children grow and develop; the concept that babies are responsible for their acts and can think and reason like an adult is all too commonly believed and must be corrected.

Education of personnel, including judges, attorneys, social workers and doctors, is necessary so that abused children are found and identified as such, and then given treatment. Parents must not be treated as criminals but rather given help so that their stress is alleviated. Equally important are the rights of children.

Social institutions such as churches and schools need to be utilized to help support families. In our mobile society where people move frequently, families can feel isolated and alone and uncared for. Homemaker services, big brothers and sisters, and parent aides, as well as community volunteers, could fill some of the gaps experienced by families who are isolated.

Preschool Assessments

Kindergarten and preschool health assessments are excellent developmental points at which to look at the physical, intellectual, and emotional growth of children. At this time, parents are increasingly aware of and concerned about the learning and thought competency of their children. They want to know that their children are ready to begin school. A child's ability to learn, see, perform appropriate gross and fine motor tasks, follow instruction, speak, communicate, and relate socially with others are all indicators of readiness for school (see Figure 13-2). The Denver Developmental Screening Test is one method used by community health nurses to look at these areas.

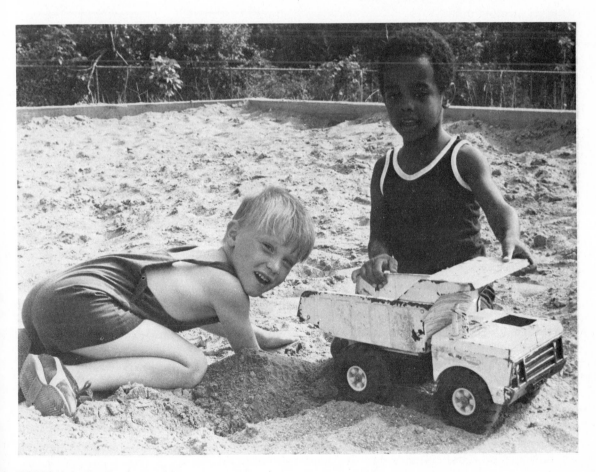

FIGURE 13-2 Healthy 5-year-olds.

Preschool assessments also provide an excellent opportunity to enforce state immunization laws so that all children receive immunizations before they are in school. Children already in school in higher grades are not covered by most state laws, so that if the law requiring immunizations is to be effective, it must be enforced at the time of preschool examinations. One large city enforced its school entrance immunizations in March 1977. Affected were 20,594 kindergarten children. Table 13-6 shows the number of immunizations before and after this enforcement took place. This is an example of the effectiveness of preventive health care among a population group vs. the effectiveness of working with one individual or one family.

The existence of a state law requiring measles vaccination for children entering school coincided with a decreased incidence of measles in that state. These laws will only be effective when they are enforced, as was done in the situation cited above (Center for Disease Control, Jan. 6, 1978, p. 7).

TABLE 13-6 Immunization Status of Entering Students before and after Enforcement of the School Entrance Law in Detroit, Michigan, March 1977

Status	At school entry		After program	
	No.	Percent	No.	Percent
Complete records:				
Adequately immunized*	6,502	31.6	15,022	75.2
Needing immunizations	5,832	28.3	4,346	21.7
Exempt under law†	20	0.1	135	0.7
No or incomplete records	8,240	40.0	482	2.4
Total	20,594	100.0	19,985	100.0

*Documented evidence of having received three doses of trivalent oral poliomyelitis vaccine (TOPV), three doses of diphtheria and tetanus toxoids and pertussis vaccine (DTP), one dose each of measles and rubella vaccine.

†Signed waiver from parents.

SOURCE: From Center for Disease Control. *Morbidity and Mortality Weekly Report.* Jan. 6, 1978, 27 (1), 7.

Day Care for Children

Societal attitudes about raising normal healthy children are changing. At one time, parents were criticized if the mother was not in the home 24 hours a day with the children. However, many mothers want to work and many of them must work: one out of three women who marry is divorced, only one job in five pays enough to support a four-member family. There are 13.5 million working mothers with 7 million preschool children (Whitehead, 1978, p. 38). Day care can help parents who want to work or have to work to deal with the stress associated with parenting and full-time employment. It may also help children from these families to obtain emotional, intellectual, and physical stimulation, as well as positive human relationships that will lay the foundation for growth in these areas. However, day care does not eliminate all the problems families must adapt to when both parents are working. Day care, for instance, does not take care of a child who is acutely ill. Thus, if a child is sick, parents need to find other resources for child care. As previously discussed, illness is common among preschool children.

GENERAL CONCEPTS OF HEALTH PROMOTION

Health promotion needs are based on the developmental tasks and common health problems of the specific population group. For the 0- to 5-year-old and parenting population, the following factors should be considered when developing a health promotion program:

1. A monitoring system to identify high-risk infants and parents

2. An organized community program to combat problems such as accidents and child abuse

3. An organized system for provision of preventive health services, such as physical examinations and immunizations

4. Health education program to meet anticipatory guidance needs of parents and children

5. Passage and revision of significant legislation, such as the enforcement of immunization laws

SIGNIFICANT HEALTH LEGISLATION

During the past 70 years there has been much federal legislation and many demonstration projects concerned with the health of infants and mothers in America. The Children's Bureau was established in 1912. White House Conferences on Children and Youth have been held every 10 years since 1910. The Shepherd-Towner Act of 1921 created maternal and child health services at the state level, supported by the federal government. Title V of the Social Security Act of 1935 provided for grants to states for maternal and child health services and services to crippled children. The Emergency Maternity and Infant Care Program existed during the 1930s. The need for community mental health programs was recognized in the 1960s. The Eighty-ninth Congress, during President Johnson's time in office (1963–1968), brought huge changes in child health legislation with the establishment of the Office of Economic Opportunity and its Headstart Program, Medicaid, and the National Institutes of Child Health and Human Development. Some of the significant current legislation follows.

Medicaid

The largest current public medical program for children is that of Medicaid (Wallace, 1975, p. 318). Title XIX of the Social Security Act mandated Medicaid which was enacted to reach high-risk, high-priority children and youth in needy families. Those eligible for Medicaid coverage include children who are members of families receiving Aid to Dependent Children or who are covered by a state's medically needy program. Medicaid benefits are covered in Chapter 4 under Governmental Health Assistance Programs.

The Early Periodic Screening, Diagnosis, and Treatment program (EPSDT) was designed to periodically assess all children under 21 in the Medicaid program (Frankenburg and North, 1974). Federal regulations are established by the Department of Health, Education, and Welfare for this screening, and the suggested schedule is at the time of hospital discharge for a new infant, 2 to 6 weeks, 2 to 4 months, 5 to 7 months, 8 to 10 months, 11 to 14 months, 17 to 19 months, 21 to 25 months, 3 to 4 years, and 5 to 6 years. The EPSDT has the following five stages:

1. Outreach and case finding, which include all of the services necessary to find, identify, inform, and assist eligible persons to utilize the EPSDT program. Federal regulations state that recipients of welfare must be informed about the program and its benefits and efforts must be made to bring eligible children into the program.

2. Screening, administering, coordinating, and developing new resources as needed, as well as evaluating and monitoring the existing screening resources.

3. Testing of children done by a trained nurse which includes an unclothed physical examination, developmental appraisal, growth measurements, anemia screening, lead-poisoning screening, tuberculosis testing, vision and hearing testing, dental screening, and the evaluation of nutritional status.

4. Compilation and reporting of results which composes a health profile for each screened individual from the findings of the testing.

5. Followthrough and treatment which ensures follow-up and treatment indicated by the testing and health profile.

Child Abuse and Neglect

The Child Abuse, Prevention and Treatment Act (Public Law 93-247) was signed into law in 1974 in response to the need for a nationwide effort to solve this complex problem. This act created the National Center on Child Abuse and Neglect as the primary place where the federal government can focus its efforts on identifying, treating, and preventing child abuse and neglect (Subcommittee on Child and Human Development, 1977, p. 589). To carry out the mandates of the act, the National Center has begun programs in four areas: demonstration and research, information gathering and dissemination, training and technical assistance, and assistance to states. In 1962, the Children's Bureau developed and promoted a model state child abuse mandatory reporting law which, in effect, states that professionals or child-care workers must report suspected child abuse to the appropriate officials. Public Law 93-247 reinforces this mandate.

The different states have acted upon the Child Abuse, Prevention and Treatment Act in various ways, and thus community health nurses must know the laws that are in effect in the states in which they are working. In Michigan, for example, the Child Protection law requires the reporting of child abuse and neglect by physicians, nurses, teachers, and other child care providers (Child Protection Law, 1975).

Maternal-Child Health Program

Title V of the Social Security Act authorized the Maternal and Child Health Program which is administered by the Health Services Administration. Each state is required to plan projects for five programs described in a rewriting of title V: Maternity and Infant Care, Intensive Infant Care, Family Planning Services, Health Services for Children and Youth, and Dental Health of Children. The programs support a wide range of health care service projects and demonstration models developed by each state under guidelines from the federal government (Committee on Labor and Public Welfare, 1975, p. 339).

Maternity and Infant Care Project

This program enables each state to promote the health of mothers and children through maternity and infant care, covering the period of pregnancy and the first year of life. Its purpose is to reduce the incidence of mental retardation and other handicapping conditions caused by complications associated with childbearing and to help reduce infant and maternal mortality by providing necessary health care to high-risk mothers and their infants. There are three types of programs authorized under this act: health care to prospective mothers, health care to infants during their first year of life, and family planning services.

Projects for Intensive Care of Infants

This section of title V authorizes grants for projects to provide necessary health care to infants during their first year of life when they have conditions or circumstances that increase the hazard to their health. Since the long-range goal of these programs is the prevention of morbidity and mortality, an effective program must begin long before the birth of the baby; it must provide improved care for mothers.

Children and Youth Projects

Comprehensive health services to children is the focus of this project. Its purpose is to provide comprehensive medical, dental, physical, and emotional care to children and youth, particularly in areas with concentrations of low-income families. Children enrolled in these projects receive continual health supervision including assessment examinations, follow-up treatment, aftercare, and preventive care.

Family Planning

Title V (section 508a) requires the provision of family planning services to recipients who will not otherwise receive such necessary health care because they are from low-income families, or for other reasons beyond their control. A wide variety of health services is offered, in addition to family planning, literature, counseling, and contraceptive devices. Most of the users of these services receive complete medical examinations with Pap smears and pelvic and breast examinations.

Dental Health of Children

Title V (section 508a) states that states must provide a program that promotes the dental health of children and youth of school or preschool age, particularly in areas that have con-

centrations of low-income families. Projects must provide preventive services, treatment, correction of defects, and aftercare.

Crippled Children's Services

Title V (section 501) of the Social Security Act authorizes annual formula grants to states to find children who are crippled or who have conditions that lead to crippling conditions. These children are then provided with medical, surgical, or other services. The state law either defines the crippling conditions to be included or directs the Crippled Children's Agency to define them. Among children currently being served, three classes of disease are predominant: diseases of the bones and organs of movement, diseases of the nervous system and sense organs, and congenital malformations.

Women, Infants, and Children Program

The United States Department of Agriculture's Special Supplemental Food program provides cash grants to make food available to pregnant and lactating women and to infants and children up to the age of 4 years. The Maternal and Child Health Program is an active and crucial participant in this program. Public Law 94-104, enacted in 1975, authorized the establishment of a National Advisory Council on Maternal, Infant, and Fetal Nutrition. The council submits an annual report to the President and Congress and makes continuing recommendations for administrative and legislative changes in programs aimed at low-income individuals at nutritional risk. The council makes recommendations for the Women, Infants, and Children (WIC) program and suggests that it serve both preventive and remedial nutritional purposes (WIC Currents, 1978, p. 11).

BARRIERS TO HEALTH CARE

Major barriers to the delivery of services have been discussed in Chapter 12. The following case situations illustrate some specific problems parents have in obtaining care for themselves and their children, ages 0 to 5 years:

Sue was 17 years old when she became pregnant. Her husband, Tom, age 18, worked as a gas station attendant. His income provided only the basic necessities of food and rent but was too high to allow them any public assistance. Sue decided to "save" money by waiting for antepartum care until near her EDC. Upon her first antepartum visit to the doctor 1 month before delivery, she was found to be severely hypertensive as well as diabetic. Her infant weighed 10 lb at birth and required 1 month's hospitalization. Sue and Tom felt that they were severely criticized by the health personnel for not receiving adequate antepartum care.

Diane and Jim Jones have four children under 5 years of age. Jim has a job-related back injury and is unemployed. The Jones have a Medicaid card and they utilize the outpatient department of a large teaching hospital in their city for medical care. They go there only when they absolutely must. The family has no car and utilizes the city bus line, which involves three transfers for the 4-mile trip. With four children, Mrs. Jones finds this most difficult, especially in cold weather. When she does arrive at the hospital, she must wait several hours and then sees a different physician each time so that she must repeatedly give her family's health histories. Mrs. Jones feels that "the people in that hospital don't care about or understand me and my kids."

THE ROLES OF THE COMMUNITY HEALTH NURSE

Roles

The community health nurse plays a number of roles in providing service to the 0 to 5 age group. The following paragraphs describe some of these roles.

Advocate-Planner

Since the children in the 0- to 5-year-old age group cannot speak for themselves, the nurse becomes an advocate. This can involve pointing out to care givers the safety hazards in the environment and urging necessary changes. On a broader level, the nurse is an advocate for the development of day-care centers in a community and publicizes the inadequacy of health and medical care for economically disadvantaged families. This role of advocate means that the nurse must be involved in the political process to correct issues such as unemployment, lack of adequate income, over-crowding, and the cycle of poverty, which can ultimately only be solved with legislative changes. Attitudes of assertiveness, a knowledge of the political process, and a willingness to take risks are necessary tools for this role.

Teacher

The community health nurse needs to be a teacher—this includes demonstrating information about child care to families and involving parents in the learning process. Helping parents to understand good nutrition for this age group, or why safety seats and belts are necessary in cars, means involvement of all concerned in the process of teaching and learning and changing values and attitudes. The community health nurse is well versed in the developmental tasks of this age group. Teaching parents about these tasks is a form of anticipatory guidance and assists in task accomplishment.

Group Worker

In order to meet the needs of the 0- to 5-year-old population, the community health nurse needs to be attuned to opportunities for group teaching and counseling. Working with the La Leche League or Parents Anonymous, a crisis intervention program set up to help or prevent damaging relationships between parents and their children, are possibilities. Other possibilities are numerous. One community health nurse, for example, had in his caseload area a huge mobile home park. Within the park, he found five families who had children in special school classes because of developmental disabilities, each of whom expressed a need for help with their child. This staff nurse helped the parents form a weekly discussion group and the results were that isolated families received mutual supportive help in the form of baby-sitting, shared meals, and problem solving about how to deal with difficult situations.

Coordinator

Coordinating community resources is another part of the nurse's role. There are numerous services available to families, and this is positive. However, families can feel uncared for and torn apart when the Department of Social Services, Medicaid Screening Clinic, the community health nurse, the school nurse, and the child guidance center all request the same information in detail, or when these same health professionals do not communicate with each other and plan different goals. Professionals need to be careful to ask the permission of a family before they share information they have regarding that family with another professional or agency. They should seek this permission as soon as they identify that families are working with multiple agencies.

Closely tied to this role is the facilitating role of the nurse. Helping families and the larger community to understand their rights as people and to understand services offered in the community all facilitate the better utilization of these services. The nurse helps families work toward desired change. In every community there are persons with ideas and skills, and all that needs to be done is to give them direction and reinforcement. Milio's *9226 Kercheval: The Storefront That Did Not Burn* is the story of how one community health nurse helped an inner-city area establish its own day-care center (Milio, 1970). This nurse found that people saw a great problem with children who were not cared for while mothers worked. She acted as a catalyst to assist in solving the problem and was a facilitator and enabler as well.

Case finder

Because of the nurse's proximity to infants and children, case finding has been a strategic role for many years. At-risk children are identified and followed periodically as they develop. Disabilities are lessened when treatment is begun early, and some can be prevented by primary intervention. A system needs to be established in each community to periodically screen all children for problems. The Early Periodic Screening, Diagnosis, and Treatment Program (EPSDT) of Medicaid is one schedule that can be followed.

Epidemiologist

Collecting data on health problems and care is an important epidemiological aspect of the nurse's role. Nurses are concerned about why parents do not use available health services and what motivates those who do. A community health nurse carried out a study to determine answers to these concerns and found that users of child health services had access to free medical care, were younger, and had more children than nonusers (Selwyn, 1978, p. 231). Reasons why people do and do not utilize health care are important elements in planning health services.

When the community health nurse visits parents after accidental poisoning incidents, the nurse can add to the epidemiological understanding of the predisposing and immediate causes of the accident and make recommendations to prevent them from occurring again. If it were the case that 75 percent of the families who have poisoning accidents have other health problems, there is evidence that this kind of stress leads to poisoning accidents.

A good record system in the health agency will help nurses to collect data on health problems, to plan interventions, and to evaluate care given. This data can provide information on changing health needs and necessary health services.

A good record system will collect data on the 0- to 5-year-old child that provides the basis for a health history upon which later happenings in the family system can be compared and built.

Clinic Nurse

Community health nurses have long worked in well-baby clinics where, at regular intervals, the health of children up to the age of 5 is assessed, immunizations are given, and parents have the opportunity to discuss concerns of growth and development. This role has been expanded to an assessment and treatment role. Nurses deal with problem behavior such as delayed play, immature social behavior, and temper tantrums. With the nurse's knowledge of child development, behavior modification, and management techniques, the roles of observer, consultant, and counselor to parents, preschool teachers, and day-care workers are valuable in dealing with minor problems that can develop into major ones.

Home Visitor

A well-known role of the nurse caring for the needs of the 0- to-5-year-old age group is that of the community health nurse who visits parents and babies in their homes. Each health department sets its own priorities and standards for the care of parents and children. This ranges from the pre- and postnatal referral of each pregnancy, in some areas, to the referral of only those mothers and infants at high risk. The broad background of community health nurses equips them with skills to help establish the standards as to which newborns and parents will be visited. The nurse who visits in the home, especially when both parents are present, is in a privileged position to closely and periodically assess the baby's, the parents', and family's development. The nurse can also identify stress, help parents deal with problems of poor bonding, provide role modeling for bonding and parenting, give anticipatory guidance, and help reinforce positive behavior. The nurse aids families in utilizing community resources as necessary. For example, when parents and a new baby with a diagnosis of spina bifida, Down's syndrome, or cleft palate come home from the hospital, it is most often the community health nurse who introduces the family to the resources of Crippled Children's Services for financial aid, to the physical therapy offered by the intermediate school program, or to the interdisciplinary diagnostic services of university-affiliated centers. This same nurse will likely be one of the persons to help parents as they go through the grief process related to having a baby who is less than "perfect." The nurse can also be alert to signs of stress within the family in this situation; living 24 hours a day with a helpless infant who has additional problems can be an overwhelming problem for some families. Homemakers, parent's aides, and parent-support groups are useful when families are in such a situational crisis.

One of the major characteristics of handicapped children, and particularly the mentally retarded, is some delay in reaching developmental milestones in self-help skills. It is sometimes assumed that these skills will develop without intervention as a result of physical growth and maturation. Often this is not the case and the child is unable to function independently. This leads to institutionalization, enormous financial and personal expenditures, and waste of human potential. With the use of behavior modification technology, most self-help skills can be attained by handicapped persons, including those who are profoundly retarded. The community health nurse is in a unique position to help families with these skills. Beginning immediately after birth with early infant stimulation is essential. The goal is that each person attain his or her own potential. The nurse can aid the family in recognizing this potential and give guidance in the process of reaching it. Time needed to exercise and teach the young child with developmental disabilities can lead to the neglect of other children. Parents and nurse must be cognizant of this situation.

SUMMARY

The years from birth to age 5 provide the foundation for a child's lifelong physical, mental, and social development. The child's health and that of the parents is inextricably interwoven; and both have health care needs that the community health nurse can help to fill.

Utilization of the developmental health promotion model to assess the needs of young children and their parents provides a positive way of involving this group in their own health care. It can also help to prevent many of the major health problems of those 0 to 5 years of age, or at least weaken their impact. This is the challenge for community health nurses!

Children are our nation's greatest resource. Decreasing infant and maternal mortality rates reflect this value as does legislation such as Medicaid, which provides health care for at least a segment of the 0- to 5-year-old population.

Appendix 13-1
Suggested Schedule for Preventive Child Health Care

Age	History*	Measurement†	Physical examination	Developmental landmarks*‡	Discussion and guidance*	Procedures†	Attending
1 month	Initial Eating Sleeping Elimination Crying At every visit mother should be asked for questions	Height Weight Head circumference Temperature Evaluation of hearing	Complete§	Eyes follow to midline Baby regards face *While prone, lifts head, off table*	Vitamins Sneezing Hiccoughs Straining, with bowel movements Irregular respiration Startle reflex Ease and force of urination Night bottle Colic "Spoiling" Accidents	PKU Urinalysis	M.D. and assistant
2 months	Health Sensory-motor development Eating Sleeping Elimination Happiness	Height Weight Head circumference Temperature	Complete or observation¶	*Vocalizes* *Smiles responsively*	Solid foods Immunizations Thumbsucking	DTP TOPV Urine screening	M.D. and/or assistant
3 months	Health Eating Sleeping Elimination Crying Other behavior	Height Weight	Complete or observation¶	Holds head and chest up to make 90° angle with table Laughs	Feeding Accidents Sleeping without rocking Coping with frustrations		M.D. and/or assistant

*May be accomplished in part by assistant if physician desires. Much of this may be accomplished in part by appropriate pamphlets or leaflets where deemed desirable.

†Usually accomplished by assistant.

‡Age given for landmarks indicates approximate age at which 90 percent of children have accomplished test. Adapted from Denver Developmental Screening Test.

§By physician. Observation of child, completely undressed, by assistant trained to observe respiration, skin, musculature, motor activities, and so forth.

¶Obvious deviations from normal must be checked by physician.

NOTE: Italicized items indicate report of parent and may be accepted as proof of accomplishment. May be obtained by assistant.

Age	History*	Measurement†	Physical Examination	Developmental landmarks*†	Discussion and guidance*	Procedures†	Attending
4 months	Health Eating Sleeping Elimination Other behavior Sensory-motor development Current living situation Parent-child interaction	Height Weight Head circumference Temperature	Complete§	Holds head erect and steady when held in sitting position *Squeals* Grasps rattle Eyes follow object for 180°	Feeding Schedule to fit in with family Attitude of father Respiratory infections	DTP TOPV	M.D. and/or assistant
5 months	Health Eating Sleeping Elimination Sensory-motor development	Height Weight Temperature	Complete or observation§	*Smiles spontaneously* *Rolls from back to stomach or vice versa* Reaches for object on table	Feeding Vitamins (if not previously mentioned)		M.D. and/or assistant
6 months	Health Eating Sleeping Elimination Other behavior Sensory-motor development	Height Weight Head circumference Temperature Evaluation of hearing	Complete or observation§	No head lag if baby is pulled to sitting position by hands	Feeding Accidents Night crying Fear of strangers Separation anxiety Description of normal micturition	DTP TOPV	M.D. and/or assistant
8–9 months	Health Eating Sleeping	Height Weight Temperature	Complete or screening§	Sits alone for seconds after support is released	Use of cup Eating with fingers		M.D. and/or assistant

*May be accomplished in part by assistant if physician desires. Much of this may be accomplished in part by appropriate pamphlets or leaflets where deemed desirable.

†Usually accomplished by assistant.

‡Age given for landmarks indicates approximate age at which 90 percent of children have accomplished test. Adapted from Denver Developmental Screening Test.

§By physician. Observation of child, completely undressed, by assistant trained to observe respiration, skin, musculature, motor activities, and so forth.

¶Obvious deviations from normal must be checked by physician.

Age	History*	Measurement†	Physical Examination	Developmental landmarks*†	Discussion and guidance*	Procedures†	Attending
	Elimination			Bears weight momentarily if held with feet on table	Fear of strangers		
	Sensory motor development				Accidents		
	Behavior			Looks after fallen object	Need for affection		
				Transfers block from one hand to the other	Normal unpleasant behavior		
				Feeds self cracker	Discipline		
10 months if last exam at 8 months	Health	Height	Complete or observation¶	*Pulls self to standing position*	Toilet training: when to start	Hemoglobin or hematocrit	M.D. and/ or assistant
	Eating	Weight		*Stands holding on to solid object (not human)*	Normal drop in appetite		
	Sleeping	Temperature					
	Elimination			Pincer grasp; picks up small object using any part of thumb and fingers in opposition	Independence vs. dependency		
	Behavior				Discipline		
	Sensory-motor development				Instructions for use of syrup of ipecac		
	Speech development			*Says Da-da or Ma-ma*			
	Current living situation			Resists toy being pulled away			
	Parent-child interaction			*Plays peek-a-boo*			
				Makes attempt to get toy just out of reach *Initial anxiety toward strangers*			
12 months	As for 10 months	Height	Complete§	*Cruises: walks around holding onto furniture*	Negativism	Tuberculin test (intradermal preferred)	M.D. and assistant
		Weight		*Stands alone 2–3 seconds if outside support is removed*	Likelihood of respiratory infections		
		Head circumference			"Getting into things"	Urinalysis	
		Temperature					

*May be accomplished in part by assistant if physician desires. Much of this may be accomplished in part by appropriate pamphlets or leaflets where deemed desirable.

†Usually accomplished by assistant.

‡Age given for landmarks indicates approximate age at which 90 percent of children have accomplished test. Adapted from Denver Developmental Screening Test.

§By physician. Observation of child, completely undressed, by assistant trained to observe respiration, skin, musculature, motor activities, and so forth.

¶Obvious deviations from normal must be checked by physician.

Age	History*	Measurement†	Physical Examination	Developmental landmarks*†	Discussion and guidance*	Procedures†	Attending
				Bangs together two blocks held one in each hand	Weaning from bottle		
					Proper dose of vitamins		
				Imitates vocalization heard within preceding minute	Control of drugs and poisons		
				Plays pat-a-cake			
15 months	As for 10 months	Height Weight Temperature	Complete or observation¶	*Walks well*	Temper tantrums	Measles	M.D. and/ or assistant
				Stoops to recover toys on floor	Obedience	Rubella and mumps may be given at this or subsequent visit	
				Uses Da-da and Ma-ma specifically for correct parent			
				Rolls or tosses ball back to examiner			
				Indicates wants by pulling, pointing, or appropriate verbalization (not crying)			
				Drinks from cup without spilling much			
18 months	As for 10 months	Height Weight Temperature	Complete§	Puts one block on another without its falling off	Reaction toward and of siblings	DTP TOPV	M.D. and assistant
				Mimics household chores like dusting or sweeping	Toilet training		
					Speech development		
21 months	As for 10 months Peer reaction	Height Weight Temperature	Complete or observation¶	Walks backward and upstairs	Manners		M.D. and/ or assistant
				Feeds self with spoon	"Poor appetite"		

*May be accomplished in part by assistant if physician desires. Much of this may be accomplished in part by appropriate pamphlets or leaflets where deemed desirable.

†Usually accomplished by assistant.

‡Age given for landmarks indicates approximate age at which 90 percent of children have accomplished test. Adapted from Denver Developmental Screening Test.

§By physician. Observation of child, completely undressed, by assistant trained to observe respiration, skin, musculature, motor activities, and so forth.

¶Obvious deviations from normal must be checked by physician.

Age	History*	Measurement†	Physical Examination	Developmental landmarks*†	Discussion and guidance*	Procedures†	Attending
				Removes article of clothing other than hat			
				Says three specific words besides Da-da and Ma-ma			
2 years	Health Eating Sleeping Elimination Toilet training Sensory-motor development Speech Current living situation Peer and social adjustment	Height Weight Temperature Hearing	Complete§	Kicks a ball in front of him with foot without support *Scribbles spontaneously — purposeful marking of more than one stroke on paper* Balances four blocks on top of one another *Points correctly to one body part* Dumps small objects out of bottle after demonstration *Does simple tasks in house*	Need for peer companionship Immaturity: inability to share or take turns Care of teeth From this point on, guidance may be indicated by the mother's answers to a questionnaire about behavior and emotional problems	Hemoglobin and/or hematocrit Urinalysis	M.D. and assistant
2½ years	As for 2 years	Height Weight Temperature	Complete§	*Throws overhand after demonstration* Names correctly one picture in book, e.g., cat or apple Combines two words meaningfully	Guidance from questionnaire answers Dental referral Perversity and decisiveness		M.D. and/or assistant
3 years	As for 2 years	As for 2 years Blood pressure	Complete§	Jumps in place *Pedals tricycle*	*Guidance from questionnaire answers*	As for 2 years	M.D. and assistant

*May be accomplished in part by assistant if physician desires. Much of this may be accomplished in part by appropriate pamphlets or leaflets where deemed desirable.

†Usually accomplished by assistant.

‡Age given for landmarks indicates approximate age at which 90 percent of children have accomplished test. Adapted from Denver Developmental Screening Test.

§By physician. Observation of child, completely undressed, by assistant trained to observe respiration, skin, musculature, motor activities, and so forth.

¶Obvious deviations from normal must be checked by physician.

Age	History*	Measurement†	Physical Examination	Developmental landmarks*†	Discussion and guidance*	Procedures†	Attending
				Dumps small article out of bottle without demonstration	Sex education		
					Nursery schools: qualifications of a good one		
				Uses plurals			
				Washes and dries hands	Obedience and discipline		
4 years	As for 2 years	As for 2 years Vision ("E" chart) Blood pressure	Complete§ Fundus examination	Builds bridge of three blocks after demonstration Copies circle and cross *Identifies longer of two lines* Knows first and last names Understands what to do when "tired" *Plays with other children so they interact—tag* *Dresses with supervision*	*Guidance from questionnaire answers* Kindergarten Use of money Dental care	As for 2 years	M.D. and assistant
5 years	As for 2 years (omit toilet training) Kindergarten	As for 2 years Vision ("E" chart) Color blindness Audiometer Blood pressure	Complete§	Hops two or more times Catches ball thrown 3 feet Dresses without supervision *Can tolerate separation from mother for a few minutes without anxiety*	Guidance from questionnaire answers Readiness for school Span of attention: how to increase it	As for 2 years TOPV DTP	M.D. and assistant

*May be accomplished in part by assistant if physician desires. Much of this may be accomplished in part by appropriate pamphlets or leaflets where deemed desirable.

†Usually accomplished by assistant.

‡Age given for landmarks indicates approximate age at which 90 percent of children have accomplished test. Adapted from Denver Developmental Screening Test.

§By physician. Observation of child, completely undressed, by assistant trained to observe respiration, skin, musculature, motor activities, and so forth.

¶Obvious deviations from normal must be checked by physician.

NOTE: Italicized items indicate report of parent and may be accepted as proof of accomplishment. May be obtained by assistant.

SOURCE: Reprinted with permission from Committee on Standards of Child Health Care, Council on Pediatric Practice, American Academy of Pediatrics, 1972. Copyright American Academy of Pediatrics 1972 and 1977.

Appendix 13-2
Accident Prevention at Various Age Levels

Typical accidents	Normal behavior characteristics	Precautions
FIRST YEAR		
Falls	After several months of age can squirm and roll, and later creeps and pulls self erect	Do not leave alone on tables, etc., from where falls can occur
Inhalation of foreign objects		Keep crib sides up
Poisoning	Places anything and everything in mouth	Keep in enclosed space when outdoors or not in company of an adult
Burns	Helpless in water	
Drowning		Do not leave alone in tub of water
SECOND YEAR		
Falls	Able to roam about in erect posture	Keep screens in windows
Drowning	Goes up and down stairs	Place gate at top of stairs
Motor vehicles	Has great curiosity	Cover unused electrical outlets; keep electric cords out of easy reach
Ingestion of poisonous substances	Puts almost everything in mouth	Keep in enclosed space when outdoors; not in company of an adult
Burns	Helpless in water	Keep medicines, household poisons, and small sharp objects out of sight
		Keep handles of pots and pans on stove out of reach and containers of hot foods from edge of table
		Protect from water in tub and in pools
		Use safety belts and car seats
2–4 YEARS		
Falls	Able to open doors	Keep doors locked when there is danger of falls
Drowning	Runs and climbs	
Motor vehicles	Can ride tricycle	Place screen or guards in windows
Ingestion of poisonous substances	Investigates closets and drawers	Teach about watching for automobiles in driveways and in streets
	Plays with mechanical gadgets	Keep firearms locked up
Burns	Can throw ball and other objects	Keep knives, electrical equipment out of reach
		Teach about risks of throwing sharp objects and about danger of following balls into street
5–9 YEARS		
Motor vehicles	Daring and adventurous	Teach techniques and traffic rules for cycling
Bicycle accidents	Control over large muscles more advanced than control over small muscles	
Drowning		Encourage skills in swimming
Firearms	Has increasing interest in group play; loyalty to group makes him willing to follow suggestions of leaders	Keep firearms locked up except when you can supervise their use
		Teach self-discipline

SOURCE: V. C. Vaughn, R. J. McKay, & W. E. Nelson. *Textbook of pediatrics*. Philadelphia: Saunders, 1975. p. 214. Adapted from: T. E. Shaffer. *Pediatric Clinics of North America*, May 1954, *1*, 426–427.

REFERENCES

Barnard, K. E., & Erickson, M. L. *Teaching children with developmental problems.* St. Louis: Mosby, 1976.

Biller, H., & Meredith, D. *Father power.* New York: McKay, 1974.

Brazelton, T. B. *Infants and mothers. Differences in development.* New York: Dell, 1969.

———. *The neonatal behavioral assessment scale.* Philadelphia: Lippincott, 1973.

Callahan, S. C. *Parenting, principles, and politics of parenthood.* Baltimore: Penguin, 1973.

Center for Disease Control. Enforcement of a state's immunization law for entering school children—Detroit. *Morbidity and Mortality Weekly Report,* Atlanta, Ga.: Public Health Service, Jan. 6, 1978, *27* (1), 7.

———. *Morbidity and Mortality Weekly Report,* Atlanta, Ga.: Public Health Service, Feb. 3, 1978, *27.*

Child Protection Law, Act No. 238, 1975. Lansing, Mich.: State of Michigan Department of Social Services, 1975.

Comer, J. P., & Poussaint, A. F. *Black child care.* New York: Simon & Schuster, 1975.

Committee on Labor and Public Welfare, Subcommittee on Health, United States Congress, Hearing before. *School-age mothers and child health act, 1975* (Nov. 4, 1975). Washington, D.C.: U.S. Government Printing Office, 1976.

Dunn, H. L. *High level wellness.* Arlington, Va.: R. N. Beatty Co., 1973.

Erickson, M. L. *Assessment and management of developmental changes in children.* St. Louis: Mosby, 1976.

Fawcett, J. Body image and the pregnant couple. *American Journal of Maternal Child Nursing,* July–August 1978, *3,* 227–233.

Foman, S. J. *Infant nutrition* (2d ed.). Philadelphia. Saunders, 1974.

Fontana, V. J. *A parent's guide to child safety.* New York: Thomas Y. Crowell, 1973.

Frankenburg, W. K., & North, A. F. *A guide to screening for the Early and Periodic Screening, Diagnosis, and Treatment Program (EPSDT).* (SRS74-24516). Washington, D.C.: U.S. Government Printing Office, 1974.

Garbarino, J. The human ecology method of child maltreatment: A conceptual model for research. *Journal of Marriage and the Family,* November 1977, *39,* 721–735.

Garner, M. K. Our values are showing: Inadequate childhood immunization. *Health Values: Achieving High Level Wellness,* May–June 1978, *2,* 129–133.

Gruis, M. Beyond maternity: post partum concerns of mothers. *American Journal of Maternal Child Health,* May–June 1977, *2,* 182–188.

Hanlon, J. *Public health administration and practice.* St. Louis: Mosby, 1974.

Hanson, R. G., & Wyse, B. W. Planning for the inevitable: Snack foods in the diet. *Family and Community Health,* February 1979, *1,* 31–39.

Harrison, L. L. Nursing intervention with the failure to thrive family. *American Journal of Maternal Child Nursing,* March–April 1976, *1,* 111–116.

Health; United States 1975. DHEW Publication No. HRA 76-1232. Rockville, Md.: Health Resources Administration, 1975.

Helfer, R. E., & Kempe, C. H. (Eds.). *Child abuse and neglect.* Cambridge, Mass: Ballinger, 1976.

Henden, D., & Marks, J. *The genetic connection: How to protect your family against hereditary disease.* Caldwell, N.Y.: Morrow, 1978.

Hoekelman, R. A., Blatman, S., Burnell, D. A., Friedman, S. G., & Seidel, H. M. *Principles of pediatrics health care of the young.* New York: McGraw-Hill, 1978.

Illingsworth, R., & Illingsworth, C. *Babies and young children.* New York: Churchill Livingstone, 1977.

Kennell, J., Voos, D., & Klaus, M. Parent infant bonding. In R. E. Helfer & C. H. Kempe (Eds.), *Child abuse and neglect. The family and the community.* Cambridge, Mass.: Ballinger, 1976.

Klaus, M. H., & Kennell, J. H. *Maternal-infant bonding.* St. Louis: Mosby, 1976.

Klaus, M. H., & Kennell, J. H. Mothers separated from their newborn infants. In J. L. Schwartz

& L. H. Schwartz (Eds.), *Vulnerable infants, a psychosocial dilemma.* New York: McGraw-Hill, 1977.

Lin-Fu, J. S. *Lead poisoning in children.* DHEW Pub. No. HSA 75-5102. Washington, D.C.: U.S. Government Printing Office, reprinted 1975.

McClelland, D. C., Constantian, C. A., Regalado, D., & Stone, C. Making it to maturity. *Psychology Today,* June 1978, *12,* 42–50, 114.

Medcom. *Year one: nutrition, growth, health.* Columbus, Ohio: Ross Laboratories, 1975.

Milio, N. *9226 Kercheval: The storefront that did not burn.* Ann Arbor: University of Michigan Press, 1970.

Miller, C. A. Health care of children and youth in America. *American Journal of Public Health,* April 1975, *65,* 353–358.

Morris, N. M., Udry, J. R., & Chase, C. L. Shifting age—Parity distribution of births and the decrease in infant mortality. *American Journal of Public Health,* April 1975, *65,* 359–362.

National Academy of Sciences. *Maternal nutrition and the course of pregnancy: Summary report.* Rockville, Md.: Department of Health, Education, and Welfare, Bureau of Community Health Services, reprinted 1975.

National Center for Health Statistics. *Accident facts 1979.* Chicago, Ill.: National Safety Council, 1979.

National Foundation for Sudden Infant Death. *Facts about sudden infant death syndrome.* 1501 Broadway, New York, N.Y. 10036.

Robertiello, R. C. *Hold them very close, then let them go.* New York: Dial, 1975.

Ross Timesaver. *WIC currents. News of women, infants, and children's programs.* May–June 1978, 4, 11. Columbus, Ohio: Ross Laboratories.

Salk, L. *Preparing for parenthood.* New York: McKay, 1974.

Schwartz, J. L., & Schwartz, L. H. (Eds.). *Vulnerable infants. A psychosocial dilemma.* New York: McGraw-Hill, 1977.

Scipien, G. M. Barnard, M. U., Chard, M. A., Howe, J., & Phillips, P. J. *Comprehensive pediatric nursing.* New York: McGraw-Hill, 1975.

Selwyn, B. J. An epidemiological approach to the study of users and nonusers of child health services. *American Journal of Public Health,* March 1978, *68,* 231–235.

Shaheen, E., Alexander, D., & Barbero, G. J. Failure to thrive: A retrospective profile. In J. L. Schwartz & L. H. Schwartz (Eds.). *Vulnerable infants. A psycho-social dilemma.* New York: McGraw-Hill, 1977.

So . . . you are going to be a father. *American Baby,* June 1976, *VXXVIII,* 35–38.

Spiegel, C. N., & Lindaman, F. C. Children can't fly. *American Journal of Public Health,* December 1977, *67,* 1143–1147.

Spock, B. *Raising children in a difficult time.* New York: Norton, 1974.

Steele, B. F. Violence within the family. In R. E. Helfer & C. H. Kempe (Eds.), *Child abuse and neglect. The family and the community.* Cambridge, Mass.: Ballinger, 1976.

Subcommittee on Child and Human Development, Committee on Human Resources, United States Senate, Hearings before. *Extension of the Child Abuse Prevention and Treatment Act, 1977* (April 6 and 7, 1977). Washington, D.C.: U.S. Government Printing Office, 1977.

Thomas, J. A. & Call, D. L. Eating between meals. *Nutrition Review,* May 1973, *31,* 137–139.

Time Magazine, July 2, 1979, *114,* 70.

Vaughn, V. C., & McKay, R. J. (Eds.), & Nelson, W. E. (Con. Ed.). *Textbook of pediatrics* (10th ed.). Philadelphia: Saunders, 1975.

Wald, L. *The house on Henry Street.* New York: Henry Holt, 1915.

Wallace, H. M. (Ed.) *Health care of mothers and children in national health services: Implications for the United States.* Cambridge, Mass.: Ballinger, 1975.

White House Conference on Children. *Profiles of children.* Washington, D.C.: U.S. Government Printing Office, 1970.

Whitehead, J. Beware of Fraiberg's apron strings. (Review of *Every child's birthright—In defense of mothering,* by S. Fraiberg) *MS.,* August 1978, *7,* 35–38.

Wilner, D. M., Walkley, R. P., & Goerke, L. S. *Introduction to public health.* New York: Macmillan, 1973.

SELECTED BIBLIOGRAPHY

Advisory Committee on Child Development. *Toward a national policy for children and families.* Washington, D.C.: National Academy of Sciences, 1976.

Barnes, K. E. Secondary prevention. The utilization of public health nurses as agents of behavioral change in the community. *American Journal of Public Health,* October 1975, *65,* 1099–1101.

Brown, M. S., & Murphy, M. A. *Ambulatory pediatrics for nurses.* New York: McGraw-Hill, 1975.

Chinn. P. L. *Child health maintenance concepts in family-centered care.* St. Louis: Mosby, 1974.

Collins, M. C. *Child abuser—A study of child abusers in self-help group therapy.* Littleton, Mass.: PSG Publishing Co., 1978.

Curry, J. B., & Peppe, K. K. *Mental retardation: Nursing approach to care.* St. Louis: Mosby, 1978.

de Mause, L. *The history of childhood.* New York: Psychohistory Press, 1974.

Dodson, F. *How to father.* Los Angeles: Nash Publishers, 1974.

Eisner, V., Pratt M. W., Hexter A., Chabot M. J., & Sayal, N. Improvement in infant and perinatal mortality in the United States, 1965–1973: 1. Priorities for intervention. *American Journal of Public Health,* April 1978, *68,* 359–364.

Erickson, M. P. Trends in assessing the newborn and his parents. *American Journal of Maternal Child Nursing,* March–April 1978, *3,* 99–103.

Finnie, N. R. *Handling the young cerebral palsied child at home* (2d ed.). New York: Dutton, 1975.

Gesell, A., Ilg, F. L., Ames L. B., & Rodell, J. L. (Rev. Ed.). *Infant and child in the culture of today.* New York: Harper & Row, 1974.

Hartman, H. *Let's play and pretend.* New York: Human Sciences Press, 1976.

Haynes, U. *A developmental approach to casefinding.* DHEW Publication No. HSA 75-5403. Washington, D.C.: U.S. Government Printing Office, reprinted 1975.

Illingsworth, R. S. *The development of the infant and young child.* New York: Churchill Livingstone, 1975.

Johnston, M., Kayne, M., & Mittleider, K. Putting more pep in parenting. *American Journal of Nursing,* June 1977, *77,* 994–995.

Kappelman, M. *Raising the only child.* New York: Dutton, 1975.

Law, S. *The rights of the poor.* New York: Avon, 1974.

Lynn, D. B. *The father: His role in child development.* Monterey, Calif.: Brooks/Cole, 1974.

Milio, N. A framework for prevention: Changing health–damaging to health–generating life patterns. *American Journal of Public Health,* May 1976, *66,* 435–439.

Morris, A. G. The use of the well-baby clinic to promote early intellectual development via parent education. *American Journal of Public Health,* January 1976, *66,* 73–74.

National Council on Family Relations. Special issue: Fatherhood. *The Family Coordinator,* October 1976, *25,* 335–520.

National Organization for Non-Parents. *Statement of principles N.O.N.* 3 North Liberty Street, Baltimore, Md., 1978.

Newbaurer, P. (Ed.). *The process of child development.* New York: New American Library, 1976.

Salk, L. *What every child would like his parents to know.* New York: Warner Paperbacks, 1973.

Sana, J. M., & Judge, R. D. (Eds.). *Physical appraisal methods in nursing practice.* Boston: Little, Brown, 1975.

Smith D. W., & Wilson, A. A. *The child with Down's syndrome. Causes, characteristics, and acceptance.* Philadelphia: Saunders, 1973.

Swendsen, L. A., Meleis, A. I., & Jones, D. Role supplementation for parents—a role mastery plan. *American Journal of Maternal Child Nursing,* March–April 1978, *3,* 84–91.

Visiting Nurse Association of New Haven. *Child health conference nurse's resource manual.* (League Exchange No. 101). New York: National League for Nursing, 1975.

White, B. L. *The first three years of life.* Englewood Cliffs, N. J.: Prentice-Hall, 1975.

Young, L. *Life among the giants.* New York: McGraw-Hill, 1966.

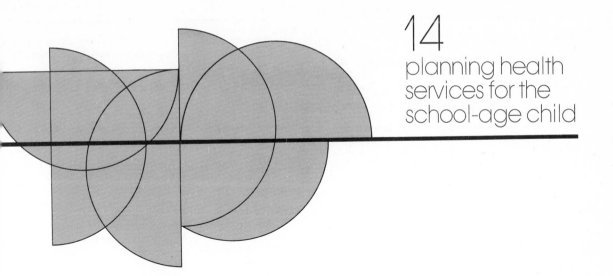

14
planning health
services for the
school-age child

During the twentieth century, a concerted effort has been made to improve the health status of all children. However, the goals of the 1930 Children's Charter which emphasized that children, regardless of their race, color, or creed (Figure 14-1), should have an environment and life experiences allowing them to develop to their fullest potential, are still far from realized.

Since the turn of the century, there have been major achievements in relation to the health status of school-age children and the services provided for them. Wallace noted in the early sixties, for instance, three particularly noteworthy advances: (1) a decrease in mortality in this age category; (2) the expansion of organized school health services; and (3) the recognition that adolescents have special problems and needs (Wallace, 1962, p. 25). Despite these accomplishments, there remain a sizable number of children who will never reach their fullest potential. Although good health care in the United States is considered a right rather than a privilege, there is still a failure to meet the health needs of specific segments of the population. Children of racial

minorities, children from poor, central-city, and rural families, and children with handicapping conditions continue to have a higher incidence of mortality and morbidity and continue to use health care services less frequently than the population as a whole (Miller, 1975, pp. 355–356). In addition, it must be emphasized that the progress noted in the 1960s is no longer being sustained. Americans in the 15- to 24-year-old age category have a higher death rate today than they did 20 years ago (Surgeon General's Report, 1979, p. 43). Even though it was recognized in the sixties that adolescents have special problems and needs, services for this developmental age group have not substantially increased since that time. In a report presented to the Surgeon General in 1979 the following data were shared to illustrate that adolescents are given little special attention by the health care sector (Hamburg, 1979, pp. 338–340):

· adolescents typically see a physician less often than younger children do and much less often than adults do;

· when adolescents are hospitalized, they are usually placed in pediatric or adult care facilities which

The Children's Charter

President Hoover's White House Conference on Child Health and Protection, recognizing the rights of the child as the first rights of citizenship, pledges itself to these aims for the children of America.

I For every child spiritual and moral training to help him to stand firm under the pressure of life

II For every child understanding and the guarding of his personality as his most precious right

III For every child a home and that love and security which a home provides; and for that child who must receive foster care, the nearest substitute for his own home

IV For every child full preparation for his birth, his mother receiving prenatal, natal, and postnatal care; and the establishment of such protective measures as will make childbearing safer

V For every child health protection from birth through adolescence, including: periodical health examinations and, where needed, care of specialists and hospital treatment; regular dental examinations and care of the teeth; protective and preventive measures against communicable diseases; the insuring of pure food, pure milk, and pure water

VI For every child from birth through adolescence, promotion of health, including health instruction and a health program, wholesome physical and mental recreation, with teachers and leaders adequately trained

VII For every child a dwelling-place safe, sanitary, and wholesome, with reasonable provisions for privacy; free from conditions which tend to thwart his development; and a home environment harmonious and enriching

VIII For every child a school which is safe from hazards, sanitary, properly equipped, lighted, and ventilated. For younger children nursery schools and kindergartens to supplement home care

IX For every child a community which recognizes and plans for his needs, protects him against physical dangers, moral hazards, and disease; provides him with safe and wholesome places for play and recreation; and makes provision for his cultural and social needs

X For every child an education which, through the discovery and development of his individual abilities, prepares him for life; and through training and vocational guidance prepares him for living which will yield him the maximum of satisfaction

XI For every child such teaching and training as will prepare him for successful parenthood, home-making, and the rights of citizenship; and, for parents, supplementary training to fit them to deal wisely with the problems of parenthood

typically are not well suited to the special characteristics and needs of adolescents;

· close to 15 percent of adolescents age 16 and 17 report no regular source of medical care, as compared to about 7 percent for children under 6;

· training opportunities for physicians in the special health needs of adolescents are limited. There are no residency positions in adolescent medicine at all, and only 55 fellowships available in this area;

· clinic services designed for adolescents are rare, although in the past several years, this situation has begun to change; where attempts have been made to provide health care in a manner compatible with the unique needs of adolescents, young people use them frequently;

· school health services and health education, if available at all, are frequently mediocre in quality, although there have recently been some promising innovations in school-based health programs; only six states and the District of Columbia require education about sexuality and family life in the schools.

Providing effective and efficient health and welfare services for all segments of the school-age population is no easy task. Demographic, vital, and morbidity statistics reveal that professionals need to deal with an array of problems when planning health and welfare services for this population group. The review of these problems which follows clearly illus-

XII For every child education for safety and protection against accidents to which modern conditions subject him—those to which he is directly exposed and those which, through loss or maiming of his parents, affect him indirectly

XIII For every child who is blind, deaf, crippled, or otherwise physically handicapped, and for the child who is mentally handicapped, such measures as will early discover and diagnose his handicap, provide care and treatment, and so train him that he may become an asset to society rather than a liability. Expenses of these services should be borne publicly where they cannot be privately met

XIV For every child who is in conflict with society the right to be dealt with intelligently as society's charge, not society's outcast; with the home, the school, the church, the court and the institution when needed, shaped to return him whenever possible to the normal stream of life

XV For every child the right to grow up in a family with an adequate standard of living and the security of a stable income as the surest safeguard against social handicaps

XVI For every child protection against labor that stunts growth, either physical or mental, that limits education, that deprives children of the right of comradeship, of play, and of joy

XVII For every rural child as satisfactory schooling and health services as for the city child, and an extension to rural families of social, recreational, and cultural facilities

XVIII To supplement the home and the school in the training of youth, and to return to them those interests of which modern life tends to cheat children, every stimulation and encouragement should be given to the extension and development of the voluntary youth organizations

XIX To make everywhere available these minimum protections of the health and welfare of children, there should be a district, county, or community organization for health, education, and welfare, with full-time officials, coordinating with a state-wide program which will be responsive to a nationwide service of general information, statistics, and scientific research. This should include:

(a) Trained, full-time public health officials, with public health nurses, sanitary inspection, and laboratory workers

(b) Available hospital beds

(c) Full-time public welfare service for the relief, aid, and guidance of children in special need due to poverty, misfortune, or behavior difficulties, and for the protection of children from abuse, neglect, exploitation, or moral hazard

For every child these rights, regardless of race, or color, or situation, wherever he may live under the protection of the American Flag.

---

trates the complex nature of the difficulties encountered when health care professionals work with school-age children.

Historically, community health nurses have assumed a major role in developing child health services. Lillian Wald initiated a special project in New York City schools in 1902 to demonstrate to city officials the value of preventive health counseling in relation to the needs of school-age children. Since that time, nursing services to meet the needs of our youth have grown steadily. Community health nurses are now working with children in a variety of settings including their homes, school environments, clinic settings, and residential facilities for special populations at risk. In order to plan nursing services for children, the community health nurse must have knowledge about their needs and an understanding of the range of services required to meet these needs.

DEMOGRAPHIC, VITAL, AND MORBIDITY STATISTICS

Knowledge and use of statistical data are essential for effective health planning. Statistical data help the community health nurse to identify how many people need nursing services

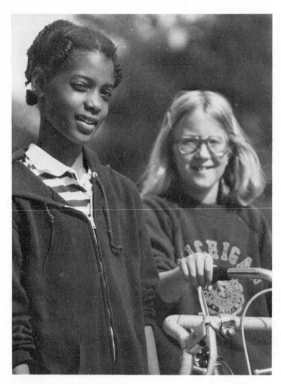

FIGURE 14-1 All children, regardless of race, color, or creed, need positive life experiences in order to develop to their fullest potential.

and what type of services can best help the population to resolve its health problems (see Chapter 11). Since health needs and services differ with age, it is important to analyze the composition of the population and the mortality and morbidity statistics specific to the particular age group under consideration.

Composition of the Population

One of the most significant characteristics of a country's population composition is age structure. It is important to examine this variable because health problems are frequently age-related, and the absolute number of people in a particular age category influences the amount of resources needed to provide adequate health care services.

The age structure of the population in the United States has been changing. Fluctuations in the birth rates since post-World War II have significantly altered the age distribution of the United States residents in the past three decades. Table 14-1 illustrates these changes since 1960. The decrease in the number of pre-

TABLE 14-1 Number of Resident Population by Age, Sex, and Race, United States, 1960, 1970, 1975, 1976, 1977*

Sex, age, and race	Unit	Year				
		1960	1970	1975	1976	1977
TOTAL						
Both sexes, all ages	Million	180.7	204.9	213.6	215.1	216.8
Male	Million	89.3	100.3	104.2	104.9	105.7
Female	Million	91.4	104.6	109.3	110.2	111.1
AGE DISTRIBUTION						
Under 5 years	Million	20.3	17.1	15.9	15.3	15.2
5 to 17 years old	Million	44.2	52.5	50.4	49.9	49.0
18 years old and over	Million	116.1	135.2	147.3	149.9	152.6
65 years old and over	Million	16.7	20.1	22.4	22.9	23.5
Median age	Million	29.4	27.9	28.8	29.0	29.4
RACIAL DISTRIBUTION						
White	Million	160.0	179.5	185.6	186.6	187.7
Black	Million	19.0	22.8	24.5	24.9	25.2
Percent of total population	Percent	11	11	11	12	12
Percent in the South	Percent	60	53	52	53	54
Persons of Spanish origin	Million	na	na	11.2	11.1	11.3

*Resident population as of July 1.
SOURCE: From U.S. Bureau of the Census. *U.S.A. statistics in brief 1978: A statistical abstract supplement.* Washington, D.C.: U.S. Department of Commerce, 1978, unnumbered pages.

school children from 11.2 percent in 1960 to 7 percent in 1977 and the increase in the 18- to 65-year-old population during the same time period are the direct result of changing birth rates. The baby boom immediately following World War II expanded the preschool population in the 1960s and is now expanding the 18- to 65-year-old population group. The declining birth rate of the 1970s is reflected in the decline of the 1977 preschool percent distribution.

Shifts in the age distribution of a population in such a short time frame present special difficulties for health professionals. This is especially true when they are attempting to predict what health services are needed for a specific age group in the future. When birth rates fluctuate, it is easy to have either an overabundance or an underabundance of health personnel and services. Health professionals in the 1950s and 1960s, for example, were underequipped to handle the number of school-age children resulting from the postwar baby boom. Today, schools have a surplus of classrooms and teachers because of the declining birth rate of the 1970s (Mazie, 1972, p. 9).

What the future holds for health care is questionable. It should not be assumed that the number of school-age children will continue to decline. Trends must be monitored carefully, because the childbearing age group (18 to 44) in the United States is increasing in size. The fluctuations in fertility in the United States over the last four decades illustrate that family-size preference has varied in response to financial and social conditions and could do so in the future (Reinke, 1972, p. 142). A difference of only one extra child per family can have a tremendous impact on the amount of services needed for our school-age population. If families average only two children in the next two decades, there will be 55 million school-age children, ages 5 to 17, in the year 2000. If, however, families average three children, there will be 80 million school-age children, ages 5 to 17, in this same year, or a 46 percent increase in the number of elementary- and secondary-school-age individuals from the year 1970 to the year 2000 (Commission on Population Growth and the American Future, 1972, pp. 22–24). Health planners for school-age children should proceed with caution when they consider reducing the quantity of services for this particular age category.

As of July 1977, there were approximately 49 million school-age children, ages 5 through 17 (roughly 22.6 percent of the United States population), who needed health services. This certainly is no small number, and it supports the need to examine carefully the common health problems of this age group and to plan *organized* health services to meet these needs. When planning for these health services, it is imperative that one analyze local as well as national statistics, because there are striking differences in the age structure in various sections of the country as a result of variations in the birth rate. In 1975, for example, the racial minority birth rate was 53.6 percent higher than that for whites (Rudov and Santangelo, 1979, p. 32). Thus, in social areas where there is a high minority population, the median age will be lower and there will be a greater need for child health services.

Community health nurses who work with the school-age population encounter a variety of physical, psychosocial, cultural, environmental, and developmental health problems and concerns. Since emphasis is placed on planning health services in this chapter, only general morbidity and mortality statistics and growth and development data will be presented here. The reader can obtain a comprehensive understanding of childhood problems and specific growth and development characteristics by referring to *Comprehensive Pediatric Nursing* (Scipien, Barnard, Chard, Howe, and Phillips, 1975) and *Principles of Pediatrics: Health Care of the Young* (Hoekelman, Blatman, Brunell, Friedman, and Seidel, 1978).

Childhood Mortality

Accidents, malignant neoplasms, congenital anomalies, homicide, and influenza and pneumonia were the five leading causes of death in children ages 5 through 14 in 1976 (latest official figures). Figure 14-2 summarizes the historical transition of childhood mortality in the United States in the past four decades. When one is reviewing any overall statistical rates such as those presented in Figure 14-2, it is important to keep in mind that these rates may vary within segments of the population. In the United States, for example, black American

children have a 30 percent higher mortality rate than white American children, and the death rate for young men is roughly three times that of young women (Surgeon General, 1979, pp. 33, 43).

It is striking to note when examining the 1976 statistics that four childhood killers—accidents, congenital malformations, homicide, and influenza and pneumonia—can be prevented; environmental, social, and behavioral factors greatly affect their occurrence. In 1976, it was estimated that approximately "50 percent of our United States deaths were due to

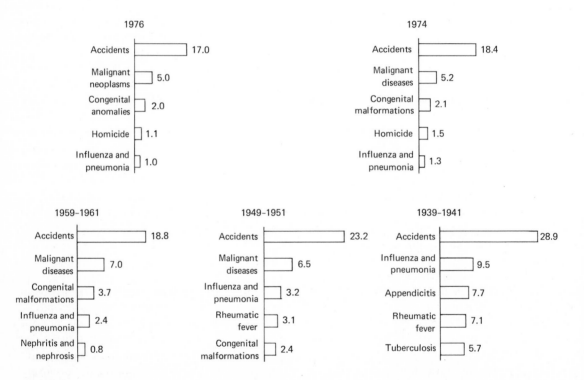

FIGURE 14-2 Five leading causes of death in children from the age of 5 through 14, 1939–1941 to 1976. Alaska and Hawaii are included for 1959–1961 and 1974. The 1949–1951 statistic for rheumatic fever includes rheumatic heart disease. (*From a report of the Harvard Child Health Project. Children's medical care needs and treatments, Volume II. Cambridge Mass.: Ballinger, 1977, p. 27. Reprinted with permission from the Ballinger Company. Data for 1976 from National Center for Health Statistics. Advance report, vital statistics of the United States, 1976. Hyattsville, Md.: Office of Health Research, Statistics, and Technology, 1979; data for 1974 from National Center for Health Statistics. Advance report, final mortality statistics 1974, Vol. 24, No. 11, Supple. 3, February 1976; data for other years from S. Shapiro, C. Schlesinger, & R. Nesbitt, Jr., 1968, p. 177.*)

unhealthy behavior or lifestyle; 20 percent to environmental factors; 20 percent to human biological factors; and only 10 percent to inadequacies in health care" (Surgeon General, 1979, p. 9).

Although a substantial decline in childhood mortality due to accidents has occurred since 1939–1941, very minimal progress has been made in reducing childhood accidental deaths since 1959–1961. Motor-vehicle, drowning, fires (burns), firearms, and poisoning accidents are some of the leading causes of premature deaths in children (National Safety Council, 1979, p. 8). Community health nurses and other health planners should carefully examine ways to promote environmental safety in order to alter this trend. Accidents have too long been the leading cause of childhood mortality.

In 1974, for the first time in the existence of our country, homicide became a major killer of children and young adults. For nonwhites ages 15 to 19, both male and female, homicide is the second leading cause of death (Hamburg, 1979, p. 343). Certainly no one factor accounts for this occurrence. Economic deprivation, family break-up, the glamorizing of violence in the media, and the availability of handguns are some important variables to consider in planning strategies to reduce childhood mortality resulting from violent causes (Surgeon General, 1979, p. 51). It is also crucial to look at societal attitudes, because studies have shown that violence is sanctioned and increasingly evident in our culture in general (Miller, 1975, p. 24; and Garbarino, 1977, p. 726). Community health nurses can no longer deal with physical health problems only. They must work closely with all agencies in the community so that a concerted effort is made to *prevent* death from homicide in our school-age population.

Poverty, poor housing, malnutrition, pregnancy at a young age, use of alcohol and cigarettes, and inadequate medical care increase the likelihood that illness, disability, or death will occur. Miller (1974, p. 355) found that the mortality rate for influenza and pneumonia in New York City was three times greater for poor nonwhite children than for their white counterparts. It has been shown that mothers in all age categories who are disadvantaged are at risk for producing an unhealthy child (Chinn, 1974, p. 80). The risk of having an abnormal birth increases as a mother's consumption of alcohol and smoking increase (Hamburg, 1979, p. 316). Young mothers and mothers who have inadequate health care are more likely to have low-birth-weight babies than other mothers. Low-birth-weight infants have a high incidence of congenital malformations. It is obvious from these facts that a preventive health program designed to reduce childhood mortality due to congenital malformations and influenza and pneumonia must include ways to eliminate poor environmental and social conditions, to expand the usage of prenatal services by young and disadvantaged mothers, and to alter unhealthy behaviors (alcohol consumption and smoking) which increase the risk for abnormal births.

Cancer, the second leading cause of childhood mortality, places a tremendous burden on the family and society. This disease kills more school-age children than any other disease. The severe nature of this condition and the prolonged treatment needed cause pain and anguish for both the child and the family. Cancer in childhood also causes financial hardship for many families, because funding for catastrophic illness is frequently not available. Health planning efforts in relation to this disease should focus on providing early detection, treatment, and supportive services, funding for research, and monies to eliminate individual financial hardships. Community health nurses can significantly assist families in coping with childhood cancer by providing hospice care services and by helping them to obtain needed resources from community agencies. The American Cancer Society, for instance, supplies dressings and equipment free of charge. Other community agencies such as the Department of Social Services and Crippled Children's Association provide funds for medical treatment.

Childhood Morbidity—Acute Conditions

The actual incidence of acute conditions in childhood is difficult to ascertain because (1) many acute conditions are not reportable; (2) reportable acute conditions are often not reported; and (3) acute illness is frequently treated at home and as a result is not brought to the attention of health professionals. Data from the national health surveys since 1956 do give estimated patterns of incidence over time. According to this survey, acute conditions are illnesses and injuries that last no longer than 3 months and have either been treated by medical personnel or have resulted in restricted activity of 1 day or more (Current Estimates from the Health Interview Survey: United States, 1977, p. 1). The major types of

acute illness for children, ages 6 through 16 years, fall into five major categories. In order of frequency, these are respiratory conditions, infective and parasitic diseases, injuries, digestive system conditions, and all other conditions. The number of days lost from school per year due to acute conditions is shown in Table 14-2. School-age children miss approximately 5 days of school per year due to these conditions.

Respiratory conditions account for over 50 percent of the reported acute illnesses among school-age children. These conditions are frequently ignored because "everyone gets a cold or an earache"; colds and earaches are "a normal part of life." However, these seemingly minor illnesses must not be disregarded. They do interfere with activities of daily living and may often lead to serious, chronic disabilities. In a study by Heazlett and Whaley (1976, p. 146), it was noted that the common cold, the respiratory condition with the highest incidence rate, affected adversely to a significant degree the perceptual and learning performance of junior high students. Otitis media, the

TABLE 14-2   Days Lost from School per 100 Children (6 to 16 Years) per Year, by Sex and Condition Group: United States, 1977

Condition group	Days lost from school in thousands			Days lost from school per 100 children per year		
	Both sexes	*Male*	*Female*	*Both sexes*	*Male*	*Female*
All acute conditions	203,500	98,181	105,319	491.2	465.0	518.5
Infective and parasitic diseases	38,132	19,284	18,848	92.1	91.3	92.8
Respiratory conditions	118,961	55,493	63,469	287.2	262.8	312.5
Upper respiratory conditions	59,822	26,636	33,186	144.4	126.2	163.4
Influenza	48,562	22,791	25,770	117.2	107.9	126.9
Other respiratory conditions	10,578	6,065	4,512	25.5	28.7	22.2
Digestive system conditions	9,399	4,478	4,921	22.7	21.2	24.2
Injuries	15,973	10,638	5,335	38.6	50.4	26.3
All other acute conditions	21,034	8,289	12,746	50.8	39.3	62.8

SOURCE: From National Center for Health Statistics. *Current estimates from the health interview survey, United States, 1977.* DHEW Publication No. PHS 78-1554, Series 10, No. 126. Hyattsville, Md.: Public Health Service, September 1978, p. 17.

third leading reason for pediatrician contact, can, if untreated, result in permanent hearing loss and/or chronic ear infection.

Infective and parasitic diseases are of concern to all health personnel because of their contagious nature. Many of them, such as scabies, impetigo, ringworm, and head lice, are still considered "diseases of the poor and unclean" even though this myth has been disproved. Children who have experienced these conditions are often socially isolated from their peers and labeled "dirty kids" even after treatment ceases. The reader will find the American Public Health Association Handbook, *Control of Communicable Diseases in Man* (Benenson, 1975), an extremely useful resource when identifying and recommending follow-up for any of these communicable conditions. It must be remembered, however, that physical care and treatment is not sufficient. The social stigma associated with these diseases is often more devastating than the disease itself. Epidemiological investigation (see Chapter 10) to determine the source of infection is essential in order to prevent further disease incidence as well as the social stigma associated with infective and parasitic diseases.

Studies have found that injuries account for roughly 25 percent of all the visits to the school health clinic (Hilmar and McAtee, 1973, p. 433; McKevitt, Nader, Williamson, and Berney, 1977, p. 278). Males have 50 percent more nonfatal injuries than females, due to differences in activities and behavior such as participation in contact sports. There are over 2 million sports-related injuries each year (Hamburg, 1979, pp. 57, 67). Better-planned sports programs in our country might substantially reduce the number of these injuries. Monitoring environmental conditions in homes and schools and promoting highway safety programs designed for the teenage driver could also significantly decrease childhood injuries.

Diseases of the digestive tract such as stomachaches, peptic ulcers, and colitis frequently have a psychosocial etiology. An astute community health nurse will assess for causes other than physical ones when working with children who have digestive tract problems. This is especially important to do when a child has recurrent unexplained abdominal pains. Some key variables to consider when physical causes for digestive conditions have been ruled out are inadequate nutrition; family conflict; separation due to death, divorce, and illness; child abuse; tense classroom atmosphere; unfavorable teacher-student relationships; poor academic achievement; unrealistic expectations for performance; and lack of peer support.

Childhood Morbidity— Chronic Conditions

Childhood chronic conditions are of special concern to health professionals for several reasons. First, these conditions may inhibit normal developmental processes and cause disability in later life. Second, the stress of chronic illness frequently affects significant others as well as the child who has the chronic condition. Last, prevention, treatment, and management services for chronic conditions are costly because of the long-term nature of these conditions and the number of persons affected by them.

The wars of our nation dramatically illustrated the need to focus attention on preventing chronic health problems in our youth. During both World War I and World War II, a significant number of men were rejected for military service because of existing chronic conditions such as dental problems, psychiatric difficulties, and orthopedic abnormalities. Despite recognition since the early 1920s that the health status of our nation's youth was far from ideal, 15 percent of the 18-year-olds were rejected for military service in 1965 because they had chronic handicapping conditions. It was believed that two-thirds of these conditions could have been prevented if they had been detected before age 15 (Travis, 1976, p. 4).

Physical examinations provided by the National Health Survey in 1963 to 1965 for children 6 to 11 years of age and in 1966 to 1970 for youth 12 to 17 years of age again revealed that a significant proportion of our school-age children have chronic health conditions such as hearing deficiencies, visual difficulties, orthopedic problems, dental caries, congenital heart and kidney diseases, and nutritional inadequacies. It was estimated from the probability sample of children examined that one out of eight children ages 6 to 11 and one out of five youth 12 to 17 years of age have one or more chronic abnormalities (Vital and Health Statistics Series 11, 1975, p. 26).

National health statistics in 1970 revealed that the leading childhood chronic abnormalities were asthma and chronic bronchitis. Although both are serious disease processes, asthma tends to limit a child's activity more than bronchitis and accounts for a higher percentage of days lost from school than any other chronic condition (*Health*, 1975, p. 399; and Report of the Harvard Child Health Project Task Force, 1977, Vol. 2, p. 36). A study of children under the care of primary physicians conducted by the Family Medicine Program of the University of Rochester–Highland Hospital in 1971 revealed similar findings (Froom, 1974, p. 77). Table 14-3 describes the prevalence of chronic illnesses in the 25,000 children, ages 0 to 14, studied in this New York project. Again, asthma was found to be the leading chronic condition among children.

It is also important to note, when examining the statistics in Table 14-3, that social problems ranked second in prevalence in this New York study. It is increasingly recognized that social problems affect all aspects of an individual's functioning. Frequently, families who experience economic and housing difficulties or dysfunctional familial conflict are unable to meet the emotional needs of their members. They are also less able to obtain adequate medical care.

Five social problems of particular concern to community health nurses who are working with school-age children are suicide, child abuse, teenage parenthood, venereal disease, and drug abuse. None of these difficulties is unique to the school-age population. However, because a sizable proportion of our youth are experiencing these problems, a discussion of them is warranted.

Suicide

Since 1960, the incidence of suicide among our youth has been steadily increasing and is now the third leading cause of death for persons ages 15 to 19 (Surgeon General, 1979, p. 50). Health professionals view suicide as a problem of extreme importance in the adolescent population, because it is an indicator that social, emotional, and physical stress is great for many youth (Powers, 1978, p. 19). Rapidly changing societal values, population mobility, and economic pressures have presented our adolescents with decision-making conflicts that result in uncertainty and stress (Figure 14-3).

The extent of our suicide problem is much greater than the recorded incidence indicates. Because suicide is often viewed as a cowardly and disgraceful act in our culture, it is frequently concealed by families and medical personnel. Many suicides are not recorded as such on the death certificate, and often it is difficult to differentiate between suicide and deaths due to accidents. The result is that the recorded incidence only reflects a proportion of the deaths caused by suicide. In addition, when one looks at the attempted suicide rate, the problem becomes even more significant because suicide attempts far exceed actual suicide deaths. Some estimates indicate that for every suicide death, there are 150 suicide at-

TABLE 14-3 Prevalence of Chronic Illness in Children under the Care of Primary Physicians in the Family Medicine Program of the University of Rochester–Highland Hospital in 1971

Chronic health problem	Age and sex						Total
	0–4		5–9		10–14		
	Male	Female	Male	Female	Male	Female	
Asthma	98	71	122	75	82	36	484
Social problems (economic, housing, parental conflict, etc.)	98	77	72	43	39	39	368
Congenital malformations (excluding heart and cleft palate and lip)	98	45	18	18	11	13	243
Epilepsy	20	19	14	24	15	11	103
Hyperkinesis	2	3	35	10	10	5	75
Congenital heart disease	15	13	5	3	3	1	40
Scoliosis	. . .	. . .	3	8	7	8	26
Diabetes mellitus	. . .	3	7	2	12	1	25
Nephritis and nephrosis	3	. . .	5	3	4	5	20
Psoriasis	2	. . .	1	6	4	3	16
Rheumatic heart disease and hypertension	1	1	. . .	7	3	2	14
All malignant neoplasms	1	4	2	2	2	1	12
Purpura and hemorrhagic conditions	1	2	2	2	2	2	11
Glaucoma	3	. . .	2	2	2	. . .	9
Schizophrenia and organic psychoses	. . .	. . .	3	1	2	2	8
Cataract	1	2	. . .	. . .	4	. . .	7
Gastric and duodenal ulcer and ulcerative colitis	. . .	1	. . .	1	3	1	6
Rheumatoid arthritis	. . .	. . .	. . .	3	2	1	6
Cleft palate	. . .	2	1	1	. . .	1	5
CNS vascular lesions	3	. . .	. . .	1	. . .	. . .	4
Total all diseases	. . .	. . .	. . .	. . .	. . .	. . .	1482

SOURCE: From J. Froom. Prevalence and natural history of chronic diseases in childhood. In G. D. Grave & I. B. Pless (Eds.), *Chronic childhood illness: Assessment of outcome*, DHEW Pub. No. (NIH) 76-877. Hyattsville, Md.: U.S. Department of Health, Education, and Welfare. Public Health Service, National Institutes of Health, 1974, p. 78.

tempts (*Journal of the American Medical Association*, 1974, p. 1246).

Adolescence is normally a period of turmoil, frequently characterized by rebellious and impulsive behavior. During times of stress, thoughts of suicide are not abnormal. These thoughts usually do not, however, result in actual suicide. Studies have shown that adoles-

cents who do commit suicide have greater problems than just the normal mood swings of adolescence. Suicidal adolescents often have a long-standing history of chronic childhood and family problems. Frequently they exhibit signs and symptoms of depression, with feelings of despair and hopelessness. Often they are crying out for help because they are deal-

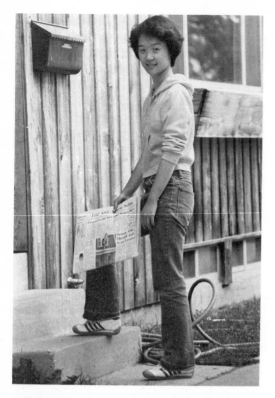

FIGURE 14-3 Accelerated societal changes have exposed American youth to increased opportunities as well as increased stresses. American youth are exposed much earlier than their previous counterparts to such things as human sexuality concerns, pressures from peers to use alcohol and drugs, and varying life-styles. Community health nurses are often in a favorable position to detect youth who are having difficulty coping with the demands of life.

to personal hygiene, crying spells without specific cause, loss of appetite, and withdrawal from extracurricular activities should not be ignored. Adolescents who feel isolated are prone to suicide. Look for the loners who lack initiative and who seemingly do not care how they relate to others. Individuals who are severely depressed or who are at odds with themselves and the people close to them are at highest risk for suicide (Surgeon General, 1979, p. 50).

Community health nurses, especially when they are functioning in the school setting, are often in a key position to detect troubled youth. When working with adolescents who are potentially suicidal, nurses must demonstrate a caring attitude and a genuine interest in learning about the adolescent's problems. Nurses must also encourage these adolescents to talk about their suicidal thoughts and plans and provide assistance so that they reach out for the help they need. Working with the troubled adolescent's family is also important. Families need supportive services and often assistance in determining how to obtain help for their child. The principles of crisis intervention (see Chapter 7) should be applied when working with these families. Prompt recognition of distressed youth may prevent suicidal behavior.

ing with overwhelming burdens such as divorce, illness, and lack of material resources to meet their basic needs, as well as changes in their social relationships (Hoekelman, Blatman, Brunell, Friedman, and Seidel, 1978, p. 667).

Problems of childhood frequently escalate during adolescence. Community health nurses should carefully observe for teenagers who suddenly have difficulty coping with activities of daily living. Changes in behavior such as a drop in school attendance, decreased attention

Child Abuse and Neglect

Since the dynamics that lead to child abuse were articulated in Chapter 13, they will not be repeated in this chapter. Limiting discussion here is not meant to imply that child abuse is not a serious problem among school-age children. Studies suggest that child abuse is reaching epidemic proportions among the school-age as well as the preschool population (Drew, 1972; Lynch, 1975; Segal, 1979). Incidence figures range from 40 to 120 new cases annually per 100,000 school-age children

(Drew, 1972). All statistics in relation to child abuse are estimates, because child abuse is seriously underreported and often not identified. All school personnel, including the community health nurse, must expand their efforts to identify undetected abuse in school-age children. Presented in Table 14-4 is a summary of physical and behavioral indicators that can assist nurses in identifying child abuse and neglect.

The problems of child abuse and neglect are compounded for professionals who work with the school-age population, because often they must deal with the lasting effects of conditions which existed during infancy and the preschool years. Longitudinal studies are beginning to report findings which indicate that there are long-term detrimental consequences of child abuse. Children who are abused during early childhood tend to have difficulty establishing trust, find it hard to relate to others, do not enjoy play, are preoccupied with many fears, have a poor self-image, and have problems with expressing feelings. They also tend to be passive individuals who are hesitant to explore their environment or to reach out to other people (Helfer and Kempe, 1976, p. 69).

Steele (1979) has found an extremely high correlation between juvenile delinquency and child abuse and neglect. He reports studies done in the Denver area which show that 80 percent of youths picked up as juvenile offenders have been abused and neglected early in life. Professionals and community citizens can no longer ignore this critical problem. To ensure that all children reach their optimal level of functioning, mechanisms must be established for early identification, reporting of actual or suspected abusing situations, and early and adequate intervention. Both health professionals and the public need educational opportunities that will increase their knowledge about child abuse and neglect and help them to intervene effectively with abusive families.

Teenage Parenthood

The birth rate for teenage women has sharply increased in the last decade. A 1976 study found that roughly 1 million teenagers, in the 15- to 19-year-old age category, had experienced a pregnancy. These teenage pregnancies in 1974 ended as follows (Alan Guttmacher Institute, 1976 pp. 10–11):

· 28 percent resulted in marital births that were conceived following marriage

· 27 percent terminated by induced abortion

· 21 percent resulted in out-of-wedlock births

· 14 percent resulted in miscarriage

· 10 percent resulted in marital births that were conceived prior to marriage

· 94 percent of teenage mothers [kept] their babies at home

· 3.5 percent [gave] their baby up for adoption

· 2.5 percent [sent] the child to live with relatives or friends

It is estimated that slightly over half, or 11 million, teenagers ages 15 to 19 have had sexual intercourse. In 1975, approximately one-half of the 15- to 19-year-olds at risk for unintended pregnancy were not receiving family planning help from either organized clinics or private physicians (Alan Guttmacher Institute, 1976, p. 45). Zelnik and Kantner (1978, p. 142) believe that if none of our sexually active teenagers used contraception there would have been an additional 680,000 teenage premarital pregnancies in 1976.

Teenagers do not use birth control measures for a variety of reasons. Many are poorly informed about their sexual development, believing that they are too young to get pregnant or not knowing how women conceive. Others find it difficult to obtain contraceptive services, feel it is morally wrong to use birth control measures, or believe that contraceptive use in-

TABLE 14-4   Physical and Behavioral Indicators of Child Abuse and Neglect

Type of CA/N*	Physical indicators	Behavioral indicators
Physical abuse	Unexplained bruises and welts:	Feels deserving of punishment
	On face, lips, mouth	Wary of adult contacts
	On torso, back, buttocks, thighs	Apprehensive when other children cry
	In various stages of healing	Behavioral extremes:
	Clustered, forming regular patterns	Aggressiveness
	Reflecting shape of article used to inflict (electric cord, belt buckle)	Withdrawal
	On several different surface areas	Frightened of parents
	Regularly appear after absence, weekend, or vacation	Afraid to go home
		Reports injury by parents
	Unexplained burns:	Vacant or frozen stare
	Cigar, cigarette burns, especially on soles, palms, back, or buttocks	Lies very still while surveying surroundings
	Immersion burns (socklike, glovelike, doughnut shaped on buttocks or genitalia)	Will not cry when approached by examiner
		Responds to questions in monosyllables
	Patterned like electric burner, iron, etc.	Inappropriate or precocious maturity
	Rope burns on arms, legs, neck, or torso	Manipulative behavior to get attention
	Infected burns, indicating delay in seeking treatment	Capable of only superficial relationships
		Indiscriminately seeks affection
	Unexplained fractures or dislocations:	Poor self-concept
	To skull, nose, facial structure	
	In various stages of healing	
	Multiple or spiral fractures	
	Unexplained lacerations or abrasions:	
	To mouth, lips, gums, eyes	
	To external genitalia	
	In various stages of healing	
	Bald patches on the scalp	
Physical neglect	Underweight, poor growth pattern, failure to thrive	Begging, stealing food
	Consistent hunger, poor hygiene, inappropriate dress	Extended stays at school (early arrival and late departure)
		Rare attendance at school
	Consistent lack of supervision, especially in dangerous activities or long periods	Constant fatigue, listlessness, or falling asleep in class
	Wasting of subcutaneous tissue	Inappropriate seeking of affection
	Unattended physical problems or medical needs	Assuming adult responsibilities and concerns
		Alcohol or drug abuse

*CA/N = child abuse and neglect.

TABLE 14-4 Physical and Behavioral Indicators of Child Abuse and Neglect (*Continued*)

Type of CA/N	Physical indicators	Behavioral indicators
	Abandonment	Delinquency (e.g., thefts)
	Abdominal distention	States there is no caretaker
	Bald patches on the scalp	
Sexual abuse	Difficulty in walking or sitting	Unwilling to change for gym or participate in physical education class
	Torn, stained, or bloody underclothing	Withdrawal, fantasy, or infantile behavior
	Pain, swelling, or itching in genital area	Bizarre, sophisticated, or unusual sexual behavior or knowledge
	Pain on urination	
	Bruises, bleeding, or lacerations in external genitalia, vaginal, or anal areas	Poor peer relationships
	Vaginal or penile discharge	Delinquent or runaway
	Venereal disease, especially in preteens	Reports sexual assault by caretaker
	Poor sphincter tone	Change in performance in school
	Pregnancy	
Emotional maltreatment	Speech disorders	Habit disorders (sucking, biting, rocking, etc.)
	Lags in physical development	Conduct and learning disorders (antisocial, destructive, etc.)
	Failure to thrive	Neurotic traits (sleep disorders, inhibition of play, unusual fearfulness)
	Hyperactive or disruptive behavior	Psychoneurotic reactions (hysteria, obsession, compulsion, phobias, hypochondria)
		Behavior extremes:
		Compliant, passive
		Aggressive, demanding
		Overly adaptive behavior:
		Inappropriately adult
		Inappropriately infant
		Developmental lags (mental, emotional)
		Attempted suicide

SOURCE: From C. Heindl, C. A. Krall, M. Salus, & D. D. Broadhurst. *The nurse's role in the prevention and treatment of child abuse and neglect.* Washington, D.C.: National Center on Child Abuse and Neglect, Children's Bureau, Administration for Children, Youth and Families, Office of Human Development Services, August 1979, p. 10.

terferes with the pleasures of sex. Some want to become pregnant to fulfill needs of love, attention, and belonging.

There is increasing evidence that psychological factors predispose women to sexual activity without the use of contraception. Aber-

nethy (1974, p. 663) completed an extensive literature review on the psychological variables that facilitate identification of teenagers at risk for unwanted pregnancy. Two key factors were prominent: family history and attitudes toward self and others. Girls who experience a family situation where there is hostility in the parents' marriage, alienation between mother and daughter, and an intimate quasi-sexual father-daughter relationship are at high risk for unwanted pregnancy. These girls have a low self-esteem, have difficulty forming meaningful relationships with women, and are promiscuous. Contraception alone does not prevent births outside of marriage. These girls need individualized counseling to increase their self-concept, especially in relation to their feminine identity.

The multiplicity and complexity of needs manifested during teenage parenthood mandate close coordination among professionals from all disciplines. Pregnancy can pose serious physical and psychosocial health problems and concerns for the teenage parents, their families, and the community at large. The involved teenagers are dealing with two developmental crises, adolescence and parenthood, which may result in adverse, long-lasting psychosocial consequences if effective intervention is not available.

Medically, both the teenage mother and her baby are at high risk. Children born to teenage parents have a much higher neonatal, postnatal, and infant mortality rate. These babies have a higher incidence of prematurity, low birth weight, and respiratory distress. The mothers tend to have more physical problems throughout their pregnancy. Considering that adolescence is a period when marked physical changes and rapid growth occurs, it is understandable that the additional stress of pregnancy increases a teenage mother's susceptibility to health difficulties. Toxemia, hypertension, nutritional deficiencies, prolonged labor, pelvic disproportion, and cesarean sections are a few complications of pregnancy common to the teenage mother (Millar, 1975, p. 17).

Parenthood in adolescence can present a number of special problems. Financially, teenagers are often not able to provide for such basic needs as food, clothing, and shelter. Frequently they need assistance from social service agencies to adequately care for themselves and their children. Because they are not prepared for a career, it is difficult for them to obtain productive employment. Often a pregnant teenager drops out of school, which increases the likelihood that future employment opportunities will be limited and that social isolation from peers will occur. In addition to peer isolation, teenage parents frequently feel rejected by their families. Dependence on welfare systems, school disruption, unstable home situations, and limited peer support often result in further pregnancies outside of marriage. Every effort should be made to ensure that teenage parents, both mother and father, are able to achieve the developmental tasks of adolescence. They need counseling which will help them to deal with the role of adolescence, as well as the role of parenthood. Their families need assistance with resolving their negative feelings so that they can help their children to handle successfully their new roles. The Adolescent Health Services and Pregnancy Prevention and Care Act of 1978 will assist professionals in providing both physical and psychosocial services to teenage parents and their families. This act was passed "to establish a program for developing networks of community-based services to prevent initial and repeat pregnancies among adolescents, to provide care to pregnant adolescents, and to help adolescents become productive independent contributors to family and community life" (Hearings before the Committee on Human Resources, 1978, p. 3).

Recently, there have been studies which indicate that individual counseling with teenage parents and their families is not sufficient to prevent further, inappropriate premarital pregnancies. Dr. Lorraine Klerman suggests that current societal attitudes have a negative impact on our young men and women and need to be changed. Specifically, she has identified four major problems. First, the absence of a sense of purpose in the general society, with a resulting lack of societal goals. Second, the lack of meaningful, well-defined roles for our youth. Third, a narrowly defined role for women. And last, the lag between sexual practices and societal attitudes toward them. Dr. Klerman firmly believes that a concerted effort should be made through education and lobbying on the local, state, and national level to alter these current attitudes. She further believes that individuals in our society will continue to pursue individual purposes and pleasures, including sex, money, and drugs, until they have societal goals to which they can commit themselves (Klerman, 1975, pp. 263–264).

Venereal Disease

One alarming consequence of the increased sexual experimentation among youths is the dramatic rise in the incidence of venereal disease in this age category. As with most social problems, hard data reflect only the tip of the iceberg. Professionals frequently do not accurately report the occurrence of venereal disease, and many nonapparent subclinical infections go untreated. From estimated reports over time, however, it is apparent that venereal disease has become epidemic in recent years.

Gonorrhea, the most frequently reported venereal disease, has steadily risen since the early 1960s. In 1978 there were 1,017,045 reported cases of this disease, a 412 percent increase since 1960. Although there has been some recent overall decline in the incidence of gonorrhea (998,795 cases of gonorrhea reported in 1979), this disease continues to increase among adolescents. The highest rate of incidence of gonorrhea occurs in young adults ages 20 to 24 years, followed by youths age 15 to 19 years (Fiumara, 1976, pp. 556–557). Gay men are especially at risk for contacting venereal diseases. "Where accurate statistics are available, every major sexually transmissible disease shows rates of infection disproportionately greater in homosexual men than in heterosexual controls" ("Sexually Transmitted Diseases," 1979, p. 278).

Besides gonorrhea, there are several other sexually transmitted diseases and complications of venereal conditions which affect youth: syphilis, chancroid, trichomoniasis, genital herpes, pediculosis pubis, and pelvic inflammatory disease are a few examples. Many young people suffer serious permanent complications from these infections. Each year, for example, an estimated 75,000 women of childbearing age become sterile because of pelvic inflammatory disease (Surgeon General, 1979, p. 49). Any community health nurse working with the school-age population must realize that the occurrence of sexually transmitted diseases is a *major* health problem in this age category. Programs that provide preventive, curative, and educative services for all children in the population served by the nurse must be planned. Use of the epidemiological process (Chapter 10) and the principles of health planning (Chapter 12) will facilitate the accomplishment of such a task.

Drug Abuse

Illegal use of drugs, like sexual experimentation and venereal disease, is sharply on the rise among youth. Of particular concern is the progressive use of drugs by our younger age groups. A 1975 survey conducted by the National Institutes on Drug Abuse (NIDA) reported several increases in drug usage, especially marihuana, barbiturates, amphetamines, and cigarettes. Among male high school seniors during the years 1969 to 1975 there was a threefold increase in marihuana and amphetamine use and a fourfold increase in the use of barbiturates. Youths age 12 to 17 increased their usage of marihuana from 14 percent in 1972 to 23 percent in 1974. Smoking of cigarettes in this same time period for this age category increased from 17 percent to 25 percent. In 1972 only 10 percent of youths age 14 to 15 years admitted to having some experience with marihuana. By 1974, this figure had more than doubled; 22 percent of the 14- to 15-year-olds admitted to some marihuana experience. These statistics are extremely significant because further evidence suggests that experimentation with cigarettes, alcohol, and marihuana frequently establishes a regular pattern for long-term usage of these drugs (Public Health Service, 1977, p. 13). One teenager in 20 has a drinking problem (White House Conference on Families, 1978, p. 562).

Drug usage varies among school-age populations across the country, but most schools consider drug usage to be on an upswing. Some schools report that only 2 percent of the students in their schools use drugs, whereas others report as high as a 65 percent usage. Evidence seems to indicate that the East Coast has a worse problem than the West Coast. One thing is certain, there is no community devoid of illegal drug usage by their youth. As with other major health problems, it is important for health professionals to survey the extent of the problem in their local community. It has been found that drug surveys conducted by the students themselves are often more accurate than those conducted by professionals (Winkel, 1974, pp. 1 and 4).

The growth in the amount of smoking among the preadult age group is thought to be due to a dramatic increase in smoking among teenage girls (National Institute of Child Health and Human Development, 1979, p. 7). The factors contributing to the increase in illegal drug usage are not as clear. One key variable, however, is availability (Winkel, 1974, p. 2). As long as illegal drugs are accessible, they will be abused. Some youth will experiment because it is the "in thing" to do. There have been studies which show that some teenagers are at high risk for drug usage and that certain family characteristics increase the probability that a teenager will use drugs. Blum (1972, pp. 93–94) reports that high-risk middle-class children come from families where alcohol is consumed, prescription and over-the-counter medications are used, permissive attitudes exist, and religion, respect for authority, child rearing, and self-control are not emphasized.

Children frequently resort to taking drugs to escape poor home environments and unhappy social situations. They use drugs to mask such feelings as sadness, boredom, hopelessness, fear, and anger. Children from homes where there is a lack of affection and discipline need extra attention and support from adults outside their home environment so that their psychosocial developmental needs will be met through supportive relationships rather than through drug usage. In order to provide the type of support needed by these youth, community health nurses must have an understanding of the dynamics associated with drug usage as well as knowledge about the developmental characteristics of this age group. Health professionals who specialize in working with clients who are drug abusers are very valuable resource persons and should be consulted when one is having difficulty handling drug problems.

DEVELOPMENTAL CHARACTERISTICS OF SCHOOL-AGE CHILDREN

Stuffed rabbit
Seven years my nocturnal security
Now neglected worn and eyeless

Lying in the memory-choked attic
Stabbed by blunt dusty shafts of sunlight
Recalling to me

Evenings of forbidden play beneath giggle-
   muffling blankets
Recalling to me the day that I grew
Too big
Too old
To sleep with innocence while hugging security.
   I'll leave you here stuffed rabbit,
   You're dead
But God, what a long slow funeral we're having!

Gregory Smith, written at age 18

All school-age children must accomplish certain developmental tasks to achieve happiness and self-fulfillment. The author of "Stuffed Rabbit," above, was describing the overall task of adolescence: "relinquishing a child's life-style and attaining an adult life-style" (Nicholson, 1980, p. 11). He was giving up secure patterns of behavior to achieve emotional independence.

Social scientists such as Duvall, Erikson, Havighurst, Freud, Piaget, and Sullivan have provided professionals with a variety of ways in which to explain human development. Havighurst's psychosocial framework seems particularly relevant for community health nurses who work with school-age children from various backgrounds because he discusses how social and cultural factors influence the growth process. His ideas are found in the text *Developmental Tasks and Education* (1972).

To work effectively with all age groups, community health nurses must have knowledge of normal growth and development processes. They must also understand how these processes affect families as well as individuals. When children, for example, become increasingly independent of parents and seek support and advice from others (peers, teachers, significant adults outside the home), parents can experience a great deal of anxiety. During these times they may need reassurance that they are not "losing" their children and an opportunity to express feelings of frustration and fear of failing as a parent. Supportive

intervention can help parents to cope successfully with stresses associated with normal growth and development.

When working with children, it is critical for all health care professionals to observe for lags in normal growth and development. Early case finding and intervention can prevent permanent disability. A comprehensive biopsychosocial and cultural assessment should be done with every child and family when the child is not performing at the appropriate developmental age level. Intervention should be started immediately if a developmental disability is confirmed.

Developmental Disabilities

Developmental disabilities are increasingly identified among our school-age children. It was estimated by the United States Office of Education in 1976 that 6.7 million children ages 6 to 19 years were handicapped by developmental disabilities (Siantz, 1977, p. 4). As of 1978, the definition for this term is found in Public Law 95-602, which reads as follows (Rehab Group, Incorporated, 1979, p. 120):

"Developmental disability" means a severe, chronic disability of a person which—

a) is attributable to a mental or physical impairment or a combination of mental and physical impairments;

b) is manifested before the person attains age 22;

c) is likely to continue indefinitely;

d) results in substantial functional limitations in three or more of the following areas of major life activity;

    i. self-care
    ii. receptive and expressive language
    iii. learning
    iv. mobility
    v. self-direction
    vi. capacity for independent living, and
    vii. economic sufficiency; and

e) reflects the person's need for a combination and sequence of special, interdisciplinary, or generic care, treatment, or other services which are of lifelong or extended duration and are individually planned and coordinated.

The major life activity for individuals ages 3 through 17 is learning or school (Boggs and Henney, 1979, p. 4). Studies estimate that as many as 9 to 20 percent of all school-age children have a learning disability (Williams, 1976, p. 515). Problems such as mental retardation, "learning disabilities," cerebral palsy, epilepsy, blindness, autism and other emotional difficulties, speech impairments, orthopedic difficulties, and deafness can affect a child's learning abilities.

As with average children, the degree to which children with developmental disabilities adjust successfully as healthy individuals varies. The nature and quality of their previous and current life experiences and their physical, emotional, and cognitive status greatly influence how well children with developmental disabilities progress. Typically, these children have different life experiences from average children and these differences are weighted in a negative direction. Clinical experience reveals that often children with developmental disabilities have deficient socializing experiences, both in quantity and quality, during childhood (Clemen and Pattullo, 1980, p. 197).

There are numerous variables that affect the socioadaptive capacity of children with developmental disabilities. Garrard (1960, p. 150) illustrated the interdependence of these variables when he discussed the needs of the adolescent with mental retardation. His findings are graphically shown in Figure 14-4. An overwhelming number of the factors depicted are influenced by environmental conditions. Few of them are inherent in the child, immutable to change (Clemen and Pattullo, 1980, p. 226).

Despite the passage of the Public Law 94-142 bill, Education for All Handicapped Children Act, on November 29, 1975, there are still many children who are not receiving the services they need to develop to their fullest potential (Figure 14-5). The states presented in Figure 14-5 have the greatest number of unserved children because they have a relatively large proportion of children who need services. Most states show the potential for serving more children in each disability area (U.S. Bureau of Education for the Handicapped, 1979, pp. 24–25). It is extremely important for health professionals to assume an advocacy role when they identify that children with handicapping conditions are not receiving the health services they need. Parents should be informed of their rights, including the mandates of Public Law 94-142.

Public Law 94-142 mandates that all handicapped children from 3 to 21 years of age be provided a free education. School systems which do not have appropriate diagnostic and therapeutic facilities and personnel are legally bound to purchase whatever is required. In addition to full educational opportunities, the other rights covered by this law are as follows:

1. Due process safeguards which assist parents in challenging decisions regarding their children

2. Education in the mainstream to the fullest extent possible

3. Assurance that tests and other evaluation materials do not reflect cultural or racial bias

4. A "child-find" plan to identify all children within the state who have special needs

Some states, such as Michigan, are even more progressive when it comes to planning services for handicapped children. The Michigan Mandatory Education law stipulates that each local school district is responsible for meeting the educational needs of handicapped persons from birth to 25 years of age. Readers

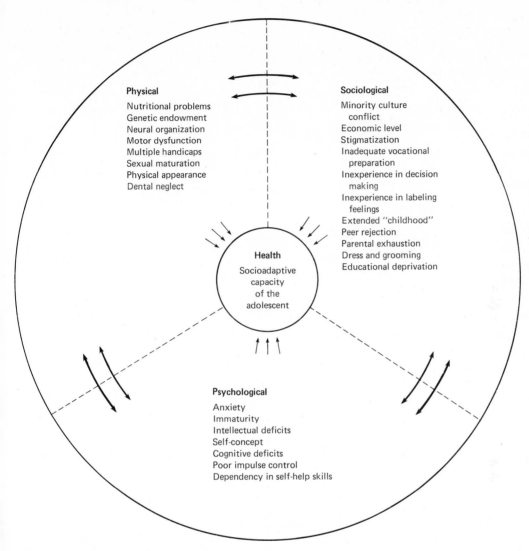

FIGURE 14-4 Factors influencing the health and socioadaptive capacity of the adolescent with mental retardation. (*Adapted from Fig. 12, Concept of multiple causation in mental retardation, in Sperling D. Garrard, Mental retardation in adolescence, Pediatric Clinics of North America, February 1960, 7(1), p. 150; by S. Clemen & A. Pattullo, The adolescent with mental retardation, in J. Howe, Nursing Care of the Adolescent, New York: McGraw-Hill, 1980, p. 226.*)

should become knowledgeable about both state and federal legislation in order to accurately inform parents of their rights.

Children with developmental disabilities, like all school-age children, need organized, comprehensive community health services designed to foster optimal growth. The coordi-

nation of services between professional disciplines cannot be overemphasized. No one community system can provide the entire spectrum of services needed by the school-age population. Lack of coordination results in duplication of efforts, inefficient use of time and energies, inconsistent messages, and deficien-

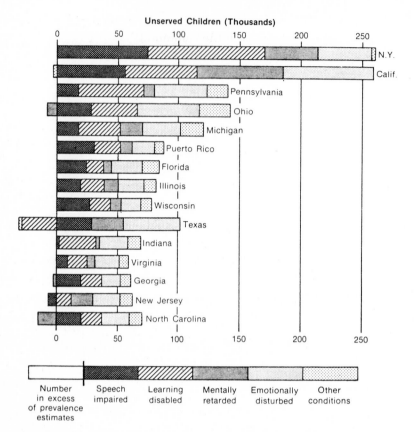

FIGURE 14-5 Potential number of unserved children in 15 states, school year 1977–1978. Fifteen highest states ranked by net unserved. The data displayed include handicapped children counted under Public Laws 89-313 and 94-142. *(From Bureau of Education for the Handicapped. Progress toward a free appropriate public education: A report to Congress on the implementation of Public Law 94-142: The education for all handicapped children act. Washington, D.C.: U.S. Department of Health, Education, and Welfare, January 1979, p. 25.)*

cies in services. One community health nurse, for example, visited a family who had a newborn infant with Down's syndrome. The nurse referred the family to the intermediate school district for diagnostic and follow-up services. The physical therapist, the occupational therapist, and the psychologist from this special service division of the educational system visited the family to assess their needs. Although each of these disciplines provided a valuable

service, it was difficult for the family to work with all of them. Alert intervention on the part of the community health nurse kept the family from rejecting the offered services.

Since most children attend school, the school is a logical environment in which to promote the health of all children. The components of an effective school health program will be elaborated on below. The reader should remember, however, that health services rendered in the school environment should be viewed within the context of the broader community. School health cannot be separated from the ecological and social conditions of the home and the community.

SCHOOL HEALTH PROGRAM

As early as 1850, the importance of health promotion activities in the school environment was stressed. At that time, Lemuel Shattuck (1850, pp. 178–179) wrote the following:

Every child should be taught, early in life, that, to preserve his own life and his own health and the lives and health of others, is one of his most important and constantly abiding duties. Some measure is needed which shall compel children to make a sanitary examination of themselves and their associates, and thus elicit a practical application of the lessons of sanitary science in the everyday duties of life. The recommendation now under consideration is designed to furnish this measure. It is to be carried into operation in the use of a blank schedule, which is to be printed on a letter sheet, in the form prescribed in the appendix, and furnished to the teacher of each school. He is to appoint a sanitary committee of the scholars, at the commencement of school, and, on the first day of each month, to fill it out under his superintendence. . . . Such a measure is simple, would take a few minutes each day, and cannot operate otherwise than usefully upon the children, in forming habits of exact observation, and in making a personal application of the laws of health and life to themselves. This is education of an eminently practical character, and of the highest importance.

There are several key concepts delineated in Shattuck's writings which have relevancy for current school health practices. Specifically, the following ideas extracted from Shattuck's comments are important to consider when establishing a school health program:

1. All citizens have the responsibility to preserve life and promote health in the community. In order to assume this responsibility, lay persons as well as health professionals need *knowledge* (sanitary sciences) and an opportunity to *apply* health principles in daily living situations. It is both logical and useful to help children in the school setting to learn healthy habits of functioning, because children spend a considerable amount of time in this environment.

2. "Sanitary examination" can prevent spread of communicable disease. Even though there has been a drastic reduction in the incidence of communicable conditions, school-age children are still very susceptible to these conditions because they are constantly exposed to them and are in environmental situations that support the spread of agents (see Chapter 10). Whenever a large number of individuals are confined in a limited space, such as a school environment, the likelihood of transmission of disease from one individual to another increases. The significance of sanitary examinations in the school setting should not be underestimated. It is also important to recognize that lay persons (children, parents, and school personnel) can learn how to observe for signs and symptoms of illness. Health care professionals do not have to routinely conduct sanitary examinations. Their time can be better spent in helping others to care for themselves.

3. Health education is an appropriate function for the school system because it provides children with skills that assist them to func-

tion effectively in society and to meet their individual health care needs. Educational curricula should be designed so that learners obtain the knowledge and skills necessary to cope adequately with the demands and stresses of situations they will be encountering after leaving the educational environment. Individuals must handle health matters constantly throughout life.

4. A "sanitary committee" or health council should be used to monitor the effectiveness of the school health program. Without such a committee, it is often found that the health component of school services is neglected.

Today, comprehensive school health programs incorporate Shattuck's ideas as well as several other activities aimed at promoting healthful living. Modern school health activities are divided into three basic interrelated categories: (1) health services, (2) health education, and (3) healthy school environment. In order to provide all the services discussed under these three categories, a school system must develop mechanisms that will facilitate interdisciplinary teamwork. Interdisciplinary coordination and collaboration is the key to successful implementation of a comprehensive school health program.

Health Services

School health services are designed to protect and promote the health of all students and all school personnel. The type of health services needed in a school setting will vary from community to community, depending on the availability of other community resources and the characteristics of the population being served. Prior to developing a school health program, health professionals, school personnel, and community citizens should jointly study the needs of their community in order to identify what specific health services should be provided in the school environment. School health services should not duplicate community services already accessible and acceptable to community citizens. Rather, they should augment community services so that the comprehensive health care needs of the school-age population are met. If, for example, a community has a shortage of physicians or families cannot afford preventive health examinations for their children, physical examination services may be provided in the school setting. In some school settings, however, these services may not be needed because the community has an adequate number of physicians or sufficient clinic services or because families are financially stable.

Regardless of the resources available in the community, certain basic health services should be provided in all school systems. Procedures should be established to meet the following objectives to detect and treat health problems which might be impeding a child's learning and to ensure that emergency health care needs are adequately handled.

1. To appraise the health status of students and school personnel on a continual basis

2. To counsel students, parents, teachers, and others regarding appraisal findings

3. To encourage health care to correct remediable defects

4. To provide emergency care for injury or sudden illness

5. To prevent and control infectious diseases

6. To identify children with handicapping conditions and to arrange for educational programs that will enhance the maximum potential of these children

To accomplish these objectives health education, health promotion, and environmental inspection activities must be integrated. Having one person in the school system responsible for coordinating this integration is essential.

Health Education

Health education is a process that helps people to make sound decisions about personal health practices and about individual, family, and community well-being. Knowledge alone does not necessarily foster appropriate health habits. In order to facilitate effective decision making in health matters, the school system should provide every child with the opportunity to acquire *knowledge* essential for understanding healthy functioning, to develop *attitudes* that foster preventive health behaviors, and to establish health *practices* conducive to effective living (Anderson, 1972, p. 223; and Stone and Rubinson, 1979, pp. 45, 48). To achieve these goals, the child, the family, and the community must be involved in the educational process. This is essential because the development of sound health habits is influenced by a variety of forces including societal norms, beliefs and attitudes of significant others, and the internal motivations and beliefs of the individual.

A *planned* series of *integrated* health educational activities based on input received from students, parents, community citizens, health care professionals, and educators is needed to ensure that health education will become an integral component of a school's curriculum. Informal health counseling with individual students and special health projects such as "know your heart" and "maturational processes" are valuable but can never adequately prepare children to make sound decisions about all the personal, family, and community health needs they will encounter. Special health projects usually have a narrow focus. When only this instructional modality is used to disseminate information about health and health-related phenomena, students become very knowledgeable about certain health needs, such as dental hygiene and nutritional requirements, but learn very little about other relevant health issues.

Unfortunately, too many school districts rely on uncoordinated, incidental methods when planning ways to handle health education in their curricula. Teachers are often requested to cover specific health topics throughout the year, but frequently they are unaware of the health content that has been presented to their students in previous years. When this happens, some concepts are repeated from one year to another and others are not covered at all. A 1967 health education project initiated by the Connecticut State Board of Education substantiated this point and also identified that students at all grade levels want health education (Byler, 1969, p. 170). The book *Teach Us What We Want to Know* summarizes the results of this 1967 project. Anyone planning health education for school-age children will find relevant guidelines for curriculum planning in this text.

Curriculum planning for health instruction is the responsibility of all professionals in the school system. The school nurse is often asked to assume a major role in organizing health education activities. A school nurse's educational preparation and clinical experience and contact with the community puts her or him in a favorable position for understanding the essential concepts of health and illness and for coordinating activities between the school and the community. It is crucial to remember, however, that a school nurse alone cannot implement a sound health education program. Without administrative support and active involvement of all teachers, it would be impossible to achieve appropriate selection and sequencing of health content throughout the grade levels or to obtain sufficient time for health educational activities.

When planning a health education curriculum, it is beneficial to have a conceptual framework for organizing the selection and sequencing of all health education activities. Many school systems throughout the United States have found the concept-oriented approach developed by the School Health Education Study in the 1960s a useful framework (Stone and Rubinson, 1979, p. 63). This study group identified 10 key concepts that should be emphasized at all grade levels. These concepts, along with subconcepts, long-range goals, and behavioral objectives for kindergarten through grade 12, are delineated in *Health Education: A Conceptual Approach to Curriculum Designs for Grades Kindergarten through Twelve* (1967). Information presented in this text provides a valuable framework for organizing curriculum-development activities. To be effectively used, however, teachers as well as health care professionals must understand the concepts being presented and must be adequately prepared to teach content related to these concepts.

Health educational activities in the school system should be aimed at promoting both physiological and psychosocial functioning. Students must be helped to analyze how normal growth and development progresses and to discuss their needs in relation to the maturational process. They should also be assisted in seeing how ineffective health practices can be altered and how they can prevent physical and psychosocial distress. In addition, it is important for children to learn how environmental forces affect the health status of all community citizens and to identify ways to promote healthy community functioning.

Healthy School Environment

Environmental factors that affect the health and well-being of children in the school setting are numerous. Psychosocial as well as physical aspects of the environment need to be monitored to ensure an optimal setting for student learning. "Healthful school living . . . embraces all efforts to provide at school, physical, emotional, and social conditions which are beneficial to the health and safety of pupils. It includes the provision of a safe and healthful physical environment, the organization of a healthful school day, and the establishment of interpersonal relationships favorable to mental health" (Joint Committee on Health Problems in Education, 1964, p. 2).

A healthful school environment has the following features:

1. An architectural design which takes into consideration the developmental characteristics of the population being served and the needs of the instructional program

2. A comfortable environment that has adequate seating, lighting, heating, ventilation, toilet facilities and drinking fountains

3. An organized safety program, including provisions for emergency care and adequate transportation

4. An established mechanism to ensure safe, sanitary conditions

5. A recreational program that allows all students to participate

6. A planned schedule of school activities which takes into account the physical and psychosocial needs of children at varying grade levels

7. An organized school lunch program which provides nutritious foods, adequate time for good personal hygiene, and sufficient facilities for comfortable eating

8. An established program that provides psychosocial counseling and consultation services for staff and students

No one professional discipline can plan and implement all the services described in the above three dimensional components—health services, health education, healthy school environment—of a total school health program. The role of nursing in the school setting will be described below. The reader should keep in mind, however, that effective teamwork is essential for successful school health programming.

THE ROLE OF THE COMMUNITY HEALTH NURSE IN THE SCHOOL HEALTH PROGRAM

Since the turn of the century when Lillian Wald placed Lina Rogers, the first school nurse, in the New York City schools, the role of nursing in the school health program has been evolving. Control of communicable disease is no longer the primary focus of nursing service. It is now recognized that the school nurse has a significant contribution to make in all aspects of the total school health program. The American Nurses' Association, in 1966, identified 20 functions and 83 related activities for staff-level school nurses (ANA, 1966, pp. 4–14). These functions and activities were designed to enhance the educability of all school-age children and to improve the health of all citizens in the United States. They were developed to ensure that the ANA's philosophy of school nursing, which follows, would be implemented in the school setting.

Philosophy of School Nursing

School nursing is a highly specialized service contributing to the process of education. That it is a socially commendable, economically practical, and scientifically sound service can be well demonstrated. It must be diligently pursued through health and educational avenues to the end that positive health among all the citizenry of this country will be a reality.

The professional nurse with her experience and knowledge of the changing growth and behavioral patterns of children is in a unique position in the school setting to assist the children in acquiring health knowledge, in developing attitudes conducive to healthful living, and in meeting their needs resulting from disease, accidents, congenital defects, or psychosocial maladjustments.

Nursing provided as part of a school program for children is a direct, constructive, and effective approach to the building of a healthful and dynamic society. (ANA, 1966, p.1. Reprinted by permission of ANA.)

School nursing is an exciting, rewarding field of nursing practice which provides numerous opportunities for creative, independent functioning. There are currently over 20,000 nurses who are members of a school health team (ANA, 1976, p. 20). Needs of the population being served, community resources, and patterns for delivery of service influence how each of these nurses functions.

Patterns for Providing School Nursing Services

Two administrative patterns are currently being used to provide nursing services in the school setting: specialized and generalized. Specialized services are provided by school nurses who are employed by the board of education. These nurses are accountable to school administrators and only work with the school-age population. Some health departments are developing special school-health units within the health department. These specialized school nurses would be accountable to the community health nursing director. Generalized services are provided by community health nurses hired by health departments or visiting nurse associations. These nurses function part-time in the school setting as part of a generalized community health nursing program. They work with all at-risk populations in their assigned area.

There is a great deal of controversy about which pattern for delivering school nursing services is most appropriate. Clinical experience has shown that both patterns can be effective. Mechanisms must be established, however, to ensure that:

· The school nurse is a sanctioned member of the school health team

· Health care for the school-age child is provided within the context of the family and the community

· The nurse serving the school-age population has an understanding of the health needs and the growth and development characteristic of the school-age child

· School health services are adequately financed by the community

· The school nurse has professional nursing supervision

The activities of generalized and specialized school nurses vary among school systems. Unfortunately, there are still many educational systems that use the nurse only to provide first aid and emergency care. A school nurse who is able to clearly articulate her or his role and functions and who demonstrates clinical expertise to all members of the school health team is more likely to be used appropriately than one who has trouble defining what it is a school nurse has to offer.

Functions of the Nurse on the School Health Team

School nurses frequently have difficulty defining what it is they have to contribute to the school health team and, thus, they are often used in a very narrow context. Traditionally, nurses are seen as the professionals who provide first aid, give injections, inspect for communicable disease, or counsel dirty children.

In any school system, the nurse must sell what she or he has to offer by demonstrating that these traditional views of nursing are very limited and not an effective way to use a nurse's talents. Described below are the various functions a nurse should implement in the school setting. Clinical experience has shown that professionals from other disciplines have a greater respect for school nurses who assume functions beyond the traditionally defined ones than for school nurses who limit their functioning to the provision of routine physical health care.

Advocacy. There still are too many school-age children who are not receiving the health care they deserve. Outreach to assist families to more effectively enter the health care system and a reevaluation of the methods for delivering services to children are needed if this trend is to be changed. Every professional, including the school nurse, must speak out for our children.

The nurse in the school setting is in a prime position to identify children who have health needs and who need more effective health care services. The school nurse must take the initiative to help the families of these children to obtain medical, socioeconomic, and emotional counseling on a continuous basis. If services are lacking, the school nurse should become actively involved in influencing funders to allocate monies for such services. It is known, for instance, that developmentally the adolescent has different needs from younger school-age children. Often, however, community services that specifically address the needs of the adolescent are lacking or inadequate. A concerned school nurse will have knowledge about the factors that affect an adolescent's use of health care (Table 14-5) and will take action to promote the development of programs designed to meet the unique needs of this developmental age group.

The school nurse should be an advocate for

TABLE 14-5 Determinants in Health Care Sought by Adolescents

Factors	Perception	Response or action
MEDICAL		
1. Actual perceived need	By adolescent	Adolescent seeks care
2. Perceived need	By family/others	Care recommended
3. Unclarified problem definition	By adolescent or by others	Randomized selection of "appropriate" service
4. Perceived threat	By adolescent	Avoidance of care
SOCIAL/ECONOMIC		
1. Age variation:		
Early adolescence	By parents	Parent seeks care
Late adolescence	By adolescents	Self-determination
2. Family background	Living unit norms	Family assessment of priority
3. Ethnic and racial background		
4. Peer group	Group norm	Group perception of service
5. Sex		
6. Place of residence	By community	Geographic access to service
7. Educational background	Classroom norm	Available knowledge of services
8. Income level	Ability to pay	Seek/avoid care
PSYCHOLOGIC		
1. The process of adolescence	Dependent upon maturational level	
2. Prior health experience	Positive/negative	
3. Prior emotional crisis resolutions	Adaptive/maladaptive	
4. Prior painful experiences	Acceptance/avoidance	Seek/avoid care
5. Parental dependence	Self-reliance/dependence	
6. Level of perception of problem	Realistic concern/fear	
7. Control	Internal/external locus	
8. Response to figures of authority	Compliance/rebellion	

SOURCE: From J. R. Gallagher, F. Heald, & D. Garell. *Medical Care of the Adolescent* (3d ed.). New York: Appleton-Century-Crofts, 1976, p. 748.

needed health services within the school system as well as within the community. It is not uncommon for the school nurse to identify environmental conditions that are unsafe, or gaps in the health education programs, or deficiencies in the delivery of personal health services. These situations must not be ignored by the school nurse because they may prevent children from reaching their maximum potential.

In order for the school nurse to successfully carry out the advocacy function in the school setting, the legal issues involved in delivering care to children must be understood. The nurse must also be knowledgeable about legislative programs that finance health care services for our youth.

Since laws and health services vary from one state to another, every nurse functioning in the school setting should become familiar with those that exist in his or her state. There are, however, some basic issues which all nurses must deal with when working with school-age children. Specifically, issues related to parental consent for the health care of minors, confidentiality in relation to the health record, laws requiring the reporting of child abuse and neglect, and legislation which mandates that children with special needs have equal educational opportunities should be examined carefully.

School-age children are minors. Parental consent is generally necessary for minors to receive health care treatment for such things as immunizations, medical treatment by a physician, and special psychological testing for learning difficulties. Children may be treated by a physician in any emergency situation without parental consent. Since, however, it is very difficult to establish what constitutes an emergency, every school should develop policies that deal with emergency situations. An emergency consent form which includes the following information should be on file for each child:

- Child's full name, address, and telephone number
- Where to reach the parents during school hours
- Who to call if the parents cannot be reached
- The name, address, and telephone number of the child's family physician
- The family's preference for hospital care
- Insurance or Medicaid numbers
- Any known allergies or chronic health problems of the child

- Parent's consent for ambulance transportation

In addition to the emergency form, every school should have a teacher who is designated as the school's primary first-aid person. This is crucial because the school nurse is often responsible for serving many school buildings and thus is frequently not available when emergencies occur. The permanent staff member assigned the responsibility for handling emergency first aid should take refresher first-aid courses as needed.

The parental consent regulations were designed to protect the rights of minors. It is increasingly recognized that children, especially adolescents, have not had access to certain health care services because they could not or would not obtain parental consent. Thus, many states have changed their laws so that minors who are emancipated or sufficiently mature to understand the consequences of their decision can obtain certain types of health care treatment without parental consent. Age stipulations for when minors can seek help on their own varies from state to state.

Laws that allow minors to seek medical treatment without parental consent usually relate to human sexuality problems, drug abuse, and mental health services. Every state now allows minors to receive medical treatment for venereal disease on their own. Several states permit physicians to diagnose pregnancy and to provide prenatal care for minors without parental knowledge. Confidential contraceptive services are available to minors in many states. Only a few states, however, have laws which stipulate that minors can obtain assistance for drug abuse or mental health problems without parental consent (Hoekelman, Blatman, Brunell, Friedman, and Seidel, 1978, pp. 526–527).

Health laws and educational laws are not necessarily the same. Youth, for instance, may receive health education relative to contraceptive practices in a medical clinic but may not be allowed to receive this same information in the educational setting. Professionals providing health care services must learn how both health and educational laws influence their practice in a particular state. Health care professionals should be advocates for change if these laws do not agree with their philosophy of professional practice.

Confidentiality in relation to a client's health record is a legal issue that concerns every health care provider in the school system. Indiscriminate sharing of school records has resulted in the passage of the Family Privacy and Education Act of 1974. This act mandates "that parents of students under 18 years of age, attending educational institutions receiving federal funds, may view their child's educational records on request and may seek expungement or correction of false or inaccurate entries. No information can be released outside of the school setting without proper parental authorization. This right devolves on students themselves once they become 18" (Hofmann, 1978, p. 531). Generalized school nurses are technically not official members of the school system, which could present a problem when they need to use the school records. Some school systems have coped with this dilemma by adopting a policy which makes the generalized school nurse an official member of the school staff.

Besides the Family Privacy and Education Act of 1974, there are several other pieces of federal legislation that influence the delivery of health care services to the school-age population. Most of these have already been described in Chapter 13 or other sections of this chapter: Medicaid, EPSDT, maternal child health, family planning, dental health, and crippled children's laws all provide funding for essential child health services. The Child Nutrition Act of 1966 and the National School Lunch Act are other federal legislative acts that provide funds for child health services. They were passed to improve the nutritional

status of children from low socioeconomic homes. Monies were allocated to strengthen and expand food lunch programs in the school setting. Unfortunately, youth who should be benefitting from these programs are not. Many families do not apply for free lunch assistance because the procedure for determining eligibility is often complex and confusing and their children may be discriminated against when they do receive free lunches (Bremner, 1974, p. 1456). A concerned school nurse should work to alter this situation if it exists in the school system in which she or he is functioning. By helping others to see the correlation between poor nutrition and illness, the community health nurse may influence people in power to support a process that facilitates rather than hinders use of federal school-lunch monies.

The Child Abuse and Neglect Act, the Education for All Handicapped Children Act, the School Age Mother and Child Acts, and Adolescent Health Services, and Pregnancy Prevention and Care Act, all of which were previously discussed, were passed to protect the rights of high-risk children. School personnel must report suspected abuse or neglect to the legal authorities. They must also provide educational services for all handicapped children and pregnant mothers if they desire to remain in school.

State as well as federal legislation is written to promote and protect the health of school-age children. Compulsory school attendance acts, immunization requirements before school entry, legislation in relation to health education in the school system, and laws that exclude ill children are some examples of state legislation that assist children to reach their optimal health status.

A knowledge of federal and state laws helps school nurses to speak out on behalf of children when services are not being provided. Laws also provide legal backing for encouraging parents to assume responsibility for acting in the best interest of their children. In addition, laws require health professionals to carry out an advocacy function when they identify that the rights of children are being abused.

Case finding. "Every child has a right to have an education which will meet his individualized needs and to have care and treatment for handicapping conditions so that he can learn more effectively" (1930 Children's Charter). Case finding is essential if these goals are to be accomplished. All personnel in the school system have a responsibility to identify as early as possible children at risk for physical, behavioral, social, or academic disabilities.

The school nurse uses a variety of methods for identifying at-risk children. Observing their appearance and behavior during their daily school activities is one way to quickly discern which students need more extensive follow-up. Many orthopedic problems, for example, have been picked up by an alert school nurse who has watched children in the school setting walk down the hall during recess. Eating lunch in the school cafeteria has helped other school nurses to identify children with poor dietary habits. Walking out on the playground during recess frequently assists school nurses in determining which children are having difficulty relating with their peers.

Incidental observations like those mentioned above are extremely valuable, but they do not replace the need for periodic, systematic health observations. The school nurse should meet with every teacher in the school system to encourage them to observe on a regular basis the health status of all students in the classroom. Teachers are the key persons in a health appraisal program. Their position in the classroom setting provides them with frequent opportunities to make significant observations of each child's health status. The school nurse can help to enhance a teacher's observational skills by discussing signs and symptoms of illness, by developing teacher

health observational forms, and by responding to teachers' concerns about a particular child's health. In-service programs for all teachers in the school system can also sharpen teachers' observational skills. One school nurse, for instance, noted a significant increase in the number of student referrals from teachers after she showed the film *Looking at Children* to the faculty in one of her elementary schools. This film was developed by Metropolitan Life Insurance Company for the purpose of promoting improved observations of children by teachers. There is no rental charge for its use and a supplementary reference pamphlet, *Looking for Health,* is also provided at no cost by Metropolitan Life.

Teachers' concerns should be taken seriously, because they observe children daily and they are likely to identify abnormal behaviors more quickly than any other member of the school health team. The authors' clinical experiences have dramatically supported this statement. One of the authors, for example, received a referral from a kindergarten teacher because a pupil in her classroom looked anemic. The teacher was also concerned because it took this child longer than most children to get up after a fall on the playground. The child was seen by his family physician and found to have a congenital heart defect, a condition that had never been diagnosed before even though the child had been seen regularly by medical personnel.

Planned comprehensive screening sessions are another way to systematically observe a child's health status. School nurses should see that such programs are developed, but they do not necessarily need to conduct all screening tests themselves. Hearing and vision technicians, school aides, teachers, social workers, nutritionists, and all other members of the health team can play a vital role in a screening program. Height and weight measurements, hearing and vision tests, dental examinations, and immunization checks have traditionally been conducted in the school settings. Recently, in many school settings, a more comprehensive screening is being done to identify children at risk. In addition to the traditional procedures, screening for scoliosis, urinary tract infections, anemia, and psychosocial difficulties is being done. Identifying the characteristics of the population being served will help the community health nurse to determine what type of screening program to initiate in the school setting in which she or he is working. Remember, though, when analyzing population data, that children from all socioeconomic backgrounds have health problems which may not be obvious to them or their families. One middle-class mother who was a nurse was very appreciative of the school's vision screening program after her 6-year-old daughter was found to have serious visual difficulties. The mother reported to the school nurse after her daughter obtained glasses that for the first time her daughter was able to see leaves on the trees. Without glasses, this 6-year-old child could only see large masses in her environment. Her mother felt bad that her daughter's eye problem had not been detected sooner.

Screening programs have identified many students in the school setting who have health problems. It is a waste of time and money to screen for defects, however, if follow-up health activities are neglected. Follow-up is a school nurse's most important function in a screening program. The school nurse can direct families to appropriate agencies for diagnostic, treatment, and rehabilitation services and can find funds for these services if necessary. The Lion's Club, for instance, frequently provides funds for glasses when the client is of school age.

Contact with students in the health clinic as well as reviewing of school records are other methods school nurses use to identify high-risk children. The school nurse should be alert to problems other than the stated concern when a child visits the health clinic. Orthopedic, vision, dental, and relationship difficulties are often identified while the nurse is putting on an adhesive bandage or comforting a crying child. Previously in this chapter, the problems of teenage parents were discussed. Too often the needs of the father are neglected. When a pregnant, unwed teenage mother visits the health clinic, the school nurse should not forget that there is another person involved in this girl's situation: single teenage fathers do need help. The school nurse can frequently help a teenage father by discussing with the mother the feelings that he might be experiencing and the services available to him for verbalizing his concerns. The nurse can also meet with the father in the clinic or home setting to identify what type of assistance he needs. In a study conducted by one social agency, it was found that 92 percent of their unwed mothers were willing to share the name of their child's father when a matter-of-fact approach was used to solicit this information (Pannor and Evans, 1975, p. 288).

Record reviews help the school nurse to discern those children who should be talked with in the school setting or families that should be visited in the home. Frequently a school nurse identifies significant health problems that should be discussed with both school personnel and families when examining school entry physicals. One school nurse, for example, noted that a kindergarten child's blood pressure was extremely high. Follow-up revealed several interesting facts: (1) the physician thought that this child's blood pressure was elevated because he was anxious about seeing a physician; (2) the child's father had hypertension; and (3) the teacher had noted that the child's ears turned bright red with physical exertion. This child was indeed hypertensive and is now under the care of a cardiac specialist, because the school nurse took the time to review health records and did not ignore health problems identified during this review.

Review of absenteeism records, along with

health records, is another way of identifying high-risk children. Studies have shown that students who are frequently absent from school have a high prevalence of health problems and are at risk for future illnesses and absenteeism. These studies have also demonstrated that families of children who have many absences from school have several health concerns (Basco, Eyres, Glasser, and Roberts, 1972; Densen, Ullman, Jones, and Vandow, 1970; and Long, Whitman, Johansson, Williams, and Tuthill, 1975). Preventive intervention services may help families as well as children when a nurse intervenes with children at risk for high absenteeism. Helping families is probably the best way to help their children. Referring them to community resources, for instance, may help these families to meet their basic human needs for clothing, shelter, and food. This, in turn, could reduce the number of illnesses experienced by their children because children usually do not function well when their nutrition is inadequate.

High-risk children are present in any school system. When school nurses discover that they are spending all of their time providing first-aid services, they should carefully evaluate their nursing practice. School nurses must regularly determine if steps have been taken to identify children in need. Sitting in the health clinic is not an effective way of delivering nursing services in the school setting.

Community liaison activities. Some of the most important factors that the school nurse must consider when working with school-age children are the beliefs, values, and resources of the community where these children reside. The health status of individuals is greatly affected by the beliefs and values which exist in the home and the community and by health resources which are available to meet their needs. The interrelationship between all of these variables cannot be ignored when health programs are being planned to resolve problems encountered by the school-age population. The problems of venereal disease and teenage pregnancies, for example, can be dealt with in the school setting only when the values and beliefs present in the home and the community allow this to happen.

School nurses have more opportunities than other school personnel to unite all of these variables. They have the freedom and flexibility to visit families in their homes and to coordinate services between the home, the school, and other community agencies. Viewing the health status of children at school often provides school nurses with data necessary for identifying health priorities and needs in the community. Health needs of school-age children tend to reflect needs of the community in general. When children lack dental care, for instance, this is frequently so because there are limited community services to meet their dental needs.

School nurses must engage in community liaison activities in order to meet the needs of all school-age children. No school system has adequate resources to handle all the health problems experienced by the children it serves. Cooperative planning and collaboration between the educational system and other community agencies who are assisting children can only serve to enhance the effectiveness of the school's total health program.

Community involvement should be sought by the school nurse during all stages of the health-planning process. Health programs conducted at school which fulfill health needs as identified by the community are far more successful than programs that ignore community priorities. Perceptions of health problems differ from community to community. Community problems as identified by one rural school district and one urban school district in the state of South Carolina are presented in Table 14-6. As can be noted, rank ordering of the communities' most pressing health problems differed in these two communities (New-

TABLE 14-6 Rank Order of Perceived Community Health Problems for Urban and Rural Respondents

Rural respondents		Urban respondents	
Problem	$\overline{X}$ (mean score)	Problem	$\overline{X}$ (mean score)
Illegitimacy	3.57	Drug abuse	3.78
Heart disease	3.43	Heart disease	3.67
Cancer	3.30	Venereal diseases	3.64
Accidents	3.18	Illegitimacy	3.56
Unemployment	3.13	Alcoholism	3.53
Alcoholism	3.12	Accidents	3.49
Nutrition	3.10	Cancer	3.48
Venereal diseases	3.02	Water pollution	3.35
Drug abuse	2.99	Consumer protection	3.15
Urban renewal	2.98	Nutrition	3.10
Availability of health services	2.83	Unemployment	3.08
Social welfare pay for elderly	2.81	Urban renewal	3.01
Consumer protection	2.80	Air pollution	2.90
Water pollution	2.80	Infant mortality	2.76
Infant mortality	2.55	Availability of health services	2.59
Air pollution	2.39	Social welfare pay for elderly	2.59

NOTE: A rating of 5 indicated a severe problem; a rating of 1 indicated little or no problem.

SOURCE: From I. M. Newman & C. Mayshark. Community health problems and the school's unrecognized mandate. *Journal of School Health*, November 1973, *93* (9), p. 563. Copyright 1973, American School Health Association, Ohio 44240.

man and Mayshark, 1973, p. 563). This study is not atypical. Practitioners regularly find that communities do have varying concerns, interests, and needs. A survey such as the one conducted by Newman and Mayshark can help school personnel to determine how to focus their health planning.

School systems may not recognize how much they can contribute to the alleviation of community health problems. Too frequently, they maintain the status quo because they fear being viewed unfavorably if their health education activities address controversial issues. The school system's perception of how the community views the value of school intervention to resolve community health problems is not always accurate. Newman and Mayshark (1973, p. 563) found in the two communities they surveyed that both urban and rural respondents felt that the school system could significantly contribute to the resolution of major community health problems. Their findings, presented in Table 14-7, clearly illustrate that

communities are aware of controversial issues. These findings further support the need for school systems to become involved in helping communities to solve controversial health concerns. Communities do want their educational systems to assist them in dealing with health as well as educational needs.

Community liaison activities can be challenging and rewarding for several reasons. Working with others in parent-teacher organizations or community agencies can strengthen the school health program. This, in turn, can increase a nurse's satisfaction because children who need help are receiving it. Community liaison activities also expose school nurses to different viewpoints, which help nurses to expand their range of alternative solutions for health problems. In addition, these activities enhance creative thinking through stimulation by others, facilitate continuity of care, and increase community participation in health programming. Community interest groups are more motivated to implement a health pro-

TABLE 14-7 Two Community Agencies Thought to Be Most Able to Contribute to the Alleviation of Major Community Health Problems

Problem	Agency	Percent response
RURAL		
Illegitimacy	Health and welfare department	50
	School	26
Heart disease	General health care system	68
	Varied responses	32
Cancer	Health department	32
	Varied responses	68
Accidents	Law enforcement	71
	School	24
Unemployment	Local, state, and federal government	69
	School	17
Alcoholism	Churches	40
	School	24
URBAN		
Drug abuse	School	36
	Health department	20
Heart disease	Health department	35
	General health care system	30
Venereal diseases	Health department	69
	School	31
Illegitimacy	Health department	43
	School	38
Alcoholism	School	27
	Health department	24
Accidents	Law enforcement	53
	School	20

SOURCE: From I. M. Newman & C. Mayshark, Community health problems and the school's unrecognized mandate. *Journal of School Health,* November 1973, *93* (9), p. 563. Copyright 1973, American School Health Association, Kent, Ohio 44240.

gram if they have participated in designing that health program. School nurses, through their involvement with groups, can gain a greater appreciation of community issues, demands, and needs.

Consultation. Nurses bring to the school setting a unique set of skills which allow them to become valuable, contributing members of the school health team. Specifically, there are three major areas where nursing differs from other disciplines in the school setting. First, nurses have been prepared to assess comprehensively all the variables which have an influence on a child's health status. Nurses' understanding of normal growth and development, as well as disease processes, provides them with the knowledge needed for identifying both physical and psychosocial health problems and for determining how to handle health concerns. Teachers frequently ask school nurses questions about disease conditions such as diabetes, epilepsy, hepatitis, or scabies. They may question if a child is ill, when to send a child home when he or she is not feeling well, or whether a child with a chronic condition should be allowed to participate in recreational activities. Children with heart problems or other chronic conditions are frequently overprotected by school personnel until medical recommendations are interpreted by the nurse. It is also not uncommon for the school nurse to encounter fear when infectious diseases are present in the school system and school personnel do not understand the etiology of communicable diseases or how to prevent the spread of these diseases. One teacher, for example, became so upset after she heard that one of her students had hepatitis that she moved the child's desk into the hall immediately and called the school nurse. She wanted the nurse to talk with her class about "what to do when they got hepatitis." The teacher was sure that everyone in the classroom would become ill, because all she knew about this condition was that it was contagious. Her anxiety was reduced once the nurse explained the etiology and the mode of transmission of this disease process and the rehabilitative needs of the ill child.

The nurse's preparation for dealing with the family as the unit of service is a second major area of uniqueness. Family problems may affect a child's functioning in the school setting and often problems of all family members need to be addressed before a child's functioning in school changes. Problem behavior such as poor school attendance, aggressive behavior, use of drugs, or withdrawal from school activities often signals that a child's family is having difficulty. The adolescent depicted in the following case situation had a high absenteeism record until the school nurse helped her mother to obtain medical care for herself.

Pattie Lynne Babcock was a 14-year-old junior high school student who was missing an average of 2 days of school per week when the school social worker referred her to the generalized school nurse. Even though Pattie only had a functional heart murmur, her mother would relate any illness she had to her "bad heart." The school social worker felt that Pattie Lynne's mother needed help with understanding how her fears were affecting Pattie Lynne's perceptions of her health. Mrs. Babcock was very receptive to the nurse visiting. She had been widowed recently and wasn't sure how "to care for Pattie Lynne properly." During the nurse's first home visit, Mrs. Babcock related that she hadn't been feeling well lately. Her heart pounded so fast at times that she feared she might have a heart attack. She had trouble with her vision but felt it was because she was getting old. Mrs. Babcock had a history of hypertension but had stopped taking "her blood pressure medication because it made her feel worse." The nurse found her blood pressure to be 210/116 and stressed the need for immediate medical follow-up. Mrs. Babcock reluctantly made an appointment with her family physician while the nurse was in the

home. She felt she had too many other things to take care of to worry about herself. Utilizing crisis intervention principles, the school nurse in this situation helped Mrs. Babcock to identify what it was she had to handle and then encouraged her to work on one thing at a time. The nurse's promise to return motivated Mrs. Babcock to seek medical care. During the nurse's second visit the following week, Mrs. Babcock reported that she was feeling better physically and was also able to verbalize that she thought she was going to die. She could identify that when she was afraid, "it was nice to have Pattie Lynne home with me." She also saw how her fear of having a heart attack altered her perceptions of Pattie Lynne's heart murmur. The school nurse continued to make home visits until Mrs. Babcock developed mechanisms to cope with the changes in her life. Like all school-age children, Pattie Lynne continued to miss a day of school periodically. Her attendance record improved dramatically, however, once the nurse assisted Mrs. Babcock in dealing with her problems.

Extensive knowledge of community resources and the referral process is the third unique skill the school nurse has to contribute in the school setting. There are many families within school systems who do not have a regular source of medical supervision. Other families have their own physician and dentist but cannot afford to use their services. One student community health nurse came back to the health department extremely disturbed following her second visit to an inner-city junior high school. She was appalled at the number of children who had obvious dental caries and questioned why their parents did not care enough about them to obtain dental care. A staff nurse suggested to her that limited financial resources might be preventing many of these families from obtaining the dental supervision they needed. When the student contacted the parents of these children, she found that in fact this was the case. After she discussed the services available at the health department dental clinic, two families requested that all of their children be referred to this resource. School personnel were appreciative of these referrals and identified several other children who needed dental assistance.

Parents and school personnel do *care*. If school nurses demonstrate that they are willing to use the unique skills they have, both families and other members of the school health team will confer with them regularly. The opportunities are endless. School nurses who reflect a genuine interest in the welfare of children and their families, a nonthreatening, accepting attitude toward other professionals seeking advice, and competency in decision making based on sound scientific principles are more likely to be used effectively than school nurses who do not demonstrate these characteristics.

Epidemiological investigation. Health services in a school setting should be designed to meet the needs of the total school population. Health counseling and instruction with individual students only reaches the tip of the iceberg in a given population. Nurses must use the epidemiological process to identify groups at risk and to plan and implement scientific health programming.

Effective school nurses organize the data they have to identify factors that influence the health status of school-age populations. The characteristics of populations are studied in order to determine the most appropriate intervention strategies to meet their needs. One school nurse utilized health records, data obtained during home visits, contact with students in the health clinic, and census tract information to substantiate the need for a breakfast program in the school system. These data revealed several significant facts. Children frequently came into the health clinic complaining of a stomachache because they had not eaten breakfast. Fifty-five percent of the children came from one-parent homes where the income was minimal. Out of the 167

children enrolled in this elementary school 110 qualified for a free lunch program. During home visits, the school nurse made numerous community referrals because families did not have adequate financial resources to meet their basic needs. All of these data were organized and shared with the school principal. Seeing the hard facts, he agreed with the nurse that federal funds should be sought to support a breakfast program in order to improve the nutritional status of students in their school district.

An epidemiological approach to school health is a prevention-oriented approach. In the above situation, the nurse worked to prevent nutritional problems such as anemia and to prevent learning difficulties in the future; children who are ill often do not learn well. Prevention is far less costly than treatment.

There are numerous situations in the school setting that require primary preventive intervention. Accidents, for example, are the leading cause of death in the school-age population. Astute school nurses may be able to identify factors that cause accidents in the school setting by analyzing their health records and by observing their school environments. Identifying commonalities among those children who receive care for accidents can result in eliminating environmental factors that increase the potential for hazardous accidents. Debris in the playground, unsupervised play, and playground equipment inappropriate to the developmental age level of children are some such factors which may need to be changed in the school setting to reduce frequent accidents.

Accurate and complete record keeping is essential if epidemiological studies are to be effective. Too often, nursing services are not well documented and it is impossible to retrieve data about what was done by the school nurse to solve a health problem. A record system must be designed to allow for complete and efficient recording of data. A cumulative record of each child's health status should be maintained and records of children with special health problems tagged. A tagging system allows for quick analysis of the needs of the population as a whole. If 50 children in a school system, for example, have problems with obesity, group counseling sessions and changes in curriculum planning may be warranted.

It is imperative for community health nurses in the school setting to evaluate the results of their interventions. When nurses work with aggregates, the epidemiological process is the tool that most appropriately helps them to examine the results of their group intervention strategies (see Chapter 10). *Until nurses begin to document what they have accomplished, they will not be used to their fullest potential.*

Health counseling. Children and youth are currently facing difficult and complex health problems and concerns. They are exposed much earlier than their previous counterparts to such things as human sexuality issues, varying life-styles, pressures from peers to use alcohol and drugs, knowledge about health problems, decisions regarding future career planning, and family disruption and disorganization. Often they have knowledge about these issues but they do not understand how to deal with them. They have a need to discuss their feelings and emotions with a nonthreatening adult. Because the school nurse does not evaluate a student's academic performance, which helps students to view her or him as nonthreatening, and because students may have physical health complaints when experiencing emotional stress, the school nurse is frequently the first member of the school health team to identify a student's need for counseling. The school nurse should take advantage of these opportunities and assist these students in obtaining the help they need.

As in other settings, the nurse in the school utilizes the family-centered nursing process to determine appropriate management goals and intervention strategies. Too often in the school setting, however, data are hurriedly collected because other children are waiting to see the nurse. Problems are missed when this is done and intervention strategies are inappropriate to the child's needs. The case situation which follows illustrates the need to collect sufficient data to diagnose a child's actual health problems and to plan a variety of intervention strategies to resolve these problems.

Lindsey Elizabeth, a first-grader, was lying on the cot in the health clinic when the community health nurse arrived for her weekly visit. The school secretary reported to the nurse that Lindsey had just come into her office crying because she had a stomachache. When asked by the school nurse how she was feeling, Lindsey sobbed and stated, "My stomach hurts." A physical examination revealed that no one spot hurt more than another and that with a little attention Lindsey stopped crying. When she was asked if her parents knew she did not feel well this morning, her answer was, "My mother doesn't love me anymore. She went away." The nurse helped Lindsey to verbalize her feelings of rejection and let her know that she understood how much it hurts to lose someone you love. A hug by the nurse assisted Lindsey in recognizing that others did care about her and so she was ready to go back to class that day. The nurse realized, however, that Lindsey had only received temporary relief from her distress. She had a conference with her teacher and ways to give Lindsey special attention were discussed. In addition, the nurse contacted Lindsey's father. He was very angry that his wife had left and found it extremely difficult to talk to his children about what was happening. Fortunately he was concerned about how his separation was affecting Lindsey and agreed to seek family counseling at a local mental health clinic. Lindsey's mother never did return home. Her father, however, learned how to deal with his anger and gradually was able to allow his children to talk about their mother. This, coupled with support from an empathic teacher, helped Lindsey to function more effectively in the school setting.

Elementary school children often verbalize their feelings more readily than do older school-age children. Since one of the developmental tasks of adolescence is to achieve emotional independence of parents and other adults, students at the junior or senior high level may test the school nurse before they share their real concerns. One such case is described below:

Noel, a 14-year-old junior high student, wandered into the health clinic during class breaks 3 weeks in a row with minor physical complaints. Finally he asked the nurse if he could talk with her alone. He wanted to know "how a person could tell if he had VD." Further discussion revealed that Noel was having nocturnal emissions and thought he had gonorrhea because he had learned in a health class that a purulent discharge occurred with this disease. Noel had never heard about nocturnal emissions and was fearful that his wet discharges at night were due to gonorrhea. He was greatly relieved when he found out that he was "normal." The nurse encouraged him to return to the clinic if he had other questions and suggested that his father might be able to talk with him about other developmental changes that occur during adolescence. The need to discuss normal developmental changes as well as to review how venereal diseases are transmitted was also shared with the teacher responsible for the eighth-grade health class.

Health counseling opportunities such as the ones described above are numerous and present in all school settings. Nurses who are attuned to the developmental needs and the social characteristics of the population they are serving will not be "Betty Band-Aid" pushers. Rather, they will take time to find out from other school personnel which students have health problems and will be alert for students who need to talk.

Health education. The ultimate goal of nursing intervention is to help the client to help himself or herself. Through health education activites in the school setting, school nurses are preparing children and their families, school personnel, and the community to make sound health decisions. They recognize that the population they serve needs adequate knowledge as well as the opportunity to explore values and attitudes about health matters before they can assume responsibility for maintaining their personal health status.

The following examples demonstrate that the nurse in the school setting has both direct and indirect responsibilities in relation to health education. Nurses utilize the principles of teaching and learning to carry out effectively their health education responsibilities:

1. *Incidental health education with students.* A second-grader was advised to keep his hands clean to avoid infection after his nail was pulled away from the skin of the right forefinger during gym class. A 14-year-old junior high girl was helped to understand body changes during adolescence after frequent visits to the health clinic with menstrual cramps. Dental hygiene was discussed with a 10-year-old boy who had several dental caries. A tenth-grader was helped to see the relationship between her frequent headaches and her refusal to wear her glasses.

2. *Incidental health education with school personnel.* A seventh-grade teacher was advised to see his family physician after several spontaneous nose bleeds. The etiology and prevention of ringworm was discussed with a first-grade teacher when she informed the school nurse that three children were absent from school because of this condition.

3. *Incidental health education with parents.* A young mother of three children, ages 5 years, 3 years, and 1 month, was given a pamphlet on breast-feeding during a nurse-parent conference. She was breast-feeding for the first time and was late for the conference because of breast discomfort. A father of a second-grader was taught to

watch for signs and symptoms of brain concussion after his son was hit on the head by a swing in the playground.

4. *Planned direct health teaching.* Child care, including such things as feeding, bathing, and dressing, was demonstrated to a group of school-age parents. Physical and emotional maturational changes were reviewed with a sixth-grade class the first time a new teacher was covering this topic with the students. What a school nurse does was discussed with first-graders. Opportunities in nursing were shared with senior high students during a career day.

5. *In-service health education.* Teachers in an elementary school were shown the film *Looking at Children* to help them identify common childhood health problems. Parents were shown the maturational films their fifth-graders were to see so that they could respond to their children's questions. A drug education workshop was conducted for junior high teachers after a sharp increase in the incidence of drug usage was noted in their school system.

6. *Curriculum planning.* Diet planning was integrated into the health class after the school nurse noted on student records that a sizable number of students had anemia or were obese. The school nurse was asked to serve on the school health committee after sharing with the school administrators several health concerns of parents she encountered while making home visits.

7. *Health instruction planning with teachers.* A resource file designed to help teachers understand common health problems was established after one school nurse received numerous requests for such information. A second-grade teacher was provided with information about dental health, was given dental models to demonstrate effective dental care, and was helped to obtain pamphlets on dental hygiene when she requested that the school nurse conduct a unit on dental care for her class. The nurse felt that the teacher knew her students better than she did and could more effectively develop teaching strategies appropriate to their needs.

The nurses in these situations all believed in the value of health education as an appropriate strategy to help clients help themselves. They involved all members of the school health team, including parents and students, so that health education would be an ongoing process, even when the nurse was not available. Health education is an essential component of any school health program. School nurses can play a very significant role in ensuring that this component is not neglected. They must, however, be careful not to assume the responsibilities of others when functioning in the school setting: health education should be *integrated* into the overall curriculum. This will never occur if the school nurse continually teaches sporadic health classes. Helping teachers to assume responsibility for health education activities is a much more beneficial approach. There may be times when a teacher is very uncomfortable with a particular topic. Demonstrating that sensitive issues can be handled effectively in the classroom setting often reduces a teacher's fears about covering this topic in the future. If, however, teachers continually ask to have the nurse present certain health topics, the need for in-service education with the teachers should be considered. It is impossible for nurses to carry out their other functions in the school setting if all their time is spent teaching in the classroom.

Home visiting. Parents are vital members of the school health team. They are ultimately responsible for the health care of their children and they greatly influence their children's health practices. Contact with parents in the home environment is a most effective way of increasing their understanding and involvement with their child's health problems. Home visits also demonstrate that the school nurse cares about parents as individuals and respects their parental rights.

At times, home visiting is the only way to obtain a comprehensive picture of a child's health status. Family dynamics do have an impact on a child's functioning. Assessment of parent-child relationships is best obtained in the client's natural setting. Observations of how the child is physically handled, of environmental conditions, and of interactions between a child, the parents, and siblings is more easily assessed in the home environment. These observations provide a different type of data from a conference with a parent in the health clinic. Parents may not be aware of how they interact with their children so that what they verbalize may not always be what is actually occurring.

Most parents do care about their children, and they desire to do the very best they can to help them develop normally. Sometimes they do not take action when their child has a health problem because they do not understand why it is necessary to do so or know what they should do to resolve the problem. At other times, health care is not obtained because the family has multiple pressures they must deal with first. Fear, guilt, and not knowing that a problem exists are some other reasons why health action is not taken. A home visit by a concerned nurse can serve as a catalyst for motivating parents to seek help for their child's health needs.

The school nurse cannot possibly visit at home every child served in the school system. Children who manifest needs or difficulties such as the following should receive priority for home visits:

1. History of many absences due to illness

2. Behavioral problems which interfere with academic functioning or which adversely affect social relationships with peers

3. Adjustment difficulties related to a chronic condition such as diabetes, epilepsy, heart defects, or obesity

4. Suspected abuse or neglect

5. Special programming needs in relation to a developmental disability

6. Lack of medical follow-up on an identified health problem

7. Pregnancy outside of marriage

8. Frequent exposure to infectious diseases

Home visiting can be rewarding and extremely beneficial. It frequently is the key which opens the door to a happier life for many children. The following case situation describes how a home visit helped one 8-year-old child to positively increase her interactions with her peers:

Tammie Baxter was referred to the school nurse because she had a very pronounced body odor. Her peers shunned her, and she appeared to be a very lonely child. Tammie's teacher had many questions about her home environment and the health status of her parents, because she had heard that Tammie's father was ill as a result of complications of diabetes. A very receptive mother answered the door when the school nurse made her first home visit. The nurse discovered that a family of seven was living in a five-room home, including a living room, a kitchen, two bedrooms, and a bath. All five Baxter children, ages 8, 6, 4, 2, and 1, were sleeping on mattresses on the floor in one bedroom. Tammie smelled like urine, not because she was ill, but because three of her siblings wet the bed at night. She had limited clothes because the family was having severe financial problems. Tammie's difficulties with personal hygiene were resolved quickly once the mother discovered how the other children were treating her. A referral was made to a community clothes closet so that Tammie could be dressed like her peers. Tammie's teacher was amazed at how quickly her personal hygiene changed. A little extra attention from the teacher also helped to alter Tammie's relationships with her classmates.

A long-term helping relationship between the Baxter family and the school nurse evolved from this one simple teacher referral. Tammie was not, however, the focus of the conversation on subsequent visits. Her father was indeed in need of medical care. Mr. Baxter was laid off from work at an industrial plant because he was showing sugar in his urine; a telephone call between the community health nurse working in the school and the industrial nurse clarified that Mr. Baxter could return to work as soon as his diabetes was under control. Several community referrals helped this family to obtain medical care.

Team participation. No one discipline can meet the needs of all school-age children. Team cooperation and collaboration are essential if children are to receive the health services they deserve. The school nurse who has a "me" philosophy rather than a "we" philosophy will quickly become frustrated and will soon recognize that it is impossible to achieve goals without the help of others.

In order for school health nurses to carry out their functions effectively and efficiently, they must provide nursing services within the framework of the total health program, working cooperatively with other school personnel. Understanding the roles of each member of the school team (Table 14-8) can facilitate planning and implementation of nursing services. The role definitions presented in Table 14-8 are only guidelines. When entering a new school system, every nurse should spend time with all of these individuals to determine how they function in that given system.

Interdisciplinary functioning can be stimulating and rewarding. For this to happen, all team members must define how they can integrate their specific skills into an effective group effort which emphasizes a common endeavor. A philosophy of care must also be delineated and goals established which are acceptable to all.

No team effort with school-age children will be successful unless the central figures on the team are the child and involved family. Planning *for* others does not work. Rather, they must be *involved* in decision making before they can internalize health beliefs and attitudes and change health behavior.

Practical Tips for Role Implementation

Implementing multiple and varied functions is a formidable task. This is especially true for the nurse in the school setting because the school's primary goal is to educate students, not to provide health care services. School nurses must demonstrate that what they have to offer will enhance a child's learning. In addition, school nurses must often deal with diverse role expectations. School administrators, teachers, parents, and students frequently define the nurse's role differently from how the nurse defines it, because they have had varying encounters with nurses in the past. It is important for school nurses to avoid panic or withdrawal when they do not initially accomplish what they have hoped to or when they experience role conflicts. It takes time to develop a meaningful role in any setting. Provided below are some suggestions for facilitating the role implementation process in the school setting:

Define Your Philosophy of Nursing Practice

If school nurses cannot articulate the role of the nurse in the school health program, they cannot expect other members of the health care team to use them as they would like to be used. Reviewing the literature devoted to school nursing and the school health policies devel-

TABLE 14-8 Role Descriptions for Some Members of the School Health Team

Discipline	Role description
Principals	School administrators who are responsible for planning and providing direction for all activities carried out to meet the goals of the school, including nursing services.
Teachers	Staff members who are responsible for the educational aspects of the school program. Teachers enhance the total school health program by conducting health education activities in the classroom and by identifying children who have physical and emotional health problems that impede learning.
Teacher consultants	Pupil personnel specialists* who have advanced training for handling educational programming for children with special learning needs such as reading problems, mental retardation, and emotional disturbances.
Teachers, homebound	Pupil personnel teachers, specially trained, to deal with physical handicaps and the educational implications of these conditions. These persons work in the home with children who have been certified by a physician as being unable to physically attend school due to a noninfectious physical disability. These individuals provide both educational instruction and counseling services for homebound students.
School social workers	Pupil personnel specialists who provide direct counseling services for a child and family, if the child is demonstrating adjustment difficulties in the school setting. School social workers apply the principles and methods of social casework to help students to enhance their social and emotional adjustment and to adapt to change. The primary purpose of their intervention is to reduce impediments to learning. These individuals are often used as resource persons by all other members of the school health team.
Screening technicians	Pupil personnel staff trained to identify particular health problems, usually vision and hearing difficulties, through the use of screening tests.
Volunteers	Lay staff who receive in-service education to carry out defined tasks for other staff members. Responsibilities should relate to the in-service training they have received. Careful selection, training, and supervision by professional staff is a must if these individuals are to be utilized successfully in the school setting.
Therapists, physical	Pupil personnel specialists who treat muscular disabilities of children upon a prescriptive order from the child's physician. Their services are designed to enable students to improve their physical health status so that their physical health problems do not impede learning.
Therapists, speech	Pupil personnel specialists who work with children who have difficulty producing and combining certain sounds in words, who are unable to speak with reasonable fluency, who speak with an abnormally pitched voice, or who have physical anomalies such as cerebral palsy. Speech therapists help children to develop normal speech patterns which help them to more effectively develop social relationships and to advance academically.
School psychologists	Pupil personnel specialists whose major responsibility is to determine the reasons for a child's inability to learn. These specialists are often known as the school diagnosticians because the primary purpose of their service is to identify or diagnose causes of learning problems. These individuals use psychological tests, such as IQ and personality tests, during the psychological assessment. Parental permission must be obtained before a child can be tested by these specialists. The amount of direct counseling a psychologist does with a child varies from one school to another. Usually, however, this person functions as a consultant to other school personnel. Psychologists in other settings are often more involved in direct counseling services.

*Pupil personnel division—a special service division of a local board of education. Personnel in this division are accountable to the superintendent of schools.

SOURCE: Adapted from special education services available to Jackson County, Jackson County Intermediate School District, Jackson, Mich.

oped by your agency will provide you with information needed to formulate a philosophy of practice with which you can feel comfortable.

Study Your Community

Understanding the needs of the population you are serving is essential. Children, families, and school personnel will respond more quickly to your suggestions if you demonstrate a sensitivity to their concerns and if you support your comments with data. Review the students' health records to identify their pressing health problems. Analyze the census tract data to determine the characteristics of the families in the school district. Talk with students and teachers as you walk around the school building. Avoid sitting in the health clinic. Leave the school setting and drive through the area in which your school is located. Do a community analysis.

Contact Key People

A school nurse who takes the initiative to contact school personnel and community groups responsible for the implementation of the school health program is more likely to become quickly involved than one who functions in isolation. Meet with the school principal before school starts. Explain your role and determine a time when you can orient teachers to the nursing services you have to offer. Find out the name of the president of the PTA and the student health council. A telephone call to these individuals may open the doors to the community and the student body.

Demonstrate Your Skills

The best way to help others to understand what it is you do is to show them what you can do. Follow up quickly on the referrals sent to you by other school personnel. Share with them the results of your interventions. A nurse who too quickly states that an activity is not the nurse's responsibility is apt to make other members of the team hesitant to use her or him. Often the nurse is requested to provide first aid or to inspect for communicable diseases because individuals making these requests are afraid to handle these situations. Respond to their concerns by first caring for the children and then providing the other school personnel with information so that they can handle these situations in the future.

Communicate with All Members of the School Health Team

Do not wait for others to come to you. Relate with teachers in their lounge and in their classroom. Ask questions about the students which will help you to determine where your services are most needed. Share in writing or in person when you have followed up on a referral. Use the bulletin board to provide health information to students. *Talk with the school secretary.* She or he probably knows the students and their families as well as any other person in the building.

Organize Your Activities

A school nurse who just lets things happen frequently does not accomplish goals. Establish a calendar of activities for the year. Be specific in regard to the goals you want to accomplish. Know when you will orient the teachers to your services, when you will provide in-service education, when you will review student records, and when you will follow up on student health problems. A tickler system (see Chapter 20) can help you to monitor student follow-up needs. *A calendar is a must.* If you do not plan your time, others will plan it for you.

Set Priorities

A nurse cannot be all things to all people. Identify what needs to be done and then determine what you can handle, considering the time you have available. Request consultation from the school health team to establish priorities significant to the needs of the population being served.

Document Your Activities

People respond favorably to concrete data. Keep a daily record of your activities. Use these records with others to substantiate what you have done, to support the need to set priorities, and to document the need for a new health program or changes in the existing health program. *Remember, changes generally do not occur when concrete data are lacking.*

SUMMARY

Traditionally, community health nurses have assumed a major role in planning health services for school-age children. Currently they work with this population group in a variety of settings such as the home, the school, clinics, and residential settings for children with special needs. A family-centered, prevention-oriented, interdisciplinary approach is the most effective way to meet the needs of school-age children, regardless of the setting in which the nurse is functioning.

As of July 1977, there were 49 million school-age children, ages 5 through 17, that needed health services in the United States. Community health nurses who work with these children encounter an array of physical, psychosocial, cultural, environmental, and developmental health problems and concerns. A well-organized comprehensive health care system which takes into consideration the developmental characteristics of children and adolescents is essential if youth are to reach their maximum potential.

Since most children attend school, the school is a logical environment in which to promote the health of all children. The role of the community health nurse in the school health program has been evolving since the turn of the century. Initially, a school nurse was seen as the professional who provided first aid, gave injections, inspected for communicable diseases, or counseled "dirty" children. Now, she or he is an advocate, a health counselor, a health educator, an epidemiologist, a consultant, a community health planner, and a coordinator. Teamwork is essential for successful implementation of these roles. The central figures on the team *must* be the school-age child and his or her family.

Working with school-age children and their families can be challenging and rewarding. A philosophy of nursing practice that stresses the need to help others help themselves and focuses on the client's strengths, reaps the nurse the most benefits.

REFERENCES

Abernethy, V. Illegitimate conception among teenagers. *American Journal of Public Health,* July 1974, *64,* 662–665.

Adolescent Health Services, and Pregnancy Prevention and Care Act of 1978. Hearings before the Committee on Human Resources U.S. Senate, Ninety-fifth Congress, second session on S. 2910, June 14 and July 12, 1978, Washington, D.C.: U.S. Government Printing Office, 1978.

Alan Guttmacher Institute. *Eleven million teenagers.*

New York: Alan Guttmacher Institute, 1976. Reprinted with permission from Alan Guttmacher Institute.

American Nurses' Association. *Facts about nursing 74–75*. New York: American Nurses' Association, 1976.

American Nurses' Association. *Functions and qualifications for school nurses*. New York: American Nurses' Association, 1966.

Anderson, C. L. *School health practice*. Saint Louis: Mosby, 1972.

Basco, D., Eyres, S., Glasser, J., & Roberts, D. Epidemiologic analysis in school populations as a basis for change in school-nursing practice—Report of the second phase of a longitudinal study. *American Journal of Public Health*, April 1972, *62*, 491–497.

Benenson, A. (Ed.). *Control of communicable diseases in man*. Washington, D.C.: American Public Health Association, 1975.

Blum, R. H. *Horatio Alger's children*. San Francisco: Jossey-Bass, 1972.

Boggs, E. M., & Henney, R. L., *A numerical and functional description of the developmentally disabled population in the United States by major life activities as defined by the Developmental Disabilities Assistance and Bill of Rights Act as amended in PL 95-602*. Philadelphia: EMC Institute, 1979.

Bremner, R. H. (Ed.). *Children and youth in America: A documentary history*. Cambridge, Mass.: Harvard University Press, 1974.

Byler, R. V. *Teach us what we want to know*. New York: Mental Health Materials Center, 1969.

Chinn, P. *Child health maintenance*. Saint Louis: Mosby, 1974.

Clemen, S., & Pattullo, A. The adolescent with mental retardation. In J. Howe (Ed.), *Nursing care of the adolescent*. New York: McGraw-Hill, 1980.

Commission on Population Growth and the American Future. *Population and the American future*. Washington, D.C.: U.S. Government Printing Office, 1972.

Current estimates from the health interview survey, United States, 1977. DHEW Publication No. PHS 78-1554. Hyattsville, Md.: Public Health Service, September 1978.

Densen, P. M., Ullman, D. B., Jones, E. W., & Vandow, J. B. Childhood indicators of adult health status. *Public Health Reports*, November 1970, *85*, 981–995.

Drew, S. K. *The child and his school: Helping the battered child and his family*. Philadelphia: Lippincott, 1972.

Examination and health history findings among children and youths 6–17 years of age, 1973. DHEW Publication No. 74-1611, Vital and Health Statistics Series 11. Hyattsville, Md.: National Center for Health Statistics, 1975.

Fiumara, N. J. Venereal diseases. In J. R. Gallagher, F. P. Heald, & D. C. Garell (Eds.), *Medical care of the adolescent*. New York: Appleton-Century-Crofts, 1976.

Froom, J. Prevalence and natural history of chronic disease in childhood. In G. D. Grove & I. B. Pless (Eds.), *Chronic childhood illness: Assessment of outcome*. DHEW Publication No. NIH 76-877. Hyattsville, Md.: U.S. Department of Health, Education, and Welfare, Public Health Service, National Institute of Health, 1974.

Gallagher, J. R., Heald, F., & Garell, D. *Medical care of the adolescent*. New York: Appleton-Century-Crofts, 1976.

Garbarino, J. The human ecology of child maltreatment: A conceptual model for research. *Journal of Marriage and the Family*, November 1977, *39*, 721–735.

Garrard, S. D. Mental retardation in adolescence. *Pediatric Clinics of North America*, February 1960, *7*, 147–164.

Hamburg, D. A. (President). *Healthy people: The Surgeon General's report on health promotion and disease prevention: Background papers 1979*. DHEW (PHS) Publication No. 79-55071A. Washington D.C.: Public Health Service, 1979.

Havighurst, R. J. *Developmental tasks and education* (3d ed.). New York: McKay, 1972.

Health, United States, 1975. DHEW Publication No. HRA 76-1232. Washington, D.C.: U.S. Government Printing Office, 1977.

Heazlett, M., & Whaley, R. The common cold: Its

effects on perceptual ability and reading comprehension among pupils of a seventh-grade class. *Journal of School Health,* March 1976, *96,* 145–146. Copyright, 1976, American School Health Association, Kent, Ohio 44240.

Heindl, C., Krall, C. A., Salus, M., & Broadhurst, D. D. *The nurse's role in the prevention and treatment of child abuse and neglect.* Washington, D.C.: National Center on Child Abuse and Neglect, Children's Bureau, Administration for Children, Youth and Families, Office of Human Development Services, August 1979.

Helfer, R., & Kempe, C. H. *Child abuse and neglect.* Cambridge, Mass.: Ballinger, 1976.

Hilmar, N., & McAtee, P. The school nurse practitioner and her practice: A study of traditional and expanded health care responsibilities for nurses in elementary schools. *Journal of School Health,* September 1973, *93,* 431–444. Copyright, 1973, American School Health Association, Kent, Ohio 44240.

Hoekelman, R. A., Blatman, S., Brunell, D. A., Friedman, S. B., & Seidel, H. M. *Principles of pediatrics: Health care of the young.* New York: McGraw-Hill, 1978.

Hofmann, A. D. Legal issues in child health care. In R. Hoekelman, S. Blatman, P. Brunell, B. F. Stanford, & H. Seidel. *Principles of pediatrics: Health care of the young.* New York: McGraw-Hill, 1978.

Joint Committee on Health Problems in Education of the National Education Association and the American Medical Association. *School health services* (2d ed.). C. C. Wilson (Ed.), Washington, D.C., and Chicago: The Associations, 1964.

Klerman, L. Adolescent pregnancy: The need for new policies and new programs. *Journal of School Health,* May 1975, *95,* 263–267. Copyright 1975, American School Health Association, Kent, Ohio 44240. This paper is the edited version of an address delivered at the 1974 Annual Meeting of the Crittenton Hastings House, Boston, Mass. Many of the ideas presented are a result of the author's work on grant MC-R-090048 from the Maternal and Child Health Service, Department of Health, Education, and Welfare.

Long, G., Whitman, C., Johansson, M., Williams, C., & Tuthill, R. Evaluation of a school health program directed to children with history of high absence: A focus for nursing intervention. *American Journal of Public Health,* April 1975, *65,* 388–393.

Lynch, A. Child abuse in the school-age population. *Journal of School Health,* March 1975, *45,* 141–148. Copyright, 1975, American School Health Association, Kent, Ohio 44240.

Mazie, S. (Ed.). *Population, distribution, and policy.* DHEW Publication No. 5258-00006. Washington, D.C.: U.S. Government Printing Office, 1972.

McKevitt, R., Nader, P., Williamson, M., & Berney, R. Reasons for health office visits in an urban school district. *Journal of School Health,* May 1977, *97,* 275–279. Copyright, 1977, American School Health Association, Kent, Ohio 44240.

Metropolitan Life. *Looking for Health.* New York: Metropolitan Life, 1969.

Millar, H. *Approaches to adolescent health care in 1970's.* DHEW Publication No. HSA 76-5014. Rockville, Md.: Department of Health, Education, and Welfare, 1975.

Miller, C. Health care of children and youth in America. *American Journal of Public Health,* April 1975, *65,* 353–358.

National Center for Health Statistics. *Advance Report, Final Mortality Statistics 1974, 24* (11), supp. 3, February 1976.

National Center for Health Statistics. *Advance report, vital statistics of the United States, 1976.* Hyattsville, Md.: Office of Health Research, Statistics, and Technology, 1979.

National Institute of Child Health and Human Development. *Smoking in children and adolescents.* DHEW Publication No. PHS 79-50066. Washington, D.C.: Department of Health, Education, and Welfare, 1979.

National Safety Council. *Accident facts.* Chicago: National Safety Council, 1979.

Newman, I. M., & Mayshark, C. Community health problems and the school's unrecognized mandate. *Journal of School Health,* November 1973, *93,* 562–565. Copyright, 1973, American School Health Association, Kent, Ohio 44240.

Nicholson, S. W. Growth and development. In J. Howe (Ed.), *Nursing care of adolescents.* New York: McGraw-Hill, 1980.

Pannor, R., & Evans, B. The unmarried father revisited. *Journal of School Health,* May 1975, *95,* 286–291. Copyright, 1975, American School Health Association, Kent, Ohio 44240.

Powers, J. *Adolescent health care services in Michigan— Needs for program modification.* Lansing, Mich.: Bureau of Personal Health Services, April 1978.

Reinke, W. (Ed.). *Health planning: Qualitative aspects and quantitative techniques.* Baltimore, Md.: Johns Hopkins, 1972.

Report of the Harvard Child Health Project Task Force. *Toward a primary medical care system responsive to children's needs.* Cambridge, Mass.: Ballinger, 1977, Vol. 1.

Report of the Harvard Child Health Project Task Force. *Children's medical care needs and treatments.* Cambridge, Mass.: Ballinger, 1977, Vol. 2. Reprinted with permission from the Ballinger Co.

Rehab Group, Incorporated. *Digest of data on persons with disabilities.* (OHDS) 79-22009. Washington, D.C.: Congressional Research Service Library of Congress, May 1979.

Rudou, M. H., & Santangelo, N. *Health status of minorities and low-income groups.* DHEW Publication No. HRA 79-627. Washington, D.C.: Office of Health Resources Opportunity, 1979.

School Health Education Study. *Health education: A conceptual approach to curriculum design grades: Kindergarten through twelve.* Washington, D.C.: 3M Education Press, 1967.

Scipien, G. M., Barnard, M. U., Chard, M. A., Howe, J., & Phillips, P. J. *Comprehensive pediatric nursing.* New York: McGraw-Hill, 1975.

Segal, J. Child abuse: A review of research. In E. Carfman, *Families today. Volume II: A research sampler on families and children.* Rockville, Md.: National Institute of Mental Health, 1979, pp. 577–606.

Sexually transmitted diseases in gay men: An insi-

der's views. *Sexually Transmitted Diseases: Journal of the American Venereal Disease Association,* October–December 1979, *6,* 278–280.

Shattuck, L. *Report of the Sanitary Commission of Massachusetts.* Boston: Dutton and Wentworth, 1850.

Siantz, M. (Ed.). *The nurse and the developmentally disabled adolescent.* Baltimore, Md.: University Park Press, 1977.

Steele, B. F. Psychological dimensions of child abuse. Paper presented to the American Association for the Advancement of Science, Denver, Colo., February 1977.

Stone, D. B., & Rubinson, L. G. The issue of school health education: Theory and practice. *Public Health Reviews,* January–March 1979, *8,* 45–79.

———. Suicide among teenagers reflects toubled society. *Journal of the American Medical Association,* Dec. 2, 1974, *230,* 1246.

Surgeon General. *Healthy people: The Surgeon General's report on health promotion and disease prevention.* DHEW PHS Publication No. 79-55071. Washington, D.C.: Public Health Service, 1979.

Travis, G. *Chronic illness in children: Its impact on child and family.* Stanford, Calif.: Stanford University Press, 1976.

U.S. Bureau of Education for the Handicapped. *Progress toward a free appropriate public education: A report to Congress on the implementation of Publication 94–142: the Education for All Handicapped Children Act.* Washington, D.C.: U.S. Department of Health, Education, and Welfare, January 1979, p. 25.

U.S. Bureau of the Census. *U.S.A. statistics in brief 1978: A statistical abstract supplement.* Washington, D.C.: U.S. Department of Commerce, 1978, unnumbered pages.

Wallace, H. *Health services for mothers and children.* Philadelphia: Saunders, 1962.

White House Conference on Families, 1978. Joint hearings before the Subcommittee on Child and Human Development of the Committee on Human Resources, United States Senate and the Subcommittee on Select Education of the Committee on Education and Labor, House of Representatives, Ninety-fifth Congress. Washington, D.C.:

U.S. Government Printing Office, 1978.

Williams, J. Learning disabilities: A multifaceted health threat. *Journal of School Health,* November 1976, *46,* 515–516. Copyright, 1976, American School Health Association, Kent, Ohio 44240.

Winek, C. *Everything you wanted to know about drug abuse . . . but were afraid to ask.* New York: Marcel

Dekker, 1974. Reprinted courtesy of Marcel Dekker, Inc.

Zelnik, M., & Kantner, J. Contraceptive patterns and premarital pregnancy among women aged 15–19 in 1976. *Family Planning Perspectives,* May–June 1978, *10,* 135–141. Reprinted with permission from Family Planning Perspectives.

SELECTED BIBLIOGRAPHY

Allensworth, D. Common intestinal parasitic infections in the school-age population. *Journal of School Health,* June 1975, *95,* 331–337.

Berlin, I. N. *Advocacy for child mental health.* New York: Brunner/Mazel, 1975.

Bryan, D. *School nursing in transition.* Saint Louis: Mosby, 1973.

Buscaglia, L. F., & Williams, E. H. (Eds.). *Human advocacy and PL94-142: The educator's role.* Thorofare, N.J.: Charles B. Slack, 1979.

Castile, A., & Jarrick, S. School health in America: A summary report of a survey of state school health programs. *Journal of School Health,* April 1976, *96,* 216–221.

Children's Defense Fund of the Washington Research Project, Inc. *Doctors and dollars are not enough: How to improve health services for children and their families.* Washington, D.C.: Children's Defense Fund, 1976.

Costin, L. *Child welfare: Policies and practice.* New York: McGraw-Hill, 1972.

Diggory-Farnham, S. *Learning disabilities: A psychological perspective.* Cambridge, Mass.: Harvard University Press, 1978.

Fricke, I. School nursing for the 1970's. *Journal of School Health,* April 1972, *92,* 203–206.

Green, A. Self-destructive behavior in battered children. *American Journal Psychiatry,* May 1978, *135,* 579–583.

Haslam, R., & Valletutti, P. *Medical problems in the classroom: The teachers' role in diagnosis and management.* Baltimore, Md.: University Park Press, 1975.

Hofmann, A. D., & Pilpel, H. F. The legal rights of

minors. *Pediatric Clinics of North America,* November 1973, *20,* 989–1004.

Jacobs, P. Fungal infections in childhood. *Pediatric Clinics of North America,* May 1978, *25,* 357–370.

Jelneck, L. The special needs of the adolescent with chronic illness. *Maternal Child Nursing,* January–February 1977, 57–61.

Klagsbrun, F. *Too young to die: Youth and suicide.* Boston: Houghton Mifflin, 1976.

Lan, S. L., Loewenstein, R., Sinnette, C., Rogers, C., & Novick L., Screening and referral outcomes of school-based health services in a low-income neighborhood. *Public Health Reports,* November–December 1976, *91,* 514–520.

Logan, B., & Dancy, B. Unwed, pregnant adolescents: Their mothers' dilemma. *Nursing Clinics of North America,* March 1974, *9,* 57–68.

McGovern, J. Chronic respiratory diseases of school-age children. *Journal of School Health,* June 1976, *96,* 344–353.

National Advocacy Project of United Cerebral Palsy Associations, Inc. *Sharing experiences in thinking, learning, doing, advocacy.* New York: United Cerebral Palsy Association, March 1977.

Noorden, G. Chronic vision problems of school-age children. *Journal of School Health,* June 1976, *96,* 334–337.

Paul, E. W., Pilpel, H. F., & Wechsler, N. F. Pregnancy, teen-agers and the law. *Family Planning Perspectives,* January–February 1976, *8,* 16–32.

Poole, C. J. Assessing the needs of the pregnant adolescent. *Washington State Journal of Nursing,* Summer–Fall 1977, 308.

Ritter, A. M. Using a teacher's health observation

form to evaluate school child health. *Journal of School Health,* April 1976, *96,* 235–237.

Robin, S., & Bosco, J. Ritalin for school children: The teacher's perspective. *Journal of School Health,* December 1973, *93,* 624–628.

Smith, E. W. The role of the grandmother in adolescent pregnancy and parenting, *Journal of School Health,* May 1975, *95,* 278–288.

Starline, K., & Shepherd, D. Symptoms and signs of cancer in the school-age child. *Journal of School Health,* March 1977, *97,* 144–146.

Thompson, V. The school nurse looks at psychogenic illnesses. *Journal of School Health,* November 1977, *97,* 519–598.

Tolar, C. The mental health of students—Do teachers hurt or help? *Journal of School Health,* February 1975, *95,* 71–75.

Wheatley, G. M. (Ed.). Childhood accidents: Prevention and treatment. *Pediatric Annals,* November 1977, *6,* 683–756.

Williams, R. (Ed.). *Textbook of black-related diseases.* New York: McGraw-Hill, 1975.

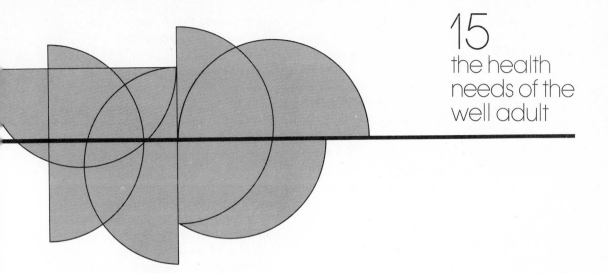

Adults are the pillars and the core of American society. They are the caretakers of the general population, and on them rests the survival of the nation. Adults are teachers, parents, workers, friends, and leaders. It is expected that they will be independent of parents, economically solvent, emotionally sound, physically strong, self-sufficient, and committed to others. In the midst of these responsibilities and expectations, they are developing as people and have their own health to maintain.

AN OVERVIEW OF ADULTHOOD

Adulthood spans the young-adult (ages 18 to 29), middlescent (ages 30 to 65), and aging (ages 65 and over) stages of life. These age ranges are arbitrary and should be viewed in terms of individual variability. The health needs of the young adult and middlescent are presented in this chapter, and the word *adult* is used here to include these two age groups. A separate chapter on aging (Chapter 18) presents health needs and services for that segment of the adult population. Maintaining the health of the adult is a complex and important task.

Developmental Tasks of Adulthood

Every developmental stage includes life goals. During childhood, a major life goal is to become an autonomous human being. The adult continues to strive for individual autonomy but also focuses on establishing generativity, self-fulfillment, and ego integrity (Erikson, 1963).

Generativity, Self-Fulfillment, and Ego Integrity

The adult is expected to establish and guide present and future generations. This extension of oneself, an ability to love and to give to others, is called *generativity* (Erikson, 1963, p. 266). It is assumed that a parent will evidence generativity in relation to his or her children. However, a parent may never reach this level of maturity if earlier developmental needs were not met. Generativity extends outside the immediate family. A person without children may be extremely generative and bring to adulthood a capacity to love and to give to others.

Adulthood is a time for achieving *self-fulfillment*. One strives to accomplish major educational, career, family, personal, and civic aspirations during this stage of life. If life aspirations are not fulfilled, adulthood can be a time of disillusionment, disenchantment, and despair.

Toward mid-to-late middlescence the adult establishes *ego integrity* (Erikson, 1963, p. 266). Establishing ego integrity involves reassessment of self. The process encompasses looking at where one has been and where one is going, as well as examining personal values, decisions, and life-styles. The person who has achieved ego integrity knows and likes himself or herself and is able to accept individual strengths and weaknesses. The person is at peace with herself or himself, is able to distinguish between the things over which she or he does and does not have control, and can accept those things that cannot be changed. Despair is likely to occur if ego integrity is not reached (Erikson, 1963, p. 266).

In order to promote wellness and to enhance an adult's self-care capabilities, the community health nurse needs to have an understanding of the processes involved in developing generativity, self-fulfillment, and ego integrity. Adults will be at varying stages of accomplishing these life goals but should be moving toward them if development is to progress and health is to be maintained. Table 15-1 identifies specific developmental tasks that help an adult to achieve Erikson's life goals. The community health nurse can facilitate growth during adulthood through anticipatory guidance, health teaching, and referral to appropriate resources. She or he must plan health promotion activities which take into consideration prevention at all three levels because individual variations in relation to wellness require preventive intervention at different levels.

The Roles of the Adult and Nursing Intervention

When one examines the developmental tasks of adulthood and the roles assumed by the adult in achieving these tasks, it can be seen that life for an adult is complex, varied, and changing. Major roles assumed by the adult are parent, grandparent, individual, spouse or companion, son or daughter, citizen, friend, leisure-time user, and worker. These roles center on the environments of home, work, and community and are not restricted exclusively to any one setting. The developmental tasks of adulthood often cross over into more than one of these roles and may not all be accomplished when one's chronological age makes one ready to assume another role.

Individual

The adult's role as an individual usurps all other adult roles. The adult is his or her own person with individual experiences. The adult must be seen as different from anyone else and autonomous.

The community health nurse working with an adult should always remember that every individual needs to define personally what is important. This concept is difficult to internalize and creates conflict for the nurse, especially when client and nurse goals differ. The nurse who recognizes that accepting the client's right of self-determination generates trust and self-esteem finds it easier to handle this conflict.

A good example of when a client's and nurse's values may differ can be seen in the contemporary issue of women's liberation. Today, many women have a career outside the home. This trend has generated feelings of anxiety and insecurity in some women who do not have outside work interests. These women may enjoy staying at home but also question if something is wrong with them because they do not have interests similar to "all" other women. A community health nurse working

TABLE 15-1 Developmental Tasks of the Adult (Ages 18–65): Major Goals—To Develop Generativity, Self-Fulfillment, and Ego Integrity

	Middlescent	
Young adult	*Middlescence I*	*Middlescence II*
Age: 18–29 years	Age: 30–50 years	Age: 51–65 years*
1. Establishing autonomy from parents or parent surrogates	1. Developing socioeconomic consolidation	1. Maintaining flexible views in occupational, civic, political, religious, and social positions
2. Choosing and preparing for an occupation	2. Evaluating one's occupation or career in light of a personal value system	2. Keeping current on relevant scientific, political, and cultural changes
3. Developing a marital relationship or other form of companionship	3. Helping younger persons to become integrated human beings	3. Developing mutually supportive (interdependent) relationships with grown offspring and other members of the younger generation
4. Developing and initiating parenting behaviors for use with own, and other's, offspring	4. Enhancing or redeveloping intimacy with spouse or most significant other	4. Reevaluating and enhancing the relationship with spouse or most significant other or adjusting to his or her loss
5. Developing a personal life-style and philosophy of life	5. Developing a few deep friendships	5. Helping aged parents or other relatives progress through the last stage of life
6. Accepting one's role as a citizen and developing participatory citizen behaviors	6. Helping aging persons progress through the later years of life	6. Deriving satisfaction from increased availability of leisure time
	7. Assuming responsible positions in occupational, social, and civic activities, organizations, and communities	7. Preparing for retirement and planning another career when feasible
	8. Maintaining and improving the home and other forms of property	8. Adapting self and behavior to signals of the accelerated aging process
	9. Using leisure time in satisfying and creative ways	
	10. Adjusting to biological or personal system changes that occur	

*In her text, Stevenson assigns the age range for Middlescence II to be 50 to 70 years.

SOURCE: Material on middlescence from J. S. Stevenson. *Issues and crises during middlescence.* New York: Appleton-Century-Crofts, 1977, pp. 18, 25.

with such women should keep in mind that the goal is to help clients to learn what is self-fulfilling for them. Work outside the home is not the only way to achieve happiness and satisfaction. The nurse should assist women who are having these conflicts to determine why they are having them; is it because they want to change their style of living or because they feel society expects them to do so? The nurse can also help these women to explore the alternatives they have for achieving self-fulfillment. The nurse should guard against stressing career alternatives over others. At times, options which have been rewarding to the nurse are emphasized; remember that varying life-styles are healthy not abnormal.

The individual needs to be prepared physically, mentally, and socially to take on the future in a manner which will promote growth and development. The changes that the adult experiences can produce frustration, confusion, and lack of direction. The nurse can help adults cope with these changes by providing supportive guidance. Familiarizing adults with the developmental tasks that they are facing, helping adults to explore how these tasks might be achieved, and emphasizing that stress is normal when one encounters new and different situations are a few examples of supportive activities which may enhance adaptation when adults are experiencing stress.

Parent/Grandparent

The generative aspect of middlescence is explicit when the roles of parent and grandparent are discussed. One extends oneself to one's children and grandchildren. However, the generative person should also extend herself or himself to others outside the family.

Parenting in the young adult years has been discussed in depth in Chapter 13. Parenting issues in the middle years often involve dealing with the developmental concerns of their adolescent children. This situation can be particularly stressful for middlescent adults because they must adapt to stresses associated with two developmental stages: adolescence and middlescence. Adolescents and young adults need to achieve independence from parents. Parents who have confronted the developmental tasks of middlescence are more likely to foster independence and relinquish control than those who have not. Middlescent parents who have not faced the developmental issues of their life period find it difficult to "let go" because their life goals still include "raising" children. The community health nurse can assist the parent in achieving this generational balance; helping each person progress along his or her developmental continuum should be the major goal.

A primary task of the parent in the middle years is launching children from the parental home. The period of *launching* is defined as the time when parents release their children from the family to lead independent lives (Knafl and Grace, 1978, p. 301). The nurse can help parents through this process by discussing with them the tasks involved in launching, along with ways to accomplish them. Assisting parents in identifying ways, other than child rearing, to achieve satisfaction is one of the most significant activities a community health nurse performs when working with launching families. Adolescents and young adults have a greater chance of achieving healthy independence when their parents support their efforts.

Duvall (1977, pp. 341–342) has discussed the tasks involved in launching as:

1. Rearranging physical facilities and resources of the home

2. Meeting the expenses of launching

3. Reallocating responsibilities among family members

4. Coming to terms with themselves as husband and wife

5. Maintaining open systems of communication within the family and between the family and others

6. Widening the family circle through release of children and obtaining new members through marriage

7. Reconciling conflicting loyalties and philosophies of life

The community health nurse can help parents to be aware of how their involvement with their children should change during launching. Parents must become less directive and allow their children to have less direct contact with them. These changes can be confusing and frustrating to the parent because launching is often a time when parents reflect on how they have raised their children. They evaluate their parenting on the basis of how their children have progressed toward financial independence and whether or not they have established a stable, happy home. Many parents do not consider a child fully launched until these two tasks have been achieved (Knafl and Grace, 1978, p. 311).

Sons are often allowed more emancipation during the launching process than daughters. Knafl and Grace (1978, p. 514) note that parents provide sons with earlier and more frequent opportunities for independent action, give them more privacy in personal affairs, and hold them to less exacting filial and kinship obligations than daughters. This pattern of functioning can cause family conflict and stress, especially if daughters are about the same age as sons. Helping parents to identify the differences in their behavior when dealing with similar issues may help them to alter their behavior.

It is important during this period that children recognize the stresses their parents may be experiencing. Too often, the focus of nursing intervention is only with the parent. Parents are made to think that what they are doing is "all wrong." Adolescents and young adults need to understand that they are not the only ones under stress and that they need to take responsibility for their actions. The rights of the parents, as well as those of the children, should be protected. This is illustrated in the following case situation:

John Michael, age 22, decided to live with his parents because he wanted to save money to buy a condominium. He expected to live free of charge and have no household responsibilities in his parents' home for the next year. His parents were experiencing financial stress because they had two other children in college and had just finished spending a considerable amount of money for John's education. Conflicts arose when John's parents did not agree with his plans. John was making an adequate

salary and they expected him to contribute financially toward family expenses, at least by paying for the food he ate. They also felt that he should assume responsibility for some of the household chores, just as he would do if he were living independently. John was angry because he wanted the freedom of adulthood without having to assume the responsibilities that went along with this freedom.

The community health nurse was involved with John's family because Mrs. Michael was a newly diagnosed diabetic. It was during her third home visit that the nurse identified the stress between John and his parents. During the visit, John's mother was tense, almost to the point of being in tears. Observing her distressed state, the nurse encouraged her to verbalize her feelings and afterward made arrangements to meet jointly with John and his parents. During this conference, the nurse requested that each family member share his or her perceptions of what was happening. Emphasis was also placed on identifying alternative ways to resolve the family conflict and on assisting each family member to see his or her needs and responsibilities.

The Michael family had always been cohesive, so John decided that he would continue to live with his parents for a period of time. He agreed to assume his share of the financial expenses and to help out with the household chores. He stated, "I never realized my parents were also under stress. They always seemed so well put together."

John's response is typical. Children often do not realize that their parents are under stress because parents try to protect them by not sharing their difficulties.

In addition to launching, grandparenting is also encountered in the middle years. Some middlescents experience significant anxiety when their first grandchild arrives because they perceive this event as a sign that they are getting "old." Other middlescents are delighted and eagerly wait for the birth of their first grandchild. Often grandparents find that they have more time to spend with their grandchildren than they did with their own children. A grandparent can greatly enhance the growth of younger generations. Duvall (1962, p. 409) states that

Children need grandparents who have come to terms with life and accept it philosophically as parents have not yet learned or have not had the time to do. When those who are at the beginning of the journey hold hands with those who have travelled a long way and know all the turns in the road, each gains the strength needed by both.

Adults who have achieved generativity, self-fulfillment, and ego integrity are more likely to hold hands with their grandchildren than those who have not achieved these life goals. The birth of a grandchild to them is not viewed as a negative sign of aging, but rather it is seen as a process which extends and expands their life.

Spouse or Companion

Adulthood is a time spent in developing and redeveloping relationships with spouse or significant others. A significant other can be anyone with whom the adult has a close, meaningful relationship. With today's many lifestyles, it is completely possible that there will be a significant other who is not a spouse. This significant other may be part of a heterosexual or homosexual relationship. Accepting various life-styles is essential if the community health nurse is to help the adult achieve self-fulfillment.

Adulthood is a time to enjoy joint activities, relax together, and spend time in a companion relationship. Once the problems associated with the raising of a family have been significantly resolved, as in later middlescence, the adult can look in new directions for ways to use physical, mental, and social energies. It is important for the couple to maintain separate interests and activities while developing, maintaining, or redeveloping complementary relationships.

Establishing satisfying sexual relationships is a major task of adulthood. It is, however, an area often overlooked or not discussed during nurse-client interactions. Clients frequently do not raise sexuality concerns unless encouraged by the health care professional to do so. Specific issues that might need to be addressed during a health interview with an adult include family planning concerns, sexual experimentation before marriage, incompatibility problems, prevention of sexually transmitted diseases, and cultural norms that inhibit the development of meaningful sexual interactions.

The human sexual and emotional responses to menopause and the climacteric can adversely affect spouse or companion relationships. The nurse can help partners to be aware of the changes that they and their mate are experiencing and encourage an emotionally supportive relationship. The adult experiencing these changes should be assisted in seeing that they are normal and do not necessarily have to interfere with sexual activities.

Son or Daughter

Adulthood is a time when children strive to develop independence as well as to maintain significant relationships with their families. It is also a period when the adult may experience role reversal with his or her own parents. As parents become aged and less able to carry out activities of daily living for themselves, the adult is placed in the position of helping aged parents progress through these later years. The adult needs to assist these aged persons without dominating their lives and without taking over decision making for them. He or she must balance this without feeling guilty for doing too little or too much and must realize that it is only possible to do one's best with the resources that are available.

The community health nurse should encourage the adult to verbalize feelings when he or she is caring for aging parents. This is especially important to do when the question of whether or not to place the parent in a nursing home or other extended-care facility arises. It is essential at this time to identify the needs of both the adult and the adult's parents and how the needs of both can be met.

During the middlescent period, it is also important to deal with the eventual death of aged parents and relatives. Burial arrangements and the handling of personal affairs should be discussed and plans should be made. In a society that does not often deal openly with death, this is not an easy task. It is far easier to avoid the topic. A great number of middlescents experience death for the first time with the loss of a parent. The death of the remaining parent has been documented as one of the most constant crisis points in the adult's life (Sheehy, 1976, p. 355). Death becomes more of a reality as one approaches middlescence, and there is often the urge to make more of one's life before it is too late. Death education and helping a family work through the grieving process are important community health nursing activities.

It is also crucial that the adult realize that when aging parents talk about death they are not emotionally disturbed. This is a normal developmental occurrence which should not be denied simply because it arouses difficult feelings. Assisting aging parents to resolve their feelings about death can help adults in accepting their own eventual death.

Citizen

During the early adult years, persons are usually involved in civic responsibilities that directly affect their families, such as membership in a parent-teacher organization, block clubs to improve their environment, and political elections when school millage is an issue. During middlescence, the individual becomes engaged to a greater degree in civic activities, because more time is freed from family re-

sponsibilities and there is stability in occupational endeavors and an increased tendency toward generative activity.

People in middlescence are accorded the highest positions in American society, including the presidency, company top executive jobs, and high military and civil positions. They are expected to take an active role in civic activities. Middlescents have much influence in the community and tend to run for federal, state, and local offices. They are sought as community leaders and often serve as community volunteers. Adults are valuable resources as volunteer staff and supporters for health projects in the community. However, the middlescent who does not experience a lessening in home and work responsibilities will have less time for such activities unless other adjustments are made. This is increasingly becoming a problem, because two-career families are frequently postponing the onset of parenthood.

The existence of people available to carry out civic activities is critical to the survival of the nation. Not having persons in leadership and volunteer positions would be a great loss for this country. Community health nurses can help make adults aware of their importance to the community. They can help adults to see the need for balancing citizen commitments and family and individual responsibilities.

Friend

Adulthood is a time of life when developing and maintaining a few deep friendships is beneficial and rewarding. It is also a time when one has decreased contact with members of the immediate family, due to mobility, death, or launching of children. Having friends that one can count on and enjoy being with helps to provide support and pleasure when family contacts are limited. Since middlescent adults have more time for leisure activities, it is often satisfying to have friends with whom they can share their activities.

The community health nurse frequently encourages the adult to mobilize additional friendship support in times of stress. Sharing ways to meet other adults with similar interests is helpful. Volunteer work with health or other community agencies, social clubs in the community, church activities, or adult discussion groups are some of the options that the nurse could explore with the adult who has limited friendships. Some adults will prefer not to develop or maintain these friendships.

Leisure-Time User

Leisure is not an easy word to define; it means many things to many people. Leisure is antithetical to work as an economic pursuit. It is a planned activity that promotes growth and is pleasurable. Table 15-2 differentiates between work and leisure activities. Internal motivation is the key factor to consider when working with clients who do not plan leisure activities.

In our society, many adults do not seriously engage in leisure-time activity. We are work oriented, and leisure activity is given a lower priority than other activities. When leisure activity does occur, it is largely in the environ-

ments of home and community. Some adults limit their leisure activities mainly to the home setting because they have a number of responsibilities that closely tie them to this environment. For the person with many responsibilities at home, leisure time may be more relaxing and fulfilling outside that setting.

Because leisure activity is a developmental task for adulthood, the community health nurse should encourage the adult to make a conscious effort to devote time to these activities. Otherwise, an important developmental area is being overlooked. People need time in which to enjoy themselves and relax. The great amount of free time that often accompanies later life will be better spent if individuals have developed leisure-time activities that are satisfying to them.

Frequently the adult needs help in examining why he or she does not engage in leisure activities. Often it will be found that many adults do not know how to use the free time they have and thus they devote all their time to work or other responsibilities. The nurse can assist these individuals by helping them to identify interests they have had in the past or would like to develop now, as well as to explore ways in which they can meet their current interests. Take for example, the case of Sara Washington:

Sara Washington was a 40-year-old divorced woman with no children. She was referred to the community health nurse for health supervision visits by her family physician following hospitalization for severe hypertension. After her divorce, Sara devoted herself to work. She was an interior designer who was well respected in her field; promotions came very rapidly. Most of her social involvements were work-related.

Sara's recent hospitalization scared her. When the community health nurse took a social history on her first home visit, she replied, "I know I can't keep working like I have been, but I get bored when I don't have something to do. There is very little social life for a woman my age in this town. My peers

TABLE 15-2 Comparison of Work and Leisure

Dimension	Work	Leisure
Decision-making control	Relatively more external	Relatively more internal
Spatial parameter	Continuity of space	Freedom of space
Time parameter	Structured time	Nonstructured time
Social structure	Permanence of structure	Transiency of structure
Activity	Defined activity	Emerged activity

SOURCE: From J. S. Stevenson. *Issues and crises during middlescence.* New York: Appleton-Century-Crofts, 1977, p. 72.

are all married or divorced themselves. Those who are divorced are like me, they work all the time."

Community health nursing intervention helped Sara to discover how much she missed contact with people on a personal level, the types of social activities she might explore, her fears about getting involved, and the middlescent's need for leisure-time activities to achieve normal growth and development. Sara had enjoyed cooking, entertaining friends, art, and drama before her divorce. Supportive encouragement by the community health nurse facilitated her getting involved once again in these activities. She especially enjoyed dance lessons and found that they provided several opportunities for socializing. "You know, when one takes the time, it really isn't that difficult to find something to do," stated Sara during one of the nurse's home visits.

Adults who have experienced a stressful life event such as divorce frequently use work to reduce their tension and anxiety. Unfortunately, this develops into a regular pattern of functioning whereby work becomes the central focus of life and leisure activity is eliminated. An astute community health nurse might prevent this from happening by providing anticipatory guidance and supportive encouragement when encountering adults during times of heightened stress.

Worker

The health of the worker and the role of the occupational health nurse are discussed in Chapter 16. Work as a major adult role is discussed here. Working is generally essential to one's economic stability and has psychological implications for the individual as well.

The young adult is in a stage of training for, and deciding upon, a career. The middlescent is often at a career peak and derives much satisfaction from her or his job; this is usually the time of maximum power and influence. The average age of American men in executive business positions is 54 years old; Americans aged 40 to 65 years old earn one-

half of the nation's income while representing only one-fourth of the nation's population (Sheehy, 1976, p. 342).

By the time a person reaches middlescence, career patterns are usually well established. It will be found, however, that some adults are in the process of changing careers or are dissatisfied with their present jobs. The community health nurse must realize that both of these situations can be difficult for the adult and may require crisis intervention services. Through the use of the nursing process, the community health nurse can help these adults to identify why they are dissatisfied with their career choice, what options or alternatives are open, and the career planning resources available in the community, including agencies like career counseling centers, state employment security commissions, and departments of vocational rehabilitation.

Job dissatisfaction is often related to other personal difficulties; stresses at work can be compounded when an adult has home pressures to handle. This was the case with Ed Sorka.

Ed Sorka was a 29-year-old husband and father of two daughters, ages 3 and 5. He became disillusioned with his job because "his boss demanded too much and gave too few rewards." Ed's wife had multiple sclerosis which was getting progressively worse. She required help with activities of daily living and found it hard to participate in social events. Ed was a devoted husband and father. All his spare time was spent with his family. He found it difficult to talk about his wife's condition or his need for leisure activities; verbalizing stress encountered at work was much easier for him to handle. When the community health nurse helped him to examine both work and home stresses, Ed discovered that he really did not want to change jobs but that he did need time for himself. Arrangements were made for homemaker services to reduce the demands on Ed's time.

Some adults change jobs or careers out of necessity and not by choice, because of changes in the job market or personal health problems. These individuals and their families can experience intense stress, especially if the adult who is changing careers derived great satisfaction from the previous work. The McSweeney family, for instance, had an increased incidence of health problems when Mr. McSweeney returned to college to prepare for another career.

George McSweeney was a 38-year-old engineer, husband, and father of three school-age children. As a result of industrial noise, he lost 50 percent of his hearing. Unable to continue functioning at his present job, he returned to college to prepare for another career. Financially, his family had few difficulties because Mr. McSweeney received workers' compensation and federal scholarship monies. The community health nurse encountered the McSweeney family after they had repeatedly taken Lisa, their 10-year-old daughter, into the emergency room for treatment of an asthmatic condition. The nurse was well received by the family because both parents were unsure of when to seek medical care for their daughter. The nurse discovered that Lisa's condition had been well under control until the family had moved and she had changed schools. In addition, she found that Mr. McSweeney was having tension headaches regularly; a medical evaluation ruled out organic problems. Lisa had fewer asthma attacks and Mr. McSweeney had fewer headaches as the family began to verbalize the frustrations associated with the multiple changes they had recently experienced.

Stress on the family system also occurs when a wife returns to work during the middlescent years. Many wives stay home during the young adult years to raise a family and to tend the home. As home responsibilities decrease, there are an increasing number of women who seek employment. Duvall (1977, p. 368) has found that the chances of wives' working are greater in the middle years than at any other time in life. Both spouses' working brings up a number of considerations. For instance, the combined incomes can give a financial flexibility that may not have existed previously. This sit-

uation gives the family more choices in relation to recreational activities and plans for the future. The wife's working can also create changes in roles and role expectations which result in stress. The husband may now be expected to assume more responsibility for household chores, meal patterns may change, and the wife may develop interests outside the home that do not include her husband. Families who have a flexible division of labor before the wife goes back to work are more likely to adjust to these changes than families whose roles are rigidly allocated prior to this time (see Chapter 6).

As the adult approaches middlescence, retirement is another area for which planning is needed. Many people look forward to retirement and see it as an opportunity for doing things that they were previously unable to do. Others dread it because they either do not want to cease working or realize that they are not financially stable enough to enjoy it. Success in retirement depends on planning for it during this period of life. Chapter 18 discusses ways in which families can plan for aging and deal with issues associated with retirement.

HEALTH AND THE WELL ADULT

Achieving health for the adult involves maintaining physical, mental, and social well-being. Most adults are considered healthy, but the well adult has many health care needs. These needs are often overlooked due to the self-sufficient nature of the adult and the caretaker role accorded to her or him by society. A combination of the two may put an adult in the position of being "too busy" or "too involved" to look after personal health care needs. It can be difficult to persuade the well adult to obtain health care and practice preventive health habits. The human body during adulthood will be briefly discussed to help illustrate some of the physical and mental changes that the adult experiences.

The Human Body in Adulthood

The human body is always undergoing physical and mental changes. During adulthood the person begins to develop an acute awareness of growing older and is faced with adjusting to a changing body image as physical alterations occur. This adjustment is difficult in American society, as the beauty and stamina of youth are prized. The incidence of chronic and handicapping conditions increases with age and these conditions can also affect how one views oneself.

There are several physical changes which occur in the human body during adulthood. Vision is usually well maintained in early adulthood, but presbyopia (farsightedness) is extremely common by middlescence. Presbyopia is caused by a decreased lens elasticity which reduces the power of accommodation. It hinders the ability of the individual to view objects at close range, and glasses may be necessary for reading or close work. After age 30, the cornea begins to lose transparency and the pupil decreases in size. These changes allow less light to be admitted to the eye and result in poor illumination (Division of Gerontology, 1957, p. 55).

Permanent sensorineural hearing loss due to aging (presbycusis) accelerates during middlescence. The person experiencing presbycusis has decreased auditory acuity for higher tones and may have difficulty engaging in normal conversation, including talking over the telephone. The duration and type of noise exposure that a person encounters during earlier life influences how soon presbycusis begins (see Chapter 16). For example, the person exposed to industrial noise and the avid hunter may experience presbycusis earlier than their counterparts because of more extensive sensorineural hearing damage during youth.

Metabolic function, the ability to combine food with oxygen to create energy, decreases during adulthood. This, coupled with the fact that the person is often becoming more sedentary, can mean increased weight. There is a decrease in metabolic activity of about 5 percent for each decade after age 25 with a resultant need for reduction in caloric intake of approximately 7.5 percent (Murray and Zentner, 1975, p. 260).

Decreasing elasticity in the blood vessels, especially the coronary arteries, predisposes the middlescent to cardiovascular disease. Many middlescents evidence the symptomology of cardiac conditions, such as shortness of breath, chest pains, and dyspnea on exertion. Incidence of death from cardiovascular disease is on the rise in adulthood.

In middlescence the female's ovarian estrogen production and menstruation cease. This event is called *menopause* and usually occurs between the ages of 40 and 50 years. This does not necessarily affect sexual functioning but does have an effect on body functioning. Once the female passes through menopause, her childbearing capabilities cease. This often has greater psychological meaning than physical significance. Some of the physical symptomology that may be evidenced during menopause are hot flashes, sweating, chills, dizziness, headaches, palpitations, and muscle cramping. Psychological symptomology include depression, change in sexual drive, and insomnia.

In middlescence, the male passes through a period called the *climacteric,* when the testes decrease, but do not cease, testosterone production. During this time, the testes atrophy slightly, sperm production decreases, and in about 20 percent of men, hypertrophy of the prostate begins (Murray and Zentner, 1975, p. 257). The male usually goes through this period between ages 50 and 60. He may or may not experience any physical symptoms. Psychological symptoms such as irritability, easy frustration, depression, and change in sexual drives are sometimes evidenced. Many people are not aware that this period exists for men and are often bewildered by male behavior during the climacteric.

Decalcification of the bones, a condition

called *osteoporosis,* begins in middlescence. When this happens, the bones become fragile and are easily broken. Vertebral compression can occur and result in backache, headache, and other problems.

As a person ages, the amount of skeletal muscle decreases and muscle cells are replaced by adipose and connective tissue. As a result of these changes, adults have decreased muscle tone, a flabbier appearance, and decreased muscle strength (Diekelman, 1977, p. 84). Exercise will help to maintain muscle tone and strength. The adult can engage in a variety of activities and sports, but it is advised that individuals check with a physician before beginning any vigorous exercise routine. The adult should exercise consistently, gradually increasing the amount to avoid overexertion.

An example of how an adult undergoing the physical changes of middlescence can be affected by these changes is seen in the following case situation.

Marge, a 50-year-old widow and mother of three daughters, ages 24, 27, and 30, is a typical example of how many people react to body changes during middlescence. She sought help at a local adult screening clinic because she perceived that the physical changes she was undergoing were making her look older than her chronological age. She wanted to maintain a youthful look and stated, "I am having a hard time getting old. I fear the physical changes and the dependency associated with aging." These thoughts were triggered when Marge's oldest daughter celebrated her thirtieth birthday.

Actually, besides the natural process of advancing chronological age, Marge was doing well. She had an established career and had just recently developed an intimate relationship with a man that could lead to marriage. She was loved and respected by her children and had frequent contact with them without interfering in their lives. Friends enjoyed being with her and described her as intellectually stimulating and fun. Marge, however, could focus only on her physical changes and was experiencing anxiety in relation to them. She was questioning whether she should terminate her relationship with

her male companion so that she would not be hurt in the future. "Men only marry beautiful women."

The community health nurse that saw Marge at the adult screening clinic made arrangements to visit her at home. This nurse utilized the principles of crisis intervention to help her sort out reality. Marge was helped to identify her strengths and to look more realistically at the changes in her physical appearance. She was assisted in seeing that she had several alternatives open to her regarding her life and that withdrawing from personal relationships could increase her social aging process. Marge gradually began to realize that if she focused on her physical appearance alone, she could lose the joys of life she had already achieved.

Marge is not atypical of the many adults with whom the community health nurse will work. The physical changes of the aging process can be difficult to handle. The development of generativity, self-fulfillment, and ego integrity helps an individual to adapt to physical changes associated with the aging process, because these life goals give meaning and direction to one's future.

Even though physical functioning changes or decreases, mental function can be maintained or increased during adulthood. Cerebral capacity begins to weaken relatively slowly, unless other factors such as cerebrovascular occlusion or depression occur. At age 70, the person can be as intellectually capable as at age 30 and has a greater experiential base than in youth to draw from when making decisions (Division of Gerontology, 1957, p. 58). General intelligence of the middlescent is greater than at any other time of life.

Selected Causes of Mortality in Adulthood

Although adults are generally considered to be physically and mentally healthy, deaths do occur during this developmental period. Table 15-3 presents selected major causes of death for the adult and points out a need for health promotion activities that will aid in identifying

TABLE 15-3 Selected Causes of Mortality for the Young Adult and Middlescent in the United States (1975)

Cause of mortality	Age group*				
	20–29	30–39	40–49	50–59	60–69
Deaths (all causes)	49,288	45,295	96,788	220,385	377,821
Malignant neoplasms (including lymphatic and hematopoietic)	3,355 (7%)	6,783 (15%)	24,045 (25%)	64,256 (29%)	102,298 (27%)
Major cardiovascular	2,527 (5%)	7,506 (17%)	31,476 (33%)	92,796 (42%)	187,369 (50%)
Accidents	20,405 (41%)	10,079 (22%)	9,310 (10%)	9,954 (5%)	9,608 (3%)
Suicide	5,926 (12%)	4,132 (9%)	4,420 (5%)	4,592 (2%)	3,354 (1%)
Homicide	7,706 (16%)	4,364 (10%)	3,199 (3%)	2,124 (1%)	1,199
Pneumonia	663 (1%)	860 (2%)	1,696 (2%)	3,514 (2%)	6,651 (2%)
Liver cirrhosis	489 (1%)	2,190 (5%)	6,219 (6%)	9,632 (4%)	8,482 (2%)
Diabetes mellitus	350	717 (2%)	1,392 (1%)	3,901 (2%)	8,208 (2%)
Emphysema	20	62	423	2,017	5,788 (2%)
Nephritis and nephrosis	182	256	506	977	1,837

*Number in age groups: 20–29 years, 37,261,000; 30–39 years, 24,611,000; 40–49 years, 22,879,000; 50–59 years, 22,516,000; 60–69 years, 17,337,000.

NOTE: Percentages were rounded to nearest whole number. Percentages less than 1 percent not given. Also, totals are not 100 percent because percentages of less than 1 and all causes of death are not listed.

SOURCES: U.S. Department of Health, Education, and Welfare (Public Service National Center for Health Statistics). *Vital Statistics of the United States 1975 (Vol. II. Mortality Pt. B).* Washington, D.C.: U.S. Government Printing Office, 1975, pp. 7-134 to 7-151; and U.S. Department of Commerce (Bureau of the Census). *Illustrative Projections of World Populations to the 21st Century.* Washington, D.C.: U.S. Government Printing Office, 1979, p. 35.

at-risk adults who may experience premature mortality. Note that although the order changes, malignant neoplasms, major cardiovascular diseases, accidents, and suicide keep repeating themselves through the adult years.

The Community Health Nurse's Role in Maintaining Health

Health is a combination of interrelated physical, mental, and social factors. The community health nurse can play a major role in maintaining adult health at primary, secondary, and tertiary levels of prevention. All three lev-els of health prevention necessitate health counseling, teaching, and utilization of appropriate resources. They all demand action on the part of the client with the nurse functioning as a facilitator. Enhancing the self-care capabilities of the client as much as possible is the nurse's major goal when working with the adult population.

Utilization of the referral process, as discussed in Chapter 9, is an integral part of the nurse's role when maintaining the health of the adult. Nurses can help adults be aware of available resources that meet their health care needs and refer them to these resources when appropriate. Many health care resources are organized to deal with acute health care episodes rather than with preventive health care measures. Several of the latter type of services, however, are available through the local health department. For example, screening, educational, and treatment services may be offered in venereal disease, tuberculosis, family planning, immunization, adult health, and antepartal clinics within this agency. Or health department personnel from mental health, nutrition, and nursing departments may provide these same types of services in other community settings.

In looking at the major causes of death for the adult, and the biological and personal changes that are occurring, the community health nurse sees that the adult has a variety of health care needs. She or he also realizes that adults are "busy" people. They are active and have responsibilities at home, at work, and in the community. They often spend so much time achieving and doing for others that their own health needs are overlooked or neglected. It is not an easy task to motivate adults to participate in health activities, especially if they consider themselves well. The well adult does not always recognize or act on health needs, or does not see the value of primary prevention activities.

The community health nurse is involved in many primary prevention activities with the adult. She or he is particularly interested in helping the adult to learn about health problems that can be prevented and about health behaviors that can promote wellness. A major primary prevention activity with adults is health teaching in relation to such things as accident prevention, nutrition, personal hygiene, health examinations, family planning, venereal disease, disease transmission, and immunizations. Such health teaching, with utilization of resources as appropriate, may help to prevent an accident, dental caries, an unwanted pregnancy, marital disenchantment, a suicide attempt, a case of tetanus, a case of flu, an in-

cident of child abuse, or a case of venereal disease. Health teaching activities help the adult to look at health in relation to present as well as future functioning.

Safety for the adult is a key factor to consider when one is developing health teaching strategies. Table 15-3 illustrated that accidents cause a significant number of deaths in this age category. Accidents happen at home as well as in all other environments. The nurse should help the adult to assess for potential safety hazards and to identify ways to correct them. Suggestions on measures to promote safety such as having stairway handrails, conveniently located electrical outlets, indirect nonglare lighting, and safe water and sewage disposal; keeping equipment in proper working order; providing easy entry and exit into bathtubs and showers; maintaining stairs and landings free from clutter; and making sure that rugs are not loose can help to prevent accidents in the home.

Health teaching with the young adult should also emphasize accident prevention. Almost 70 percent of all the deaths in this age category are from violent causes (accidents, suicide, and homicide). Over 40 percent are from accidents, and many of these accidents involve motor vehicles. Just being aware of these astounding statistics may have an effect on the risk-taking behavior of the young adult. Many young adults do not take the threat of accidental injury seriously. The "it won't happen to me syndrome" encourages risk-taking behavior, such as fast driving, that could possibly have been avoided. The young adult should be made aware of the possible consequences of this type of behavior, as well as the advantages of using safety measures such as seat belts. Lecturing does not facilitate change in persons in this developmental age group. They must be given the message that they are responsible for making personal health decisions and for the consequences of their health actions.

In order to prevent conditions from occurring, nurses can assist adults in looking at their own personal health habits. Smoking, excessive intake of alcoholic beverages, lack of sufficient rest, and not eating a well-balanced diet all have an impact on an individual's present and future health status.

On the secondary prevention level, the nurse can again stress the importance of medical, dental, and ophthalmological examinations for early diagnosis and treatment of disease. Secondary preventive health measures for the adult include practicing self-examination of the breasts and other self-check measures, yearly Pap smears, and adherence to prescribed medical and dental regimens. The adult should be encouraged in close self-monitoring for conditions for which he or she has a familial or individual predisposition, such as cardiovascular accidents, diabetes, cancer, or hypertension. The adult should utilize health resources available to and appropriate for himself or herself, such as those previously discussed.

Tertiary prevention health activities that the nurse may utilize with the adult are largely related to rehabilitation activities which minimize the degree of disability of the condition. These activities are discussed in Chapter 17, where the nurse's role in rehabilitation of the handicapped adult is covered. They often involve interdisciplinary functioning and focus on encouraging client compliance with prescribed medical and dental regimens, as well as exploring ways to promote coping behaviors.

It should be stressed that the physical, mental, and social components of health are interrelated. When one aspect of health is affected, the others are also affected. Thus, when planning preventive activities on all three levels, it is important for the community health nurse to take into consideration the client's psychosocial needs as well as the physical ones.

Significant Legislation Affecting Adult Health

Much of the legislation that influences the adult also makes an impact on other age groups. The Social Security Act of 1935 and its amendments provide many maternal-child health programs, which are discussed in Chapters 4 and 13. The Social Security Act also provides for Medicaid and Medicare, for which the medically indigent or terminally ill adult may qualify. The Public Health Service Act of 1944 and its amendments have helped to provide adult health care services such as the cancer, heart, and stroke amendments of 1965 and 1970. These amendments provide funds for research, prevention, and early diagnosis and treatment for "killer" conditions that primarily attack the adult population.

Possibly one of the most significant pieces of legislation that addresses the adult population is the Occupational Safety and Health Act of 1970, which is discussed in Chapter 16. It deals with maintaining the health of the adult in the workplace and focuses on maintaining wellness.

As with the other age categories, legislation is often passed to help the poor and disadvantaged. The adult years have been neglected ones in terms of health care structured particularly for them. The very dearth of legislation aimed at providing preventive health services for this particular age group dramatically demonstrates this neglect.

SOME CRISES OF ADULTHOOD AND NURSING INTERVENTION

Life comprises a series of *major life events* (see Table 6-6). Major life events are ones that have a significant impact on how well an individual is able to accomplish life goals. The number, duration, and type of these events will vary from individual to individual. A major life event for one person may not be considered a major life event for another.

Unlike children, who have parents or others to support and guide them through the experience of major life events, the adult often does not have support available during times of heightened stress; or the adult may not use the help that is available because dependency is feared. This happens especially when one is immature and cannot accept oneself. A mature adult recognizes his or her strengths and values interdependency. However, because our society emphasizes self-sufficiency during adulthood, even a mature adult may experience feelings of insecurity when seeking assistance from others.

Examples of some major life events for most adults are leaving the parental home, obtaining job education and training, pursuing a career, marriage, childbearing, child rearing, child launching, providing for an aging parent, pursuing leisure-time activities, and experiencing the death of a parent. Other major life events that some adults experience include divorce or separation, loss of a child, loss of a job, development of a chronic health condition, and career changes. If these events occur in rapid succession, the adult may have difficulty adapting and experience crisis.

An example of what can happen when major life events occur in rapid succession is seen in the Stephen Johns case situation:

In a period of less than 10 years, Mr. Johns, 28 years old, left home to enter college, completed a college education, entered a career, married, had a child, changed jobs, moved to a new residence, became divorced, moved to another residence, changed jobs again, and experienced the death of a parent. These were all significant life events for Mr. Johns, and the rapid succession of their development left him in a confused and disorganized state. Because he began to question whether his life had meaning, he sought counseling through a local mental health clinic. Through work with a psychiatric nurse therapist, Mr. Johns was able to establish

life goals and to take action to achieve these goals. This made him comfortable about himself as a person, and gave direction and meaning to his life.

Mr. Johns is not atypical. Although major life events may not always be experienced this rapidly, or in this magnitude, many significant stresses do occur during adulthood. While experiencing these stresses, adults are also trying to achieve a balance between their responsibilities to family and society, to develop as individuals, and to maintain health. These tasks in themselves produce stress. Thus, when sudden or unexpected situational difficulties arise, such as divorce, death, or changes in job and residence, the individual is at risk for crisis.

It is important for the community health nurse to recognize that the crisis state may be experienced at any time throughout adult life. When mobilizing coping mechanisms during times of stress, the adult has many life experiences from which to draw. These experiences, however, do not necessarily prepare one to handle all the threatening events that occur throughout adulthood. At each developmental stage there are new or different events requiring adaptation. The following quote from Knafl and Grace (1978, p. 265), for instance, vividly portrays the pressures one deals with during middlescence:

He (the middlescent) realizes that the choices of the past have limited his choices in the present. He can no longer dream of infinite possibilities. He is forced to acknowledge that he has worked up to or short of his capabilities. Goals may or may not have been reached; aspirations may have to be modified. The possibility for advancement becomes more remote. He will have to go on with ever-brighter, ever-younger men and women crowding into competitive economic, political and social arenas. In the United States success is highly valued, and is measured by prestige, wealth or power. To be without these by middle age causes stress, and the likelihood of achieving them diminishes with age.

When working with the adult in crisis, it is important for the community health nurse to deal with the current realities of the situation. The individual should be helped to look at the circumstances that precipitated the crisis and modify them to reduce future occurrences. The nurse should be supportive of the client without leveling judgment. She or he should help the client and family to assess the resources and support systems they have available and to make plans for the immediate future. As discussed in Chapter 7, the mastery of a crisis provides opportunities for personal growth and development.

A major goal of community health nursing practice in relation to crisis is prevention. In order to achieve this goal, the community health nurse must recognize early signs and symptoms of heightened stress (see Chapter 7) and must help individuals who are experiencing these symptoms to mobilize appropriate coping mechanisms. Depression is frequently a symptom experienced by an adult who has intensified stress. Encountering clients who are depressed is a common occurrence in community health nursing practice. At times, the client is able to resolve the depressed state by utilizing the supportive assistance of the community health nurse and significant others, such as family, friends, relatives, and lovers. At other times, additional mental health counseling is necessary.

Persons who are depressed often are not aware that their condition exists. They know that they do not feel right but frequently seek help for minor physical problems. That is why it is so important for the community health nurse to systematically collect a complete health history (see Chapter 8) when working with adult clients. If data are collected only in relation to the client's physical health complaint, depression will be missed.

Depression is not always a sign that the individual is experiencing a crisis. Depression is a normal state in life. All persons have times when they feel low and discouraged. Depression becomes a problem when it is chronic and affects the person's ability to cope with the events of daily living.

Freud saw depression as aggression turned inward. Others see depression as a state that occurs when the person loses a valued object, such as a person, material resources, or status. A contemporary view of depression is that it is a chronic frustration stemming from environmental stresses beyond an individual's coping ability and resources (Akiskal and McKinney, 1973, p. 21).

Depression can be evidenced by somatic symptoms. Feeling tired, listless, having sleep disturbances, anorexia, abdominal discomfort, weight loss, or constipation are common symptoms experienced by depressed clients (Ayd, 1961, p. 26). It is important for the community health nurse to realize that many medical problems as well as psychological difficulties cause depression. Some of these are hypertension, hyperparathyroidism, pernicious anemia, hypoglycemia, intracranial tumors, multiple sclerosis, and systemic lupus erythematosus. Any chronic or painful condition has the potential for causing depression. Depression is often characterized by withdrawal from others, loss of appetite, insomnia, difficulty in concentration, and a general disinterest in people and things (Peplau, 1975, p. 1773).

When working with clients who are depressed, the community health nurse should help to structure or restructure their environment into something positive and hopeful (Cole, Schatzberg, and Frazier, 1978, p. 185). The depressed person should be given a chance to air complaints and grievances and assistance which will help her or him to deal with problems. The nurse should remember that depressed persons may be angry at themselves or think that others have failed them. It may be difficult for them to develop a trusting relationship with another person. Thus, it is important to recognize that when a depressed client withdraws from the nurse-client interaction, it does not necessarily mean he or she does not want help. It probably means that the client is afraid to trust others.

Clients who are depressed are frequently unable to see any positive alternatives in their lives because they dwell on their failures. It is critical that the nurse help the client to see the alternatives to the current situation. Depressed clients can feel an intense sense of hopelessness. They feel immobilized, as if there were no solution to the situation. If persons can see that there are alternatives, the atmosphere of hopelessness is diluted.

When visiting depressed clients, the community health nurse needs to extend empathy without being sympathetic. Sympathy serves to reinforce the person's depressed state. The nurse should encourage the client to be an active participant in the therapeutic process rather than a passive sufferer. The nurse must remember that the client will need support to be active, since it can be difficult for the person who is depressed to take action. Helping the client to recognize strengths and assets, instead of focusing on the negative aspects of the situation, frequently assists the client to assume greater independence.

Maintaining two-way communication between the client and nurse is essential. People who are depressed generally like feedback on what is going on (Cole, Schatzberg, and Frazier, 1978, p. 195). They like to know that someone has listened to them and is available for support and assistance. Unfortunately, all too often the depressed client is excluded from social contacts. Family, friends, and even professionals do this frequently because they are trying to protect the client or themselves from further hurt or stress. Excluding the client who is depressed does not help and only serves to reinforce his or her weaknesses and feelings that no one cares.

Depressed individuals who are assessed to be potentially suicidal should be referred for psychotherapy. Some nurses are afraid to assess for suicide potential because they fear their questioning may precipitate a suicide attempt. Suicide is not prevented by avoiding conversation about it. Rather, it is prevented by helping clients get the assistance they need to deal with stresses in their daily lives.

Helping clients who are depressed can be discouraging because progress is very slow and the client appears to resent any assistance received. When working with such clients, community health nurses find it especially helpful to talk with peers and supervisors about the feelings that they are experiencing and about alternatives for enhancing client action. Sometimes others who are not directly involved in the nurse-client interaction can better identify progress made than those who are.

There are numerous life events that can precipitate depression and crisis in the adult years. A few examples of these events will be shared below. It should be remembered that depression will continue to exist until the individual is able to successfully mobilize coping mechanism that enhance growth. Most chronic depressions are related to unresolved psychosocial difficulties. Crisis is self-limiting; chronic depression is not.

Changing Jobs or Careers

The case situations presented earlier in the chapter on the worker role illustrate that making a decision to alter one's work role can result in crisis and indecision. During this time, a major reorganization is required in one's life and the stresses encountered should not be underestimated. The adult's perceptions of the situation should be ascertained. Does the individual see it as a new and challenging adventure or as a threat to personal and economic security? The community health nurse should be especially sensitive to the distresses that occur when an individual is changing jobs or careers not because he or she wants to but because it is necessary. Change is not easy. It can result in a more satisfying life or it can result in dissatisfaction, depending on how the client views what is happening. Support, encouragement, or concrete assistance through referral can facilitate individual growth and development and make the change more rewarding.

Chronic Illness

As discussed in Chapters 10 and 17, chronic illness is a major health problem in the American population. An overview of the nurse's role with the adult who has a chronic illness is given here.

When the adult is afflicted with a chronic health condition, major changes in family life may occur. The extent of these changes varies, depending on the degree of disability encountered and the adult's perception of the event. Role reversal, changes in sexual behavior, and alterations in self-image are a few examples of the problems experienced by clients who have developed debilitating chronic illness during adulthood. The adult who is not progressing well along the developmental continuum may regress, become depressed, or become dependent when chronically ill. He or she may resist treatment and techniques to make recovery faster, or become self-absorbed, not relate to others well, and use the illness as an escape from responsibility (Knafl and Grace, 1978, p. 275).

Community health nurses must understand the difficulties encountered when one is chronically ill before they can effectively work with clients who have chronic conditions. The nurse must believe that the well-adjusted adult will want to resume the normal level of independence and functioning as soon as possible and she or he must provide the support needed for the individual to do so. The nurse can assist the client and family by making them aware of what is happening in the course of the client's condition, giving anticipatory guid-

ance, and encouraging them to take an active role in health care decision making.

It is important for the community health nurse to maintain a therapeutic role with the chronically ill adult. It is easy for the nurse to fall into a pattern of encouraging clients to meet societal expectations of self-sufficiency, minimal dependency, and support to those around them. The nurse must realize that the chronically ill adult needs adequate support from others to deal successfully with his or her condition. The nurse should not make unrealistic promises of recovery or an optimistic prognosis; there may be no guarantee that treatment will improve the level of disability. False hopes prevent the client from confronting the crisis.

Use of both the educative and problem-solving approaches to nursing intervention is often essential when one is working with families who are dealing with a chronic condition. These families frequently need increased knowledge in order to realistically evaluate the changes which are occurring and which may occur in the future. These families also need to problem-solve in order to determine the most appropriate ways for them to adapt to changes, especially permanent ones. Chronic illness, for instance, can be both emotionally and financially draining. Different coping mechanisms must be mobilized to reduce tension and to maintain financial stability. The possibility of death may also be a matter for the nurse to think through with chronically ill adults and their families. Families should be allowed to express their fears whether or not they are realistic and be encouraged to prepare for death if the client's situation warrants such action. Reading materials written by Kübler-Ross (1974, 1975) can enhance a community health nurse's skill in working with clients who are dying.

The hospice care movement is gaining popularity in this country (Amado, Cronk, and Mileo, 1979, p. 522). Hospice care is designed to keep the chronically ill person who is terminal at home as long as possible. A family-centered, multidisciplinary approach is used in this movement, with an emphasis placed on improving the quality of life for both the client and the client's family during the final stages of dying. Community health nurses are regular participants on this interdisciplinary team, and thus they must be prepared to deal with the concerns of dying clients and their families. It is becoming increasingly important for community health nurses to be skilled at caring for this group of people.

When working with any chronically ill adult, the community health nurse will more than likely utilize the referral process. There are a variety of community resources, such as the Lost Chord Club, the Multiple Sclerosis Association, the Cancer Society, Goodwill Industries, the Division of Vocational Rehabilitation, and the Department of Social Services, which will help clients and their families to adapt to chronic illness. It is critical, when working with clients who are chronically ill, for the community health nurse to know about resources that will help the client with his or her rehabilitation process.

Marital Crises

It is not uncommon for the community health nurse to encounter families who are experiencing marital disenchantment, separation, or divorce. There has been "an increase in the divorce rate to the point that two out of every five marriages in the United States end in divorce" (White House Conference on Families, 1978, p. 288). Marital crises occur throughout adulthood and should not be considered a problem of youth. During middlescence, for instance, spouses find that they have more time together, and if they are unable to re-establish intimacy or reinforce it, they may become disenchanted with their marital relationship. In addition, the sexual changes (menopause and climacteric) that occur during middlescence can also adversely affect the way in which spouses relate in the marital relationship.

Marital crises (disenchantment, separation, and divorce) have an impact on all family members. Adults as well as children need to make major changes. Experiencing feelings of uncertainty, betrayal, insecurity, failure, and loss is common during this time. As with all crises, the primary focus of the community health nurse with clients who have marital stress is on helping the clients to achieve homeostasis. Adaptation could require divorce or separation, but it also may occur through renegotiation and alteration of family patterns which are dysfunctional. A therapeutic approach that encourages problem solving rather than blaming can best facilitate successful adaptation during this time of crisis.

Anticipatory guidance activities by the community health nurse may be instrumental in preventing marital crises. Preparing young adults to handle the stresses of parenthood or middlescent couples to deal with the conflicts during launching, for instance, may decrease the amount of distress experienced at these times.

Helping adults handle life crises such as those described above can be rewarding as well as challenging. Confusion, crisis, stress, and depression are all normal parts of life. If the adult has a supportive environment and assistance from others, he or she is better able to achieve health. Community health nurses are often in a favorable position to provide the extra assistance needed to adapt during times of crisis and stress.

SUMMARY

The adult is a significant member of our population and one who is often overlooked as having health needs. This group, which financially supports other age groups, is vulnerable to some unique pressures and stresses because adults are expected to be self-sufficient. It is often hard for them to admit that they have health problems or are experiencing stress.

The role of the nurse in helping adults achieve their developmental tasks is an important one. Understanding the growth process is essential in dealing with it effectively. It is easier for the adult to grow and to maintain health when he or she knows about health behaviors that enhance wellness and prevent stress. The major goal of the community health nurse when working with adults is to help them to increase their self-care capabilities.

REFERENCES

Akiskal, H. S., & McKinney, W. T. Depressive disorders: Toward a united hypothesis. *Science*, Oct. 5, 1973, *182*, 20–29.

Amado, A., Cronk, A. A., & Mileo, R. Cost of terminal care: Home hospice versus hospital. *Nursing Outlook*, August 1979, *27*, 522–526.

Ayd, F. J., Jr. *Recognizing the depressed patient*. New York: Grune & Stratton, 1961.

Cole, J. O., Schatzberg, A. F., & Frazier, S. H. *Depression*. New York: Plenum Press, 1978.

Diekelman, N. *Primary health care of the well adult*. New York: McGraw-Hill, 1977.

Division of Gerontology, University of Michigan. *Aging in the modern world*. Ann Arbor, Mich.: University of Michigan, 1957.

Duvall, E. M. *Family development* (2d ed.). New York: Lippincott, 1962.

———. *Family development* (5th ed.). New York: Lippincott, 1977.

Erikson, E. H. *Childhood and society* (2d ed.). New York: Norton, 1963.

Knafl, K. A., & Grace, H. K. *Families across the life cycle*. Boston: Little, Brown, 1978.

Kübler-Ross, E. *Death: The final stages of growth*. Englewood Cliffs, N.J.: Prentice-Hall, 1975.

———. *Questions and answers on death and dying*. New York: Collier Books, 1974.

Murray, R., & Zentner, J. *Nursing assessment and health promotion through the life span*. Englewood Cliffs, N.J.: Prentice-Hall, 1975.

Peplau, H. E. Mid-life crises. *American Journal of Nursing*, October 1975, *75*, 1761–1775.

Sheehy, G. *Passages: Predictable crises of adult life*. New York: Dutton, 1976.

Stevenson, J. S. *Issues and crises during middlescence*. New York: Appleton-Century-Crofts, 1977.

U.S. Department of Commerce. *Illustrative projections of world populations to the 21st century*. Washington, D.C.: U.S. Government Printing Office, 1979.

U.S. Department of Health, Education, and Welfare. *Vital statistics of the United States 1975*. Volume II. *Mortality*, Pt. B. Washington, D.C.: U.S. Government Printing Office, 1975.

White House conference on families, 1978. Joint hearings before the subcommittee on Child and Human Development of the Committee on Human Resources, U.S. Senate and the Subcommittee on Select Education of the Committee on Education and Labor, House of Representatives, Ninety-fifth Congress. Washington, D.C.: U.S. Government Printing Office, 1978.

SELECTED BIBLIOGRAPHY

Albrecht, S. L. Reactions and adjustments to divorce: Differences in the experiences of males and females. *Family Relations*, January 1980, *29*, 59–68.

Anderson, J. E. *Psychological aspects of aging*. Washington, D.C.: American Psychological Association, 1956.

Arlin, M. Controversies in nutrition. *Nursing Clinics of North America*, June 1979, *14*, 229–245.

Ball, M. Issues of violence in family casework. *Social*

Casework, January 1977, *58,* 3–12.

Bell, R. R. *Marriage and family interaction* (4th ed.). Homewood, Ill.: Dorsey, 1975.

Braun, S. (Ed.). *Catalog of sexual consciousness.* New York: Grove Press, 1975.

Brothers, J. D. *Better than ever.* New York: Simon & Schuster, 1975.

Burns, K. R., & Johnson, P. J. *Health assessment in clinical practice.* Englewood Cliffs, N.J.: Prentice-Hall, 1980.

Clark, H. H. *The law of domestic relations in the United States.* St. Paul, Minn.: West, 1968.

Diekelman, N. L. The choice is health or illness. *American Journal of Nursing,* August 1976, *76,* 1272–1273.

Dignan, M. B., Hall, M. B., & Hastings, D. W. Effect of increased access to health care on mortality from cardiovascular disease in rural Tennessee. *Public Health Reports,* March–April 1979, *94,* 186–192.

Flynn, J. P. Recent findings related to wife abuse. *Social Casework,* January 1977, *58,* 13–20.

Gulbrandsen, M. W. Guide to health assessment. *American Journal of Nursing,* August 1976, *76,* 1276–1277.

Havighurst, R. J. *Developmental tasks and education.* New York: McKay, 1972.

Hendrix, M. J., LaGodna, G. E., & Bohen, C.A. The battered wife. *American Journal of Nursing,* April 1978, *78,* 650–653.

Hite, S. *The Hite report: A nationwide study of female sexuality.* New York: Dell, 1976.

Hudson, M. She's 22, dealing with catastrophic illness. *American Journal of Nursing,* August 1976, *76,* 1274–1275.

Langley, R., & Levy, R. C. *Wife beating: The silent crisis.* New York: Simon & Schuster, 1977.

Levin, L. S., Katz, A. H., & Holst, E. *Self-care: Lay initiatives in health.* New York: Prodist, 1979.

Lynch, J. J. *The broken heart: The medical consequences of loneliness.* New York: Basic Books, 1977.

Mahan, K.: A sensible approach to the obese patient. *Nursing Clinics of North America,* June 1979, *14,* 229–245.

Masters, W., & Johnson, V. *Human sexual response.* Boston: Little, Brown, 1966.

McGrary, A. *A well model approach to care of the dying client.* New York: McGraw-Hill, 1978.

Merino, H. Z., Judson, F. N., Bennett, D., & Schaffnit, T. R. Screening for gonorrhea and syphilis in gay bathhouses in Denver and Los Angeles. *Public Health Reports,* July–August 1979, *94,* 376–379.

Michigan Women's Commission. *Domestic assault.* Lansing, Mich.: State of Michigan, 1977.

Neugarten, B. L. (Ed.). *Middle age and aging.* Chicago: University of Chicago Press, 1968.

Neugarten, B. L., Berkowitz, H., & Associates. *Personality in middle and late life.* New York: Atherton Press, 1964.

Newman, B., & Newman, P. *Development through life: A psychosocial approach.* Homewood, Ill.: Dorsey, 1975.

Oelbaum, C. Hallmarks of adult wellness. *American Journal of Nursing,* September 1974, *74,* 1623.

Roznoy, M. S. How to take a sexual history. *American Journal of Nursing,* August 1976, *76,* 1279–1280.

Rudov, M. H., & Santangelo, N. *Health status of minorities and low-income groups.* DPHEW Publication No. HRS 79-627. Pittsburgh, Pa.: Centers for Health, Education and Social Systems Studies, 1979.

Williams, R. A. *Textbook of black-related diseases.* New York: McGraw-Hill, 1975.

Williamson, J. B., Boren, J. F., & Evans, L. (Eds.). *Social problems: The contemporary debates.* Boston: Little, Brown, 1974.

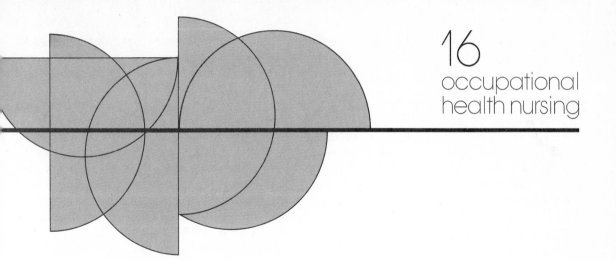

The first census in 1790 showed the United States to be an agricultural nation with limited industry. The Industrial Revolution, which began in the late 1800s and early 1900s, rapidly changed this fact. Between 1870 and 1910 the population in the United States rose 132 percent and the number of persons working in industry rose almost 400 percent, from 3.5 million to 14.2 million workers (Morris, 1976, p. 109). Today there are over 6 million workplaces in the United States, and in excess of 80 million workers. The working population cuts across all economic and social levels. Workers may be men or women, young or old, urban or rural, and they have a variety of characteristics, conditions, traits, and ethnic or religious backgrounds. There exists no stereotype for the American worker. The health of these workers is important not only to the workers and their families, but to the economic security of the nation as well. The working population is basically a well population. The health professionals dealing with this group place emphasis on primary prevention and early diagnosis and treatment. This chapter will deal with promoting the health of workers through services provided by the nurse working in the occupational health setting.

OCCUPATIONAL HEALTH IN THE UNITED STATES

Work is a major means of establishing individual and national economic security. Historically, wages have been a major worker concern. Health is often considered by the worker only when poor health, injury, or disability impedes his or her ability to work. The first recorded strike in the United States was over wages, not health issues. In 1786, the printers of Philadelphia went on strike to secure a minimum wage of $6 a week [U.S. Department of Labor (USDL), 1976, p. 1]. By the mid-1800s other worker concerns were emerging, and workers rallied for shorter work days, child labor laws, and health and safety measures. In 1850, at the urging of workers, Massachusetts became the first state to study occupational safety. It was not until 1903, however, that the federal government issued a report on occupational safety (USDL, 1977, pp. 15–16).

In the early twentieth century the emergence of labor unions and the formation of the U.S. Department of Labor placed new emphasis on the rights of the worker. At this time, the health of the worker became a primary concern for several reasons. The workers were concerned because if they were not healthy, their economic livelihood was threatened. The employer wanted a healthy worker because an unhealthy one threatened the economic stability of the workplace. Both the worker and the employer agreed on the value of maintaining worker health. A major point of difference was what happened when an employee became ill, injured, or disabled due to work-related conditions.

At the turn of the century, many workplaces did not offer sick-time benefits. A worker was often subject to dismissal for missing time from the job because of illness or injury. Many workers went to work ill to keep their jobs. If the illness, injury, or disability was job-related, the employees thought that the employer should compensate the worker. This view, however, was not always shared by the employer. In fact, it had to be proved that the employer was negligent before the worker could receive financial compensation for medical care or lost wages. When workers' compensation was granted, it was usually for amounts much smaller than the employee's wages, and was hardly enough on which to exist.

The worker gradually took a firm stand on the right to be compensated for job-related illness, injury, or disability and as a result, workers' compensation legislation was developed. These initial workers' compensation acts met with much resistance from employers and many acts were found to be unconstitutional. In 1911, New Jersey passed the first workers' compensation act to be upheld by the courts.

By 1948, all 48 states and the territories of Alaska and Hawaii had enacted workers' compensation legislation. The primary function of this legislation was, and is, to compensate the worker for illness, injury, or disability related to the job. It places liability for workplace illness, injury, and disability on the employer. Workers' compensation is administered by the individual states and, thus, the benefits vary from state to state. Workers' compensation legislation, its cash benefits for loss of wages, and its health and disability components are discussed in detail in Chapter 4.

At about the same time that labor unions and the Department of Labor were emerging, health professionals began to appear in industry. Their numbers were scant, and they were usually employed at the discretion of the owner or operator of the workplace. Their primary function was to provide emergency care for on-the-job illness and injury.

In 1887, the Homestake Mining company sponsored the first industrially financed medical department in the United States (USDL, 1977, p. 15). It was not until 1895 that the first occupational health nurse, Ada Mayo Stewart, was hired by the Vermont Marble Company. Miss Stewart was employed to give care to company employees who were sick and to go into the schools of the employees' children to teach health. From one occupational health nurse in 1895, the field has grown to more than 20,000 occupational health nurses practicing in the United States. Recent government studies show that another 20,000 to 30,000 are needed in the workplace (American Public Health Association, 1975, p. 89).

Almost 50 years after Miss Stewart began her work in occupational health nursing, the American Association of Industrial Health Nurses was founded in 1942. At its founding, the association was composed of about 300 nurses from 16 states (Martin, 1977, p. 10). Today that organization is known as the American Association for Occupational Health

Nurses and has a membership of greater than 9000 nurses drawn from all states (Martin, 1977, p. 11). The change in name occurred on January 1, 1977, and reflected the trend toward the placement of nurses not only in large industries but also in other occupations such as banking, communication centers, retail stores, airlines, and construction sites. The primary goal of this association is to promote health in the workplace, wherever that workplace may be.

The beginning of the twentieth century also brought with it a pioneer of occupational medicine, Dr. Alice Hamilton. In 1910, Dr. Hamilton was named to chair the first Occupational Disease Commission in the United States, sponsored by the state of Illinois. Dr. Hamilton chose lead poisoning as the subject of her primary study. Her studies of industrial hazards were so impressive, and her advocacy for the rights of the worker so staunch, that in 1911 she was asked to head a similar commission for the federal government (Martin, 1977, p. 13).

Dr. Hamilton became internationally recognized for her studies in industrial health and her prolific writings in the field. Today her writings are classics in the area of occupational medicine. She died in 1970, the year that the first federal occupational safety and health act was passed in the United States, leaving behind a great legacy in occupational medicine.

Occupational health nurses, occupational physicians, and countless workers have stressed the hazards involved in the workplace. As late as 1968, the then–Surgeon General, Dr. William Steward, told Congress that U.S. Public Health Service studies showed 65 percent of United States industrial workers to be exposed to toxic or harmful conditions in their workplaces (Stellman and Daum, 1973, pp. xiii–xiv). The same year, President Lyndon Johnson proposed an occupational health law. That law was defeated by Congress.

TABLE 16-1 Legislative Overview of Occupational Health in the United States— Some Firsts

Year	Significant events
1836	First restrictive child labor law enacted in Massachusetts. At that time two-fifths of all employees in New England factories were children from 7 to 16 years old.
1877	State legislation requiring factory safeguards (Massachusetts).
1879	State legislation requiring factory inspections (Massachusetts).
1886	State legislation requiring reporting of industrial accidents (Massachusetts).
1904	National Child Labor Committee organized.
1910	State legislation requiring formation of an Occupational Disease Commission (Illinois).
1911	Workmen's Compensation Act passed and not declared unconstitutional (New Jersey).
1911	Federal Occupational Disease Commission.
1912	Children's Bureau placed in the Department of Labor.
1913	U.S. Department of Labor given cabinet status.
1935	Social Security Act passed establishing the federal-state unemployment insurance program.
1936	Federal legislation setting occupational safety and health standards and minimum age limitations for workers employed in government contract work where the contract exceeded $10,000 (Walsh-Healy Act).
1938	Federal legislation setting a minimum age for child labor: 16 years old for general work and 18 years for hazardous work, applicable to most industrial settings (Fair Labor Standards Act).
1948	All states have workers' compensation acts.
1965	Federal legislation extends to suppliers of government services the same protection as had been embodied in the Walsh-Healy Act of 1936 (McNamara-O'Hara Act).
1966	Federal legislation requiring mandatory inspections and health and safety standards in the mineral industry (Mine Safety Act).
1969	Federal legislation that sets mandatory health and safety standards for underground mines (Coal Mine Health and Safety Act).
1970	Federal legislation to ensure occupational safety and health (Occupational Safety and Health Act).

Occupational Health Legislation in the United States

Occupational health and safety legislation did not come early in the history of United States industry. Many European nations were much more expeditious in developing such legislation. By 1884, Germany had already enacted a law which provided for a comprehensive system of occupational health, including compensation for occupational illness, injury, or dis-ability irrespective of who was responsible for the condition occurring (McCall, 1977, p. 21). Many Americans thought that legislation in the workplace would endanger the free enterprise system. Occupational safety and health legislation gradually began, but it was not until 1970 that the United States had a comprehensive occupational safety and health program. Table 16-1 presents a historical overview of the significant legislation relative to occupational health in the United States.

OCCUPATIONAL SAFETY AND HEALTH ACT OF 1970 (PUBLIC LAW 91-596)

The primary piece of legislation making an impact on occupational health and safety in the United States today is the Occupational Safety and Health Act of 1970. This act made the health of employees a public concern. It was late in evolving, but it is here now.

Intents and Mandates of This Act

The intents of this act were to (1) prevent placing toxic substances in the workplace, (2) regulate exposure to toxic and dangerous substances already in the workplace, and (3) compensate workers for occupational illness and injury. To carry out these intents, the act had specific mandates:

1. Formation of the:

   a. *Occupational Safety and Health Administration (OSHA).* Sets and enforces standards for occupational safety and health. Under the jurisdiction of the Department of Labor.

   b. *National Institute for Occupational Safety and Health (NIOSH).* Researches and recommends occupational safety and health standards to OSHA. Under the jurisdiction of the Department of Health, Education, and Welfare.

   c. *Occupational Safety and Health Review Commission.* A commission to advise OSHA and NIOSH on the legal implications of their rules, regulations, and actions. Appointed by the President.

   d. *National Advisory Council on Occupational Safety and Health.* A consumer and professional council to make occupational safety and health recommendations to OSHA and NIOSH. Appointed by the President.

   e. *National Commission on State Workers' Compensation Laws.* A temporary evaluative commission to study and make recommendations on the adequacy of state workers' compensation laws to the President. Appointed by the President and recommendations made to the President. Official termination date: October 30, 1972.

2. Establishment of federal occupational safety and health standards.

3. Imposition of fines and sentences for violation of federal occupational safety and health regulations.

Under the Occupational Safety and Health Act, an employee can request that OSHA inspect the workplace for a suspected hazardous condition; OSHA must respond. The employee's name must be kept confidential at his or her request. When OSHA comes to investigate the workplace, the employees have the "walk-around" right, which enables an employee or representative to walk around with the OSHA investigators on the inspection. The act also requires employers to keep records of work-related deaths, injuries, and illnesses for OSHA review. Under the act, states can develop their own occupational safety and health administrations as long as the state standards meet or excel the federal standards.

Some Problems with the Act

There are a number of areas in the act that have proved to be problematic. Consequently, the act has not been as effective as planned. Many of the problems center on the following areas.

Funding. The funding for the act has been grossly inadequate. The amount of money appropriated for OSHA and NIOSH in 1976 was less than $1 per United States citizen per year. This rate of funding greatly affects the ability of both OSHA and NIOSH to staff and train people to carry out the intents and mandates of the act. With the 1200 compliance officers that OSHA had in 1976, they would only be able to visit each workplace covered under the act once every 50 years.

Coordination of services. The services of OSHA and NIOSH have not been well coordinated in the past. These two agencies are under the jurisdiction of two different federal departments and the fact that one researches standards (NIOSH) while the other sets and enforces them (OSHA) has often complicated the issue. The two agencies have not always been in agreement on standards and regulations.

Fines and sentences. The fines and sentences set forth by the act are usually too low to serve as an incentive to employers to improve working conditions. Sentences have usually not been imposed. Employers are generally more concerned with the monetary amounts of employee lawsuits than with OSHA fines and sentences.

Economic impact statements. Economic impact statements became policy in 1975. They are an occupational cost analysis study of a proposed OSHA standard or regulation. If the workplace can show that it would not be economically feasible for them to comply with a standard or regulation, they can appeal the proposed regulation. OSHA must then prove that the standard or regulation would not be detrimental to the economic stability of the workplace. The workplace often has better resources to finance such studies than does OSHA.

Scope of the problem. The scope of the problem is enormous: it has been estimated that there are more than 15,000 toxic agents in industry today, with standards existing for less than 500 of them (Stellman and Daum, 1973, p. 6). It is also estimated that every 20 minutes a new and potentially toxic chemical is introduced into U.S. workplaces (Serafini, 1976, p. 755). Presently, OSHA is able to put out standards at the rate of 100 each year.

Legal challenges. Through the legal system, various industries and groups are challenging the right of OSHA to set and enforce occupational safety and health standards. It will be of great interest to the American worker how these legal challenges are decided.

Lack of trained personnel. There are great shortages of professionals trained in occupational medicine and industrial hygiene, which affects their ability to implement and evaluate the mandates of the act. Figure 16-1 shows the availability and deficits of occupational health personnel in 1973; the picture has not changed

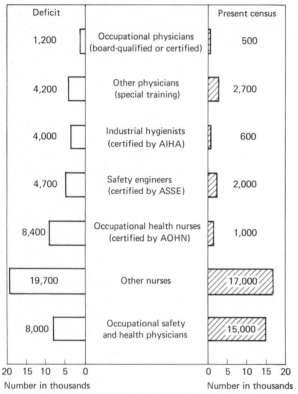

Deficit		Present census
1,200	Occupational physicians (board-qualified or certified)	500
4,200	Other physicians (special training)	2,700
4,000	Industrial hygienists (certified by AIHA)	600
4,700	Safety engineers (certified by ASSE)	2,000
8,400	Occupational health nurses (certified by AOHN)	1,000
19,700	Other nurses	17,000
8,000	Occupational safety and health physicians	15,000

20 15 10 5 0   0 5 10 15 20
Number in thousands   Number in thousands

FIGURE 16-1 Availability of occupational health personnel: 1973. AIHA = American Industrial Hygiene Association, ASSE = American Society of Safety Engineers, and ADHA = Association of Occupational Health Nurses. [*From Edward M. Dolinsky. Health maintenance organizations and occupational medicine. Bulletin of the New York Academy of Medicine, 1974, 50 (10), p. 1126.*]

significantly since then. It is hoped that with the advent of federally subsidized programs in occupational medicine, these deficits will be corrected.

What the Act Means to the Occupational Health Nurse

The Occupational Safety and Health Act of 1970 has many implications for the occupational health nurse. It means that the occupational health nurse needs to be increasingly aware of occupational hazards and must be able to pinpoint these hazards in the workplace. The increased emphasis on identifying hazards in the workplace will require that nurses become involved in carrying out a variety of epidemiological studies of the work environment.

The nurse needs to be knowledgeable about OSHA regulations and be prepared to assist in OSHA investigations. Frequently it is the nurse who accompanies the OSHA investigators as they go throughout the workplace.

The increased demands placed on the nurse under this act and the many primary responsibilities that the nurse assumes in occupational health make it imperative that the nurse have adequate educational and experiential preparation for the job.

THE OCCUPATIONAL HEALTH NURSE

The nurse working in this area of community health nursing needs special preparation for this role.

Qualifications of the Occupational Health Nurse

The American Nurses' Association recommends that an occupational health nurse be a graduate of an accredited school of professional nursing and have current registered nurse licensure (ANA, 1960). It is also rec-

ommended that the occupational health nurse have courses in industrial and social law, industrial psychology, industrial health, statistics, research, and business management. Previous work experience and membership in professional organizations is suggested.

Most undergraduate nursing programs do not offer clinical experience in occupational health nursing. There was little opportunity to study occupational health nursing on the master's level or higher until the recent establishment of educational resource centers (ERCs) in occupational safety and health. These centers were funded by the National Institute for Occupational Safety and Health of the Department of Health, Education, and Welfare. They have an interdisciplinary focus, as well as a specific core curriculum component for each discipline.

Educational resource centers are located in major universities and offer training and graduate degrees to health professionals interested in occupational health. They are located at Harvard University, New York University, Johns Hopkins University, University of North Carolina, University of Illinois, University of Cincinnati, University of Minnesota, University of Iowa, Texas University, University of Utah, University of Arizona, and the University of Washington. It is expected that these centers will provide nurses with the opportunity to obtain advanced education in occupational health. It is hoped that more nursing programs offering specialist education for nurses interested in occupational health will be developed and implemented.

The American Association of Occupational Health Nurses has offered certification in occupational health nursing since 1972. Certification is processed through the association and involves a combination of work experience, university course hours, and a written exam.

Objectives of Occupational Health Nursing

Simply stated, the primary objectives of the occupational health nurse are:

1. To protect the worker from occupational health and safety hazards

2. To help facilitate the worker and family to adapt to health and welfare needs

The occupational health nurse accomplishes these objectives through several specific nursing functions. These nursing functions involve primary, secondary, and tertiary aspects of prevention. The nurse engages in activities ranging from health promotion and prevention of disease to early diagnosis, treatment, disability limitation, and restoration. All of these activities are carried out in a therapeutic milieu involving employee, employee's family, and occupational health service personnel. In carrying out these objectives, the occupational health nurse must have a holistic philosophy which focuses on the employees' physical, emotional, and social needs.

Functions of the Occupational Health Nurse

The functions of the occupational health nurse fall into three categories: administrative, direct nursing care, and health education and promotion. The occupational health nurse will carry out a variety of these functions on a day-to-day basis in the workplace.

Administrative

Administrative functions consume a large part of the occupational health nurse's time. These functions involve operation of an occupational health service, evaluation of the occupational health service, maintenance of worker occupational health records, development and maintenance of an occupational health nursing policy and procedure manual, training of auxiliary health personnel, coordination of emergency procedures, cooperation with federal and state occupational health regulatory bodies, and participation in student educational placement programs. Although these functions are not all-inclusive, they are representative of the administrative functions carried out by the nurse in the occupational health setting.

Since many workplaces do not have full-time medical staff, the occupational health nurse is often the most accessible health care worker. It has been estimated that two-thirds of all occupational health nurses work without the direct supervision of a physician or another nurse. This puts the occupational health nurse in a position where much independent action is required. The nurse in this setting will often function in a relatively independent role. It is important, however, for all nurses to recognize that professional supervision and peer collaboration are essential to good nursing practice. Professional collaboration can be obtained from nurses such as peers in other industrial settings, members from the Occupational Health Nursing Division of the American Nurses' Association, and the director of nursing from the local health department.

Among the primary administrative functions mentioned are operating the occupational health service at the workplace and maintaining the records of the health service. These are important tasks that should not be underestimated. The occupational health service is the primary source for health care within the workplace. Health services are often initiated there and referred elsewhere as necessary. There are supplies to be ordered for such a service and equipment to keep in repair. The records kept by such a service are invaluable. These records would include individual employee records and records on appropriate workplace health statistics or information. Employee records should contain all employee contacts with the health service from preemployment physical through termination physical. This would include each employee visit to the health service along with results of screening tests and periodic health reviews. The reason for each employee visit, treatment, and plan of care should be carefully recorded. The Occupational Safety and Health Act requires logging of specific illness and injury for review. These records are in addition to the records of the health service.

The nurse should also keep records of other health statistics or information as related to the workplace. This would include what areas of the workplace appear to have higher than expected illness or injury rates, what kind of illness or injury occur, time of occurrence, and other applicable data. Potential stressors, hazardous or potentially hazardous equipment, and known and suspected irritants should all be logged and closely watched for their effect on the worker. It is through careful epidemiological collection of data that hazards in the workplace are pinpointed and solutions found. An example of this is illustrated in the following situation.

An occupational health nurse suspected an area of the plant in which she worked to be a higher-than-average noise area. After obtaining permission from plant management to do periodic audiometric testing on the workers in this area, along with testing on a control group, she began to follow up on her suspicion. Employees in both areas were tested every 6 months. Over a period of time the nurse was able to show that the workers in the suspected area had increasingly abnormal audiograms and the control group did not. The workers themselves had not noticed any change in levels of hearing, but the audiograms told the story. The results of the study were shared with management and the workers, and corrective measures were taken. The comparative aspect of screening tests, coupled with knowledge regarding protective measures and substance control, can do a great deal to further the health of the worker.

Evaluation of the occupational health service is often largely the administrative responsibility of the nurse. Through evaluation, the services' strengths and weaknesses can be assessed and the appropriate measures taken. The recommendations coming from this evaluation are often done collaboratively with the physician and management. The nurse becomes an advocate for workers' rights and services in this situation.

The occupational health nurse may work with students. Primarily this involves graduate and undergraduate nursing students in educational experiences. However, as occupational health has expanded, the nurse is often found facilitating the studies of other students in fields such as industrial hygiene, audiology, toxicology, and medicine. Participating in these student experiences is enriching not only for the student but also for the nurse.

One administrative task that is presently in a state of flux is that of cooperating with federal and state occupational health regulatory bodies. There are many new regulations, procedures, pieces of equipment, and occupational reviews as a result of the 1970 occupational safety and health legislation. It is frequently the occupational health nurse who participates in the regulatory reviews of the workplace and the implementation of occupational safety and health regulations. The nurse is a logical person for this type of participation because of the daily contact she or he has with the worker and the workplace. The nurse is often the first health professional to recognize danger areas and substances in the workplace that could be creating health problems for the worker. Any time that the nurse works in a regulatory review process, she or he must be able to point out the advantages of such a review to both employer and employee.

Direct Nursing Care

The direct nursing care given by the occupational health nurse centers on occupational illness and injury but may also involve nonoccupational illness and injury. Occupational injuries such as abrasions, lacerations, fractures, sprains, bruises, concussions, burns, and puncture wounds are all treated by the nurse. Care of occupational injuries requires a good background in first aid and emergency procedures. These injuries can range from minor to major, and may include occupational death. Each year in the United States there are more than 14,000 deaths due to accidents on the job, and at least 2.2 million disabling occupational injuries (Ashford, 1976, p. 3; Stellman and Daum, 1973, p. 3). Studies by the U.S. De-

partment of Labor estimate that at least 25 million serious injuries and deaths in the workplace go uncounted each year (Stellman and Daum, 1973, p. 3). These figures are staggering and show that there is much to be done to minimize injury in the workplace.

Occupational illness, including occupational disease, is a serious matter. It is estimated that as many as 100,000 deaths occur each year in the United States as a result of occupational disease and illness (Ashford, 1976, p. 10). Occupational illness is evidenced in many ways. Hypertension, nausea, dizziness, asbestosis, silicosis, cancer, mercury poisoning, as well as many other conditions are evidenced in occupational illness. The occupational illness dealt with most frequently by the nurse is dermatitis, but occupational injury accounts for the most time lost from the job.

Mass psychogenic illness is a newly researched occupational illness. It is evidenced when a number of workers show the same symptoms over the same period from a cause that appears to be job-related but for which no identifiable cause except a psychological one can be found. Since 1974, the National Institute for Occupational Safety and Health has done extensive study of mass psychogenic illness which indicates that it occurs regularly in the workplace. Symptoms may vary from individual to individual, but usually they include headaches, nausea, chills, blurred vision, muscular weakness, and breathing difficulty (Colligan and Stockton, 1978, p. 94). Women are more frequently involved than men. Mass psychogenic illness has regularly been connected with stressful job situations, and it is one of many occupational illnesses with which the nurse will work.

Colligan and Stockton (1978, pp. 93–99) cite many examples of mass psychogenic illness. One such example involved a large industrial city on the Great Lakes where workers stood at an assembly line packing frozen fish into boxes. Someone on the assembly line stated that he smelled a strange smell, and within minutes many workers were falling ill from the smell. Most of the victims became nauseated and dizzy, and some appeared very ill. An epidemiological investigation was done, but no apparent reason was found for the illness. Within a short period of time the workers recovered.

The occupational health nurse will also work with nonoccupational injuries and illnesses. These are incurred outside the work setting but present themselves at the work setting. The occupational health nurse will generally treat these conditions initially and refer the client for further treatment.

Among the nonoccupational conditions that the employee may present within the workplace and which the nurse should be cognizant of are the problems of alcoholism and drug abuse. If an employee comes to work intoxicated or under the influence of drugs, and the employer allows the individual to remain, workers' compensation laws in many states would rule in favor of the worker in the event of occupational injury. For the safety of the worker, and the liability of the employer, employees who are unfit to work should not be permitted to stay. In some cases the worker's supervisor will make the decision regarding fitness for work, and in other cases the nurse or physician will. Unfortunately, most non-job-related conditions are not being dealt with effectively in the workplace. The challenge exists for the occupational health nurse to influence management to initiate effective treatment programs dealing with all health problems of employees.

Physical examinations are another part of direct nursing care. The nurse will be responsible for carrying out certain aspects of the physical examination such as vital signs, baseline screening procedures, and health and occupational histories. In some cases, an employee's job or job placement will depend on the outcome of the physical examination.

Screening procedures are often done by the occupational health nurse. Many workplaces provide special training for the occupational health nurse in audiometrics, electrocardiograms, vision screening, and pulmonary function analysis. Other screening measures involve periodic blood pressure measurement, urinalysis, hematocrit, hemoglobin, and vision testing. The importance of these screening measures cannot be underestimated; they often provide baseline and subsequent data for the study of occupational injury and illness. Screening is only valuable if there is adequate follow-up.

Rehabilitation services are another direct nursing care function. The nurse will often be involved in occupational, physical, and medical therapy rehabilitation plans. Many of these rehabilitation plans will have aspects that are to be carried out in the workplace on a regular basis for a given period of time.

Emergency care is probably the most dramatic of the occupational health nurse's direct nursing care functions. The occupational health nurse must be skilled in cardiopulmonary resuscitation, first aid, and emergency care techniques. The nurse frequently has to make a decision and take action immediately; she or he is usually the first health professional in the workplace to have contact with the ill or injured worker.

The direct nursing care functions of the occupational health nurse are diverse and demand a high level of nursing skill, professional flexibility, and independence. To carry out these direct nursing care functions, the nurse must be able to assess both the worker and the workplace. An assessment guide for nursing in industry is included in this text (Appendix 16-1).

Health Education and Promotion

Through health education, the nurse has the opportunity to greatly affect the health of the worker. However, the nurse is heavily involved in the administrative and direct nursing care functions of the job and often has little time available for the function of health education. This situation exists not only because of management's influence, but also because nursing has not taken the initiative to develop health education programs.

Health education includes employee in-service programs on health and safety. It also involves health and safety counseling on a one-to-one or small-group basis. The Occupational Safety and Health Act of 1970 requires that workers be told of the hazards they are exposed to in the workplace, and making the worker aware of these hazards is often left to the occupational health nurse. The nurse may also do group and individual health education on a variety of health-related conditions; the nurse works closely with alcohol and drug abuse programs in the workplace. Discussing with an employee how a given condition such as diabetes will affect the employee's job and daily living is another aspect of this function.

An important aspect of health education is the interpretation of health and welfare benefits to the employee. This means interpreting what is offered through the employer and also what is available through the community. The nurse can be instrumental in initiating a referral to counseling services or procuring services for family members of an employee. Thus, the occupational health nurse must establish and maintain close working relationships with community health and welfare agencies. Clinical experience has demonstrated that when an occupational health nurse assists an employee in meeting family needs, there is less job-related injury and illness.

Another important task of health education and promotion is assisting the worker to see work as a developmental task and using anticipatory guidance for meeting some of the possible crises and challenges that may arise in one's work career.

Looking at Work as a Developmental Task

Developmental tasks have been discussed throughout this text. Work is a developmental task of adulthood and crosses over the age groups of young adult, middlescence (Stevenson, 1977, pp. 18, 25), and aging. As presented in Chapters 15 and 18, developmental tasks as related to work are:

1. Young adult

   a. Advancing self-development and the enactment of appropriate roles in society

   b. Integrating personal values with career development and socioeconomic constraints

2. Middlescence I

   a. Developing socioeconomic consolidation

   b. Assuming responsible positions in occupational, social, and civic activities, organizations, and communities

3. Middlescence II

   a. Maintaining flexible views in occupational, civic, political, religious, and social positions

   b. Keeping current on relevant scientific, political, and cultural changes

   c. Preparing for retirement and planning another career when feasible

4. Aging

   a. Adapting to retirement-level income, often a sharp decline

The occupational health nurse should be aware of the developmental tasks associated with work and should help the worker to achieve task fulfillment. Work is a part of one's overall development throughout life.

SELECTED HEALTH PROBLEMS OF WORKERS

The health problems presented in this chapter are not all-inclusive. There are many health stressors in the workplace. Many of these stressors are *chemical, physical,* or *biological.* Less subtle stressors such as fatigue, boredom, and monotony are also very prevalent. These stressors are seen as the effects of the environment on humans and are termed *ergonomic stressors.* Although this chapter speaks largely to physical and chemical stressors, the other stressors should not be overlooked. Many occupational exposures can cause serious health problems for the worker and family. In some cases these stressors can cause direct harm to the worker's family. Some occupational exposures can result in fatalities. Almost every day one can pick up the newspaper and read about the effects of various occupational stressors on the worker. This is not surprising, since at last estimate there were thought to be at least 15,000 toxic chemical agents in industry, with more being introduced. Ensuring the health of the worker is one of our great national challenges. The occupational health nurse plays a major role in safeguarding worker health.

Occupational illness and injury are major national concerns; the hardships experienced by individuals and their families is inestimable. One cannot place a dollar estimate on the inability of a worker to communicate with his or her family as a result of occupational deafness. From a financial viewpoint, it is estimated that almost $10 billion is lost annually in the United States to illness and injury on the job through wages, medical expenses, insurance claims, and production delays (Ashford, 1976, p. 17). Approximately 25 million workdays are lost each year in the United States to absenteeism from the job; that is the equivalent of 100,000 worker years. The occupational health nurse can make an impact on these statistics through the preventive aspects of occupational health nursing.

The stressors in the workplace that cause occupational illness and injury are extensive. These stressors are listed by category with some examples of each.

1. Chemical: liquids, gases, dusts, particles, fumes, mists, and vapors

2. Physical: electromagnetic and ionizing radiation, noise, pressure, vibration, heat, and cold

3. Biological: insects, mold, fungi, and bacteria

4. Ergonomic: monotony, fatigue, repetitive motion, and boredom

Studying the effects of these stressor agents in relation to occupational disease and injury is difficult and involves a number of factors. A primary problem is that sometimes there is no immediate, observable effect of the stressor. Long latency periods may exist between contact with the stressor and stressor effects. In diseases with long latency periods, the worker may have already left the job where contact with the stressor occurred. This makes it difficult, if not impossible, to trace the condition back to the occupational stressor.

It can be difficult to ascertain if the stressor was from the ambient (normal) environment or the work environment. How can the miner with emphysema prove that mine work rather than a heavy smoking habit was the primary factor in causation?

Many occupational stressors are not visible to the human eye. If something cannot be seen, it is often difficult to conceptualize and prove that it is causing damage. People are less suspicious, or minimize the hazards, of those things they cannot visualize.

It is important for the nurse in the community, as well as the occupational health nurse, to be aware of the hazards of the workplace, since many workplace problems may first be evidenced or recognized at home or in the community at large. Symptoms of many occupational conditions may go unnoticed in the workplace. Family, friends, and community may be aware of, or be affected by, an occupational health problem long before the workplace is aware of it. The nurse in the community has the potential for early detection of the effects of occupational stressors. Often when individuals seek medical care, they are not questioned about their jobs or occupational histories. Thus, occupational stressors are not correlated with the client's symptomology. An astute nurse who recognizes the significance of correlating symptomology with occupational hazards may prevent further disease progression.

The following are examples of some specific occupational stressors and health problems of workers.

Mercury

Lewis Carroll's Mad Hatter in *Alice in Wonderland* was no figment of the imagination and no exception; many hatters in Carroll's day went mad from mercury poisoning. For a long period of time, especially in the 1800s, felt and fur hats were in fashion. Hat makers used a mercury and nitric acid solution to shape the fabric, and mercury was vaporized in the process. Mercury poisoning can cause central nervous system damage and ultimately brain damage. Many workers who inhaled mercury vapors went mad. The felt and fur industries were a major source of occupational mercury poisoning in the United States until about 1940, when a substitute chemical was found for mercury. Mercury has been recognized as a poison since as far back as the ancient Roman Empire.

Characteristics

Mercury is a silvery white metal that is liquid at room temperature. It was one of the first metals known, mined by the Romans about 415 B.C. (NIOSH, *Working with Mercury*, 1973).

In the workplace, mercury poisoning usually results from worker exposure to low levels of mercury over long periods of time (NIOSH, *Occupational Exposure*, 1973, p. 21).

Mercury is absorbed through the skin, gastrointestinal tract, and lungs. The primary source of mercury poisoning is inhaled mercury vapor. Excessive exposures to mercury vapor can produce either an acute (short-term) or chronic (long-term) disease. The symptoms of acute mercury poisoning include tightness in the chest, difficulty breathing, coughing, and chest pain (NIOSH, *Working with Mercury*, 1973). Acute poisoning is rare but does result from accidental exposure to mercury or its compounds.

Chronic mercury poisoning is much more common in the workplace and results from mercury accumulating in the body over a period of time. It is evidenced by emotional disturbances such as personality change, disturbed sleep, and irritability along with tremors, particularly tremors of the hands. Other symptoms can include gingivitis, loss of appetite, increased salivation, and kidney disturbances. In the advanced stages of chronic mercury poisoning, the kidneys, liver, brain, heart, and lungs may be severely involved. High concentrations of mercury accumulate in the kidney, and kidney damage may result in a nephrotic syndrome characterized by edema, proteinuria, and the presence of casts or cells in the urine (NIOSH, *Occupational Exposure*, 1973, p. 20). Mercury can also cross the placenta, where it can have teratogenic effects on the unborn child.

Mercury in the Workplace

Today mercury has many uses, some of which are as a herbicide, mildew preventer, dental filling substance, seed protector, and metal purifier (Montague and Montague, 1971). It is estimated by NIOSH that at least 150,000 Americans are significantly exposed to mercury at work.

Dentists and dental assistants are at higher-than-average risk of contracting mercury poisoning because of the use of mercury in the silver amalgam of dental fillings. A recent study of 19 dental offices with 303 workers showed that all the offices were contaminated with mercury at levels up to 30 times the recommended federal standard (Dickens, 1977, p. 16). The 1976 death of a Kentucky dentist was attributed to mercury poisoning (Dickens, 1977, p. 15).

A study was done by researchers at the University of Michigan in 1975 where 142 volunteers from plants using mercury in small amounts were tested (USDL, *Mercury,* 1975). Workers on the average had 5 years' exposure to mercury. They were asked to do fine motor tasks such as finger and toe tapping, button pressing, and pencil flipping. A control group was used that had not been exposed to mercury. Tests showed that workers exposed to mercury had more trouble performing small, fast, repetitive movement than the control group. The exposed workers also had slower tapping rates and more frequent muscle tremors. The findings indicated that even low levels of mercury affect the motor control centers of the brain.

Mercury can cling to clothing and other items and can be carried from the workplace on the skin or under the fingernails of the worker to the home and other community settings. This mercury carried from the workplace can vaporize or be ingested, exposing others to its hazardous effects. These modes of transmission make the personal hygiene of the mercury worker an important matter. Workers should have separate clothes for the workplace, and these clothes should not leave the workplace. Workers exposed to mercury should shower, with special attention to handwashing, before leaving the workplace. Anyone dealing with mercury must wash his or her hands thoroughly before eating or smoking. No food or tobacco should be kept or used in any area where there is mercury (USDL, *Mercury,* 1975).

Mercury vapors have no odor, so it is important to monitor the workplace air frequently when mercury is being used. An adequate ventilation system is essential, and respirators should be used as a filtering mechanism. The amount of mercury that a worker is inhaling can be measured by having the worker wear a sampling device around the neck.

Every worker exposed to mercury (Table 16-2) should have at least a yearly physical examination; the worker can be monitored for mercury during this physical. Since mercury is accumulated in the kidneys, urinalysis done on a regular basis will show how much mercury is in the worker's body. Effective control of mercury, as well as other hazardous substances, requires an awareness by the worker of the potential health hazards, knowledge of the workplace, and implementation of effective preventive measures.

Standard

The OSHA mercury standard is 0.1 mg of mercury per cubic meter of air per 8-hour workday. (NIOSH has recommended a new mercury standard for OSHA consideration: 0.05 mg of mercury per cubic meter of air per 8-hour workday.)

Asbestos

The working population in the United States presently exposed to asbestos has been conservatively estimated at 200,000. Asbestos is encountered to some extent in almost every kind of industry.

Characteristics

Asbestos, a fibrous mineral silicate, is virtually indestructible. It is resistant to chemical action

TABLE 16-2 Workers Frequently Exposed to Mercury

Amalgam makers	Fur processors
Bactericide makers	Gold extractors
Barometer makers	Histology technicians
Battery makers, mercury	Ink makers
Boiler makers	Insecticide makers
Bronzers	Investment casting workers
Calibration instrument makers	Jewelers
Cap loaders, percussion	Laboratory workers, chemical
Cap makers, percussion	Lamp makers, fluorescent
Carbon brush makers	Manometer makers
Caustic soda makers	Mercury workers
Ceramic workers	Miners, mercury
Chlorine makers	Neon light makers
Dental amalgam makers	Paint makers
Dentists	Paper makers
Direct current meter workers	Pesticide workers
Disinfectant makers	Photographers
Disinfectors	Pressure-gauge makers
Drug makers	Refiners, mercury
Dye makers	Seed handlers
Electric apparatus makers	Silver extractors
Electroplaters	Switch makers, mercury
Embalmers	Tannery workers
Explosives makers	Taxidermists
Farmers	Textile printers
Fingerprint detectors	Thermometer makers
Fireworks makers	Wood preservative workers
Fungicide makers	
Fur preservers	

SOURCES: Adapted from W. M. Gafarer (Ed.). *Occupational diseases: A guide to their recognition*. Washington, D.C.: U.S. Government Printing Office, 1964, pp. 175–176; and National Institute for Occupational Safety and Health. *Occupational exposure to inorganic mercury*. HSM 73-11024. Washington, D.C.: U.S. Government Printing Office, 1973.

and temperature changes and is fireproof. Asbestos fibers are extremely small: fibers that can be seen by the human eye consist of thousands of fibrils. There are approximately 1 million asbestos fibrils to an inch and it takes an electron microscope to make an individual asbestos fibril visible.

Asbestos enters the body through inhalation. Once the fibers are inhaled they lodge in the lung, and the body is unable to destroy them. The body attempts to isolate the fibers by surrounding them with fibrous tissue, and the result is that over a period of 20 to 30 years the fibers are surrounded by a thick wall of scar tissue. The elasticity of the lung is decreased, and the person generally evidences shortness of breath, expectoration, and loss of weight. The resultant disease state is called *asbestosis,* which is defined as a diffuse, interstitial, nonmalignant, scarring of the lungs (USDL, *Occupational Exposure to Asbestos,* Federal Register, 1975, p. 47653).

Persons with asbestosis live at the brink of pulmonary incapacity and often die of complications from a simple cold, bronchitis, or pneumonia (Page and O'Brien, 1973, p. 21). Modern medical treatment of acute infections has lessened the severity of the infection, and now many victims of asbestosis are living longer and dying of asbestos-induced cancer of the lung, intestine, and a rare form of cancer, *mesothelioma,* that involves the lining of the chest or abdomen. Mesothelioma usually covers the entire lining surface and cannot be surgically removed. Asbestosis and mesothelioma are truly industry-specific diseases.

Asbestos in the Workplace

Asbestos fibers float in the air and can thereby move from the air in the workplace to the outside air. Asbestos fibers will cling to most clothing, and can be carried from the workplace in that manner.

Asbestos is used primarily as an insulator

and fire retardant. It has been found in a number of spackling, patching, insulation, and taping compounds used in home repair and construction. Measurements have indicated that home repair and construction work involving the use of these materials may result in exposure to asbestos at concentrations sufficient to produce disease and in excess of current OSHA standards ("Spackling Compound," 1976, p. 8).

A number of older buildings in this country are insulated with asbestos. Because of the now-recognized asbestos hazards, many buildings insulated with asbestos are having insulation replaced, and in recent years a number of schools have closed to replace the asbestos insulation. Every time an old building is razed, there is the chance that asbestos fibers will be released into the ambient air; this is a serious matter considering the apparently high toxicity level of asbestos.

A 1964 review of mesothelioma cases in London, England, showed that out of 70 diagnosed cases, 31 were asbestos workers, 9 cases lived with an asbestos worker, and 11 cases lived near an asbestos plant. There was an asbestos relationship with 51 of the 70 diagnosed mesothelioma cases.

A recent study showed that 40 percent of the family contacts of asbestos workers at a New Jersey plant had the kinds of abnormalities in their lungs common to asbestos workers ("Spackling Compound," 1976, p. 8). In some cases the worker had only been in the plant for a few days and had had minimal contact with asbestos. Cases of asbestosis and mesothelioma have been diagnosed where the person had had only short exposure, as little as 1 day, to asbestos. It is obvious that not only the worker is at risk, but also his or her family, friends, and community.

Dr. Irving Selikoff of Mt. Sinai School of Medicine in New York City has studied asbestos extensively. He did a classic study of 632 men who were members of the New York City and Newark locals of the asbestos workers union on December 31, 1942 (Stellman and Daum, 1973, p. 350). The study looked at the workers' mortality rates and causes of mortality over the last 20 years. Each of the workers in the study had at least 20 years' exposure to asbestos. Dr. Selikoff and his associates found that asbestos workers had 15 times the expected rates of cancer of the respiratory tract, 5 times the expected rates of cancer of the stomach, at least twice the expected rates of many other cancers, and high death rates from asbestosis and mesothelioma. More recent studies by Dr. Selikoff and Dr. James Holland predict that 5 to 7 percent of the estimated 1 million Americans who have been employed as asbestos workers will develop mesothelioma (Chen, 1977). His studies cite a further danger, the indication that asbestos acts as an absorption agent within the body to attract all toxic substances.

Work precautions to prevent the inhalation of asbestos and the release of asbestos fibers into the workplace are essential. Workers can wear masks to filter out asbestos fibers, and protective clothing can be worn that does not leave the workplace. Asbestos can be wetted down to prevent floating fibers, plastic drop cloths can catch the fibers and then be discarded each day, ventilation systems can be installed to entrap fibers, and asbestos materials can be appropriately enclosed. It is recommended that employees working with asbestos (Table 16-3) have at least yearly physical examinations where lung studies are done, including x-rays.

Standard

The OSHA asbestos standard is 2 fibers per cubic centimeter of air per 8-hour workday. (The OSHA proposed standard is 0.5 fibers per cubic centimeter of air per 8-hour workday.)

TABLE 16-3 Workers Frequently Exposed to Asbestos

Acoustical product makers	Herbicide users
Acoustical installers	Laboratory hood installers
Air filter makers	Metal workers, alloy makers
Agricultural workers	Metal workers, blast furnace
Appliance makers	Metal workers, coke oven
Asbestos plant workers	Office workers (air conditioned)
Asbestos product workers	Oil well workers
Asphalt mixers	Paint makers
Bookbinders	Petroleum refinery workers
Brake lining makers	Pipefitters
Brake lining installers	Pipe insulators
Building demolition workers	Pipeline workers
Carpenters	Plastic workers
Caulking compound makers	Plasterers
Caulking compound users	Printers
Clutch facing makers	Pump packing maker
Construction workers	Railroad shop workers
Cosmetics makers	Roofers
Dock workers	Roofing materials makers
Electrical workers	Rubber compounders
Fireproofers	Scientific equipment makers
Firemen	Shingle makers
Furnace filter makers	Ship builders
Garage workers, automobile	Shipyard workers
Garage mechanics, automobile	Talc makers
Gasket makers	Talc miners
Herbicide makers	Textile workers, rayon makers
	Undercoaters
	Ironing board cover makers

SOURCES: Adapted from Jeanne M. Stellman and Susan M. Daum, *Work is dangerous to your health.* New York: Vintage Books, 1973, pp. 368–419; and U.S. Department of Health, Education, and Welfare. *A guide to the work-relatedness of disease.* Washington, D.C.: U.S. Government Printing Office, 1976, p. 24.

Noise

The fact that workers in noisy environments lose their hearing has been known for at least the last 200 years. By the early twentieth century boilermakers' deafness, caused by boilermakers' riveting inside a metal boiler, was an occupational hazard of considerable magnitude (Lawrence, 1978, p. 22). It has been estimated that 1 to 2 million workers in the United States are at risk for occupational hearing loss and that there may be 100,000 to 200,000 occupationally noise-deafened people in the United States. It is estimated that 1.7 million workers in the United States between the ages of 50 and 59 have significant occupational hearing loss (Olishifski and Harford, 1975, p. 7). Estimates show that 14 percent of the working population are employed where the noise level is in excess of the federal noise standard (Olishifski and Harford, 1975, p. 7). Federal efforts to regulate effectively occupational noise were begun about 1955 (NIOSH, 1972, p. II-1).

Characteristics

Noise is defined as unwanted sound or sound out of control. Noise is variable, is not transported over great distances by the atmosphere, and dies out rapidly once the generation process stops. There is little protection from noise, and noise levels are increasing due to greater mechanization at home and work. In the workplace, machines are becoming larger, faster, and unfortunately noisier.

Noise can have many adverse effects. These include hearing loss, disruption of sleep and relaxation, interference with speech activity, decreased ability to do complicated tasks, and general annoyance. It can trigger changes in cardiovascular, endocrine, and neurological functions. An extremely loud noise, such as a sonic boom, may even cause physical damage to buildings and structures. The most common effect of noise is, tragically, hearing loss. Persistent exposure to enough continuous or impact noise will cause hearing loss. Whereas impact noise damages hearing instantly, continuous noise does it over a period of time and extends the damage over a broader range of hearing.

Olishifski and Harford (1975, p. 234) list many factors that affect the degree and extent of noise-induced hearing loss:

1. Intensity or loudness of the noise (decibel measurement)

2. Type of noise (frequency, continuous, or intermittent)

3. Time period of exposure each day

4. Total work duration (years of employment)

5. Individual susceptibility (tender or tough ears)

6. Age of worker

7. Coexisting hearing loss and ear disease

8. Distance of ears from the noise source

9. Position of ear with respect to the noise source

To understand noise-induced hearing loss, it is important to understand the process of hearing. The ear consists of external, middle, and inner components. The external ear consists of the pinna (external ear), external auditory canal, and the eardrum membrane (tympanic membrane). Sound waves pass through the external auditory canal to the eardrum membrane, where they are converted to mechanical vibration. These vibrations are carried to the middle ear. The middle ear is primarily composed of three bones—malleus (hammer), incus (anvil), and stapes (stirrups)—and the oval and round windows. The middle-ear bones provide amplification of sound vibrations and transmit them to the oval window where they travel to the inner ear. It is in the

ear's cochlea that vibrations are changed to nerve impulses (auditory nerve) via the organ of Corti. The nerve impulses are then transmitted to the brain and sound is heard. The cochlea is an extremely small, snail-shaped structure extending for two and one-half turns. It is smaller than a standard aspirin. Its small size should not be deceiving; it is very important.

Noise causes hearing damage by impairing or destroying the organ of Corti and the receptor mechanism in the cochlea. The organ of Corti has approximately 30,000 nerve fibers, which are activated to send the signals to the brain and produce sound.

The tensor tympanic and stapedius muscles in the middle ear appear to protect the inner ear from damaging noises and severe sound pressure levels. These muscles are two of the smallest muscles in the body. Both muscles contract on sensing significant noises and stiffen up the membranes of the oval window and tympanic membrane. The amplitude of the noise vibration is reduced by this membrane stiffening, and the sound pressure level, or shock, to the inner ear is reduced. This reflex is referred to as the middle ear's *aural reflex*. The protection provided by these muscles is not adequate against impulse or impact noises, because it takes about 100 milliseconds for the muscles to respond, and impulse noises are produced in a time period of usually less than 100 milliseconds. Therefore, impulse noise enters the inner ear and damages the cochlea before any aural reflex or muscle contraction occurs. This means that hearing losses due to high impulse noises are unavoidable without ear protection. Such noises are often encountered in the workplace.

High-level, steady-state noise can therefore be less damaging than a lower-level impulse noise that occurs faster than the time needed for aural reflex protection. People dancing to disco music of 110 to 115 dBA, where the noise peaks are cut off by electronics amplification, could be receiving far less damage to their hearing than someone working on a job where there is natural impulse or impact noise with unreduced peaks. Lower-noise-level jobs with greater hazards for impulse or impact noise could be in industries having bottling machines, machine shops, air compressor rooms, and punch presses.

Sound measurement. Noise is measured in decibels (dB), a parameter obtained for any given sound by computing a logarithmic ratio of the present sound pressure to a reference pressure equal to the weakest audible sound thought to be perceived by the human ear. A 120-dB increase would represent a sound which is 1 million times as intense as the reference pressure. Whenever a sound pressure is 10 times greater, it can be called 20 dB greater. The decibel is $\frac{1}{10}$ of a bel. The bel is a parameter for measuring noise and is named after its inventor, Alexander Graham Bell. Bell was attempting to invent a voice machine for his deaf wife but failed. The failure was not entirely disastrous, for the result was the telephone.

Frequency is a property of sound that is measured in cycles per second (cps) called a *hertz* (Hz). A high-frequency sound is shrill and a low-frequency sound is a deep murmur. As people lose hearing, they will generally have varying amounts of hearing ability at different frequencies. A worker may be able to hear low- and middle-frequency sounds and communicate, but will not be able to hear high-frequency sounds.

Threshold shift is a term used to describe hearing-level variance. It means that hearing sensitivity has shifted by rising, or more often by dropping. It can be a temporary shift or a permanent shift. It is generally agreed that physiological hearing damage begins at exposure to noise levels of 85 dBA. The dBA noise measurement scale consists of dB noise values that have been corrected to equal the sensitivity of the human ear at normally audible frequencies. The dBA measurement was developed for measuring only the sounds the human ear can hear and is used in noise regulations.

Hearing sensitivity. The range of sound which the ear can hear is limited. The extreme range of audible frequencies, or the minimum audible field, usually found only in young people, is from 16 Hz to almost 20,000 Hz. Some of these frequencies are perceived at lower intensities than others.

The most sensitive hearing is in the area of normal speech which is in the 500- to 3000-Hz frequency range. Discomfort is encountered at about 120 dB and the pain threshold is slightly above 140 dB.

Occupational Noise

It has been determined that an industrial noise hearing loss is represented by a notch at approximately 4000 Hz on audiograms (Figure 16-2). This notch is often referred to as the industrial noise or industrial acoustic trauma notch. The inner ear damage related to this hearing loss has been determined to be located at the first turn of the cochlea (AIHA, 1975, p. 34). More specifically, the damage is located at approximately 12 to 15 mm from the oval window, or base of the cochlea. The person suffering from this loss may initially complain of tinnitus, which is a ringing in the ear. Many such persons are unaware of any hearing loss, and by the time a hearing loss is noticed, which may be years later, the person is experiencing difficulty communicating. Most workers are unaware of the continuing hearing damage until the damage is severe and permanent. The 4000-Hz notch is indicative of industrial noise hearing loss. The audiogram presented in Figure 16-2 shows such hearing loss and is characteristic of industrial noise hearing loss.

A successful hearing conservation program

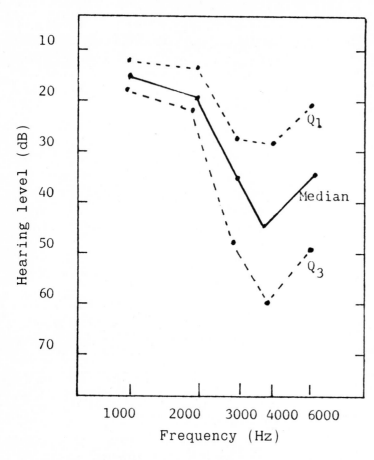

FIGURE 16-2 Noise-induced permanent threshold shift after 4 years on the job based on 8 hours of exposure per day. [*Adapted from American Industrial Hygiene Association. Industrial Noise Manual (3d ed.). Akron, Ohio: American Industrial Hygiene Association, 1975, p. 35.*]

in industry consists of five basic components (Lacy, 1978, p. 18):

1. It provides noise surveys for analyzing the workers' environment for excess noise exposure.

2. It utilizes administrative and engineering controls for reducing noise levels.

3. It performs audiometric testing on each prospective employee and continues to measure an employee's hearing periodically.

4. It furnishes hearing protection for employees working in noisy areas.

5. It provides continual educational programs

to encourage the employees' cooperation in hearing conservation.

The success or failure of an occupational hearing conservation program will depend largely on the occupational health nurse. It is the nurse who obtains the workers' medical and occupational history, carries out the audiometric testing, refers employees with ear complaints or poor audiograms to the physician, counsels the employees regarding industrial noise, and fits or supplies the employee with appropriate hearing protection devices.

An industrial hearing conservation program reduces noise levels primarily in three ways. The first approach is to reduce the noise at the source. Examples of this are the design and production of quieter engines, manufacturing processes, industrial machinery, and home appliances.

A second approach is operational in nature. This involves enclosure of machinery with sound-absorbing materials and noise abatement changes. In general, the primary noise sources in industry are the machines, including high-speed equipment, looms, and stamping operations.

The third approach is personnel protection through the wearing of devices such as earplugs or earmuffs. Earmuffs are, in general, much more effective than plugs.

In some cases, a combination of approaches is needed. Also, employee contact time with noise can be limited in any given work period. The simplest solution is to put distance between the noise source and the individual worker. Table 16-4 lists workers who are frequently exposed to dangerous noise levels.

OSHA Noise Standard

Permissible Noise Exposures

Duration per day, hours	Sound level (dBA)
8	90
6	92
4	95
3	97
2	100
1½	102
1	105
½	110
¼	115

Asbestos, mercury, and noise are examples of problems encountered in the occupational setting. The occupational health nurse, in such situations, uses the nursing and epidemiological processes to identify primary, secondary,

and tertiary preventive services that could promote health and reduce disability. Serafini's assessment guide (see Appendix 16-1) provides a theoretical foundation for comprehensively analyzing the needs and strengths of population groups in the occupational environment, as well as environmental character-

TABLE 16-4 Workers Frequently Exposed to Noise

Boiler room workers	Ordinance manufacture workers
Chemical products manufacture workers	Paper manufacture workers
Construction workers	Paper products manufacture workers
Corrugated paper manufacture workers	Petroleum refiners
Demolition workers	Plastics manufacture workers
Earth-moving equipment operators	Power plant operators
Electrical equipment manufacture workers	Primary metal processors
Engine room workers	Printers
Fabricated metal produce manufacture workers	Quarry workers
	Rubber manufacture workers
Farm equipment operators	Shipbuilders
Food processors	Steel makers
Foundry workers	Stone products industry workers (cement mills)
Furniture manufacture workers	Stone workers
Glass manufacture workers	Textile manufacture workers
Lumberers	Transport equipment operators
Metal farmers	Truckers
Metal workers	Tunneling workers
Miners, open pit	Wood products manufacture workers
Miners, underground	

SOURCE: Adapted from U.S. Department of Health, Education, and Welfare. *A guide to the work-relatedness of disease.* Washington, D.C.: U.S. Government Printing Office, 1976, pp. 49–50.

istics which facilitate or inhibit healthy living. In addition to using this guide, reviewing the health problems of the well adult, discussed in Chapter 15, will help the reader to identify other significant health problems an occupational nurse encounters in the work setting.

MIGRANT FARM WORKERS

Increasingly, it is being recognized that the well adults among the migrant work force have some unique health problems, as well as major barriers to the utilization of health care resources. In addition, it is found that these workers and their families are not protected by many of the laws which govern the health and welfare conditions of other workers. For these reasons, the authors of this text have included a discussion of migrant workers and their related health concerns. It is hoped that the emphasis placed on the needs of the migrant worker will stimulate the reader to become involved in advocating for needed health and welfare reforms for the migrant worker and family.

Being a migrant farm worker poses many occupational health problems. There are over 3 million farm workers in the United States and almost one-half of these are migrant farm workers. Migrant farm workers will often make less than $3000 in gross annual wages (Law, 1974, p. 158). Most of the workers and their families live in chronic poverty.

Migrant farm workers represent a large, mobile supply of cheap labor. Their work is characterized by low wages, long hours, few benefits, and poor working conditions. They move from place to place to meet the nation's agricultural demands. Many are unable to vote because of their mobility. They are the working poor, but without many of the benefits that other workers have.

The living conditions in migrant camps are often substandard, with resultant health problems. The meals provided for migrant farm workers are frequently not well balanced, the housing is generally crowded and inadequate, and living conditions are often not sanitary.

The migrant farm worker has been excluded from protection by much state and federal legislation. Law (1974, pp. 159–163) states that most migrant workers are excluded from the minimum-wage–maximum-hour and child labor provisions of the Fair Labor Standards Act, all are excluded from the National Labor Relations Act, most are excluded from collecting unemployment insurance and workers' compensation, and they are also discriminated against in the Social Security Act. A few states have made provisions for the migrant worker, but provisions are sparse, and the migrant farm worker has little legislative protection.

Until recently migrant farm workers were not part of organized labor. Now some have unionized under either the United Farm Workers of America or the International Brotherhood of Teamsters. However, these two union groups are often in conflict.

Child Labor

Child labor has all but disappeared from U.S. industry, but estimates of the number of working migrant children are high. Growers continue to seek child labor because it is inexpensive and available. Families allow it because of the additional income it brings. Working may keep migrant children from school and other childhood activities. Working migrant children are often subject to the same job hazards and health problems as adults, such as long hours and hazardous or faulty equipment.

Migrant Education

Many children of migrant farm workers never enter high school, and of those who enter, few graduate. The mobility of these children and their families and the seasonal nature of farm work necessitates frequent school changes, leaving school early in the school year, and not returning until late in the fall. Local school authorities are often lax in enforcing school attendance regulations for migrant children. As a result, many migrant farm workers' children are poorly educated, making it difficult for them to escape from their present living conditions. There is a Migrant Education Branch in the Office of Education, Department of Health, Education, and Welfare to facilitate and oversee migrant education.

Access to Local Services

Although the migrant worker may qualify for federal aid programs, restrictive local and state policies often limit the access the migrant has to the health and welfare services within these boundaries. Migrant workers may be subject to rejection and hostility from the community in which they are working.

Migrant workers may be unfamiliar with local resources, personnel, and other individuals. Workers tend to stay together rather than mix in a community that does not welcome them or provide resources to them. Migrant workers generally have no voice in community planning and decision making and often do not feel any major attachment other than economic to the community in which they work.

In 1969, a Supreme Court decision (*Shapiro v. Thompson*, 394 U.S. 618) ruled that a state could not exclude persons from welfare benefits because they were not residents of that state or had not resided in that state for a specific period of time. This was a great help to the migrant worker, because many of them became eligible for health and welfare services, such as food stamps.

The Department of Labor provides many benefits for migrant farm workers and their families. Programs such as child care, economic development, housing subsidies, training, health services, legal aid, transportation, and others are provided for eligible migrant farm workers.

Health

The migrant farm worker represents a unique occupational health problem. Not only is the work often hazardous to health, but the living conditions associated with the work also present several health problems. Historically, the migrant farm worker has had minimal access to the health care system.

The Health Revenue Sharing Act of 1975 (Public Law 94-63) authorized grants to public and other nonprofit agencies for cost sharing in the establishment and operation of migrant family health service clinics. These projects offer a comprehensive range of health services, such as diagnosis and treatment, dental services, preventive care, and health counseling. Services not available at these centers are often supplemented by referrals to other agencies and groups.

The migrant worker is cut off from a stable community. The transient nature of the migrant worker's employment makes it difficult to establish regular routes for health care. The pay base of the work does not allow sufficient funds for health care services, and many migrants are not covered under private health insurance plans. Migrant workers are often not aware of the health care services in the area where they reside and have limited access to them.

Farm workers have a disproportionate number of occupational illnesses and injuries. In 1971, the National Safety Council did a study that showed farm employees suffered 16 percent of all occupational deaths, and 9 percent of all occupational disabling conditions, yet they accounted for only 4.4 percent of the work force (Ashford, 1976, p. 521). Migrant workers are subject to more occupational illness and injury than other farm workers. Only workers in mining and construction exceed the death rates of agricultural workers, and agricultural death rates have risen in recent years. A major problem with estimating occupational illness and injury among migrant farm workers is that few reliable statistics are kept. However, two types of occupational hazards for the farm worker which have been documented are (1) farm machinery and (2) pesticides and other chemicals.

Ashford (1976, p. 522) stated that migrant farm workers experience (1) a life expectancy 20 years lower than the average American, (2) an infant mortality rate 125 percent higher than the national average, (3) death rates from influenza and pneumonia 200 percent higher than the national average, and (4) tuberculosis rates 250 percent higher than the national average. These statistics indicate the magnitude of the health problems facing the migrant worker and his or her family.

The stresses a migrant worker must face are ones to which many of us have never been exposed. The poor working and living conditions, minimal health services, decreased educational opportunities for their children, and low wages all contribute to a poverty beyond what most Americans know. The migrant farm worker is largely concerned with immediate, day-to-day survival, and plans for the future are almost a luxury.

The nurse working with migrant farm workers and their families can greatly facilitate their obtaining health care. The nurse needs firsthand knowledge of community resources, health care facilities, and occupational hazards. The nurse can assist the migrant family in obtaining necessary services and is often in a position to be an advocate for their rights. Migrant health is a vast and challenging field.

SUMMARY

Maintaining the health of the working population is an extremely important task of all health care professionals. The health of well adults influences not only the status of the worker as an individual, but also the health of society as a whole.

Nursing plays a very significant role in promoting the health of the well-adult population. The occupational health nurse provides key services in an occupational health program. In the past, there has been little education in institutions of higher learning which prepared

nurses for a specialty in occupational health nursing. Recently, however, educational research centers, through NIOSH funding, have been established in schools of public health and schools of nursing to prepare nurses for roles in occupational health.

Occupational health nursing is an exciting, expanding field, that hopefully will gain the interest of many new graduates. It is a challenging field and part of the nursing role of the future.

APPENDIX 16-1

Assessment Guide for Nursing in Industry: A Model

1. Community in which industry is located

    a. Description of the community

    (1) Size in area and population

    (2) Climate, altitude, rainfall

    (3) Pollution (noise, radiation, etc.)

    (4) Housing

    (5) Transportation

    (6) Schools

    (7) Sanitation

    (8) Protection: fire, police, etc.

    (9) Trends

    b. Population

    (1) Age distribution

    (2) Sex distribution

    (3) Ethnic and religious composition

    (4) Socioeconomic characteristics

    c. Health information

    (1) Vital statistics

    (2) *Disease incidence and prevalence*

    (3) *Health facilities available*

    (4) Community resources

2. The company

    a. Historical development

1. Just as industry affects the community, so the community affects industry.

    a. Use three or four key descriptive words.

    (1) How far do the employees travel to work and are the workers neighbors?

    (2) Are there times or seasons that are more hazardous than others?

    (3) Can the worker's dermatitis or hearing loss be attributed to the community or is it work related?

    (4) Is there adequate, safe housing in the area? Must the worker spend too great a percentage of his or her salary on housing?

    (5) Is there safe, adequate transportation to work as well as to a hospital or school?

    (6) Do children have to be bused to school or attend overcrowded classes?

    (7) Are roaches and rats common to the area?

    (8) Are the workers and the industry protected?

    (9) Is the area becoming more urban? Residential? Rundown? Deserted?

    b. How alike or different is the population of the industry from that of the community?

    (1) Are the families of child-rearing age or of retirement age?

    (2) Are there more men or more women?

    (3) Are there certain customs or languages that are predominant in the community?

    (4) What is the level of education of the community? What is the mean community income?

    c. Is it an ill or well community?

    (1) What is the infant mortality rate, birth rate, average life expectancy? Usually the local health department has this information.

    (2) *What are the leading causes of morbidity and mortality?*

    (3) *What physical facilities and professional services are available?*

    (4) Are there day-care centers, drug rehabilitation facilities, Alcoholics Anonymous groups, etc.?

2. The official name and address of the company.

    a. Get a perspective on how, why, and by whom the company was founded and compare it with the present situation.

b. Organizational chart

c. Policies

    (1) Length of the work week

    (2) Length of work time

    (3) *Sick leave*

    (4) *Safety and fire provisions*

d. Support services (benefits)

    (1) Insurance programs

    (2) Retirement program

    (3) Educational support

    (4) Safety committee

    (5) Recreation committee

e. Relations between worker and management

f. Projection for the future

3. The plant

    a. General physical setting

    (1) The construction

    (2) Parking facilities and public transportation stops

    (3) Entrances and exits

---

b. What is the formal order of the system and to whom will the nurse be responsible?

c. If there is a policy manual, try to obtain a copy. Are the workers aware of the manual?

    (1) How many days a week does the industry operate?

    (2) Are there several shifts? Breaks? Is there paid vacation?

    (3) Is there a clear policy, and do the workers know it?

    (4) Is management aware of situations or substances in the plant which represent danger? Are there organized fire drills? *The Federal Register* is the source of information for federal standards and serves as a helpful guide.

d. What is the attitude of management concerning worker benefits?

    (1) *Is there a system for health insurance and life insurance, and is it compulsory?* Does the company pay all or part? *Who fills out the necessary forms?*

    (2) Are the benefits realistic?

    (3) Can the worker further his or her education? Will the company help financially?

    (4) The programmed Red Cross First Aid course is excellent. For information consult your Red Cross. *If there is no committee, do certain people routinely handle emergencies?*

    (5) Do the workers have any communication with or interest in each other outside the work setting?

e. This is difficult information to get, but it is important to know how each perceives the other.

f. If the company is growing, workers may see themselves as having a secure future; if not, they may be worried about their job security. How will plant expansion affect the need for nursing services?

3. Draw a small map to scale, labeling the areas. When an accident occurs, place a pin in the exact location on your map. Different-color pinheads can be used for keeping statistics.

    a. What is the gross appearance?

    (1) What is the size and general condition of buildings and grounds?

    (2) How far does the worker have to walk to get inside?

    (3) How many people must use them? How accessible are they?

(4) Physical environment

(5) Communication facilities

(6) Housekeeping

(7) Interior decoration

b. The work areas

(1) Space

(2) Heights: workplace and supply areas

(3) Stimulation

(4) Safety signs and markings

(5) Standing and sitting facilities

(6) Safety equipment

c. Nonwork areas

(1) Lockers

(2) Hand-washing facilities

(3) Rest rooms

(4) Drinking water

(5) Recreation and rest facilities

(6) Telephones

(7) Ashtrays

4. The working population

a. General characteristics

(1) *Total number of employees*

(4) Comment on heating, air conditioning, lighting glare, drafts, etc.

(5) Are there bulletin boards, newsletters?

(6) Is the physical setting maintained adequately?

(7) Are the surroundings conducive to work? Are they pleasing?

b. Get permission to examine them. Use *The Federal Register* as a guide.

(1) Are workers isolated or crowded?

(2) *Falls and falling objects are dangerous and costly to industry.*

(3) Is the worker too bored to pay attention?

(4) Is danger well marked?

(5) Are chairs safe and comfortable? Are there platforms to stand on, especially for wet processes?

(6) Do the workers make use of hard hats, safety glasses, face masks, radiation badges, etc.? Do they know the safety devices the OSHA regulations require?

c. Where are they located? Is there easy access?

(1) If the work is dirty, workers should be able to change clothes. Are they taking toxic substances home?

(2) If facilities and supplies are available, do workers know how and when to wash their hands?

(3) How accessible are they and what condition are they in?

(4) Can a worker leave the job long enough to get a drink of water when he or she wants to?

(5) Can a worker who is not feeling well lie down? Do workers feel free to use the facilities?

(6) Can a worker receive or make a call? Does a working mother have to stay home because she can't be reached at work?

(7) Are people allowed to smoke in designated areas? Is it safe?

4. Include worker and management, but separate data for comparison.

a. Be as accurate as possible, but estimate when necessary.

(1) Usually, if an industry has 500 or more employees, full-time nursing services are necessary.

(2) General appearances

(2) Heights, weights, cleanliness, etc.

(3) *Age and sex distribution*

(3) Certain screening programs are specific for young adults whereas others are more for the elderly. Some programs are more for women; others are more for men. Is there any difference between day and evening shift? Are the problems of the minority sex unattended?

(4) Race distribution

(4) Does one race predominate? How does this compare with the general community?

(5) Socioeconomic distribution

(5) Great differences in worker salaries can sometimes cause problems.

(6) Religious distribution

(6) Does one religion predominate? Are religious holidays observed?

(7) Ethnic distribution

(7) Is there a language barrier?

(8) Marital status

(8) Widowed, single, divorced people often have different needs.

(9) *Educational backgrounds*

(9) *Can all teaching be done at approximately the same level?*

(10) Life-styles practiced

(10) Are certain life-styles frowned upon?

b. Type of employment offered

b. What percentage of the work force is blue-collar and what percentage is white-collar?

(1) Background necessary

(1) What educational level is required? Skilled vs. unskilled?

(2) Work demands on physical condition

(2) Strength needed: sedentary vs. active.

(3) Work status

(3) Part-time vs. full-time; overtime?

c. Absenteeism

c. Is there a record kept? By whom? Why?

(1) *Causes*

(1) *What are the five most common reasons for absence?*

(2) Length

(2) Absenteeism is costly to the employer. There is some difference between one 10-day absence and ten 1-day absences by the same person.

d. Physically handicapped

d. Does the company have a policy about hiring the handicapped?

(1) Number employed

(1) Where do they work? What do they do?

(2) *Extent of handicaps*

(2) Are they specially trained? Are they in a special program? Do they use prosthetic devices?

e. Personnel on medication

e. Know what medication and where the employee works.

f. Personnel with chronic illness

f. At what stage of illness is the employee? Where does the employee work? Will he or she be able to continue at this job?

5. The industrial process

5. What does the company produce and how?

a. Equipment used

   (1) General description of placement

   (2) Type of equipment

b. Nature of the operation

   (1) *Raw materials used*

   (2) Nature of the final product

   (3) Description of the jobs

   (4) Waste products produced

c. Exposure to toxic substances

d. Faculties required throughout the industrial process

6. The health program

a. Existing policies

   (1) Objectives of the program

   (2) *Preemployment physicals*

   (3) First-aid facilities

   (4) *Standing orders*

   (5) *Job descriptions for health personnel*

b. Existing facilities and resources

   (1) Trained personnel

   (2) Space

a. Portable vs. fixed; light vs. heavy.

   (1) Mark each piece of large equipment on the scale map.

   (2) Fans, blowers, fast moving, wet or dry.

b. Get a brief description of each stage of the process so that you can compare the needs and abilities of the worker with the needs of the job.

   (1) *What are they and how dangerous are they? Are they properly stored?* Check *The Federal Register* for guidelines on storage.

   (2) Can the workers take pride in the final product or do they make parts?

   (3) Who does what? Where? Label the map.

   (4) What is the system for waste disposal? Are the pollution control devices in place and functioning?

c. Describe the toxins to which the worker is exposed and the extent of exposure. Include physical and emotional hazards. Remember that chronic effects of industrial exposure are subtle; a person often gets used to having mild symptoms and won't report them. *The Federal Register* contains specifications for exposure to toxins and some states issue state standards.

d. The need for speed, hearing, color vision, etc., can help determine the types of screening programs necessary.

6. Outline what is actually in existence as well as what employees perceive to be in existence.

a. Are there informal, unwritten policies?

   (1) Are they clear?

   (2) Are they required? Are they paid for by the company? Is the information used to deselect?

   (3) What is available? What is not available?

   (4) Is there a company physician who is responsible for first aid or emergency policy? If so, work closely with him or her in planning nursing services.

   (5) If there are no guidelines to be followed, write some.

b. Sometimes an industry that denies having a health program has more of a system than it realizes.

   (1) *Who responds in an emergency?*

   (2) Where is the sick worker taken? Where is the emergency equipment kept?

(3) *Supplies*

(4) *Records and reports*

(3) *Make a list and describe the condition* of each item.

(4) What exists? The Occupational Safety and Health Act requires that employers keep three types of records: a log of occupational injuries and illnesses, a supplemental record of certain illnesses or injuries, and an annual summary (forms 100, 101, and 102 are provided under the act). Good records provide data for good planning.

c. *Services rendered in the past year*

(1) Care needed

(2) Screening done

(3) Referrals made

(4) Counseling done

(5) Health education

c. Describe as specifically as possible.

(1) Chronic or acute? Why?

(2) Where? By whom? Why?

(3) By whom? To whom? Why?

(4) Often informal counseling goes unnoticed.

(5) What individual or group education was offered by the company?

d. *Accidents in the past year*

d. Including those occurring after work hours, as some of these accidents may be directly or indirectly work-related.

e. *Reasons employees sought health care*

e. List the five major reasons.

SOURCE: From P. Serafini. Nursing assessment in industry. *American Journal of Public Health*, August 1976, *66*, 755–760. (Author is now P. Serafini Blanco.)

REFERENCES

American Industrial Hygiene Association. *Industrial noise manual* (3d ed.). Akron, Ohio: American Industrial Hygiene Association, 1975.

American Nurses' Association (Occupational Health Nursing Section). *Functions, standards and qualifications for occupational health nurses.* New York: American Nurses' Association, 1960.

American Public Health Association. *Health and work in America: A chart book.* NIOSH No. 210-75-0045. Washington, D.C.: U.S. Government Printing Office, 1975.

Ashford, N. A. *Crisis in the workplace.* Cambridge, Mass.: M.I.T., 1976.

Chen, E. Fatal cancer in asbestos workers high. *Detroit Free Press*, March 1977.

Colligan, M. J., & Stockton, W. The mystery of assembly-line hysteria. *Psychology Today,* June 1978, 93–99, 114–116.

Dickens, D. Dental offices—Open wide to mercury hazards. *Job Safety and Health,* July 1977, *5*, 15–20.

Dolinsky, E. M. Health maintenance organizations and occupational medicine. *Bulletin of the New York Academy of Medicine,* October 1974, *50*, 126.

Gafafer, W. M. *Occupational diseases: A guide to their recognition.* Washington, D.C.: U.S. Government Printing Office, 1964.

Lacy, S. E. Dow nurses make hearing conservation a reality. *Occupational Health and Safety,* January 1978, *47*, 18–20.

Law, S. *The rights of the poor.* New York: Avon, 1974.

Lawrence, M. Researchers seek to pinpoint physiological mechanisms of noise-induced hearing loss. *Occupational Health and Safety,* January 1978, *47*, 22–24.

Martin, G. New roles for the occupational health

nurse. *Job Safety and Health,* April 1977, *5,* 9–15.

McCall, B. How West Germany protects its workers. *Job Safety and Health,* July 1977, *5,* 21–25.

Montague, K., & Montague, P. *Mercury.* San Francisco: Sierra Club, 1971.

Morris, R. (Ed.). *The American worker.* Washington, D.C.: U.S. Government Printing Office, 1976.

Page, J. A., & O'Brien, M. W. *Bitter wages.* New York: Grossman Publishers, 1973.

National Institute for Occupational Safety and Health. *Occupational exposure to inorganic mercury.* HSM 73-11024. Washington, D.C.: U.S. Government Printing Office, 1973.

National Institute for Occupational Safety and Health. *Occupational exposure to noise.* Washington, D.C.: U.S. Government Printing Office, 1972.

National Institute for Occupational Safety and Health. *Working with mercury in industry.* Washington, D.C.: U.S. Government Printing Office, 1973.

Olishifski, J. B., & Harford, E. R. *Industrial noise and hearing conservation.* Chicago: National Safety Council, 1975.

Serafini, P. Nursing assessment in industry. *American Journal of Public Health,* August 1976, *66,* 755–760. (Author is now P. Serafini Blanco.)

Spackling compound, a toxic warning. *Carpenter,* February 1976, p. 8.

Stellman, J. M., & Daum, S. M. *Work is dangerous to your health.* New York: Vintage Books, 1973.

Stevenson, J. S. *Issues and crisis during middlescence.* New York: Appleton-Century-Crofts, 1977.

U.S. Department of Health, Education, and Welfare. *A guide to the work-relatedness of disease.* Washington, D.C.: U.S. Government Printing Office, 1976.

U.S. Department of Labor. *Important events in American labor history. 1778–1975.* Washington, D.C.: U.S. Government Printing Office, 1976.

U.S. Department of Labor. *Labor firsts in America.* Washington, D.C.: U.S. Government Printing Office, 1977.

U.S. Department of Labor. *Mercury.* OSHA 2230. Washington, D.C.: U.S. Government Printing Office, 1975, unnumbered pages.

U.S. Department of Labor. Occupational exposure to asbestos. *Federal Register,* 1975.

SELECTED BIBLIOGRAPHY

Brodeur, P. *Expendable Americans.* New York: Viking Press, 1974.

Burleen, O. The nurse and industrial hygiene. *Occupational Health Nursing,* April 1976, *24,* 7–10.

Freeman, R. B. *Community health nursing practice.* Philadelphia: Saunders, 1970, chap. 21.

Goldstein, D. H. The occupational safety and health act of 1970. *American Journal of Nursing,* August 1971, *71,* 1535–1538.

Goldwater, L. J. *A history of quicksilver.* Baltimore: New York Press, 1972.

———. Mercury in the environment. *Science Academy,* January 1971, *224,* 15–21.

Hamilton, A. *Industrial poisons in the United States.* New York: Macmillan, 1925.

——— & Hardy, H. *Industrial toxicology* (2d ed.). New York: Hoeber-Harper, 1949.

Martin, F. N. *Introduction to audiology.* Englewood Cliffs, N.J.: Prentice-Hall, 1975.

McCord, C. P. *A blind hog's acorns.* Chicago: Cloud, 1945.

———. What happened at Gauley bridge 1930–1935? *Industrial Medicine and Surgery,* April 1961, *30,* 145–149.

———, Holden, F. R., & Johnston, J. Basophilic aggregation test in the lead poisoning epidemic of 1934–35. *American Journal of Public Health,* October 1935, *25,* 1089–1098.

National Institute for Occupational Safety and Health. *Occupational exposure to asbestos.* Washington, D.C.: U.S. Government Printing Office, 1972.

National Institute for Occupational Safety and Health. *Occupational health and safety for agricul-*

tural workers. Washington, D.C.: U.S. Government Printing Office, 1976.

National Institute for Occupational Safety and Health. *The yard of occupational health nursing.* USPHS Publication No. 2176. Washington, D.C.: U.S. Government Printing Office, 1971.

Neal, P. A., Jones, R. R., Bloomfield, J. J., Dallavalle, J. M., & Edwards, T. I. *Study of chronic mercurialism in the hatter's, fur-cutting industry.* Public Health Bulletin 234. Washington, D.C.: U.S. Government Printing Office, 1937.

Sataloff, J., & Michael, P. L. *Hearing conservation.* Springfield, Ill.: Charles C Thomas, 1973.

Scott, R. *Muscle and blood.* New York: Dutton 1974.

U.S. Department of Health, Education, and Welfare. *Community health nursing for working people.* USPHS Publication No. 1296. Washington, D.C.: U.S. Government Printing Office, 1970.

U.S. Department of Labor. *All about OSHA.* Washington, D.C.: U.S. Government Printing Office, 1976.

U.S. Department of Labor. *Lead.* OSHA 2234. Washington, D.C.: U.S. Government Printing Office, 1975.

U.S. Department of Labor. *Vinyl chloride.* OSHA 2225. Washington, D.C.: U.S. Government Printing Office, 1975.

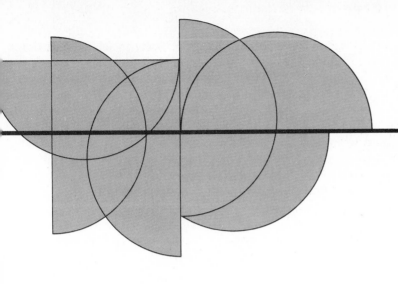

17
the adult who
is handicapped

When one is working with people who are handicapped, it must be remembered that first they are people and, secondary to that, they have a handicapping condition.

From early in recorded time people have noted the handicapping conditions among them. Handicapping conditions were recorded as early as 384 B.C. by Aristotle (Buscaglia, 1975, p. 171). Later Hippocrates, Galen, and others studied such conditions and sought answers to why they existed.

Throughout history societies have dealt in various ways with members who were handicapped. Attitudes toward the handicapped have ranged from acceptance to rejection and from understanding to fear. The Elizabethan Poor Law of 1601 equated handicapping conditions with crime, and under this law people who were handicapped were often disenfranchised, publicly punished, and imprisoned (Sussman, 1966, p. 3). The classic story of the *Hunchback of Notre Dame* clearly illustrates society's reaction to disfigurement during the eighteenth century.

Although being handicapped is no longer considered criminal, in contemporary American society people who are handicapped are often labeled and separated from the mainstream of the general population. An example

of this is the placing of people who are mentally retarded in institutional settings.

Community health nurses have historically worked with people who are handicapped. However, prior to the twentieth century few severely handicapped people lived into adulthood because they succumbed early in life to a variety of illnesses and conditions. Due to recent advances in medical, pharmaceutical, and industrial technology, the handicapped are living longer, and the community health nurse is having increased contact with adults who are handicapped. Also, the emerging trend in the United States to maintain people who are handicapped in the community finds the community health nurse working with the handicapped in the community instead of in institutional settings.

Two terms that the community health nurse is likely to hear when working with the adult who is handicapped are *normalization* and *mainstreaming*. These terms are used in this chapter and are briefly explained here.

Mainstreaming is the phenomenon of having the person who is handicapped integrated into the everyday life of the community. The person functions in the "mainstream" of the community and is not separated from community activities as is the case with the person who is institutionalized.

Normalization refers to the practice of assisting persons who are handicapped to live as "normal" a life as possible. They are aided and encouraged to participate in the same activities as other members of the community, such as adhering to laws, working, housekeeping, riding buses, driving, going to school, and shopping to the best of their ability.

Both mainstreaming and normalization reflect a humanistic philosophy that could alter the way in which people who are handicapped are treated. Successful implementation of these concepts requires careful planning and adequate support services so that clients are not asked to compete in "normal situations" without the help they need to do so.

DEFINITION OF A HANDICAP

A *handicap* is defined as a condition that substantially limits one or more of an individual's major life activities (U.S. Department of Health, Education, and Welfare, 1978; President's Committee on Employment of the Handicapped, *Affirmative Action,* 1978). Major life activities are communication, ambulation, self-care, socialization, education, vocational training, transportation, housing, and employment (President's Committee on Employment of the Handicapped, *Affirmative Action,* 1978).

A handicap involves alteration of body functions or parts and can be categorized as (1) physical (i.e., blindness, deafness, hypertension, cancer, and amputation) or (2) mental (i.e., mental illness and mental retardation). A person who is handicapped can have one or a combination of the above categories of handicaps.

A handicapping condition can cause secondary handicaps. An example is a person who, because of severe hypertension, evidences a cerebrovascular accident (CVA). As a result of the CVA, the person becomes paraplegic and has decreased mental capabilities. The person would now have physical and mental handicapping conditions secondary to hypertension.

Handicapping conditions include, but are not limited to, alcoholism; cancer; cerebral palsy; deafness; drug addiction; epilepsy; heart disease; mental or emotional illness; mental retardation; multiple sclerosis; muscular dystrophy; orthopedic, speech, or visual impairment; and perceptual handicaps such as dyslexia, minimal brain dysfunction, and developmental aphasia (President's Committee on Employment of the Handicapped, *Affirmative Action,* 1978). The U.S. Attorney General has ruled that alcoholism and drug addiction qualify as handicapping conditions if they limit one or more of life's major activities.

Handicapping conditions may be congenital or acquired. Congenital handicapping conditions are evidenced from birth, whereas acquired handicapping conditions are evidenced after birth.

By definition, to be termed a handicap, a condition must be limiting, and the degree of limitation imposed by the handicap can be discussed in terms of disability. To determine the level of disability, the individual's ability to perform major life activities would be evaluated. For the purpose of this text, the assessed degree of disability would be classified as follows:

LEVEL I: Partial disability characterized by slight limitation in one or more of the major life activities.

LEVEL II: Partial disability characterized by moderate limitation in one or more of the major life activities.

LEVEL III: Partial disability characterized by severe limitation in one or more of the major life activities.

LEVEL IV: Total disability characterized by complete dependency on others for activities of daily living and economic support.

Most chronic handicapping conditions of adults can encompass the entire disability range. For example, an individual with cerebral palsy may evidence any of the levels of disability with capabilities ranging from independence to complete dependence. The level of disability will largely determine the functional capacity the individual is able to attain.

In 1972 more than 15 million Americans between the ages of 20 and 64 had a handicapping condition that limited their ability to work (U.S. Department of Health, Education, and Welfare, *Work Disability,* 1977). The chances of developing a handicapping condition increase with age, but it cannot be said that only older people have handicapping conditions. Figure 17-1 illustrates the increasing incidence of handicapping conditions with age.

ADJUSTMENT TO THE HANDICAP

Adjustment to a handicap is a complex process and is influenced by both individual and societal variables. It is a combination of these variables that determines the adjustment a person makes to a handicap.

Societal Attitudes toward People Who Are Handicapped

Societal attitudes toward people who are handicapped will play a major role in an individual's adjustment to a handicapping condition. Societal attitudes toward the handicapped are influenced by the following variables (Safilios-Rothschild, 1970, p. 4):

1. *Beliefs regarding the value of physical and mental integrity.* The values held in regard to physical and mental integrity will greatly affect the acceptance of handicapping conditions and the services rendered to people who are handicapped. The values placed on physical and mental integrity are usually high, and the higher the value placed, the more likely there is to be prejudice against those who are physically and mentally handicapped. It should be remembered that physical and mental deviations may have meanings totally unrelated to the person who is handicapped but reflecting an individual's preconceived ideas regarding the condition.

2. *Beliefs in relation to illness.* There is often a difference between the role given someone who is acutely ill and one who is chronically impaired. If a chronic condition is severely limiting, there is a tendency to separate the person from the mainstream of society through institutional, nursing home, or extended-care placement. If the condition is only mildly to moderately limiting, the person is often expected to perform "normally." The attitude also exists that because a condition has become chronic and has existed for a long time, it is more bearable.

3. *Beliefs regarding condition occurrence.* If it is believed that the individual had a high degree of responsibility in the occurrence of the handicapping condition, less aid is generally accorded that person. Obesity and alcoholism are examples of this.

4. *The role of the government in alleviating social problems.* If a society does not believe that

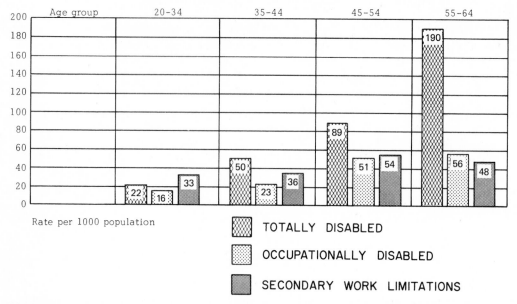

FIGURE 17-1 Age and the adult who is handicapped. *(Social Security Administration. Work disability in the United States, Washington, D.C.: U.S. Government Printing Office, 1977.)*

the government should assume an active role in alleviating social problems and subsidizing those who cannot otherwise support themselves, there may be little public assistance to people who are handicapped.

5. *Beliefs regarding the origins of poverty.* Many people who are handicapped frequently fall below the poverty level. If a society believes that poverty is generally a matter of self-will, there will likely be less assistance to the handicapped.

6. *The rate of employment and economic development.* When unemployment is high, preferential hiring practices are often accorded the nonhandicapped individual. Also, if an economy is unstable, there is less inclination to financially subsidize those who are handicapped.

Studies have been done on the emergent societal attitudes toward people who are handicapped. Buscaglia (1975) described a study involving nonhandicapped people view-

ing nonhandicapped people (1) in a wheelchair, giving one the impression of being handicapped, and (2) out of a wheelchair. Seen in the wheelchair, the nonhandicapped individual was described as helpless, hopeless, and of decreased value; however, the same person, out of the wheelchair, was described positively. The same type of responses occurred with a nonhandicapped person viewed (1) with leg braces and (2) without leg braces. Other studies have shown that even people with handicapping conditions showed negative attitudes toward people with handicapping conditions and showed preferential feelings toward people with the same handicap as they had (Dixon, 1977, p. 308). People often become tense and uncomfortable when dealing with people who are handicapped. Handicapping conditions, as human deviations, can pose a threat to one's self-image.

People who are handicapped are often relegated to inferior societal positions and are not granted the same basic rights and privileges as others. Handicapping conditions have been used to justify separation of people from the mainstream of the community, as has been the case with many institutionalized mentally handicapped people. Many people encourage the handicapped to interact with each other, rather than with nonhandicapped people, because they think that this will give them a better chance of being accepted (Safilios-Rothschild, 1970, p. 110).

It is not uncommon to find that there are inadequate residential, educational, occupational, medical, or social programs to meet the needs of the person who is handicapped in the community. When services do exist, they are often fragmented, of questionable quality, and poorly monitored. This pattern of inadequate service provision for the handicapped is due for a change.

The community health nurse can help to eliminate societal prejudices that exist toward the handicapped. She or he can be instrumental in getting health legislation passed which reflects a humanistic philosophy toward individuals who need special services to maximize their potential. Through health education activities, the nurse can aid health care professionals, clients, and others to gain a realistic understanding of the nature of handicapping conditions and an appreciation for the strengths as well as needs of individuals who have handicaps.

Health education activities in the school setting are especially beneficial in changing attitudes toward individuals who have handicaps. It is not uncommon for children in elementary classrooms to encounter peers who deviate from the normal. A sensitive teacher and school nurse can help these children to accept peers who are different and to understand why these differences have occurred.

Individual Variables Influencing Adjustment to the Handicap

In addition to the societal variables, there are individual variables that influence adjustment to a handicapping condition. The following are significant individual variables:

1. The stage the individual has reached in the grief and mourning process associated with the handicap

2. Age at which the handicapping condition occurred

3. Rapidity of onset of the handicapping condition

4. Level of disability caused by the handicapping condition

5. Visibility of the handicapping condition

6. Value of the handicapped area

7 Attitudes regarding self

8. Attitudes of significant others

9. Rehabilitation services available and utilized

Psychological research has explored human adjustment to handicapping conditions and determined that definite stages of grief and mourning are experienced (Vargo, 1978, p. 32; Bower, 1977, p. 10). The following is a summation of the grief and mourning process that a person goes through in adjusting to a handicap:

DENIAL: The individual is not prepared to accept the reality and ramifications of the handicap and denies the existence of the handicap.

ANGER: The individual realizes that the handicap is real, the loss becomes real, and feelings of hostility, anger, and bitterness arise in response to the handicap.

BARGAINING: The individual attempts to barter and deal his or her way out of the handicap.

DEPRESSION: The individual realizes the permanency of the condition and experiences feelings of rejection, worthlessness, and despair.

ADJUSTMENT: The individual becomes self-accepting and is capable of coping with the various aspects of the handicap. The goal of this stage is rehabilitation.

Handicapping conditions that occur after the development of a self-image are frequently more difficult to handle than others. A child born without an arm will have a different adjustment process than the child who loses an arm at age 5 or the adult who loses an arm at 50. The internalized body image of the adult makes it difficult to accept, much less incorporate, drastic alterations of body structure (Safilios-Rothschild, 1970, p. 80).

The rapidity of a condition's onset is also critical to adjustment. If a condition develops gradually, as does rheumatoid arthritis, the adjustment time is lengthened and there is an opportunity to develop skills, resources, support systems, and coping mechanisms. If the occurrence is sudden, as with a traumatic injury, there is little or no adjustment time. Any person needs time to adapt to a condition, and rehabilitation techniques may need to be delayed until adaptation can take place. Sudden change is often difficult to incorporate into one's body image (Safilios-Rothschild, 1970, p. 88).

The level of disability associated with a condition will have a great deal to do with the adjustment the person is able to make to the condition. Generally, the higher the level of disability, the more difficult it is to adjust to the handicap. An individual with a paralyzed hand will likely have less difficulty in adjustment than a paraplegic or a person who is severely mentally retarded. The level of disability will be a major determinant of the functional capacity the individual is able to attain.

The level of disability has an impact on the person's ability to accomplish the age-specific developmental tasks discussed throughout this text. They include such things as establishing an occupation and a companionship life-style, utilizing leisure time, and taking part in civic activities. The person who is handicapped is often impeded in accomplishing or maintaining these developmental tasks.

The visibility of the condition affects the adjustment made to it. People generally have stronger reactions to visible than to invisible signs and symptoms. Even handicapped persons have more negative attitudes about handicaps with visible physical ramifications, such as an amputation, than toward handicaps without, such as hypertension (Goldberg, 1977). Any visible condition will generally elicit more discriminating individual and societal responses than a nonvisible or slightly visible condition.

The value of the handicapped part is of major importance. A person becomes more upset when something happens to a part of the body that is highly valued. The value placed on body parts will vary from individual to individual; however, some parts seem to have a higher value than others. Facial disfigurement illustrates well the value placed on certain body parts. Although facial disfigurement causes few physical limitations, it is one of the most difficult handicapping conditions to adjust to because of the high value placed on facial characteristics (Safilios-Rothschild, 1970, p. 126).

The attitudes held about oneself and the attitudes about oneself held by significant others are critical to the outcome of a handicapping condition. If such attitudes are negative, their impact can be detrimental to the outcome of the condition. Community health nurses, and others in therapeutic roles, should build upon the positive attitudes found and help the client and significant others to analyze why negative attitudes exist. Since attitudes have an important effect upon an individual's social and psychological adjustment to his or her handicap, it is crucial for the community health nurse to identify attitudes that may hamper successful adaptation.

Rehabilitation services play a key role in handicap outcome. Handicap adjustment is impeded if rehabilitation services are not available, appropriate, or accessible. Rehabilitation is an extremely important concept and will be discussed in a separate section of this chapter.

AREAS OF MAJOR CONCERN FOR PEOPLE WHO ARE HANDICAPPED, THEIR FAMILIES, AND HEALTH PROFESSIONALS

People who are handicapped are at a definite disadvantage in contemporary society. As they try to keep up with the rapid pace, and increased social, educational, and occupational demands, a number of concerns emerge.

Education

Approximately 40 percent of the adults who are handicapped have a high school diploma, whereas almost 70 percent of their nonhandicapped counterparts have high school diplomas (Posner, 1978, p. 15). Lack of education makes it difficult for the adult who is handicapped to find a job. Lack of education stems not from a lack of interest among the handicapped in seeking education, but from a lack of provision of such education by the public. It was not until the 1970s that states began enacting mandatory education laws for people who were handicapped. Prior to this time, if a person did not fit into the existing school district programs, and most individuals who were handicapped did not, the school district was not responsible for the education of this person. As mandatory education programs for the handicapped evolved, they often applied only to children; the adult who was handicapped was frequently excluded. The Federal Education for All Handicapped Children Act of 1975 (Public Law 94-142) instituted education for children who were handicapped from age 3 to 18 as of September 1, 1978, and encompassed people from age 3 to 21 as of September 1, 1980. After age 21 the federal law does not mandate educational programs for the adult who is handicapped. Some states, such as Michigan, have state education laws for the handicapped that provide more educational services than the federal law. In Michigan, people who are handicapped have a right to a free public education from birth through age 25.

What happens to a person's educational training program after he or she reaches the age where the mandatory education laws no longer apply is a contemporary educational dilemma. By law, the handicapped adult who applies for college, job training, or adult basic education must be considered on academic and other school and work records, not on the basis of his or her current handicap. An educational program may not (U.S. Department of Health, Education, and Welfare, 1978):

- Ask a person who is handicapped to take a preadmission test that inadequately measures his or her academic level because no special provisions were made for the fact that the person is blind, deaf, or otherwise handicapped

- Inquire about any handicapping condition before admission unless trying to overcome the effects of prior limitations on enrollment of handicapped students and the person volunteers the information

- Limit the number of handicapped students admitted

Colleges are not required to lower academic standards or alter degree requirements for people who are handicapped. However, if the college is receiving federal subsidy, it may be required to modify teaching methods and provide teaching aids as necessary to accommodate the student who is handicapped.

The previously discussed factors in relation to education were largely a result of the Rehabilitation Act Amendments of 1974 (Public Law 93-516). These amendments stated that no otherwise qualified handicapped individual in the United States would, solely by reason of his or her handicap, be excluded from participation in, be denied the benefits of, or be subject to discrimination under any program or activity receiving federal assistance (Park, 1977, p. 11). Many educational facilities, including colleges and universities, receive federal assistance.

A number of people who are handicapped utilize homebound instruction. Home study programs can offer the person who is handicapped an opportunity to learn a skill or train for a number of careers (President's Committee on Employment of the Handicapped, *Careers for the Homebound,* 1978). The U.S. Department of Education recognizes the Accrediting Commission of the National Home Study Council (1601 Eighteenth Street, N.W., Washington, D.C. 20009) and its handbook *Directory of Accredited Home Study Schools* as a valid resource for locating quality schools of home study (President's Committee on Employment of the Handicapped, *Careers for the Homebound,* 1978).

Vocational rehabilitation has been an important part of the education and training of adults who are handicapped since the enactment of the first federal Rehabilitation Act in 1920. The state-federal vocational rehabilitation programs that resulted from this act remain the largest public programs providing rehabilitation services to the adult who is handicapped. In order to qualify for these programs the person must be of an employable age, at least 16 years old, have a physical or mental disability that constitutes an employment handicap, and be able to become employable as a result of vocational training. These programs encompass the following (Terry, Benz, Mereness, Kleffner, and Jensen, 1961, p. 51; and President's Committee on Employment of the Handicapped, 1976, p. 92):

1. Early location of people in need of rehabilitation services

2. Evaluation of the individual's rehabilitation potential

3. Physical or mental restoration services including medical and surgical treatment, psychological care, dental care, physical and occupational therapy, and speech and hearing services

4. Telecommunications, sensory, and other technological aids and services

5. Vocational counseling

6. Vocational training

7. Financial assistance to provide maintenance and transportation during training and job recruitment

8. Occupational licenses, tools, equipment, and initial supplies

9. Employment placement service

10. Follow-up on job performance and retraining as necessary

To apply for vocational rehabilitation services, a person should contact the local office of the state Department of Education, Division of Vocational Rehabilitation Services. It is through these offices that programming can be initiated.

Financial Stability

An adult who is handicapped is financially responsible for himself or herself. He or she may, however, be eligible for federal or state assistance programs. Most of the financial assistance available to the adult who is handicapped comes from either the state department of social services (DSS) or the federal Social Security Administration (SSA). Under the DSS the adult is eligible for all forms of categorical aid such as General Assistance (GA), and Aid to Families of Dependent Children (AFDC). Under the SSA the adult may qualify for Supplemental Security Income (SSI) or be eligible for other social security benefits. To qualify for SSI under the aid to disabled category the person must have a physical or mental impairment resulting from anatomical, physiological, or psychological abnormalities which are verified by medical diagnosis (U.S. Department of Health, Education, and Welfare, *Key Federal,* 1977, p. 47). Supplemental Security Income is used extensively by the adult who is handicapped for financial subsidy and may be applied for through the local SSA office.

It is not mandatory that the adult who is handicapped apply for financial assistance. Many times the family of the handicapped adult totally or partially supports the person. This may work for an indefinite period of time, but there is great likelihood that this method will eventually prove inadequate. The community health nurse should encourage the adult who is handicapped, and his or her family, to explore the different funding possibilities available to them. Local DDS and SSA offices can be contacted for specific information regarding funding mechanisms available.

When an adult who is handicapped is able to work on the same job, sheltered employment excluded, for a period of 9 or more consecutive months, he or she is considered to have shown capability for gainful employment and may permanently lose SSI eligibility under the disabling condition(s) existing prior to the employment. The person would have to evidence an additional disabling condition to requalify for SSI. An example of this would be a person who is mentally retarded and who has worked for 1 year as a dishwasher in a local restaurant. If he loses his job after a year, he will not qualify for SSI under a mental retardation classification. The person would have to evidence a qualifying, disabling condition in addition to the mental retardation to requalify for SSI. The person may qualify for unemployment insurance, but these benefits would soon be exhausted.

Since SSI is widely used as a source of financial support for the adult who is handicapped, the loss of SSI eligibility can seriously affect a person's financial stability. An adult who is handicapped and his or her family would want to look seriously at the implications of competitive employment on future financial stability, and specifically at SSI eligibility.

Figure 17-2 presents median income for the person who is handicapped in relation to that for the nonhandicapped population. It dramatically illustrates that financial stability of the person who is handicapped is a serious concern.

Employment

America's work ethic makes employment a central part of life. Work has a great deal to do with how people identify themselves, as well as how they are identified by others (Rosow, 1976, p. 29). Work situations for the adult who is handicapped are limited and will be largely dependent on the presenting handicap. Adults who are handicapped are found in competitive, modified, and sheltered employment. *Competitive employment* is work with

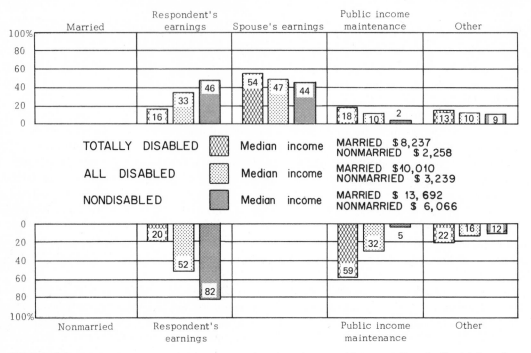

FIGURE 17-2 Source of income and the person who is handicapped (by percentage). *(Social Security Administration. Work disability in the United States. Washington, D.C.: U.S. Government Printing Office, 1977.)*

nonhandicapped members of the work force on an equal basis, such as a job on the assembly line at an automotive factory. *Modified employment* is work done with nonhandicapped members of the work force in a work environment that has been modified to meet the needs of the handicapped worker. *Sheltered employment* is work that is open only to the handicapped and is done under direct supervision and guidance. The Association for Retarded Citizens and Goodwill Industries frequently sponsor sheltered workshops. The Wagner-O'Day Act of 1938, and its amendments of 1971, provided for special preference in bidding on government contracts to sheltered workshops for the severely handicapped.

There are few federal, state, or local incentives for employers to hire the handicapped.

Since 1978 the Internal Revenue Service has allowed tax incentives for businesses employing people who are handicapped in the form of tax credits for employment of the handicapped and deductions for the cost of removing architectural and transportation barriers for handicapped employees. The Small Business Administration is permitted to make loans to people who are handicapped to establish, acquire, or operate a business when other loans are not available on reasonable terms. This was enabled through the Loans to the Handicapped law of 1972 (Public Law 92-595). The legislation also allowed loan assistance to certain businesses that employ individuals who are handicapped.

The Rehabilitation Act of 1973 required that federal agencies, and federally contracted agencies, take action to hire and promote handicapped persons. The act stated that any employer receiving federal assistance may not discriminate against the handicapped employee in recruitment, hiring, promotion, demotion, transfer, layoff, firing, or rehiring. An employer receiving federal assistance is required to take reasonable steps to accommodate the handicapped worker. This includes obtaining a reader if the person is blind, an interpreter if the person is deaf, and adequate workspace if the person needs a wheelchair or other equipment (U.S. Department of Health, Education, and Welfare, 1978).

A handicapped job applicant or employee has the same rights and privileges as nonhandicapped applicants and employees. A person's handicap must not be considered in employment unless it keeps him or her from performing adequately at the work (U.S. Department of Health, Education, and Welfare, 1978).

If a handicapped person believes that he or she has been discriminated against in relation to a federal job, the person should file a complaint with a federal job information center. If he or she believes that promotion has been denied in a federal agency because of this handicap, the handicapped person should contact the equal opportunity officer in the agency (U.S. Department of Health, Education, and Welfare, 1978). If a person thinks that an agency contracted with the federal government is discriminating against the handicapped, he or she should file a complaint within 120 days of the alleged violation with:

Veterans and Handicapped Division
Office of Federal Contract Compliance
  Programs
Department of Labor
Washington, D.C. 20210

Individuals whose earnings or productive capacity is impaired by physical or mental deficiency can qualify for employment at less than minimum wage. This is often an acceptable alternative for employers. For the person who is handicapped, it is often more acceptable than not working. The Secretary of Labor must certify such employment, and filing for certification is done through the Regional Director of Wage and Hour Division of the Department of Labor (U.S. Department of Health, Education, and Welfare, *Key Federal*, 1977, p. 34). Wages paid to a worker who is handicapped cannot be less than 50 percent of the wages that are being paid to the nonhandicapped worker. Those qualifying must be engaged in work which is related to training or diagnostic evaluation and be handicapped to the extent that they cannot engage in competitive employment.

A major drawback to obtaining employment for the handicapped is the unavailability of transportation for them to a work setting. Many people who are handicapped cannot drive or do not have cars. Public transportation, such as buses, trains, trolleys, and subways, is often inadequate. Many people who are handicapped must rely on friends, relatives, Dial-a-Rides, taxis, and public and voluntary transportation services. This shortage of transportation for the handicapped has an impact not only on employment, but on social, recreational, medical, and educational opportunities as well. Recent federal legislation has mandated that the person who is handicapped cannot be denied the use of public transportation because of his or her handicap.

Medical and Dental Care

People who are handicapped cannot be excluded from state and federally funded programs such as Medicaid and Medicare. In fact, many people who are handicapped qualify for one or both programs and receive services through them. A large number of doctors, dentists, and other health care professionals choose not to work with people who are handicapped, especially those who are mentally handicapped. Even with adequate funding the handicapped may be unable to find a private health care provider and it is difficult for them to obtain other medical or dental care. The community health nurse can be instrumental in procuring health services for the person who is handicapped. Once the services are found, there are often such problems as funding and transportation to be dealt with. Transportation to medical and dental appointments is sometimes facilitated if the person has Medicaid, since Medicaid may provide funds for transportation to medical appointments.

Health insurance on a private basis is difficult for persons who are handicapped to obtain because they are considered high-risk (Figure 17-3).

The cost of medical care for the person who is totally disabled is frequently at least three times that of the nonhandicapped population (Social Security Administration, 1977). Many of these costs are not covered by insurance since people who are handicapped are less likely to have comprehensive insurance coverage (Social Security Administration, 1977). Figure 17-3 clearly illustrates this point. It is obvious from the data presented in this figure that individuals who are handicapped may need help in obtaining financial assistance for their health needs.

Social and Recreational Programs

There are few social and recreational programs that are designed to include people who are handicapped. Many buildings where these programs are offered are physically inaccessible to the person who is handicapped; there may be no wheelchair ramps or wide doorways for wheelchairs to go through. Some adults who are handicapped, especially adults who are mentally retarded, often find great enjoyment in participating in social and recreational activities planned especially for them. Other

adults who are handicapped, such as the severe diabetic, often mix freely in social and recreational activities that nonhandicapped adults enjoy. Whatever the level of disability, people who are handicapped are social beings and should have social programs and activities available to them.

As well as being a person with social needs, the adult who is handicapped is a person with sexual needs. Depending on the handicap, the person may or may not have regular sexual functions. This lack or impairment of function does not nullify the need. Sexuality is the area of greatest concern to many handicapped. If one has had normal sexual function for years, and then has this function lost or impaired, the emotional significance can be great. People who are handicapped need sensitive, nonjudgmental and empathic guidance and counseling in the area of sexual fulfillment. If a professional does not feel capable or comfortable to deal with this area, outside resources should be considered. The sexuality of the person who is handicapped needs to be recognized. Avenues of expression and fulfillment of sexual needs must be found.

Guardianship

Once the age of majority is reached, a person is legally responsible for himself or herself unless a legal guardian has been appointed. Any responsible adult can petition for guardianship of another person through probate court. The court decides if a guardian should be appointed, who is an appropriate guardian, and whether the guardian should be plenary (complete) or partial. Partial guardianship is not allowed in all states. What partial guardianship implies is that the person is able to carry out some functions alone but needs assistance in carrying out other functions. Delineation of the guardian's functioning is provided specifically by the court. If the court does not deem a guardian necessary, no guardian is ap-

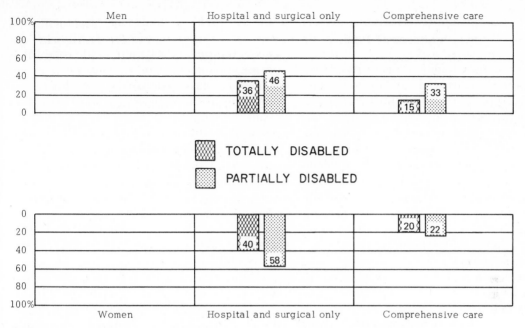

FIGURE 17-3 The person who is handicapped and health insurance. *(Social Security Administration. Work disability in the United States. Washington, D.C.: U.S. Government Printing Office, 1977.)*

pointed and the person is responsible for making his or her own decisions. Also, until guardianship is applied for, generally none is appointed by the court. Guardians are frequently appointed for people who are mentally handicapped, but guardians may be appointed for other adults who need assistance in carrying out the activities of everyday life.

Parents are "natural" guardians of their own minor children and can make legal decisions for them. Parents are *not* natural guardians of their adult offspring who are handicapped and cannot make legal decisions for them without having legal guardianship. Many parents are unaware of this fact, which can present a problem when their adult offspring needs medical care or other social services. If the adult who is handicapped is unable to make a rational decision, medical care may be denied until a legal guardian is appointed.

Anticipatory guidance with parents or significant others can prevent this from happening.

Handling guardianship issues is difficult for many families. Families who have adult offspring who are handicapped frequently experience a crisis when they realize that their offspring are not able to make rational decisions at the age of maturity. Parents at this point can no longer avoid the reality that their offspring may never develop the skills to function independently. Feelings of sadness and hopelessness at this time are not uncommon. It is crucial for the community health nurse and other health care professionals to recognize the distress these parents are experiencing and to provide consistent support during this critical transition period. Helping these families to identify the strengths their adult offspring have, as well as the potential for benefiting from experiences that are developmentally within their reach, frequently reduces their anxiety and increases their ability to plan for the future.

When helping a family to deal with guardianship issues, it is crucial for the community health nurse to focus on the entire family system. Siblings are often asked at this time to make a commitment to assume responsibility for the care of an adult sibling who is handicapped after the parents are no longer able to do so. This can stimulate feelings of fear, shame, guilt, or hostility, especially if the siblings do not want to make this commitment. Families frequently need assistance in analyzing what is best for all family members.

At times, community health nurses have found that some families assume that adults who are handicapped are unable to care for themselves just because they are handicapped. It is important to remember that not all adults who are handicapped need guardians. In fact, most of them do not.

Community Residential Opportunities

People who are handicapped reside in a number of types of residential placements. Many people who are handicapped with low disability levels live independently or in semi-independent living situations. They may be financially independent and reside in these placements on their own, or they may be receiving some form of financial assistance. The recruitment, funding, placement, and monitoring aspects of residential placements for people who are handicapped varies from state to state and even from county to county.

The available community placements are geared to the level of disability of the person and encompass independent living, living in the household of another, foster care, group homes, nursing homes, public medical care facilities, state residential facilities, emergency placement situations, and respite care situations (McGuire and Guernsey, 1978). Respite care is a form of residential placement with which many people are not familiar. It involves temporary 24-hour-a-day care for a person during a period of time when a permanent caretaker is unable to care for her or him. This inability to care for the person may result from caretaker illness, vacation time, or personal or other reasons. Whatever the reason, it is legitimate for the caretaker to request time away from his or her charge. Unfortunately, there are few agencies that provide respite care and it is difficult to obtain. When respite care is offered, it is usually through state residential facilities on a sliding-scale fee assessment. When respite care is offered privately, the fees are frequently prohibitive.

One needs to be sure that the placement selected is appropriate for the person involved. In selecting residential placement for the person who is handicapped, one should carefully evaluate the facility and establish placement objectives for the individual. If the placement objectives, such as amount of personal freedom and educational goals, are not being met, the agencies responsible for licensing and monitoring the facility should be contacted promptly and notified of the deficiencies (McGuire and Guernsey, 1978). These licensing and monitoring agencies will vary from state to state.

In many areas restrictive zoning regulations do not allow the development of group homes for people who are handicapped. Zoning laws have changed in some states to become more liberal in regard to community placement of people who are handicapped (McGuire and Guernsey, 1978). Restrictive zoning policies in the past led to clustering of community residential facilities in areas where zoning policies were not restrictive. These areas were often the less desirable residential areas. The geographic clustering of facilities should be looked at when considering a residential facility (McGuire and Guernsey, 1978). If people who are handicapped are to be integrated into the mainstream of the community, they should not be clustered together in settings apart from the mainstream of the community.

In recent years there has been a major return to the community of people who resided in institutional settings, particularly people who are mentally handicapped. An example of what this has involved is evidenced by the decrease in population of state institutions for the mentally ill and mentally retarded in the state of Michigan. In 1960 the population of these institutions was 30,320 and by 1975 the population was 11,450, a decrease of 62 percent (Mastin, 1976, p. 2). This trend toward decreasing institutional populations and returning people to the community is being seen across the nation. The Michigan Department of Mental Health, in August 1979, made an even greater pledge to return institutionalized people who were mentally retarded to the mainstream of local communities. This has many implications for the community health nurse; a major one is that the nurse will be working in the community with increasing numbers of people who are handicapped and facilitating their use of community services.

Prior to community placement, the adult who is handicapped, his or her family, and the community must be prepared to deal with any needs of the individual who is returning to the community setting. If this preparation is not done, many problems can ensue. If not adequately prepared for community placement, the person will have difficulty adapting to this new situation, will not fit into the mainstream of the community, and will likely be returned to a more restrictive setting.

If the community is not prepared to work with the person who is handicapped, placement often becomes difficult. Many communities have gone to court to prevent, remove, or restrict residences for the handicapped. The community health nurse can do much to help educate the community and its leaders regarding the needs of a person who is hand-

icapped. Actively participating on community advisory boards established to facilitate community placement programs provides many opportunities to influence community leaders and to educate the public.

Families, like the handicapped adult and the community, need assistance in dealing with the deinstitutionalization process. Frequently they need help to reestablish their relationship with their adult offspring, especially if this individual has been institutionalized for several years and they have not had much contact with her or him. Often families must reevaluate all the decisions that were made in relation to the future of an adult who is handicapped. If the handicapped member returns home, the family may again have to decide how to ensure adequate care, as well as deal with increased physical, mental, social, and economic responsibilities. If he or she returns home or to another setting in the community, such as an adult foster care home, the family may have to deal with feelings of guilt and inadequacy in regard to the original placement, concern regarding financial and parental responsibility, and uncertainty as to the appropriateness of the placement. An example of the dilemma that this transition from institution to community can pose with a family is seen with Mrs. Bartel.

Mrs. Bartel, a 75-year-old widow on social security, was being seen by the community health nurse for hypertension. Mrs. Bartel's blood pressure was unusually high on this home visit and she seemed openly troubled. When the nurse asked her if something was upsetting her, she began crying and stated that her 52-year-old son, who was moderately retarded and had been in the local institution for 35 years, was now being considered for community placement in an adult foster care home. She had received a letter inviting her to a case conference to discuss this placement, but she had no way to get there. Mrs. Bartel was worried that her son was not being appropriately placed and that she would be expected to pay for the community placement. With

An Overview of Legislation and Voluntary Efforts for the Handicapped in the United States

1798 U.S. Congress established a marine hospital to provide for disabled seamen (England had established such a facility in 1588).

1902 Goodwill Industries was originated by a minister, Dr. Edgar Helms. Provided employment opportunities for people who were handicapped.

1918 Federal Board of Vocational Rehabilitation was established. Provided vocational rehabilitation services to the disabled veterans of World War I.

1918 Massachusetts became the first state to establish public provisions to aid in the vocational rehabilitation of disabled citizens.

1920 The first Vocational Rehabilitation Act (Public Law 565) was passed. Services under the act were primarily for physically disabled military personnel. This act was administered by the Vocational Rehabilitation Administration.

1935 Social Security Act was passed. It resulted in increased federal appropriations to states for vocational rehabilitation with direct relief provided for the disabled.

1943 Amendments to the Vocational Rehabilitation Act of 1920 broadened vocational rehabilitation services to include facilitating a disabled person to engage in competitive employment and included such services as diagnosis, medical and surgical treatment, prescriptions, hospitalization, books, tools, and occupational equipment.

1943 Baruch Committee on Physical Medicine was established by the son of Dr. Simon Baruch, a confederate army surgeon and pioneer in the field of physical medicine. The committee supported research and scholarship in physical medicine.

1945 Joseph Bulova School of Watchmaking established a training program in watchmaking for people who were handicapped. Forerunner of many companies offering employment and training opportunities to the handicapped.

1947 The Department of Rehabilitation and Physical Medicine was started at New York University College of Medicine at Bellevue Hospital under the direction of Dr. Howard Rusk. The first comprehensive program in rehabilitation at Bellevue was made possible by a grant from the Baruch committee. This department served as a model for the development of rehabilitation centers all over the world.

1953 Establishment of the Department of Health, Education, and Welfare with the Office of Vocational Rehabilitation as a part.

1954 Federal provisions made to support training and education programs for professional rehabilitation personnel in the form of scholarships, stipends, research, and construction grants.

1956 Amendments to the Social Security Act gave benefits to workers and their families during periods of extended disability.

1965 Amendments to the Vocational Rehabilitation Act of 1920 provided for increased flexibility in financing and administrating state rehabilitation programs and for assisting in the expansion and improvement of private services and facilities of rehabilitation, with a state-federal payment sharing plan of 25 to 75 percent. The word *handicapped* was substituted for *physical disability*. The Federal Board of Vocational Education was established.

1965 Medicaid and Medicare established by federal law.

1968 Architectural Barriers Act (Public Law 90-480) passed. The act stated that almost any public building, with the exception of some military facilities, constructed or leased by federal funds must be ac-

---

Mrs. Bartel's permission, the nurse contacted the case conference coordinator and shared her concerns. It was arranged for the nurse on the community placement team to visit with Mrs. Bartel and the community health nurse to discuss the situation.

The nurse visited and explained the process of community placement to Mrs. Bartel. She arranged for her to visit John's tentative foster home so that she could meet the people there. She assured Mrs. Bartel that John's needs would be met and that there would be no charge to her for the placement. The nurse assured Mrs. Bartel that she would be able to visit John, that his placement would be regularly monitored, and that a change in placement would be made if necessary. After visiting the adult foster

cessible to the physically handicapped. The act affected many educational settings and was enforced by the Architectural Barriers Compliance Board. It required that all construction after 1968 using federal funds ensure building accessibility to handicapped persons with no exceptions allowed.

1971 Developmental Disabilities Act (Public Law 91-517) passed. The act stated that each state would receive federal funds to establish and maintain services which are required by developmentally disabled children and adults. These services include diagnosis, evaluation, treatment, personal care, special living arrangements, training, education, sheltered employment, recreation, counseling, protective and sociolegal services, information services, transportation services, and follow-up services.

1971 Urban Mass Transportation Act (Public Law 91-453) passed. The act stated that special efforts would be made in federally funded mass transportation to include utilization by persons who are handicapped.

1973 Rehabilitation Act of 1973 (Public Law 91-453) and amendments of 1974 (Public Law 93-516).

1973 Social Security Act of 1935 amendments eliminated previous categories of Aid to the Blind, Aid to the Aged (Old Age Assistance), and Aid to the Disabled under which direct financial assistance was given to people who were handicapped. Supplemental Security Income was established as of January 1, 1974, under which the aged, blind, and disabled could qualify.

1974 Numerous transportation legislation including the following:

1. Amtrak Improvement Act (Public Law 93-140) stated that the Amtrak corporation must ensure that the handicapped would not be denied transportation because of the handicap on any Amtrak train. Provisions did not apply to commuter and short-haul service.

2. Federal Aid Highway Act (Public Law 93-87) stated that funding could not be approved for any state or federal highway not granting reasonable access for the movement of the physically handicapped across curbs.

3. National Mass Transportation Act (Public Law 93-503) stated that mass transit funds could not be approved unless the rates charged persons who are handicapped were reduced rates from regular fare. Federal Bus Act (Public Law 93-37) stated that all federally funded projects to improve bus transportation must include plans to facilitate usage by people who are handicapped.

1975 Education for All Handicapped Children Act (Public Law 94-142) passed. Enables by September 1, 1980, a free, appropriate public education to all persons aged 3 to 21 years old regardless of handicapping condition involved.

1977 Reorganization of the Department of Health, Education, and Welfare with creation of the Office of Human Development. The Administration for Handicapped Individuals (AHI) is under the Office of Human Development and oversees (1) Rehabilitation Services Administration, (2) President's Committee on Mental Retardation, (3) Architectural and Transportation Barriers Compliance Board, (4) White House Conference on Handicapped Individuals, (5) Developmental Disabilites Office, and (6) Office of Handicapped Individuals.

1977 Federal Aviation Act of 1958 amended (Public Law 95-163) to provide special rates (reduced) on a space-available basis to persons with severe visual or hearing impairments and other physically or mentally handicapped people as defined by the Civil Aeronautics Board, as well as any attendant required by such persons.

---

home, Mrs. Bartel said, "I wish I had had this choice 35 years ago. I would never have placed John in the institution. I know I cannot take care of him, but here it is more like a home. He will have a more normal life and I am happy for him. I will be able to die in peace."

The community health nurse, by utilizing

available resources, was able to help ease this transition for Mrs. Bartel and aid in her adjustment to her son's deinstitutionalization. Concerns like Mrs. Bartel's are not uncommon.

Persons residing in state residential facilities, such as state institutions for people who are mentally retarded or mentally ill, are usually eligible for state funding for community placement as they leave the facility. Persons who reside at home rather than in an institutional setting, often have a difficult time finding funding for necessary services, including residential services, when they are needed. It seems ironic to put caretakers, who had not previously used the state residential system, at a disadvantage for procuring community placement when they are no longer able to care for a family member. Some states are taking concrete action to correct this discrepancy.

The federal government is also providing assistance so that individuals who are handicapped can find adequate housing in the community. The Housing and Urban Development Act of 1965 (Public Law 89-117) provides funds so that the Department of Housing and Urban Development can subsidize rent for individuals who are handicapped and who have an income below a certain level. Also under this act, a group of individuals who are handicapped may be categorized as a family for the purposes of qualifying for low-income family housing.

LEGISLATION

In addition to helping the individual who is handicapped with housing, federal legislation has provided financial assistance for many community services for the handicapped. A historical overview of federal legislation and voluntary efforts in the United States for the person who is handicapped is presented herein. Note particularly how legislation in the last decade has increased.

REHABILITATION

Rehabilitation is defined as the process of restoring an individual to the fullest mental, social, vocational, and economic usefulness possible, with a resultant integration of the individual into society as a full and equal member (Terry, Benz, Mereness, Kleffner, and Jensen, 1961, p. 13; Safilios-Rothschild, 1970, p. 287). It has been described as a bridge spanning the gap between usefulness and uselessness (Terry, Benz, Mereness, Kleffner, and Jensen, 1961, p. 13). The concept of rehabilitation becomes very important when one realizes that medical cure does not exist for most of the chronic handicapping conditions that exist today.

The need for rehabilitation services became increasingly apparent after both world wars. World War II left more than 265,000 American soldiers with combat injuries, including more than 5000 amputees (Krusen, 1964, p.

2; Safilios-Rothschild, 1970, p. 133). The American government and voluntary agencies operating on behalf of these disabled veterans established rehabilitation services for them. Once services were established for veterans, the door was open for their establishment among the general public.

Comprehensive rehabilitation programs combine the use of medical diagnosis and treatment with physical and occupational therapy, and sociological, psychological, and financial counseling and services. These programs offer a multidisciplinary approach that includes physicians, nurses, social workers, psychologists, vocational therapists, physical therapists, and others.

There are a number of established rehabilitation centers and programs across the country. The vocational rehabilitation component of a comprehensive rehabilitation program should not be underestimated for the adult who is handicapped. Vocational rehabilitation has been discussed previously in this chapter under "Education" and should be reviewed at this time by the reader.

Settings for rehabilitation include the home, rehabilitation centers, nursing homes, outpatient rehabilitation facilities, hospitals, and community living facilities. Rehabilitation services are often fragmented, and there is minimal continuity of care. A problem in procuring adequate rehabilitation services is that many medical care facilities are not oriented to a rehabilitation philosophy, but instead stress an acute, temporary-care orientation. It is important that the rehabilitation facility have a staff with a strong philosophy of rehabilitation and have the cooperation and financial assistance for the program from community and other organizations. Rehabilitation is a long-term process and demands a high level of commitment from all involved.

The Rehabilitation Process

The rehabilitation process follows the same steps as the systematic nursing process. It involves data gathering, formation of diagnosis and rehabilitation prognosis, goals, plans, follow-up, and ongoing evaluation. Records are kept and discharge planning is done as the process proceeds. The plan of care developed for the rehabilitation process is done in conjunction with the client, family, and significant others, and has both rehabilitation facility and home care aspects.

Individual motivation is critical to the outcome of the rehabilitation process. The process is facilitated when the client is motivated toward rehabilitation. Motivation is increased if the client believes that rehabilitation will result in increased independence and that the rehabilitation program is realistic. It is important for the nurse to discover and utilize methods that promote belief in the rehabilitation activities.

The individual may have to change his or her whole mode of life, including role orientation, economic support system, and body image, during the rehabilitation process (Terry, Benz, Mereness, Kleffner, and Jensen, 1961, p. 30). The client must also be willing to participate in the demanding process of rehabilitation. The client must make the efforts necessary to improve his or her condition, endure the therapeutic procedures, overcome possible distaste for appliances, and be willing to face the prospect of having to carry out activities independently (Hirschberg, Lewis, and Vaughn, 1976, p. 55).

The problems of the person who is handicapped do not end with rehabilitation. In fact, rehabilitation may often accentuate some of the problems because it will restore the person to a level where it will be necessary to deal with the nonhandicapped population on his or her own. The person often needs help in seeing the value of becoming part of the mainstream of society. This frequently is a difficult task because society is often not able to accept the person who is handicapped, either socially or emotionally, even after successful rehabilitation.

NURSE'S ROLE WITH THE ADULT WHO IS HANDICAPPED

Rehabilitation should be the major focus when one is working with an adult who is handicapped. Rehabilitation nursing services deal with restoring the individual to previous levels of activity and functioning. The nurse is a vital member of the rehabilitation team and must work with the whole client, not just the condition; she or he must stress the client's abilities and encourage the client to start or maintain a treatment regimen (Colorado Department of Public Health, 1966, p. 1).

Community health nurses carry out a variety of functions on a rehabilitation team. They utilize the family-centered nursing process to facilitate decision making and diagnosis during the planning phase of the rehabilitation process. They actively engage in coordination activities so that all community agencies involved in a rehabilitation program for a client provide consistent direction and support. They work directly with clients to enhance their skills and abilities to cope with activities of daily living. They provide support and encouragement for clients and their families so that discouragement does not result in discontinuation of the rehabilitation process.

The community health nurse is often in a key position to help a client accept or initiate a rehabilitation program. She or he frequently encounters clients in the home environment who are unaware of the services available to them in the community setting. In addition, the nurse often sees families during a time of crisis when they have to make decisions regarding how to deal with family situations that have altered as a result of the changing needs of an adult who has become handicapped.

Nurse's Responsibility to the Client in Rehabilitation Nursing

The community health nurse's primary responsibility in rehabilitation is to the client. This responsibility includes the following requirements (Terry, Benz, Mereness, Kleffner, and Jensen, 1961, p. 58; Colorado Department of Public Health, 1966, p. 7):

1. Understanding and accepting the client as a person who has the same physical, emotional, and social needs as other people

2. Understanding the emotional factors in long-term conditions and the effect they

have on the client, his or her family, and society; for example, the influence of emotional factors on the client's motivation for recovery

3. Being aware of the areas of major concern to the client and family

4. Knowing community resources and referring the client and family to community resources as necessary

5. Knowing and applying good nursing care and rehabilitation nursing techniques as determined by the individual rehabilitation needs of the client, for example, skin care, oral hygiene, range of motion exercises, transfer and walking activities, bowel and bladder training, proper body alignment, and positioning and usage of rehabilitation equipment

6. Teaching the client, family, and appropriate others the specific aspects of the rehabilitation program so that the program will progress as rapidly as possible

7. Reinforcing client activities

8 Sharing information regarding the rehabilitation process with the client and family

9. Partaking in the establishment, implementation, evaluation, and follow-up of the individual's rehabilitation program

10. Remembering that through attitudes and actions the nurse can influence the client's attitudes and actions involving his or her condition.

In almost every component of a client's rehabilitation program, the community health nurse is put in a position of teacher and counselor. She or he guides the client, offers support, and advises on care alternatives. In all these situations, the nurse must be aware of the fact that the person who is handicapped is often in need of a variety of services and frequently at a disadvantage to obtain such services. It is often the nurse who helps the client who is handicapped and his or her family to become aware of resources available, to utilize such resources, and to evaluate the effectiveness of the services provided by the resources. Few other health professionals offer as comprehensive and thorough service to people who are handicapped.

Allowing for meaningful expression of feelings that may range from despair and hopelessness to unrealistic optimism is one of the most significant functions of a community health nurse when working with individuals who are handicapped (Safilios-Rothschild, 1970, p. 90). The nurse must be equipped to deal with this range of feelings. It must be recognized by the nurse that she or he may have a variety of personal feelings, both positive and negative, which can inhibit or enhance the ability to function effectively with a client who is handicapped. Community health nurses have frequently found it extremely beneficial to have peer support meetings in which they have the opportunity to examine their feelings in relation to client needs and progress when working with clients who are handicapped.

The client should always be the central person on the rehabilitation team, for it is the client who must assume the primary responsibility in the rehabilitation process. Health care professionals can provide support, guidance, and concrete assistance. They cannot alter the client's behavior on a long-term basis. Only the client can do this.

Nurse's Responsibility to the Rehabilitation Team

The community health nurse plays an important role on the rehabilitation team. As a part of this team, she or he has the responsibility to (Terry, Benz, Mereness, Kleffner, and Jensen, 1961, pp. 57–58):

1. Develop, revise, implement, and evaluate the rehabilitation plan of care with other members of the rehabilitation team, the client, and his or her family

2. Understand the functions and skills of all the members of the rehabilitation team

3. Participate in ongoing exchange of information between team members regarding the rehabilitation program, and work cooperatively with other members of the team

4. Assist in the promotion, stimulation, and coordination of team care

5. Know what resources are available to the client in the community and make appropriate referrals to such resources

6. Recognize that the rehabilitation potential of the individual is dependent on the individual and that rehabilitation team efforts will need to work with this factor

The Nurse, Affirmative Action, and Advocacy for the Person Who Is Handicapped

The nurse is the health professional most familiar with the health care system in its totality, including its gaps and inequities. Sometimes the gaps and inequities in the system can be coped with, but sometimes they need to be challenged.

The person who is handicapped is often at risk in the system. The handicapped person finds it difficult to advocate for herself or himself and fears retaliation if he or she does. It is frequently someone other than the person who is handicapped who is in the best position to advocate for change.

Client advocacy among health professionals is a relatively new phenomenon. Many health professionals hesitate to put themselves in advocacy positions for clients for some of the following reasons:

1. Advocacy is an unfamiliar role. Professionals have generally not been trained to be

advocates and are not used to undertaking such a role. The person assuming an advocacy role is not conforming to the established system and may be pressured to conform. The advocate may find advocacy difficult, awkward, and uncomfortable.

2. Fear of reprisal. There are many ways that an individual can be punished for advocacy actions. Often the greater the impact of the advocacy action, the greater the risk of reprisal. The advocate must be aware of the possibility of reprisal and must decide the possible outcomes of his or her behavior.

3. The symbiotic snarl. It can be difficult for the professional to remain separate from the professional role and place himself or herself in the role of advocate, especially if the advocate role is in conflict with the professional one. It is difficult to take stands contrary to the stand of other professionals in the field or contrary to the organization for which one works.

4. Apathy, or the old "why bother" approach. If one is not personally and directly affected, why deal with the situation at all? The status quo is okay; let time be the deciding factor. The "let them help themselves" philosophy is evidenced here.

5. Lack of support. If one finds oneself standing alone, or almost alone, it is often difficult to take a firm stand on any position. If one lacks the support of significant others, the stand also becomes difficult.

6. Change implications. Professionals realize the implications of changing a situation. To encourage change, to take a stand, is often to encourage stress. Are we willing to give up a system, possibly a stable one, to invoke an unstable one?

Health professionals and the organizations they represent have many frequently used excuses for not advocating on behalf of the client in addition to the ones listed. Excuses such as not enough time, not enough money, no one to help, not wanting to get involved on an emotional level, and the system not being ready for such a change all enter in. It is relatively easy to show empathy with these excuses as most of us have probably used them at one time or another. Taking or not taking an advocacy stand often boils down to one common denominator—one's philosophy in life. If one believes that all people are equal, and as such desire equal rights and treatment, the question of advocating or not advocating becomes almost secondary whenever one sees an individual's rights being violated or ignored.

One should not underestimate the impact that a nurse can have on the system as an advocate. As has been mentioned previously, the nurse is usually familiar with the gaps in the system and also with how the system works. A recent example of this was the case of a nurse working with a local association of parents of retarded children. The parents were increasingly aware of instances of suspected abuse to their children in the institutional setting in which they resided. The parents had talked with the institution administration and felt they were not receiving adequate information; some of the parents felt intimidated. The parents were concerned about the implications of their actions on their institutionalized children. If they continued to press for information, they were worried about reprisals. If they did not press for information, they were worried that the situation would get worse. A nurse who was a member of the association was able to take action because she did not fear reprisal and she had the support of the parent group.

The nurse met with the parents and the institution administration. Upon assessing that the administration was resistant to change, the nurse examined the laws existing in the state regarding child abuse. One section of the law clearly stated that an institution must be independently investigated when there were suspected cases of child abuse or neglect. By obtaining legal counsel, and working with the established grievance procedure for state mental health clients, the community health nurse was able to help incur change in the system. The state now has impartial investigations of all cases of child abuse in state institutions, and parents or guardians have access to the results.

The advocacy efforts of this community health nurse had many positive effects. Reporting procedures for institutional cases of suspected abuse and neglect have been clearly written and implemented in this state. The state legislature recently appropriated a large sum of money to be used in further protection and advocacy services for people who are developmentally disabled. In addition, the general public has become increasingly aware of the needs of people who are mentally handicapped.

Nurses are in a position to correct public misconceptions about people who are handicapped. They can work with people to gain greater acceptance of individuals who are handicapped in whatever setting they reside. The nurse can be instrumental in promoting a positive attitude toward the handicapped by the general public.

SUMMARY

The adult who is handicapped is confronted with the same developmental tasks as the normal adult. Societal, individual, and family attitudes and variables, however, often make it more difficult for an adult who is handicapped to work toward and accomplish developmental tasks. Comprehensive rehabilitation services which involve the client and the client's family and significant others can help adults who are handicapped to achieve a meaningful life in our society.

The community health nurse is frequently in a key position to assist clients who are handicapped to obtain services that will enhance their abilities to handle activities of daily living. A sensitivity to the needs of this population group and an awareness that there are individual differences among clients who are handicapped are essential if the community health nurse is going to function effectively with clients who have special needs.

Increasingly, health care professionals are recognizing the value of advocacy in obtaining essential services for clients in the community health setting. Legislation in the last decade reflects a more positive attitude toward individuals who are handicapped.

REFERENCES

Bower, F. L. (Ed.). *Distortions in body image in illness and disability.* New York: Wiley, 1977.

Buscaglia, L. F. (Ed.). *The disabled and their parents: A counseling challenge.* Thorofare, N.J.: C. B. Slack, 1975.

Colorado State Department of Public Health. *Elementary rehabilitation nursing care.* Washington,

D.C.: U.S. Government Printing Office, 1966.

Dixon, J. K. Coping with prejudice: Attitudes of handicapped persons toward the handicapped. *Journal of Chronic Diseases,* May 1977, *30,* 307–321.

Goldberg, R. T. Rehabilitation research on disability: New horizons. *Journal of Rehabilitation,* July–August 1977, *43,* 14–18.

Hirschberg, G. G., Lewis, L., & Vaughan, P. *Rehabilitation* (2d ed.). Philadelphia: Lippincott, 1976.

Krusen, F. H. *Concepts in rehabilitation of the handicapped.* Philadelphia: Saunders, 1964.

Mastin, P. (Chairperson). *Final report of the joint legislative committee to study community placement in Michigan.* Lansing, Mich.: State of Michigan, 1976.

McGuire, S. L., & Guernsey, C. *Residential placement opportunities in Michigan for people who are mentally retarded.* Lansing, Mich.: Michigan Association for Retarded Citizens, 1978.

Park, L. The law says. . . . *Disabled U.S.A.,* 1977, *1*(4), 11–13.

Posner, B. Less than equal. *Disabled U.S.A.,* 1978, *1*(5), 14–15.

President's Committee on Employment of the Handicapped. *Affirmative action to employ handicapped people.* Washington, D.C.: U.S. Government Printing Office, 1978.

President's Committee on Employment of the Handicapped. *Careers for the homebound.* Washington, D.C.: U.S. Government Printing Office, 1978.

President's Committee on Employment of the Handicapped. *A handbook on the legal rights of handicapped people.* Washington, D.C.: U.S. Government Printing Office, 1976.

Rosow, J. M. Disadvantaged people and the changing market place. *Journal of Rehabilitation,* March–April 1976, *42,* 28–31.

Safilios-Rothschild, C. *The sociology and social psychology of disability rehabilitation.* New York: Random House, 1970.

Social Security Administration. *Work disability in the United States.* Washington, D.C.: U.S. Government Printing Office, 1977.

Sussman, M. B. (Ed.). *Sociology and rehabilitation.* Washington, D.C.: American Sociological Association, 1966.

Terry, F. J., Benz, G. S., Mereness, D., Kleffner, F. R., & Jensen, D. M. *Principles and techniques of rehabilitation nursing* (2d ed.). St. Louis: Mosby, 1961.

U.S. Department of Health, Education, and Welfare. *Key federal regulations affecting the handicapped 1975–76.* Washington, D.C.: U.S. Government Printing Office, 1977.

U.S. Department of Health, Education, and Welfare. *Work disability in the U.S.* Washington, D.C.: U.S. Government Printing Office, 1977.

U.S. Department of Health, Education, and Welfare. *Your rights as a disabled person.* Washington, D.C.: U.S. Government Printing Office, 1978.

Vargo, J. W. Some psychological effects of physical disability. *American Journal of Occupational Therapy,* January 1978, *32,* 31–34.

SELECTED BIBLIOGRAPHY

Ballard, J., & Zettel, J. Public law 94-142 and section 504: What they say about rights and protections. *Exceptional Children,* February 1977, *44,* 177–184.

Bower, F. L. (Ed.). *Distortions in body image in illness and disability.* New York: Wiley, 1977.

Campbell, J. Reorganization at HEW. *Disabled U.S.A.,* 1977, *1*(4), 6.

Clements, H. R. NISH finds its niche. *Journal of Rehabilitation,* May–June 1977, *43,* 16–24.

Cull, J. G., & Hardy, R. E. *Rehabilitation facility approaches in severe disabilities.* Springfield, Ill.: Charles C Thomas, 1975.

Epstein, R. L., & Lawrence, A. M. First questions on the HEW handicap regulations. *Hospitals,* October 1977, *51,* 57–60.

Goldin, G., Perry, S. L., Margolin, R. J., & Stotsky, B. A. *Dependency and its implications for rehabilitation.* Lexington, Mass.: Lexington Books, 1972.

Horton, M., & Schechter, D. Tax incentives for business-women and men. *Disabled U.S.A.,* 1978, *1*(7), 13.

Maloney, S. Section 503 conference . . . A new day for handicapped people. *Journal of Rehabilitation,* May–June 1976, *42,* 14–15.

Mayo, W. J. Contributions of pure science to progressive medicine. *Journal of the American Medical Association*, May 1925, *84,* 1465.

Moersch, M. S. Developmental disabilities. *American Journal of Occupational Therapy*, February 1978, *32,* 93–99.

Myers, J. S. (Ed.). *An orientation to chronic disease and disability.* New York: Macmillan, 1965.

National Health Education Committee. *The killers and cripplers.* New York: McKay, 1976.

Remarks of Joseph Califano, Jr. (Secretary of Health, Education, and Welfare), before the NRA National Conference, Washington, D.C., September 10, 1977. *Journal of Rehabilitation*, November–December 1977, *43,* 31–33.

Rubin, S. E. A national rehabilitation program evaluation and training effort: Some results and implications. *Journal of Rehabilitation*, May–June 1977, *43,* 28–31.

Rusk, H. A., & Taylor, E. J. *Living with a disability.* Garden City, N. Y.: McGraw-Hill, 1953.

Spellane, B. F. Look who's enforcing section 503: Simple modification can make the difference. *Disabled U.S.A.*, 1978, *1*(7), 4–6.

Strauss, A. L. *Chronic illness and the quality of life.* St. Louis: Mosby, 1975.

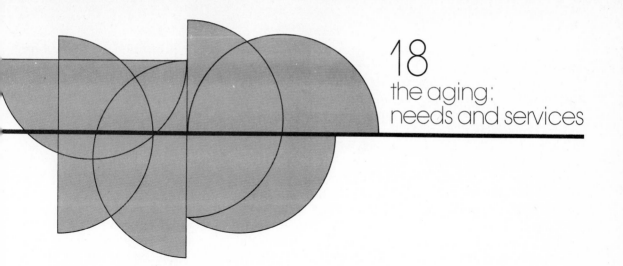

Meet Will and Ariel Durant: he is 92 years old and she is 75. They have spent a lifetime studying and writing about people and events as historians and philosophers. Together they wrote the 11-volume *Story of Civilization,* and one of the volumes, *Rousseau and Revolution,* was published when he was 82 and she was 65. It won them the Pulitzer Prize. Their *Age of Napoleon* came out the week of Mr. Durant's ninetieth birthday. In his ninety-first year and her seventy-fourth, they published their *Dual Autobiography.* At the age of 92 Mr. Durant says that "he feels his disintegration every day. He accepts it as natural and desirable. Death is the greatest invention that life ever made. It allows new life to have room to operate" (Proctor, 1978, p. 12).

The description of the Durants' attitudes toward life and its approaching end are in direct contrast to the concept of acute loneliness and unproductiveness in old age held by many people of all ages. One can't help but wonder why some people are old and weary at 65 and others, like Will and Ariel Durant, are vigorous and productive long after age 65. Examining some concepts of aging sheds light on this question and helps us to better prepare ourselves for this part of our own life cycle, as well as to better care for aging clients.

AGING DEFINED

The aging process is a series of complex changes that occur in all living organisms. It is a process that continues over a lifetime at different rates among people. The rate varies among populations and among individuals of the same population. It also varies within individuals, since different body systems do not age at the same rate.

The term *aged* is often used to describe persons who have achieved a certain chronological age in a given population. The reasons for using age 65 to designate the beginning of old age in the United States are basically legislative and social. In some poorer nations of the world, a person 40 years old is considered aged.

Older people are as varied as people in any other age group, and caution must be used when they are discussed as a group. Myths and stereotypes result from the habit of expecting people to act in certain ways simply because they have reached a specific chronological age. They are then expected to act more or less alike: "People about 70 usually like to move to retirement homes." This is a stereotype that research refutes!

Aging is a very gradual process. People generally learn that they are "old" through the way people treat them. In the youth-oriented and productive culture of the United States, we tend to expect very little of older people. Mandatory retirement at age 65 or 70, for instance, does not take into consideration the performance and creativity of people beyond this point.

Vigorous! Active! Attractive! Independent! These words for many people describe a person of 20 or 30 or 40 but hardly one 60 or 70. The American view of aging does not allow us to automatically associate such positive words with this time of life. The advantages of youth are constantly emphasized through our entire societal structure, so that Americans invest money and energy in staying young as long as possible.

Ultimately our professional nursing care, our social interactions, our personal decisions, and our decisions as citizens are affected by this viewpoint. The course of our own aging is influenced by our attitudes, for people are likely to age in a manner that fulfills their expectations.

This pessimistic view of aging is serious because Americans are living longer today than ever before. Mortality rates among the elderly have been declining during the past several years and even without further reductions in mortality, persons currently reaching their sixty-fifth birthday will, on the average, live 16 more years (*Health, United States*, 1977, p. 3). In 1900 there were 3.1 million people 65 years and over in the United States. By 1975 there were 22.4 million elderly people. Population projections estimate 31.8 million elderly people by the year 2000 and 55.0 million by 2030. Since mortality rates are declining at all ages, the number of people surviving into old age could be even greater than these estimates (*Health, U.S.*, 1977, p. 4). The economic and social implications for society are great because there are increasing numbers of aging people for whom to care.

OTHER PERSPECTIVES ON AGING

Because the negative view of aging is so pervasive and because the numbers of aging persons are growing, health professionals including gerontologists, behavioral scientists, and biologists are seeking new concepts of aging. There *are* positive roles for aging people and recognition needs to be given to the positive as well as the negative aspects of this period of life. Productiveness like the Durants' should become the usual rather than the unusual.

Biological View

It is the biological aspect of aging that has fostered our culture's negative feelings about ag-

ing. Gray hair, wrinkles, stooping, pigmented skin, forgetfulness, and deafness are all visible signs and point to a physical deterioration of the body. Sensory loss occurs, responding to ideas and instructions takes longer, social relationships are less intense, and the time of growth, reproduction, and active work are past. There is no urgent reason for accomplishing one task rather than another.

However, what about aging people like Will and Ariel Durant? Are we justified in saying that physical deterioration brings concomitant mental deterioration? Or have our cultural views on aging turned this state of life into a deteriorating process?

Other Cultures' Views of Aging

History, anthropology, and art imply that aging has not always been equated with deterioration. "The notion that aging is an irreversible biological process which leads to negative mental and social consequences is a relatively new idea in history" (Manney, 1975, p. 8).

The Chinese philosopher Confucius, speaking to his followers about aging, said, "At fifteen my mind was bent on learning. At thirty, I stood firm. At forty I was free from delusions. At fifty, I understood the laws of Providence. At sixty, my ears were attentive to the truth. At seventy, I could follow the promptings of my heart without overstepping the moon."

Other cultures have said that aging leads to deterioration or growth, depending upon a person's inner resources, dedication, strengths, attitudes toward aging, and some luck. This period of life can give a person insight, knowledge, and freedom if it is seen as a manageable process with developmental tasks that need to be accomplished (Figure 18-1).

Developmental Tasks of Aging

Duvall (1977, p. 390) discusses eight developmental tasks of aging persons:

1. Finding adequate housing in their own home, apartment, retirement community, or with children

2. Adapting to retirement-level income, often a sharp decline

3. Organizing enjoyable daily routines which may involve having a spouse home all day for the first time

4. Protecting physical and emotional health at a time when physical energy is declining

5. Continuing enjoyable marital and sexual relationships which can continue and even increase in enjoyment

6. Providing for relationships with family members such as children and grandchildren

7. Remaining active in community activities when it is physically and financially possible

8. Feeling a sense of worth as a person, of which independence is a valuable part

Three Concepts Basic to a Positive Philosophy of Aging

Manney has presented three concepts about aging that are important to understand if care givers are to develop a positive philosophy about aging.

1. Aging has no chronological rules. The notion of "older" people is a demographic one because no matter how we look at it, aging varies in its onset and course.

2. The processes of aging are interrelated. Society's attitudes toward older people and the roles it assigns them affect intellectual per-

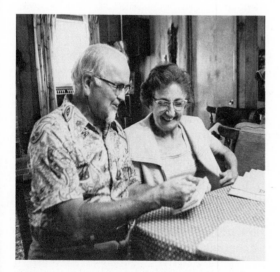

FIGURE 18-1 A healthy, happy aging couple.

formance, motivation, and interest in learning. Mandatory retirement typically cuts an individual's income in half. This affects the person's ability to obtain health care, to eat well, and to visit friends and family, as well as to maintain adequate housing.

3. Aging is a developmental process. Old age cannot be studied apart from middle age, adulthood, adolescence, childhood, and infancy. At each stage there are losses and gains. The gains and losses of old age do not arise immediately at age 65 and they do not stay the same until death. Aging is a part of the life cycle, which is constantly changing.

DEMOGRAPHY OF AGING PERSONS

A knowledge of the numbers and location of persons 65 and over is helpful in planning for their health needs. As was indicated earlier in this chapter, their numbers are very large and growing.

Within the age group 65 years and over, those 65 to 74 are getting fewer in number while the group 75 years and over is getting larger. By the year 2000 it is expected that 45 percent of the population 65 years and over will be 75 years and over (*Health, U.S.,* 1977, p. 4). The percentage of persons who are over 75 is important in evaluating health status and estimating needs for care because the prevalence of chronic disease and impairments, as well as the utilization of medical services which increase with age, increases more rapidly beginning about the age of 75.

The ratio of men to women is very low in the elderly population because death rates for men at every age are higher than for women. Among people 65 years and over, there are 69 men per 100 women. At age 85 there are only 48 men per 100 women.

In the 1970 census, 5 percent of those 65 and over were residents of institutions by age 85. However, at any given time the vast majority (95 percent) of the elderly are not in institutions. Most remain in their homes. In the past decade the proportion of elderly maintaining their own household has increased and those classified as living with relatives has decreased. In 1975, among U.S. citizens over 65, 21.3 million elderly were not in institutions, 5.8 million lived alone, 11.4 million were married, and 4.1 million lived with relatives or nonrelatives. Seventy-seven percent of the men were married with their wives present and 38 percent of the women were married with their husbands present. Widowhood was the status of 51 percent of the women.

Those 65 years and over face financial problems. In 1974 men 65 years and over had a median income of $4500. This was nearly double the $2400 median income of women the same age. Social security benefits were the main source of income for most elderly people who lived alone.

And, finally, older people like younger ones are likely to be living in a metropolitan area. Only 21 percent of those over 65 live in counties that have an urban population of fewer than 20,000 people.

Aging, world wide. The increase of aging persons in the United States has accompanied the increase world-wide. With advances in medicine and the decrease in the birth and death rates, this trend is expected to continue (United Nations, 1975, p. 16).

As Table 18-1 shows, there were about 291 million persons 60 years of age and over in 1970, world-wide. This will increase to about 585 million by the year 2000—an increase of over 100 percent. The world's population will enlarge by about 80 percent in that time.

TABLE 18-1   World Population 60 Years and Over: Estimates for 1970 and Projections for 1985 and 2000 by Major Regions

Regional	Year	Total population	Population 60 years and over	
			Number	*Percentage of total population*
World total	1970	3,631,797,000	290,697,000	8.0
	1985	4,933,463,000	406,750,000	8.2
	2000	6,493,642,000	584,605,000	9.0
More-developed regions	1970	1,090,297,000	153,741,000	14.1
	1985	1,274,995,000	188,602,000	14.8
	2000	1,453,528,000	231,105,000	15.9
Less-developed regions	1970	2,541,501,000	137,024,000	5.4
	1985	3,658,468,000	218,474,000	6.0
	2000	5,040,114,000	353,917,000	7.0

SOURCE: United Nations Department of Economics and Social Affairs. *The aging: Trends and policies.* New York: United Nations Publication, 1975, p. 17.

COMMON HEALTH PROBLEMS

It is important to remember that aging by itself does not mean illness. People who are 80 often are healthier than those who are 70 because only the healthiest will live that long. However, aging does mean increased risks of sickness, disability, widowhood, isolation, financial stress, and not being valued in our society; and, of course it means that death is near.

Mortality rates, the oldest and most available measure of health, have declined considerably for older people. From 1950 to 1975 the death rates for persons over 65 decreased by 13 percent. Most of this decline has been recent with 11 percent of the decrease having occurred after 1965.

Table 18-2 shows the death rates for the 10 leading causes of death among persons 65 and over. There have been declines in two of the three leading causes of death, heart disease and cerebrovascular accidents. The death rates for cancer have been rising.

As is shown in Table 18-2, the leading cause of death among the elderly is heart disease. It is responsible for 44 percent of the deaths of people over 65. Malignant neoplasms are the cause of another 18 percent of deaths. The third leading cause is cerebrovascular disease, which accounts for 13 percent of the deaths. Together, these three diseases make up the cause of death for 75 percent of all people over 65 (*Health, U.S.,* 1977, p. 8).

Other major pathologic conditions besides cancer, heart disease, and stroke seen in elderly persons are Parkinson's disease, osteoarthritis, rheumatoid arthritis, and diabetes. All of these conditions are chronic and require skilled nursing interventions to avoid concomitant problems such as immobility, dependence, and resulting custodial care.

A high prevalence of chronic conditions does not necessarily mean a high prevalence of disabling conditions. About 47 percent of noninstitutionalized elderly people in 1975 were limited in activity due to chronic conditions, but these limitations varied tremendously. Two chronic conditions caused half of

TABLE 18-2 Death Rates for the 10 Leading Causes of Death among Persons 65 Years and Over, by 1975 Rank Order for Both Sexes and for Each Sex Individually: United States, 1950, 1965, and 1975*

| | | | | Deaths per million resident population 65 years and over | | |
| | | | | | 1975 | |
Cause of death	ICDA code	1950	1965	Both sexes	Male	Female
All causes		6270.3	6118.3	5432.4	6702.7	4550.9
Diseases of heart	390–398, 402, 404, 410–429	2860.9	2823.9	2403.9	2933.0	2036.7
Malignant neoplasms	140–209	865.5	901.4	961.1	1301.1	725.2
Cerebrovascular diseases	430–438	923.8	901.0	729.7	740.5	722.1
Influenza and pneumonia	470–474, 480–486	191.3	213.7	187.1	239.2	150.9
Arteriosclerosis	440	....	....	123.0	119.8	125.2
Diabetes mellitus	250	121.1	122.9	112.9	102.8	119.9
Accidents	E800–E949	210.8	155.0	109.6	140.6	88.1
Motor vehicle accidents	E810–E823	43.1	38.9	25.3	38.7	16.0
All other accidents	E800–E807, E825–E949	167.7	116.1	84.3	101.9	72.1
Bronchitis, emphysema, and asthma	490–493	....	....	80.5	152.5	30.5
Cirrhosis of liver	571	34.9	34.5	36.6	58.1	21.6
Nephritis and nephrosis	580–584	....	....	23.2		
Suicide	E950–E959	30.0	22.8	....	36.8	
Hernia and intestinal obstruction	550–553, 560	37.6	35.6	....	....	20.5
All other causes		....	....	664.9	878.4	510.1

*Data are based on the National Vital Registration System.

NOTE: Cause of death titles and numbers are based on the Eighth Revision International Classification of Diseases, adapted for use in the United States. Because of decennial revisions in the classification and changes in rules of cause-of-death coding, there is lack of comparability for some causes from one revision to the next. In some instances data are omitted for earlier years because the appropriate subcategories are not available. Data for influenza and pneumonia should not be interpreted for trends since they are influenced by epidemics which cause large fluctuations in data for a single year.

SOURCES: Adapted from National Center for Health Statistics. *Vital statistics of the United States,* Washington, D.C.: U.S. Government Printing Office, Vol. II, for data years 1950 and 1965; data for 1975, Rockville, Md.: Health Resources Administration, Department of Health, Education, and Welfare, to be published.

the 47 percent limitations referred to above: heart disease and rheumatism (*Health,* U.S., 1977, p. 11).

Problems with communication often complicate work with elderly clients.

Mr. Mendoza was a client 83 years of age who had a permanent tracheostomy as a result of cancer of the larynx. He was almost completely deaf. His wife, also 83, was blind, and before his surgery had depended greatly upon her husband. They were active, independent people who cared for their home alone. The Mendozas were childless and had lost most of their friends by death. The weeks after the surgery were extremely difficult for them. Skilled intervention by the community health nurse helped them to find ways to remain independent. Referrals to community resources, where they were able to obtain an artificial plastic larynx and speech therapy to use it, were especially beneficial.

Mental disorders such as acute (reversible) and organic brain syndrome, depression, paranoia, and schizophrenia can be seen in working with the elderly. The myth that "aging equals mental deterioration" as well as the complex relationship between physiological and psychiatric elements make this a complex subject. Burnside (1976) has done a beautiful job of describing the differences among these conditions as well as the nursing care involved.

The end of aging, of course, is death, and both nurses and the aged must come to terms with this fact. Kübler-Ross's (1969) five stages of grief are well known, and knowledge of them provides a structure for the nurse to guide and support clients and involved families. Aging people see loss continually. It is a theme that is constantly with them.

In America we tend to ignore death. We place a high value on progress, growth, youth, and physical strength, and we often give little meaning to old age and death. The nurse's capacity to give care depends on the personal feelings of the nurse about death, the nurse's educational preparation, and the support he or she receives for nursing care.

Problems among the Aging as Seen by the Residents of One State

In 1974, 3000 of Michigan's noninstitutionalized citizens aged 60 and over were interviewed to determine their perceived problems and needs. The major categories examined were neighborhood characteristics, housing, transportation, nutrition, health, social supports, employment, retirement, earnings and expenditures, government services, consumer protection, general problems, and demographic characteristics.

Table 18-3 is a summary of the top 11 problems that were found among the persons surveyed. The respondents as a whole believed that income, crime, health care, transporta-

TABLE 18-3   Concerns Which 3000 Michigan Residents over 60 Believe Face Older Americans

Concerns	Percent of entire sample concerned
Income	38
Crime	31
Health care	24
Transportation	21
Nutrition and food	15
Consumer protection	
Spare time activities	11–12
Housing	
Employment opportunities	
Age discrimination	8
Getting more education	5

SOURCE: From *The Michigan comprehensive plan on aging.* Office of Services to the Aging, Policy and Program Analysis Division. Lansing, Mich. 1974, p. xix.

tion, and nutrition were the top concerns for aging persons in Michigan. Difficulty with services and businesses misleading consumers, spare-time activities, and housing composed the second major area of concern.

Old age does bring health problems. But as nurses, we need to look for the wellness of old age rather than becoming immersed in its pathology. Weissman (1974, p. 93) wrote, "Does old age make sense? Not if we insist upon seeing it as total calamity, decrepit and demented. But if growing older is a destiny, then we become what makes sense, and nothing else, and we are what makes sense, nothing else."

HEALTH PROMOTION NEEDS

The high prevalence of chronic conditions, impairment, and limitation of activity among aging people often leaves those younger with the impression that elderly people view themselves as being in poor health.

Good health does not necessarily mean that there is no disease present. It does mean that if there are disease conditions, they do not significantly interfere with an individual's functioning. In predicting behavior, the individual's definition of health may be as important as the actual health status.

Table 18-4 shows that many elderly people feel they are in good health. Two-thirds of noninstitutionalized people rated their health as good or excellent in 1975 (*Health, U.S., 1977*, p. 12). People who do rate their health as poor tend to have more activity-limiting chronic conditions and more frequent acute conditions than others.

Normal Changes of Aging

Aging does bring normal body changes that need to be accommodated. Listed in Table 18-5 are major physical changes along with the implications for these changes. Elderly people as well as nurses caring for elderly people must take these changes into account if a client's health potential is to be maximized. For instance, smooth muscle weakness and muscle atrophy causing constipation are part of aging, to be sure, at differing rates for different persons. Diet can be changed to accommodate the constipation that may result so that the client does not need to use laxatives. Fluids and bran products are helpful suggestions. Another change that comes with aging is thinning of the vaginal walls in women and atrophy of the testes in men. The results are not asexual aging people but persons who have sexual experiences different from earlier years. Sexual needs continue throughout life and the aging need information, counseling, and encouragement to fulfill these needs. Community health

TABLE 18-4 Percent Distribution of Assessment of Health Status as Reported in Health Interviews for Persons 65 Years and Over, According to Selected Demographic Characteristics: United States, 1975

Demographic characteristic	All health statuses*	*Health status, percent distribution*		
		Excellent	Good	Fair	Poor
Total	100.0	28.6	40.3	21.5	8.6
SEX AND AGE					
Male	100.0	28.1	40.0	21.4	9.4
65–74 years	100.0	28.5	39.8	21.5	9.3
75 years and over	100.0	27.5	40.3	21.3	9.8
Female	100.0	28.9	40.6	21.6	8.0
65–74	100.0	29.2	41.4	21.5	7.2
75 years and over	100.0	28.6	39.3	21.8	9.4
COLOR					
White	100.0	29.4	40.8	21.0	7.8
All other	100.0	20.6	35.5	26.7	16.3
REGION					
Northeast	100.0	27.3	44.4	21.2	6.2
North Central	100.0	27.1	43.2	21.6	7.1
South	100.0	27.6	35.4	23.5	12.4
West	100.0	35.3	38.4	18.0	7.5
RESIDENCE					
Metropolitan	100.0	30.6	40.5	20.1	7.8
Nonmetropolitan	100.0	24.4	40.0	24.7	10.3
FAMILY INCOME†					
Less than $5000	100.0	23.3	38.7	24.9	12.2
$5000–$9999	100.0	29.8	41.3	21.4	6.8
$10,000–$14,999	100.0	31.6	42.7	19.9	5.1
$15,000 or more	100.0	38.7	40.3	13.9	5.8

*Includes unknown health status.

†Excludes unknown family income.

SOURCE: National Center for Health Statistics, Division of Health Interview Statistics. In *Health, United States, 1976–1977*. DHEW Publication No. HRA 77–1232. Washington, D.C.: U.S. Government Printing Office, 1977, p. 12.

nurses are in a unique position to provide this counseling: there is literature available to help professionals with this task (Stanford, 1973; Weg, 1976).

Finch (1976) has written about the changes that come with aging and has compared those that are the result of aging and those that are secondary to disease. The latter are reversible changes. The concept is exciting because if aging is not necessarily a deteriorating process, a great deal of rehabilitation can be accomplished among aging people. For example, it is often taken for granted that aging people lose intellectual function as well as the ability to remember past events. Studies have demonstrated that those most prone to these problems are persons with high blood pressure and other vascular diseases (Finch, 1976, p. 92). Loss of memory is *not* synonymous with aging.

Most of the deaths among elderly people result from disease conditions which have existed for many years or from personal habits or environmental factors that likewise have existed for many years (*Health, U.S.*, 1977, p. 9). Preventing such deaths must start early in life. Coronary heart disease may be altered with a program of exercise, proper diet, absence of smoking, and protection from stress. People, beginning when they are young, must realize that they have a responsibility for their own health which goes beyond medical care.

The community health nurse, when working with well adults in occupational and clinical settings and in the home environment, is in a key position to help youth to see the value of taking responsibility for maintaining their health. She or he can help youth to recognize the long-term detrimental consequences of poor health habits and can assist them in establishing a preventive health maintenance program that will decrease their risks for future health problems.

Belloc (1973) found a significant relationship between life expectancy and the following seven health practices: no smoking of cigarettes, 7 hours of sleep nightly, eating breakfast daily, keeping one's weight down, no or moderate alcohol intake, daily exercise, and no eating between meals. These are all habits over which individuals have control but they need to be begun before the age of 65 to be truly effective.

Safety

Accidents, one of the top 10 causes of death among elderly people, can be decreased at any age by modifying living conditions. Falls are the leading problem in this category, followed by motor vehicle accidents and fires. Inhalation of food with subsequent obstruction, poisoning, and drowning also kill a very small number of elderly people. Accident rates are higher among those who are limited in their activities. Also, most accidents occur at home.

Safety precautions for the home environment that need assessing are proper lighting and handrails, especially on stairs; elimination of cords, slippery rugs, and linoleum; a method of obtaining help quickly in emergencies; avoidance of sedation other than for sleeping after other alternatives have been explored; distinct labeling on medications; and frequent reevaluation of the older person's ability to drive motor vehicles.

The contributing factors to accidents are physiological as well as environmental. Slowed reaction time, uncertain gait, and changes in hearing and vision are examples of physiological factors.

"An attitude conveying safety as an area in which the older adult can exert some control and live sensibly will reinforce a sense of responsibility" (Combs, 1978, p. 1341).

Nutrition

Loss of teeth, dryness of the mouth, decreased activity of the senses, decreased efficiency of the digestive and excretory system, reduced

TABLE 18-5 Physical Changes with Age

Change	*Implications*
SKELETAL SYSTEM	
1. Calcification of vertebral ligaments	1. Postural change
2. Fibrocartilaginous atrophy; muscle atrophy	2. Loss of muscle power; contractures; paralysis; decreased respiration efficiency
3. Osteoporotic bone change	3. Diminished weight bearing; spontaneous fractures
4. Ossification of joint cartilage	4. Joint stiffness; ankylosis
GASTROINTESTINAL SYSTEM	
1. Atrophy of mucosal linings; diminished production of hydrochloric acid (achlorhydria)	1. Delayed gastric emptying; decreased secretion of enzymes; impaired absorption; diminished food appeal
2. Smooth muscle weakness; muscle atrophy	2. Decreased excretory efficiency; incontinence; constipation; diminished peristalsis
RESPIRATORY SYSTEM	
1. Increase in residual lung volume	1. Distressed breathing; fear, anxiety; CO_2 retention; limited mobility
2. Muscle atrophy	2. Impaired ventilation, reduced ability to cough or deep breathe
3. Thickened membranes, alveoli, and capillaries	3. Impaired diffusion of O_2; diminished lung resiliency; impaired circulation
NERVOUS SYSTEM	
1. Atrophy of brain surface and brain cells	1. Behavioral changes: diminished emotions; disrupted self-image; less adaptability; confusion; disorientation; narrowing of interests
2. Atrophy of tendon reflexes	2. Stimuli-response change
3. Spinal cord synapse degeneration	3. Diminished overall coordination of neuromuscular, circulatory, glandular systems; increased susceptibility to shock
GENITOURINARY SYSTEM	
1. Muscle weakness; muscle atrophy	1. Retention; guilt or embarrassment; incontinence
2. Kidney: reduced filtration; reduced blood flow; atrophy of glomeruli, tubules, nephrons; interstitial fibrosis	2. Urine retention; infection; pain, fear, anxiety; urinary stones; polyuria; nocturia; diminished excretion of toxic substances; diminished bladder capacity
3. Increased bladder-urethra infection	3. Urinary stasis

SOURCES: Linda Davis, Institute of Gerontology, as Consultant to Relocation Preparation Program, Pennsylvania Department of Public Welfare. References utilized: I. Rossman. Human aging changes. In I. M. Burnside (Ed.), *Nursing and the aged.* New York: McGraw-Hill, 1976; D. C. Kimmel. Biological and intellectual aspects of aging. In *Adulthood and aging.* New York: Wiley, 1974, chap. 8, pp. 369–376; M. Jennings, M. Nordstorm, & N. Shumake. Physiologic functioning in the elderly. *Nursing Clinics of North America,* June 1972, 7, 237–246;

TABLE 18-5 Physical Changes with Age (*Continued*)

Change	Implications
4. In females, atrophy of ovarian, uterine, vaginal tissues; thinning of vaginal walls	4. Decreased lubrication; loss of fertility; need for increase in stimulation time
5. In males, diminished spermatogenesis; decreased number of sperm; atrophy of testes; enlargement of prostate	5. Increased time for erection; reduced intensity of sensation; reduced volume and viscosity of seminal fluid; reduced force of ejaculation

NUTRITION AND METABOLISM

1. Vitamin deficiencies: lack of vitamin B, inflammation of mucous membranes of the mouth; lack of vitamins C and K, capillary fragility	1. Discomfort; decreased food appeal; multiple bruises; disturbed self-image; fear, anxiety
2. Metabolic rate decrease—estimated at 1 percent per year after 25	2. Changes in nutrition, drug reaction, hypothermia
3. Depletion of water	3. Increased stress in excretion; constipation
4. Increased proportion of body fat	4. Less muscle mass, weakness; storage of nutrients in body fat
5. Mineral intake deficiency	5. Malnutrition; bone demineralization
6. Teeth: diseased, lost, ill-fitting dentures	6. Dehydration, malnutrition
7. Decreased digestive enzymes gastric acidity, saliva	7. Impaired digestion; swallowing stress; cracking of mucous membranes of the mouth

CARDIOVASCULAR SYSTEM

1. Protein degeneration; lipofuscin accumulation	1. Diminished cardiac output—decreased blood flow to brain, heart, kidneys, liver
2. Fibrosis of blood vessel lumen; calcification of arteries; elongation of arteries	2. Increased systolic blood pressure; vasal sluggishness
3. Thickening of vessel membranes	3. Impaired tissue nourishment; impaired removal of waste; edema
4. Increased perivascular fibrosis tissue	4. Increased peripheral resistance to blood flow; edema

SKIN AND CUTANEOUS TISSUE

1. Atrophy of sweat glands, hair follicles, subcutaneous tissue	1. Decreased perspiration; balding; increased susceptibility to trauma, abrasions, bed sores; inability to regulate body temperature
2. Deposits of melanin	2. "Age spots"
3. Thickening of connective tissue	3. Finger- and toenail thickening and hardening

and Marcia Cameron. *Views of aging: A teacher's guide.* Ann Arbor, Mich.: Institute of Gerontology, University of Michigan–Wayne State University, 1967, pp. 146–148.

NOTE: Listed in the left-hand column are major physical changes associated with normal aging; among these are changes often compounded by chronic disease. In the right-hand column are implications of these changes. It is often helpful to take these implications into account in day-to-day dealings with older persons.

income, and loneliness may all affect an aging person's nutritional status. Extensive deficiencies in the intake of protein, calcium, iron, and vitamins C and A are present in the older population as a result of limited income and the inability to prepare adequate meals (Berger, 1976, p. 113).

The aging person's physical, emotional, and economic status must be the basis for nutritional counseling. A 3-day diet recall by the client can be used by the nurse to evaluate what the person is consuming. Salaried homemakers and nutritionists from extension services can assist in counseling, meal preparation, and budgeting for food. "Spending down" for food is difficult when food prices increase and income remains static. Ingenuity with dried legumes, beans, whole cereal grains, poultry, fish, dried fortified milk, and organ meats is necessary. Fixing these foods in such a way that they are simple to prepare as well as simple to eat is another challenge.

Overnutrition with resulting atherosclerosis, obesity, and diabetes also needs to be evaluated. A diet rich in fats, sweets, and alcohol, along with inefficient use of labor-saving devices are problems for some older people. These problems can be adjusted with proper nutritional intake and exercise.

There are physical barriers to proper nutrition that need to be considered. Lack of transportation to big stores where clients can use food stamps or get their money's worth, physical disabilities such as foot problems, hearing and vision difficulties, inability to carry many packages, as well as fear for personal safety are all barriers that the nurse needs to consider.

Eating with a neighbor may reduce the work and loneliness involved in eating. Meals-on-Wheels, meals at special senior centers, and friendly visitors and volunteers are of some help in this area. Special food-preparation techniques such as cooking larger quantities and freezing in freezer dinner trays may also be an aid.

Physical Examinations

Annual physical examinations, dental examinations, and hearing and vision checks need to continue into the aging period. Unfortunately, they are not currently part of Medicare coverage.

These actions cannot slow down aging, but they can help to detect disease early, minimize the effects of existing problems, and prevent further complications. Health habits such as sleep, exercise, alcohol, and cigarette consumption need to be examined and discussed with clients so that they understand the relationship of these habits to health.

Medications

The elderly account for 25 percent of all drugs used. The physiological changes that come with aging alter responsiveness to drugs that an elderly person may ingest (Gotz and Gotz, 1978). Among this group of people, changes in behavior and mental status are often attributed to age, senility, and depression, and a drug reaction may go unrecognized (Kayne, 1976).

Older people frequently have chronic disease conditions that require long-term multiple-drug therapy. Errors of omission and commission in self-administration of drugs are not at all uncommon.

The community health nurse is in an excellent position to help clients avoid medication errors. During home visits, a 24-hour medication history is essential. "Let's take yesterday, starting with when you woke in the morning. What was the first medicine you took?" "How much?" "How many times a day?" "What are you taking the medicine for?" Checking a client's medication and assessing changes needs to be done on each visit. An alert student nurse made a visit to an 84-year-old woman and discovered an error in the client's dosage of digitalis. The very independent client was somewhat deaf and during a phone call to the doctor described symptoms which the doctor felt necessitated cutting the digitalis dosage in half. The client tripled the dosage. During a 24-hour medication check, the student realized the mistake just as the client was beginning to experience symptoms of drug toxicity.

Preparation for Retirement

There is a strong correlation between successful retirement and good health. There is also a strong correlation between successful retirement and retirement planning (Diekelmann, 1978). Planning for retirement must begin well before retirement occurs.

A Louis Harris poll was commissioned by the National Council on Aging to help to determine how aging people felt they could best prepare for retirement (Harris, 1975). Eleven areas of preparation for retirement were uncovered:

1. Making certain medical care will be available
2. Preparing a will
3. Building up savings
4. Learning about pensions and social security benefits
5. Buying one's own home
6. Developing hobbies and other leisure-time activities
7. Deciding whether to move or to stay where one lives
8. Planning new part-time or full-time jobs
9. Talking to older people about what it's like to grow old
10. Enrolling in retirement counseling and preparation programs
11. Moving in with relatives or children

In the following four areas, the older public felt less prepared than they would like to be:

1. Building up savings
2. Preparing a will
3. Planning new part-time or full-time jobs
4. Enrolling in retirement counseling and preparation programs

The poll showed that the least prepared in these 11 areas for retirement were those with incomes under $3000 (28 percent of those over 65) and especially blacks. A Senate report printed in 1971 stated that most blacks over 65 are less well educated and have lower incomes, more illness, earlier deaths, poorer housing, and fewer choices as to where they will live and work than others over 65 (Dancy, 1977, p. 11).

Life-Cycle View of People's Needs

Manney has constructed a life-cycle view of older people's needs which is accompanied by the system of services that responds to these needs. This chart (Table 18-6) appears to show a continuum of loss in the lives of aging persons. The lines on the chart indicate that services continue throughout the life-span but that priorities for services change. Services can be arranged so that people can compensate for their losses and live the fullest lives possible for themselves.

Role reorientation, needed during the 50- to 65-year-old period, includes services such as recreation, education and employment, opportunities for volunteer work, and preventive health care.

Social intervention, beginning during the 65- to 75-year-old period, includes income maintenance programs such as social security, Medicare, Medicaid, and housing and transportation assistance.

Personal intervention, beginning with age 75 to 85, maximizes the individual's personal independence. Dresen (1978) has elaborated on the need for autonomy in an aging person's life and has discussed ways in which this can be accomplished, such as using the family network, homemakers, home health aides, friendly visitors, Meals-on-Wheels, and intergenerational living.

Finally, at the end of life the aged person may become almost completely dependent on others and require either institutional care or complete care by the family.

TABLE 18-6　A Life-Cycle View of Older People's Needs

50–65	*65–75*	*75–85*	*85–death*
Departure of children from home, career stabilization, nagging health problems	Retirement, income problems, widowhood, chronic health problems, death of friends	Further loss of health, friends, strength; threat to independence	Serious loss of health, critical income need, dependency

Role reorientation _____
　　　Social intervention _____
　　　　　Personal intervention _____
　　　　　　　Personal maintenance _____

SOURCE: From James D. Manney, *Aging in American society.* Ann Arbor, Mich.: Institute of Gerontology, University of Michigan—Wayne State University, 1975, p. 14.

CONSIDERATIONS IN HEALTH PROMOTION IN THE AGED

The community health nurse takes into consideration multiple variables when planning health promotion activities for the aged. She or he utilizes the principles of primary, secondary, and tertiary prevention and knowledge of the natural life history of a disease or condition when identifying nursing services that will maximize the aged person's potential for growth.

Primary prevention activities that the community health nurse may plan when working with the aged may include measures to promote accident prevention, health instruction relative to adequate nutrition, teaching regarding avoiding exposure to infectious diseases and the need to maintain immunization levels, and counseling to prepare aging persons and their families for significant life changes such as retirement and loss of family and friends through death.

Community health nurses have found it to be particularly important to assess for environmental factors that foster accidents when working with the aged. Steffl (1976, pp. 466–468) has identified several significant primary prevention changes that can be made in the home environment and other settings to reduce accidents in the aging population. These are:

1. Good lighting, especially on landings and stairwells.

2. Handrails on both sides of staircases and halls or at least on one side, designed to show when top and bottom steps have been reached.

3. Top and bottom steps and risers painted in easily seen colors, and use of nonskid treads.

4. Elimination of loose extension cords, small mats, sliding rugs, slippery linoleum.

5. Use of rubber-backed nonskid rugs and nonskid floor waxes.

6. Tacking down edges of rugs or using wall-to-wall carpeting.

7. Advising use of corrugated soles on shoes.

8. Adequate lighting from the bedside tables to the bathroom with baseboard light. Easily available switches and flashlight at bedside.

9. Levers rather than door knobs.

10. Telephone at bedside.

11. Elimination of casters on chairs, rickety tables, sharp-cornered furniture, and high beds.

12. Advising against looking up when climbing stairs or making sudden movement of the head to the side, since this may interfere with the blood supply to the brain and cause fainting.

13. Avoidance of sedation.

14. Distinct and complete labeling of medications, including large letters indicating if it is for internal or external use, and good illumination of the medicine cabinet in order to avoid errors in self-administered medicine.

15. Avoidance of smoking in bed.

16. Distinct markings of dials on stoves.

17. Use of controls outside the tubs and showers.

18. Complete instructions on accident prevention to all personnel in hospitals and other institutions.

19. Use of grab rails and nonskid mats or emery strips in the tub.

20. Use of high sinks, high toilet seats, and high refrigerators to prevent undue bend-

ing of the head, which may cause dizziness and falls.

21. Careful training in use of wheelchairs.

22. Careful feeding of aged people in institutions to prevent aspiration and asphyxiation in presence of poor gag reflex.

23. Avoidance of large bowls of food for same reason as above.

24. Frequent reevaluation of capability for driving a motor vehicle. To be checked are such things as type of medication being used, type of underlying chronic illness, understanding of new rules and new signs. Curtailment of driving at night and in bad weather or on high-speed routes.

25. Pedestrian escort in bad weather or even in good weather, depending on the person's physical and mental capabilities.

26. Frequent testing of vision and hearing and immediate treatment of eye, ear, and foot abnormalities to prevent stumbling, etc.

Although primary prevention is the ultimate goal of community health nursing practice, the needs of clients frequently reflect situations that require counseling in relation to the secondary and tertiary levels of prevention. Secondary prevention activities that the community health nurse may be involved in center on early diagnosis and treatment. They include encouraging and facilitating regular medical and dental care, obtaining periodic screening for conditions to which the person is predisposed (e.g., hypertension and diabetes), adherence to medical treatment regimens, and carrying out of self-monitoring activities such as self-examination of the breasts and assessing for the danger signs of other types of cancer.

Tertiary prevention involves rehabilitative, restorative activities. The community health nurse is often involved in helping elderly persons to carry out a physical or speech therapy program and to adjust activities of daily living to their changing physical and mental functioning.

SIGNIFICANT LEGISLATION

Politicians have begun to grasp the value of supporting programs to benefit the elderly. They are a large group and represent 17 percent of the vote (Butler and Lewis, 1977, p. 279). The National Council of Senior Citizens and the American Association of Retired Persons are two of the largest organizations for older people. These two groups, along with the activist Gray Panthers, have lobbied on the state and national level for more favorable legislation for aging people.

Nearly every department or agency within the federal government conducts some program which relates directly to the concerns of the aging. The following is a partial list of such activities and legislation (Subcommittee on Aging, 1972, pp. 149–150):

1. Department of Health and Human Services:

   a. Social and Rehabilitation Service:

   (1) Administration on Aging—State and community service programs, training in the field of aging, nutrition services.

   (2) Assistance Payments Administration—old age assistance payments.

   (3) Medical Services Administration—medical payments for people with low incomes under the Medicaid program.

   (4) Community Services Administration—social services for recipients of old age assistance and other needy individuals.

   (5) Rehabilitation Services Administration—vocational rehabilitation services.

   (6) Office of Research, Planning, and Training—research and demonstration projects in a wide range of areas.

   b. Public Health Service:

   (1) National Institutes of Health—research into the biological and psychological aspects of aging.

   (2) Health Services and Mental Health Administration—health services and mental health programs.

   c. Social Security Administration—benefits under the old-age, survivors, and disability insurance program, health insurance protection under the Medicare program, research relating to economic security for the aged.

   d. Office of Education—research and training activities, Library Services, University Community Services, and Adult Education.

2. Department of Labor:

   a. Manpower Administration—jobs for low-income older persons in Operation Mainstream.

   b. Employment Standards Administration—enforces the Age Discrimination in Employment Act.

3. Department of the Treasury: Assistance relating to the tax problems of senior citizens provided by the Internal Revenue Service.

4. Department of Defense: Payments under the military retirement program.

5. Department of the Interior: Issues a Golden Eagle Passport allowing use of national parks at no cost.

6. Department of Agriculture:

   a. Food and Nutrition Service— Food Stamps and Food Distribution Program.

   b. Extension Service—educational programs including nutrition education, housing and continuing education.

   c. Farmers Home Administration—loans for housing.

7. Department of Housing and Urban Development:

    a. Office of Housing Production and Mortgage Credit—low-rent public housing, Section 236 program, rent supplements, congregate housing, Section 235 program, nursing and intermediate care facilities.

    b. Office of Housing Management—services in housing for the elderly.

    c. Office of Community Development—programs for the elderly in Model Cities and grants for neighborhood centers under the Neighborhood Facilities program.

    d. Office of Community Planning and Management—development of a national urban growth policy and new community projects.

8. Department of Transportation: Urban Mass Transportation Administration provides funding to assist in providing mass transportation facilities and services for elderly persons.

9. Federal Trade Commission: Action against unfair and deceptive practices such as in the unwarranted sale of hearing aids.

10. Office of Economic Opportunity:

    a. Office of Operations: Senior Opportunities and Services and Community Action agency multi-generational programs.

    b. Office of Legal Services: Legal problems of the elderly poor.

    c. Office of Health Affairs: Emergency Food Assistance and Comprehensive Health Services.

11. Veterans' Administration:

    a. Department of Medicine and Surgery—comprehensive health care for older veterans.

    b. Department of Veterans' Benefits—compensation, pension, and dependency and indemnity compensation.

12. Action: Volunteer service opportunities through VISTA, Peace Corps, SCORE (Service Corps of Retired Executives), ACE (Active Corps of Executives), Foster Grandparent Programs, RSVP (Retired Senior Volunteer Program).

13. Railroad Retirement Board: payments under the Railroad Retirement program.

14. General Services Administration: enforcement of Architectural Barriers Act requiring Federal buildings and structures built with Federal aid to have ready access by handicapped.

15. Civil Service Commission: administers the Civil Service Retirement program and provides protection of older workers from age discrimination.

16. Department of Commerce: enforces the Flammable Fabrics Act.

17. Advisory Commission on Intergovernmental Relations: property tax relief studies.

18. Library of Congress: Division for the Blind and Physically Handicapped provides talking books and braille books.

Unfortunately, the old adage "What is everyone's business is no one's business" very often applies to the elderly. Services for the aging are spread so thinly over the entire government establishment that many individuals fall through the cracks.

There are several legislative programs that are especially significant for the aging, and these will be discussed.

Older Americans Act

Congress passed the Older Americans Act (OAA) in 1965. It has since been amended several times. The act provides funds for service, research, and training. It is carried out by the Administration on Aging of the Department of Health and Human Services. The act has three titles that are of interest to those who work with the aging.

Title III of the OAA gives funds to states to establish state agencies on aging and, in turn, to help states to establish local area agencies on aging. These area agencies plan and coordinate programs for aging persons in certain areas of each state. The area agency on aging in a given community can be identified by calling the Federal Information Center, located in the telephone directory under "United States Government."

Title IV of the OAA provides grant money for research and demonstration projects that have either regional or national value.

Title V of the act provides grant money for the specialized training of persons who want to work with the aging.

Medicare

Medicare, a legislative program passed in 1966, is administered by the Social Security Administration, Department of Health and Human Services. It is a health insurance program that is available to almost every person over 65.

There are two parts to Medicare:

1. Part A provides hospital insurance that helps to pay for care when an aging person is in the hospital. It also pays for some health-related services after the person leaves the hospital. There is no monthly premium for part A, though clients do have to pay a small part of the total cost of their hospital stay.

2. Part B provides supplementary medical insurance which costs a small monthly premium. It covers doctor's services, outpatient hospital services, skilled home health services, medical services, physical therapy, and speech pathology services. The exclusions in part B are numerous and significant. Routine physical examinations, eye refractions, immunizations, hearing examinations, prescription drugs, false teeth, and eyeglasses are among those items not covered by Medicare.

Medicaid

Medicaid is a medical assistance program that helps pay the medical bills for low-income people. Each state administers its own Medicaid program and thus eligibility requirements and benefits differ. Generally, an elderly person may receive Medicaid if he or she receives public assistance payment. Medicare and Medicaid may be received concurrently.

All state Medicaid programs pay for at least the following services to people who are 65 and older: inpatient hospital care, outpatient hospital services, lab and x-ray services, skilled nursing home services, physicians' services, and home health services.

BARRIERS TO HEALTH CARE

The mindset of care givers, of aging people, and of our culture toward aging is a barrier to health care. Until we all see aging as a natural and even beautiful part of the life cycle, we will not "age gracefully." People do have at least some control over their own health and they may need assistance in recognizing this. Developing healthy ways of living and planning for the years after retirement when we are young means that life after 65 or 70 can be both healthy and enjoyable. We have to believe that this is the case, however, and believe that people can still be productive and valuable as they age.

There are two outstanding barriers to achieving health care in this age group, aside from the attitude that "to be old is to be sick, lonely, and tired."

Transportation

Studies have shown that transportation problems cause a considerable barrier for aging persons (Rossman and Burnside, 1975, p. 106). Getting to health care facilities, service agencies, or grocery stores may be impossible without a car or public transportation. The inability to drive or physically to get around due to mobility limitations contributes to the problem. In some communities, Dial-a-Ride and the Red Cross have provided some transportation to solve this problem.

Income

Even though the prices of food, medicine, doctors' visits, and gas rise, most elderly people must live on a fixed income. Poverty breeds mental illness, malnutrition, and anemia in old age. To enjoy retirement one must have money to pursue hobbies, to travel, and to visit children, grandchildren, and friends. Some federal programs that provide limited resources for increasing income in old age include Green Thumb, Foster Grandparents, Food Stamps, Supplemental Security Income, and Medicaid. (See Chapter 4.)

ROLE OF THE COMMUNITY HEALTH NURSE

Care of aging persons holds unique challenges for community health nurses, such as helping elderly people who lack a feeling of self-worth to find it, helping them to maintain independence, and assisting them to be contributing citizens, as well. Some of these challenges are the result of the special economic, biological, and psychological characteristics of people who have lived a long life.

Basically, the main role of community health nurses with aging persons has been that of working in the area of health maintenance and prevention of disease and disability. An example of this role is health teaching and counseling about the use of medications.

Underlying this role are many other ones that the nurse must participate in if comprehensive care is to be given. Some of these are discussed below.

Evaluating Available Services for the Aging

Four community health nurses in a city of 30,000 people were asked to assess the needs for further services to the elderly in their community. Because of their knowledge of currently available services as well as their contacts with clients, the nurses were in an excellent position to be able to evaluate services for this population group.

Table 18-7 shows the services that elderly people of the community, as well as the community health nurses, felt were needed. It then compares the way in which these two groups rank the needs with each other. The table demonstrates that aging people desire services that will help them to remain independent in the community. Nurses want aging people to have recreational centers and church relationships. The elderly desire the services of the community health nurse or visiting nurse as well as home-delivered meals. In summary, the expansion of programs to include more prevention and maintenance activities by nurses receives *more* support from clients than from nurses. Perhaps we have underestimated the importance of our role with aging persons! As with other age groups, the community health nurse needs to ascertain the services that clients need, in addition to those they are already receiving. The survey

TABLE 18-7 Ranking of Services According to Need for Provision of Additional Resources by Public Health Nurses and Individuals 65 or Over

Service	*Rank assigned by public health nurses*	*Rank assigned by the elderly*
Ambulance service	21	23
Hospital service	17	20
Access to physicians	23	21
Nursing and custodial homes	16	14
Services of a public health or visiting nurse	14	9*
Homemaker–health aide services	9*	8*
Meal and nutrition services, such as group meals, home-delivered meals	10*	5*
Availability of large print (books, records, tapes, etc.)	19	13
Services to deliver books, tapes, and records to shut-ins	20	18
Social and recreational center for, or including, older people	3*	16
Church relationships with older people	5*	15
Education or training in subjects of special interest to older people	8*	19
Employment service for older people in the community who wish to work	6*	12
Handyman service	12	7*
Help for older people in finding housing	11	6*
Information and referral service	13	10*
Legal help for those who cannot afford to pay	2*	2*
Preretirement training programs	15	22
Program of reassurance by regularly scheduled telephone calls to the elderly	7*	4*
Senior citizens club	18	11
Transportation services	1*	1*
Visiting program to older people in their homes, hospitals, nursing homes, retirement homes	4*	3*
Agency or organization that offers older people opportunities to volunteer their services	22	17

*Services ranked in the top 10 in terms of priority for provision of additional resources.

SOURCE: From Pat M. Keith. A preliminary investigation of the role of the public health nurse in evaluation of services of the aged. *American Journal of Public Health*, April 1976, 66, p. 379.

discussed here is one way of accomplishing this.

Political Involvement

Good nursing care must involve a knowledge of the political system and how to work within it. Many of the services that aging clients need, such as an adequate income and transportation, can be obtained only when caring people work to obtain them on the local, state, and federal levels. Nurses need to learn to know their legislators, inform them of the needs in the community, and help to organize aging people into power groups. Only with this kind of action will major changes take place.

Home Visiting

Home is an extremely significant place to most older people. It is a place where things are familiar and where one is able to remain independent and have a sense of autonomy. A home visit is a very useful way of making an individualized assessment of the needs and strengths of older people. The needs can be met by making necessary referrals to available services and by working out solutions with clients. The physical environment, interpersonal relationships, and the client's physical and psychological capabilities need to be assessed. Remnet (1976) has constructed tools to assess these different areas.

Helping with the Decision of Institutionalization or Home Care

The home assessment may show that the aging person needs help to remain at home. Most people prefer home care to institutionalization, which separates them from familiar patterns.

There are many support services that the nurse can mobilize. Butler and Lewis (1977, p. 215) have summarized the range of these services (Table 18-8). Few communities will have all of these services.

If the home assessment indicates that care outside the home is needed, the community health nurse can be a resource person for help in this decision. The nurse has the opportunity to help the family work through this difficult, often guilt-producing situation as well as to help in choosing a good institution. This is not an easy situation because the community health nurse is helping to make radical changes in the lives of clients and families. There are three kinds of long-term care facilities for the aging person, often referred to as *institutional care:*

1. *Home for the aged*—for those over 65 years of age who need a minimum of care which is often characterized as "supervised living" or "residential care"

TABLE 18-8 Support Services

Mental health intake, screening, and evaluation

Mental health care

Physicians' services

Nursing services

Homemaker–home health aides

Physical therapy

Occupational therapy

Speech therapy

Inhalation therapy

Dental care

Nutrition service (Meals-on-Wheels, group dining, food distribution programs)

Health education

Laundry services

Social services:

    Information and referral

    Financial support

    Legal services

    Personal needs (transportation, telephone reassurance, grooming, shopping, companions, friendly visitors, pets)

    Family "respite" services

    Night sitters (for short-term illnesses)

    Home safety

    Chore services (handyman) or home maintenance repairs

    Recreation (community center, senior center)

    Employment and volunteer work (VISTA, Senior Aides, SCORE, Peace Corps, Foster Grandparent, Green Thumb, etc.)

    Education (home library service, academic courses)

Religious support (clerical or pastoral counseling, "practical" ecumenism)

Police assistance

Outpatient care in clinics, community mental health center, day hospitals, day-care centers

Multipurpose senior centers

Protective services

Screening before hospital admission

SOURCE: From R. N. Butler and M. I. Lewis. *Aging and mental health* (2d ed.). St. Louis: Mosby, 1977, p. 215.

2. *Basic home*—for those who need assistance in eating and bathing or who need routine nursing care, perhaps including the administration of medication

3. *Skilled home*—for those with serious health problems who need 24-hour nursing care and supervision

Various sources of money are used to pay for nursing home care:

1. Medicare is a federal insurance program administered by the U.S. Social Security Administration.

2. Medicaid is a state program for persons with limited income and assets which is administered by the Department of Social Services. Information can be obtained from county offices of the Department of Social Services.

3. Blue Cross/Blue Shield offers certain health insurance plans that have a convalescent care rider paying for up to 720 days of skilled nursing care. This information can be obtained from the Blue Cross/Blue Shield insurance representative.

4. Other private insurance plans may also pay for nursing home care.

5. *Private pay* applies to individuals who are financing the total cost of their nursing home care.

A provision of the 1972 Social Security Act gives consumers the right to ask any Social Security or Welfare office for the records of deficiencies found in government inspections of all Medicare- and Medicaid-funded nursing homes. Full reports of these inspections can be obtained at Social Security offices.

Local health and welfare councils, such as Citizens for Better Care of Michigan (1975), publish assessment guides that are useful to families and nurses in looking at the different levels and types of institutions available for the full care of aging persons.

The decision to institutionalize a person is often a crisis for the family and the client. The nurse has an excellent opportunity to offer support. Helping the family to continue supporting the aging client in the institution is important also.

SUMMARY

Aging persons have unique characteristics. The views of our culture about aging have to change if aging people are to receive high-quality care. Some of the common health problems of this group stem from the negative view held by young people and by older persons themselves. Old age may be a positive part of life if it is planned for and if good health habits are begun early in life. One of the health promotion needs is that of preparation for retirement. Significant legislation, including the Older Americans Act, Medicare, and Medicaid, are of great help to aging people, but many people "fall between the cracks" and are not helped by them. Two major barriers to achieving health among the aging are lack of transportation and limited income. Community health nurses can play a significant role in meeting the health needs of this group. This begins with the nurses' understanding of how they themselves view aging. Involvement in the political process is essential if the system of health care of the aging is to be improved.

REFERENCES

Belloc, N. B. Relationship of health practices and mortality. *Preventive Medicine*, March 1973, *2*, 67–81.

Berger, R. Nutritional needs of the aged. In I. M. Burnside (Ed.), *Nursing and the aged*. New York: McGraw-Hill, 1976.

Burnside, I. M. (Ed.) *Nursing and the aged*. New York: McGraw-Hill, 1976.

Butler, R. N., & Lewis, M. I. *Aging and mental health. Positive psychosocial approaches* (2d ed.). St. Louis: Mosby, 1977.

Cameron, M. *Views of aging: A teacher's guide*. Ann Arbor, Mich.: Institute of Gerontology, University of Michigan–Wayne-State University, 1967.

Citizens for Better Care of Michigan. *A guide for the use of public information about nursing homes*. 960 E. Jefferson, Detroit, Mich., 1975.

Combs, K. L. Preventive care in the elderly. *American Journal of Nursing*, August 1978, *78*, 1339–1341.

Dancy, J., Jr. *The black elderly. A guide for practitioners*. Ann Arbor, Mich.: Institute of Gerontology, University of Michigan–Wayne State University, 1977.

Diekelmann, N. Pre-retirement counseling. *American Journal of Nursing*, August 1978, *78*, 1337–1338.

Dresen, S. E. Autonomy: A continuing developmental task. *American Journal of Nursing*, August 1978, *78*, 1344–1346.

Duvall, E. M. *Marriage and family development* (5th ed.). Philadelphia: Lippincott, 1977.

Finch, C. B. Biological theories of aging. In I. M. Burnside (Ed.), *Nursing and the aged*. New York: McGraw-Hill, 1976.

Gotz, B. E., & Gotz, V. P. Drugs and the elderly. *American Journal of Nursing*, August 1978, *77*, 1347–1351.

Harris, L., & Associates. *The myth and reality of aging in America*. Washington, D.C.: National Council on Aging, April 1975.

Health, United States, 1976–1977. DHEW Publication No. HRA 77-1232. Washington, D.C.: U.S. Government Printing Office, 1977.

Jennings, M., Nordstorm, M., & Shumake, N. Physiologic functioning in the elderly. *Nursing Clinics of North America*, June 1972, 7, 237–246.

Kayne, R. C. Drugs and the aging. In I. M. Burnside (Ed.), *Nursing and the aged*. New York: McGraw-Hill, 1976.

Keith, P. M. A preliminary investigation of the role of the public health nurse in evaluation of services of the aged. *American Journal of Public Health*, April 1976, *66*, p. 379.

Kimmel, D. C. Biological and intellectual aspects of aging. In *Adulthood and aging*. New York: Wiley, 1974, chap. 8.

Kübler-Ross, E. *On death and dying*. New York: Macmillan, 1969.

Manney, J. D. *Aging in American society. An examination of concepts and issues*. Ann Arbor, Mich.: Institute of Gerontology, University of Michigan–Wayne State University, 1975.

National Center for Health Statistics. *Vital statistics of the United States*. Washington, D.C.: U.S. Government Printing Office, Vol. 11, for 1950–1965 data; Rockville, Md.: Health Resources Administration, Department of Health, Education and Welfare, to be published for 1975 data.

Office of Services to the Aging, Policy and Program Analysis Division. *The Michigan comprehensive plan on aging*. Lansing, Mich.: State of Michigan, 1974.

Proctor, P. Durants on history from the ages, with love. *Parade*, Aug. 6, 1978, p. 12.

Remnet, V. L. The home assessment: A therapeutic tool to assess the needs of the elderly. In I. M. Burnside (Ed.), *Nursing and the aged*. New York: McGraw-Hill, 1976.

Rossman, I. *Human aging changes*. In I. M. Burnside (Ed.), *Nursing and the aged*. New York: McGraw-Hill, 1976.

——— & Burnside, I. M. The United States of America. In J. C. Brocklehurst (Ed.), *Geriatric care in advanced societies*. Baltimore: University Park Press, 1975.

Stanford, D. All about sex after middle age. *American Journal of Nursing*, April 1977, 77, 608–611.

Steffl, B. M. Prevention measures and safety factors for the aged. In I. M. Burnside (Ed.), *Nursing and the aged.* New York: McGraw-Hill, 1976.

Subcommittee on Aging of the Committee on Labor and Public Welfare. *Legislative history of the older Americans comprehensive services amendments of 1972.* Washington, D.C.: U.S. Government Printing Office, December 1972.

United Nations, Department of Economics and So-cial Affairs. *The aging: Trends and policies.* New York: United Nations Publication, 1975.

Weg, R. B. Normal aging changes in the reproductive system. In I. M. Burnside (Ed.), *Nursing and the aged.* New York: McGraw-Hill, 1976.

Weissman, A. D. Does old age make sense? Decisions and destiny in growing older. *Journal of Geriatric Psychiatry,* January 1974, *7,* 93.

SELECTED BIBLIOGRAPHY

Arling, G. The elderly widow and her family, neighbors and friends. *Journal of Marriage and The Family,* November 1976, *38,* 757–770.

Bell, B. D. (Ed.). *Contemporary social gerontology. Significant developments in the field of aging.* Springfield, Ill.: Charles C Thomas, 1976.

Burnside, I. M. (Ed.). *Psychosocial nursing care of the aged.* New York: McGraw-Hill, 1973.

Busse, E. W., & Pfeiffer, E. *Behavior and adaptation in late life.* Boston: Little, Brown, 1977.

de Beauvoir, Simone. *The coming of age.* New York: Putnam, 1972.

Diekelmann, N. *Primary health care of the well adult.* New York: McGraw-Hill, 1977.

Hain, M. J., & Chen, S. P. C. Health needs of the elderly. *Nursing Research,* November–December 1976, *25,* 433–439.

Hess, B. B. (Ed.). *Growing old in America.* New Brunswick, N.J.: Transaction Books, 1976.

Hess, P. A., & Day, C. *Understanding the aging patient.* Bowie, Md.: Robert J. Brady Company, 1977.

Jacobs, J. J. *Older persons and retirement communities.* Springfield, Ill.: Charles C Thomas, 1975.

Kalish, R. A. *Late adulthood: Perspectives on human development.* Monterey, Calif.: Brooks/Cole, 1975.

Lawton, M. P. *Planning and managing housing for the elderly.* New York: Wiley, 1975.

Lowenthal, M. F. *Lives in distress.* New York: Basic Books, 1964.

McCuan, E. R. Geriatric day care. A family perspective. *The Gerontologist,* December 1976, *16,* 517–521.

Mendelson, M. A. *Tender loving greed.* New York: Vintage Books, 1974.

Percy, C. H. *Growing old in the country of the young.* New York: McGraw-Hill, 1974.

Reichel, W. (Ed.). *Clinical aspects of aging.* Baltimore: Williams & Wilkins, 1978.

Rosenfield, A. *Prolongevity.* New York: Knopf, 1976.

Shanas, E., & Maddox, G. L. Aging, health and the organization of health resources. In R. Binstock & E. Shanas (Eds.), *Handbook of aging and the social sciences.* New York: Van Nostrand Reinhold, 1976, pp. 592–615.

Silverstone, B., & Hyman, H. K. *You and your aging parent.* New York: Pantheon Books, 1976.

Treas, J. Family support systems for the aged: Some social and demographic considerations. *The Gerontologist,* December 1977, *17,* 486–491.

Weaver, J. L. *National health policy and the underserved.* St. Louis: Mosby, 1976.

White, M. J., & Johnson, D. M. Changes in nursing students' stereotypic attitudes toward old people. *Nursing Research,* November–December 1976, *25,* 430–433.

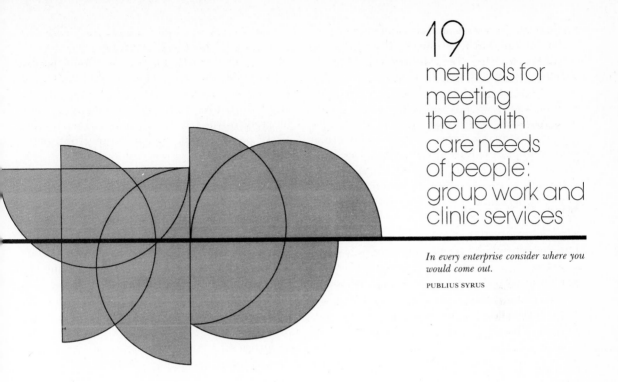

19
methods for meeting the health care needs of people: group work and clinic services

In every enterprise consider where you would come out.

PUBLIUS SYRUS

"There are many ways to skin a cat" is one way of saying that a goal can be reached by numerous routes. This axiom applies to meeting the health care needs of people in community health nursing. The nurse who visits people in their homes is taking one route. As discussed in Chapters 13 and 18, nurses visit parents of newborns to help them with the unique tasks that accompany parenthood and they visit aging people to help them with changing developmental tasks. Other routes, explained in Chapters 14 and 16, are the school nursing role and the occupational health nursing role.

In this chapter, two more methods of meeting people's health care needs are presented: group work and clinic services. Both methods can be used by nurses to provide primary, secondary, and tertiary preventive services to population groups so that they achieve their maximum level of functioning. Both methods focus on groups of people rather than on the nurse-to-family approach utilized in home visits. Clients come to the nurse rather than the nurse serving the family members in their own personal environment.

GROUP WORK IN COMMUNITY HEALTH NURSING

Community health nurses have long worked with groups of people to meet health care needs effectively. In this context *group* is de-

fined as a gathering of people who are together for a specific reason. An example of the use of group work in community health nursing practice is a parent effectiveness training class. Parents in this situation come together to discuss ways to rear children effectively. A gathering of people at a bus stop is not defined as a group.

Community health nursing agencies frequently utilize the group intervention strategy. Community health nurses focus on delivering services to populations in census tracts and on caseloads rather than on individual clients only. Thus, needs common to an area are more readily apparent, particularly if caseload analyses are done. One community health nurse who served a large trailer park realized that she continually received numerous referrals from the intermediate school district to visit families with children who had developmental delays. She formed a parent support group to serve the many primary and secondary health needs of this population.

The History of the Group Approach to Health Care Needs

Kurt Lewin is generally considered to be the founder of modern group process (Luft, 1970, p. 2). His research during World War II was aimed at increasing work production as well as changing food consumption patterns. Lewin found that group discussion and group decision helped people to change their ideas much more effectively than lectures or even individual instruction (Lewin, 1947). Giving people information did not motivate them to change personal attitudes and behavior. Rather, discussion in groups helped persons to become involved and to conceptualize ideas. Group participants learned something about their own behavior in group settings, and the information gained became more relevant to their personal lives.

Another development in the group approach to health was group psychotherapy. It became a part of the treatment plan of psychologists and psychiatrists in the 1920s and 1930s, but it was not until the 1960s that group process and group psychotherapy came together (Loomis, 1979, p. 5). During the decade of the 1960s, the encounter group movement proliferated and the differences between sensitivity groups and psychotherapy groups blurred. It was realized that everyone, not just "sick" people, could benefit from group process.

The terms *group process, group dynamics,* and *group interaction* all refer to the way groups work. The study of group process is not a clearly organized science, but it is a growing field. Groups are formed for a variety of purposes such as losing weight, controlling drugs and smoking, and giving support during divorce and death. Nurses are part of a group on the health team and in professional associations, in choirs, parent-teacher organizations, League of Women Voters, and synagogues. Clearly, group work is an integral part of life in the United States today.

Advantages and Disadvantages of the Group Approach

The definition of community health nursing states that promoting and preserving the health of populations is its goal. Thus, nurses are constantly looking at ways of helping people to look critically at their own health behavior. Telling people about healthy behavior is not enough—the low immunization levels of children discussed in Chapter 13 is verification of that statement. There must be a way of helping people to value preventive health practices so that they will change their health behavior. Lewin's work, among many others, gives evidence that groups help to accomplish this. The main reason for using the group approach is that different kinds of people with similar concerns can work on these concerns together. Feelings of isolation and aloneness that are so often a part of crisis can be worked through. "I'm not the only one who feels this way, and that's sure a relief" becomes a frequent comment.

It must be emphasized that the group approach will not meet all clients' health needs in community health nursing. Some people will never feel secure enough to leave their own familiar surroundings, to find transportation, to have the needed energy and skill to become part of a group. There are people who lack the social expertise, experience, and motivation required to become involved in a group. This behavior can be learned, but it requires patience and skill on the part of the nurse to teach it. An overwhelmed 17-year-old single mother with two children under 2 years of age who has exhibited poor bonding behaviors with her newborn probably needs an intense one-to-one relationship with a nurse before she can profit from a group discussion about parenting.

Nurses gain valuable information about a family when they see individual family members interacting with each other in their own surroundings. A data base on the family system as discussed in Chapter 6 is very difficult to collect when the client is a member of a larger group. Situations that warrant a family-centered nursing approach are best handled in the home environment.

Some people like to function in groups; others do not. These differences need to be respected because what an individual expects to receive from a group experience will largely determine what he or she learns.

Luft has summarized the advantages of group vs. individual productivity and problem-solving as follows (1970, p. 30):

1. There are definite advantages and disadvantages to group versus individual problem-solving and productivity.

2. When a problem demands a single over-all insight or an original set of decisions, an individual approach may be superior to a group effort.

3. Problems calling for a wide variety of skills and information or the cross-checking of facts and ideas seem to call for a group approach. Feedback and free exchange of thinking may stimulate ideas that would not have emerged by solo effort.

4. If goals are shared, then there is greater likelihood for cooperative effort; when the group goal is not shared by members, morale and productivity may suffer. Consequently, when the goal is decided upon by group discussion and participation, there is greater likelihood of full member involvement.

5. The greater the group members' desire for individual prominence and distinction, the lower will be their friendly sharing or group morale.

6. When members decide on the need for group effort, the smaller the size of the group the better it will function, provided that the necessary diversity of skills and group maintenance resources are present.

7. A group may be a source of strong interpersonal stimulation; a group will also generate its own conformity pressures. In order to decide between group and individual work, these two sets of forces (stimulating and binding) should be kept in mind.

8. A society which places highest value on the worth and freedom of the individual also encourages the strongest independent thought, independent work, and independent responsibility. An inherent goal of a sound group in such a society is the reaffirmation of true independence while meeting group needs concerning tasks and morale.

How Community Health Nurses Utilize the Group Approach

Loomis (1979, pp. 3–11) has discussed six ways that groups can be used to meet the biopsychosocial health needs of clients: support, task accomplishment, socialization, learning–behavior change, human relations training, and psychotherapy–insight and behavior change.

Support. This text focuses on the developmental needs of clients throughout the life cycle. Many people are healthy, but during periods of rapid development and change, they need help to manage the maturational and situational crises that can occur. La Leche League groups and classes of expectant parents come under this category. Primary prevention of problems is the thrust of support groups because they help those participating to develop healthy methods of dealing with potentially difficult situations.

Task accomplishment. Large complex tasks need more than one person to carry them out. The interdisciplinary team of a health department which includes nurses, physicians, environmentalists, nutritionists, and physical therapists is one example of how meeting the health care needs of people is accomplished by a group.

Clients in a group can help each other to accomplish goals as well. One large senior citizen's center uses retired volunteer physicians, nurses, and lay people to carry out monthly health screening. The workers *are* needed and *feel* needed, and the clients screened feel that they are helped "by people who understand them."

Socialization. The situational and maturational crises of death, divorce, and retirement produce pain and isolation. Parents Without Partners, Welcome Wagon Clubs, and senior citizens' activity clubs provide fellowship for those experiencing common needs. As with support groups, clients can learn to develop new ways of dealing with these developmental and situational crises.

Learning–behavior change. Having a new colostomy and coping with a new diagnosis of diabetes or leukemia are situational crises common to the community health nurse. Clients must learn completely new methods of functioning and living with irrigations, diet, and approaching death. Groups composed of clients with common problems provide support as well as teach new methods of coping. Ostomy clubs, Weight Watchers, and Parents Anonymous are examples of learning–behavior change groups.

Human relations training. The National Training Laboratory (now the NTL Institute for Applied Behavior Science) was established in Maine in 1947 to look at informal experimental methods of teaching group process (Luft, 1970, p. 4). It was designed as a 3-week workshop for professional people who wanted to deal more effectively with coworkers. T-groups or skills-training groups grew from the NTL. The subsequent encounter group movement was another later outgrowth. The purpose of these human relations groups is education. Such groups usually meet for a specific number of hours with the purpose of learning cognitively and affectively about human relations. Assertiveness training, body workshops, emotive therapy, and sexuality workshops are all kinds of human relations training groups. They have grown rapidly and their effectiveness depends greatly upon the skills of the leader. Before community health nurses refer clients to them or attend them, they should investigate the quality and preparation of the leader.

Psychotherapy–insight and behavior change. Therapy groups are conducted to treat clients. Usually these clients are people who are discontented and want to change something about their lives. Such groups are usually led by people with graduate degrees in nursing, medicine, or psychology. This group classification is different from the other five because "it focuses on the goal-directed alteration of how the client relates to himself and others in an overall way. Psychotherapy may include altering specific behaviors or learning new ways of relating to other people, but it also includes specific assistance with how one feels about oneself."[1] The reason for mentioning this kind of group is to facilitate the referral process for the community health nurse who has clients who need psychotherapy.

Developing a Group

Before nurses think about using the group approach to meeting health needs, they must be familiar with the policies of their employing agency. Some agencies will not permit nurses to form groups under their auspices. Others will actively support group efforts if they are compatible with agency philosophy and resources. The nurse must also know whether or not her or his workload can support the added responsibility of group work. This can be ascertained by discussion with the nurse supervisor. Chapter 20 deals more fully with this aspect of the nurse's role, that is, dealing with caseload management issues.

Since community health nurses work with populations such as a county, a city, or a township, common needs that can be met by a group may be expressed by clients, staff nurses, or others (for example, school officials). If the client and the nurse are so inclined, almost any health need can be met by the group process except those for which clients need one-to-one relationships (Loomis, 1979, p. 19). The very young single mother referred to earlier is a client whose needs may not be met by the group process. Frequently it can be useful to combine group and individual intervention strategies. One nurse had a family in her caseload which included a child with spina bifida and paraplegia. The nurse visited the home to assess family functioning and the environment, as well as to help the mother with the child's daily routine. The nurse also referred

the parents to a group at the intermediate school, where they received support from families with similar problems.

Once a need that is common to a number of people has been established, the potential group members need to be contacted. The nurse should discuss with them the objectives of what can be accomplished in a group. The important principle involved is that the nurse must have objectives in mind for the group, that the client must have needs in mind, and that the two should be congruent. This principle is also valid when the nurse is considering a referral to an already established group; it must meet the needs of the client. For example, a support group for new parents would probably not be helpful for a client with severe postpartum depression.

To facilitate this principle, Loomis has suggested the use of a health care contract when working with groups (Loomis, 1979, p. 109). A contract is a written statement of the mutual expectations of both client and nurse for each other. Chapter 8 discusses contracting with families and the same principles can be applied to groups. Contracts provide a basis for evaluation of the progress that takes place; the key question to consider is have we or have we not met the objectives we set out to achieve?

The setting plays a crucial role in groups. Several questions, such as those below, should be asked in order to determine whether a particular setting is appropriate.

- Is the group meeting in a place that is easily accessible, that can be reached by public transportation or personal cars easily?

- Is the meeting place near the population being served?

- Is the location of the meeting place safe after dark?

- Does the meeting room provide privacy and warmth?

[1]M. E. Loomis. *Group process for nurses.* St. Louis: Mosby, 1979, p. 11.

· Can participants sit in a circle?

· Will the facility be consistently available?

Besides the setting, there are many other factors to consider when developing a group. The size of the group is a major consideration. Though there are no clear rules, 5 to 15 people usually facilitate good communication. When the group should meet is another important variable. If it is composed of mothers, mornings may be fine. Wage earners, on the other hand, are likely to be free only in the evenings. The frequency and length of meetings and child care arrangements are other issues that need to be decided by nurse and clients. If small children are to be brought along with clients, there needs to be a place with equipment and a caretaker provided. None of these details have a right and wrong answer, but it is essential that clients know them and help to plan them.

Many nurses are hesitant to use the group approach to nursing care because they lack experience with this intervention strategy. Careful planning, staff development activities which facilitate the understanding of group dynamics, and guidance from professionals comfortable with this process will reduce fear.

The Life of a Group

It is helpful for nurses who lead groups to understand that a group goes through phases. Table 19-1 is a summary of these phases, which include the initiation phase, the working phase, and the termination phase. The table includes the goals, the group strategies, and leader behaviors for each phase.

The Functions of the Community Health Nurse as Group Leader

Effective leadership is fundamental to a positive group experience. Marram says that there are four basic leadership functions that are

TABLE 19-1   Summary of Group Phases

Group phases	Goals	Group strategies	Leader behaviors
Initiation	Orient group. Facilitate trust.	Introduces self and students. Describes objectives and purpose of group. Orients group to time limitations and behavior expected of each student. Encourages questions and discussion of group activities.	Reduces group anxiety. Sets limits. Deals with anger without becoming defensive. Displays trust.
Working	Encourage problem solving.	Presents group with problem-solving situations, games, or opportunities. Intervenes only to facilitate problem solving.	Shares control of group. Directs problem solving.
Termination	Initiate termination. Facilitate separation.	Initiates discussion of termination. Allows for group regression and encourages reminiscing and expressions of warmth, anger, and depression. Accepts and encourages distancing devices and final separation.	Facilitates and accepts angry feelings. Accepts warm feelings. Accepts regression. Accepts separation.

SOURCE: From H. J. Knopke & N. L. Diekelmann. *Approaches to teaching in the health sciences.* Reading, Mass.: Addison-Wesley, 1978, p. 135, Table 10-1. Reprinted with permission.

appropriate for nurse group leaders (Marram, 1978, pp. 124–127):

1. The leader facilitates benefits of group membership. People join groups for the reasons discussed earlier and the leader can help the group to meet expected objectives by outlining a direction for the group and interpreting group objectives.

2. The leader maintains a viable group atmosphere by keeping relationships within the group pleasant or relatively secure. Group members need to feel free to be present and to be able to discuss what concerns them. Being able to experience new behaviors is also important to growth.

3. The leader oversees group growth by keeping members attuned to the objectives and by clarifying issues in terms of how they relate to the objectives. The leader also needs to periodically help the group evaluate the progress they have made toward their objectives.

4. The leader regulates individual members' growth within the group setting. People will move toward objectives at different rates of speed and some members may need more specific objectives than others. The leader is concerned not only with the progress of the group toward objectives but also with the growth of individuals within the group.

To succeed in implementing leadership responsibilities in a group, a nurse must have an awareness of how people interact with each other. Community health nurses must utilize basic interviewing and communication skills in all settings, and group work is no exception. People want to be able to communicate and this can be facilitated by asking open-ended questions, asking direct questions, and using other techniques such as reflection and role playing. Games and audiovisual aids are different methods that can be used to stimulate interaction between group members.

Nurses who are interested in working with groups but who have never done so should ask for supervision and a preceptor to help them with the process. Effective communication with group members and agency personnel, careful scheduling, and attention to small details of organizing the group can help this to be a successful experience.

USING CLINIC SERVICES IN COMMUNITY HEALTH NURSING

Another route community health nurses use to meet the health care needs of people is clinic services.

Clinics, often called *ambulatory health services,* are centers that examine and treat ambulatory clients on an outpatient basis. They are frequently operated under the auspices of a larger institution such as a hospital, medical school, health department, church, or community organization. Defining their services is difficult because they vary from one institution to the next.

The clinic setting offers a wide range of preventive health services. Clinics may provide only primary intervention: this is usually the major focus in immunization clinics. Or clinics may provide screening, diagnosis, and treatment, such as venereal disease clinics, which find the disease, administer appropriate antibiotics, and locate contacts of the infected client for screening.

Clinics may serve only specific populations. Well-baby clinics usually provide assessment for children from birth to 5 years of age, and family planning clinics usually serve females of childbearing age. Other clinics may serve anyone who comes, any time, with any problem, as do walk-in clinics of large teaching hospitals and neighborhood health care centers. Emergency rooms function as ambulatory clinics in many towns where there are no other resources.

The type of care provided may be episodic, where only the immediate needs of the clients are handled, or they may be comprehensive and provide three levels of preventive services: preventive diagnostic, therapeutic, and rehabilitative services.

Fees may be assessed in some clinics. Some have a sliding-scale assessment where clients pay what they can afford. Others are free.

Outpatient care systems (hospital outpatient departments and publicly financed health centers) are the fastest-growing service in the nation's health care systems. Between 1962 and 1973, outpatient visits increased from 71 million to 164 million (U.S. Comptroller General, 1975, p. i). The greatest impact has come from the poor who look to outpatient clinics for primary health care. This is a result of the insufficient numbers of physicians in inner cities to serve the medical needs of this population.

The Beginnings of Nurses in Clinics

Community health nurses have long worked in clinics. Beginning with the era of Lillian Wald, they have had to assume a considerable amount of responsibility, make independent judgments, and use skill in teaching clients. These competencies especially fitted them to work in the relatively independent clinic setting.

One of the earliest demonstrations of the role of the community health nurse in clinics was in 1949, in a large Veterans' Administration Pulmonary Disease Clinic in Los Angeles (Brown, 1971, p. 227). The nurses employed in the clinic worked with tuberculosis clients. They conducted health education sessions based on the needs of the individual clients. They

also served as liaison agents between the clinic and the health departments of the area. In cooperation with the Tuberculosis and Health Association of Los Angeles County, the nurses conducted a survey of the knowledge of and attitudes toward tuberculosis of a large number of clients who attended the clinic.

The expanded role of the nurse, discussed in Chapter 2, has aided community health nurses in more adequately meeting the health care needs of people in clinics. The area of maternal and child health services is an excellent illustration of where community health nurses meet needs utilizing this role. In well-child conferences (defined as a comprehensive evaluation of the emotional, physical, and social gains of a child who is developing normally), nurses do physical examinations, take histories, evaluate neurological, physical, social, and mental aspects of growth and development, and do nutrition counseling. In a setting like this, community health nurses have the opportunity to obtain information on other family members and do case finding. Referrals to other community agencies or for home visits by community health nurses are often made in this way.

Location of Clinic Facilities

The community health nurse may have the opportunity to help plan where ambulatory care facilities will be located and how they will be designed. There is much literature on this subject, but there are several basic principles that will be mentioned.

Location of a clinic affects the way it will be utilized. Some clients are affected more than others by the locations, namely the poor and the old. Difficulty and expense of access are important, so a knowledge of the possible transportation alternatives is important. Accessibility also involves appointment delay time, waiting time, hours when the clinic is open, services offered, health care given, and client relationships. The clinic should have a physically professional and competent appearance as well.

A population group that is fairly homogeneous in sociodemographic terms will not necessarily be homogeneous in the kinds of health care that it desires. Some clients are interested in easy accessibility; others choose a health care site based upon what they feel is good-quality care (Skinner, Price, Scott, and Gorry, 1977, p. 439).

Planning Clinic Facilities

As is the case with developing groups, it is critically important that specific needs and objectives for a clinic be written before planning begins. Prospective clients should be part of the planning team to help ensure that clients' needs can be met through the clinic. One objective for an immunization clinic might be "that all children from birth to 5 years in Smith County will be completely immunized." Prospective clients on planning committees can help to plan clinic locations and times that facilitate reaching this objective.

The steps of the planning process for clinic facilities include the following (Giglio, 1977, p. 14):

Step 1. Define service areas for the clinic which are geographical clusters of the population. Generally service areas are most conveniently defined as census tracts. A census tract contains 4000 to 7000 people, usually three to nine blocks. Chapter 13 describes health systems areas (HSA). Each HSA must assemble and analyze the following data:

1. Status (and determinants) of the health of the residents of its health service area—prevalence and incidence rates can be used to define "status," and measures of relative and attributable risks can help to describe "determinants."

2. Status of the health care delivery system and its use by residents.

3. Effect the area's health care delivery system has on the health of residents—prevalence and incidence rates measured over time and at different levels and quality of service help to measure effectiveness.

4. Number, type, and location of resources.

5. Patterns of utilization by residents.

6. Environmental and occupational exposure factors affecting the immediate and long-run health of residents.

Thus, HSAs should provide valuable data about defining the service area for a clinic.

Step 2. Determine relevant population data which will determine clinic utilization. Census data describes populations in terms of age, sex, race, and economic and social status. The characteristics which significantly affect utilization are sex, age (under 17, 17 to 44, 44 to 63, over 64), and ability to pay. Secondarily, level of education, income, and race are important. The numbers of people in each category should be determined for the coming year and for the next 5 years.

Step 3. Estimate current and projected need. Need is difficult to estimate because a need for one person is not a need for another, and as the health system grows, its services generate new demands. Estimates of demand can be based on *Current Estimates from the Health Interview Survey,* published by the National Center for Health Statistics, Public Health Service (see Table 19-2). These data are limited because they reflect visits to physicians only. If other services are included, such as pediatric nurse practitioner services, the potential numbers in each age category should be multiplied by the actual visits per year to find the estimated need expressed in terms of total visits per year.

TABLE 19-2 Visits per Year to Physician per Population Group

	Under 17	17 to 44	45 to 64	Over 64
Male	4.5	3.5	4.9	6.4
Female	4.0	6.2	6.1	6.8

SOURCE: From R. J. Giglio. *Ambulatory care systems. Volume II: Location, layout, and information systems for efficient operations.* Lexington, Mass.: D. C. Heath, 1977, p. 17.

Planners should have estimates for the current population and for 5-year projections.

Step 4. Current and projected demand. Since need is defined as demand, planners generally can use the figures found in step 3 to serve as demand. However, ability to pay can change these figures: some people in an HSA may be near the poverty line but be ineligible for Medicare and Medicaid. Their visitation value should be reduced 20 to 40 percent. Individuals with more than 12 years' education should have their visitation rates increased 10 percent.

Step 5. Prepare distance tables and timetables. The location of the proposed clinic should be marked on a map and travel time should be estimated. This is a very difficult task since some people will use mass transit, which involves waiting, and others will not perceive distances accurately. Potential clients can help planners with this problem.

Step 6. Evaluate potential sites. Step 5 should be expanded to all potential sites for the clinic so that all possible alternatives are considered.

One health department decided to open a well-baby clinic because they felt that a rural portion of a large county was underserved. Their first move was to send a staff nurse for preparation as a pediatric nurse practitioner. The steps of the planning process were not logically followed and though there actually were no other facilities for well-child care in

the area, the clinic closed because of a lack of clients. It was extremely isolated with no public transportation available, and thus clients did not use the services.

The Role of the Community Health Nurse in the Clinic

The community health nurse can function in various ways to meet the health needs of populations in the clinic setting.

Manager

The role of manager was the main nursing function in clinics for many years. Nurses attended to the many details necessary in order for clinics to run smoothly: distributing client caseload, following up clients with problems, bringing needed reports to physicians, preparing clients physically for exams, performing procedures, supervising aides and practical nurses, and carrying out clerical work. Although all this is necessary, the nurse should perform *nursing* activities, that is, helping clients when they are unable to help themselves. The nurse should supervise other members of the health team as described in Chapter 20 so that they can carry out these other functions. This means that the nurse will understand the different levels of functioning of team members and utilize them appropriately. Clerks and aides as well as as volunteers can be valuable assets in the clinic. They can weigh and measure babies, file and pull records, label and carry specimens to the laboratory, act as receptionists, and take temperatures. Smooth flow of clients from waiting to examining rooms is important and can be done by aides. The community health nurse must understand that she or he is responsible for the care that these team members give. The nurse's supervision of team members is fundamental to the care given clients in the clinic setting.

Group Leader and Teacher

Many clinics have as one of their most important functions group sessions in which information is discussed that is designed to promote health. One example is an ostomy information clinic which disseminates information and helps clients to cope with problems related to their ostomies (Yahle, 1975, p. 457). Another example is a prenatal education program located in a large hospital in New York. The prenatal clinic of the hospital serves 800 clients annually and the prenatal education class capitalizes on the waiting time within the clinic system (Hawkins, 1976, p. 226). The concepts presented earlier in this chapter on developing and leading a group are applicable to the nurse's role in clinics as group leader and teacher.

Practitioner

The expanded role of the nurse has provided nurses with physical assessment skills. They are also able to identify the current health status of clients, including emotional and physical components, and to plan interventions with clients. One adolescent health care clinic offers physical, mental, social, and emotional support to clients between 12 and 19 years old (Sheffield, 1976, p. 93). As with other adolescent clinic populations, many of the clients served in this clinic have psychosocial problems. An interdisciplinary team meets weekly to discuss client needs and to propose alternative solutions which they discuss with the client.

Evaluator

An integral part of working in the clinic setting is evaluation. Are the objectives of the clinic being met? If this is the immunization clinic in Smith County, are children upon school entrance at age 6 completely immunized? Are the numbers of clients being served increasing or decreasing? If the number of clients being served is changing, is it because the health service area population is changing or because clients feel that they are not being served adequately? The way clients feel about the care they receive determines whether or not they will use the health facility. Some method of client contact on a regular basis, either questionnaire or interview, provides data concerning this factor. Knowing who is served also means that a record system will be in operation so that numbers of visits and kinds of visits can be tabulated easily. A good record system will also provide for continuity of care from one visit to the next and yet not be overly time-consuming.

The Future of Clinics

The health care system in the United States is expensive and physician- and disease-oriented, as well as poorly distributed. Clearly, changes need to be made. Garfield (1970) has suggested that a new system be developed that regulates the flow of clients into health centers in a manageable way. His system separates sick clients from well clients by health testing at the point of entry into the health care system (see Figure 19-1). After testing, the client is referred for either sick care, health care, or preventive maintenance. Garfield thinks that National Health Insurance will result in an uncontrolled flood of well, worried-well, early-sick, and sick people into health centers on a first-come, first-served basis that has little relation to need. The result will be an overloaded health care system. His proposal for regulating the flow of clients takes care of this problem.

Although Garfield proposes a physician-dominated delivery system, the possibilities for nurses to function in an innovative system can be exciting if nurses realize the necessity of helping to plan for the future. The health systems agencies of Public Law 93-641, as de-

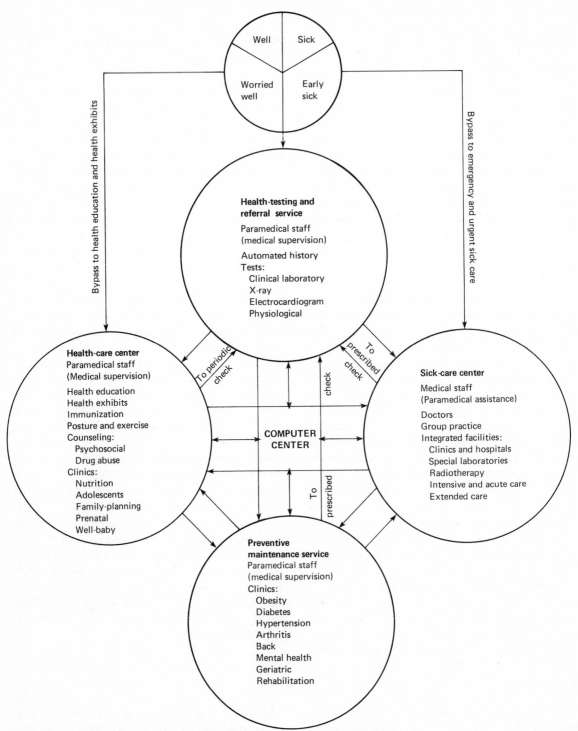

FIGURE 19-1 Proposed health care delivery system with a health-testing service as a new method of entry. (*From S. R. Garfield. The delivery of medical care. Scientific American, April 1970, 222, p. 22.*)

scribed in Chapter 12, provide one mechanism for this planning.

A Final Comment on Group Work and Clinic Services

As adequate finances for health care delivery become a scarcer commodity, health care agencies are moving in the direction of using clinics and groups to meet the needs of people. One large health department in the Midwest uses clinics almost exclusively; home visits to families are a rare occurrence. At a time when each home visit is costing taxpayers up to $60, it is not difficult to see why this is happening.

It is important to remember that no one method will meet everyone's health needs and that nurses need "in every enterprise to consider where you would come out." Families generate as well as help to solve health problems, and this important aspect can be lost in group and clinic work. However, clinics and groups do have a place in health care, and each will likely increase in number. Remember, though, to start with the needs of clients to decide what route to use to assist them. This kind of choice contributes to the challenge, excitement, and creativity of community health nursing.

SUMMARY

Nurses can use many routes to meet the health care needs of clients. Group work and clinic services are two possible routes. Advantages and disadvantages of the group approach are many and nurses need to be familiar with them. Understanding the methodology used to develop a group, the phases of a group, and the functions of the nurse as a group leader is essential if the nurse is going to function effectively in a group setting.

Clinics have long been a place where community health nurses have served varied populations. The location aspect of clinic facilities plays an important part in how well they are utilized. Clinic services need to be well planned if they are to be effective. Thus, it is crucial for the community health nurse to be familiar with the planning process.

The community health nurse carries out multiple roles and functions in the clinic setting—manager, group leader and teacher, practitioner, and evaluator. The nurse's major function is to assist clients to help themselves.

The nurse must learn to appropriately delegate tasks to other members of the health care team, so that she or he has sufficient time to work with clients.

Increasingly, health care agencies are using clinics and groups to meet the needs of populations in the community. It is known, however, that a more effective and efficient health care delivery system must be established if the needs of all are to be met. Garfield has proposed that a new system which regulates the flow of clients into health centers in a more manageable way be developed. He believes that National Health Insurance may cause an overload in the health care system and that planning is crucial to avoid this problem. Garfield's proposal, like so many health care proposals, has not defined an active role for nursing. Nurses must become involved in planning for the future so that a viable role for nursing is built into health care proposals such as the the one suggested by Garfield.

REFERENCES

Brown, E. L. *Nursing reconsidered. A study of change. Part 2: The professional role in community nursing.* Philadelphia: Lippincott, 1971.

Garfield, S. R. The delivery of medical care. *Scientific American,* April 1970, *222,* 15–23.

Giglio, R. J. *Ambulatory care systems. Volume II: Loca-*

tion, layout, and information systems for efficient operations. Lexington, Mass: D. C. Heath, 1977. Reprinted by permission of the publisher.

Hawkins, M. M. Fitting a prenatal education program into the crowded inner city clinic. *American Journal of Maternal Child Nursing,* July–August 1976, *1,* 226–230.

Knopke, H. J., & Diekelmann, N. L. *Approaches to teaching in the health sciences.* Reading, Mass.: Addison-Wesley, 1978.

Lewin, K. Group decision and social change. In T. M. Newcomb and E. L. Hartley (Eds.), *Reading in social psychology.* New York: Holt, 1947.

Loomis, M. E. *Group process for nurses.* St. Louis: Mosby, 1979.

Luft, J. *Group process. An introduction to group dynamics* (2d ed.). Palo Alto, Calif.: Mayfield Publishing Company, 1970.

Marram, G. P. *The group approach in nursing practice* (2d ed.). St. Louis: Mosby, 1978.

Sheffield, R. Teen health service employs team approach. *Hospitals,* Dec. 16, 1976, *50,* 93–98.

Skinner, T. J., Price, B. S., Scott, D. W., & Gorry, G. A. Factors affecting the choice of hospital-based ambulatory care by the urban poor. *American Journal of Public Health,* May 1977, *67,* 439–445.

U.S. Comptroller General. *Outpatient health care in inner cities: Its users, services and problems.* MWP 75-81. Washington, D.C.: Department of Health, Education, and Welfare, 1975.

Yahle, M. E. An ostomy information clinic. *Nursing Clinics of North America,* September 1975, *11,* 457–467.

SELECTED BIBLIOGRAPHY

Brois, D. P., & Mullin, K. R. Cluster clinics create flexibility. *Hospitals,* Feb. 1, 1976, *50,* 117.

Burnside, I. M. *Working with the elderly. Group processes and techniques.* North Scituate, Mass.: Duxbury Press, 1978.

Davis, M. Z., Kramer, M., & Strauss, A. L. *Nurses in practice. A perspective on work environments.* St. Louis: Mosby, 1975.

DesRoches, H. B., & Hughett, B. G. A hospital and a health center establish a group-home program. *Hospitals,* Aug. 16, 1977, *15,* 79–80.

Hinds, M. W. Gonorrhea screening in family planning clinics. When should it become selective? *Public Health Reports,* July–August 1977, *92,* 361–364.

Hughes, C. B. An eclectic approach to parent group education. *Nursing Clinics of North America,* September 1977, *12,* 469–479.

Menning, B. E. Resolve—A support group for nurses. *American Journal of Nursing,* February 1976, *76,* 258–259.

Morris, A. G. The use of the well-baby clinic to promote early intellectual development via parent education. *American Journal of Public Health,* January 1976, *66,* 73–74.

Myers, S. A. Diabetes management by the patient and a nurse practitioner. *Nursing Clinics of North America,* September 1977, *12,* 415–426.

Parsons, J. A new approach to group learning. *Journal of Continuing Education in Nursing,* 1978, *7,* 5–9.

Peterson, L. D., & Green, J. H. Nurse managed TB clinic. *American Journal of Nursing,* March 1977, *77,* 433–435.

Plant, J. Teaching hospital nurtures growth of community oncology clinics. *Hospitals,* March 16, 1978, *52,* 151.

Ruddock, R. Working with groups. *Nursing Mirror,* March 2, 1978, 38–40.

Segal, G. S. Verbal behavior and group process. *Health Education,* September–October 1977, 13–14.

Shaw, M. E. *Group dynamics. The psychology of group behavior.* New York: McGraw-Hill, 1976.

Strow, C., & MacKreth, R. Family group meetings. Strengthening a partnership. *Journal of Gerontological Nursing*, January–February 1977, *3*, 30–35.

Sweeney, B. Learning groups: Survival level, growth level. *Journal of Nursing Education*, August 1975, *14*, 20–26.

Szasz, T. S., & Hollander, M. H. A contribution to the philosophy of medicine. *Archives of Internal Medicine*, 1956, *116*, 585–592.

Vorzimer, J. J. *Coordinated ambulatory care: The POMR*. New York: Appleton-Century-Crofts, 1976.

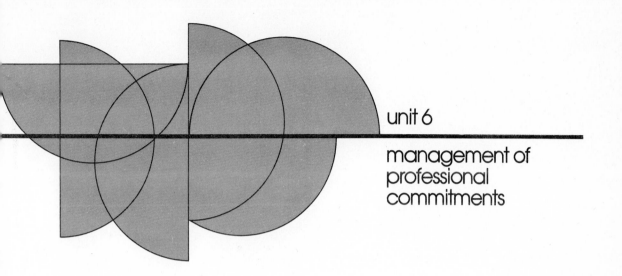

unit 6

management of
professional
commitments

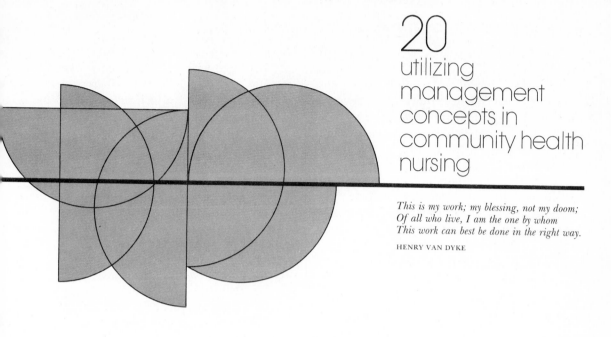

20
utilizing
management
concepts in
community health
nursing

This is my work; my blessing, not my doom;
Of all who live, I am the one by whom
This work can best be done in the right way.
HENRY VAN DYKE

The community is a challenging setting which provides much professional independence for the community health nurse. An outstanding characteristic of community health nursing is the independence of its practitioners. In any one day, a community health nurse may decide what families to visit and in what order they will be visited. During that day, the nurse may make a nursing diagnosis and carry out nursing interventions without nursing supervision, without a doctor's order, or without even talking to another nurse. That day, he or she may also receive new referrals and make decisions on their priority. Furthermore, the nurse may be carrying out nursing care indirectly through delegation to registered nurses, licensed practical nurses, or home health aides. When these health personnel are caring for clients under the nurse's supervision, the nurse is responsible for the care given by them.

This independence and delegation in com-munity health nursing practice must be accompanied by knowledge of management concepts. Knowledge of management concepts helps the community health nurse to provide care, directly and indirectly, to families and population groups. Understanding management helps the nurse to evaluate the quality of health services that the client receives. Available resources, such as finances and personnel, need to be managed so that maximum productivity, efficiency, and quality of care are achieved.

This chapter will briefly analyze concepts of management and then examine how community health nurses can utilize them. A limited discussion of the historical development of management thought will also be shared. Knowledge of the evolution of management concepts provides the information an individual needs in order to formulate a personal philosophy of management.

THE HISTORICAL DEVELOPMENT OF MANAGEMENT CONCEPTS

There are numerous leaders in the field of management who contributed to its development. To list them all here would be an almost impossible task. When reviewing the development of management thought, however, one can see that modern concepts of management have evolved over time. Historically, emphasis was placed on analyzing the functions and processes of management tasks, without taking into consideration the needs of the worker (see Chapter 16). Today, there is a trend for managers to apply systems concepts (see Chapter 6) in the work environment in order to determine how to maintain employee satisfaction and to increase productivity and efficiency.

Frederick Taylor is the founder of the scientific management movement. His belief was that the planning of tasks needed to be separated from their performance. In relation to this thought, he felt that managers should be responsible for the planning and controlling of tasks and that employee's should assume responsibility for production. He conducted time and motion studies to determine the best way to accomplish tasks, to develop work standards, and to identify how to divide the work between managers and employees. Taylor's book, *The Principles of Scientific Management,* was published in 1911 (Kazmier, 1974, p. 4). This book provides a more detailed description of his ideas.

Henri Fayol expanded on Taylor's thoughts by identifying a composite of very well defined functions and tasks for managers. In 1916 he published his ideas about management, which were that managers had five basic functions: planning, organizing, command, coordination, and control (Longest, 1976, p. 39). With some minor changes in this list, these functions are still used by most authorities on management.

Significant criticism of management occurred during the first half of the twentieth century, because managers emphasized task performance without looking at worker satisfaction. As a result of this criticism, modern management trends which stressed the importance of examining employee needs emerged. The classic Hawthorne experiment conducted by Elton Mayo clearly demonstrated to management the value of looking at employees as people.

The Hawthorne studies of the Western Electric Company during the 1920s and 1930s applied the principles of psychology, social psychology, and sociology to the understanding of organizational behavior. The researchers of this study started out investigating the relationship between physical conditions of work and employee productivity; however, they found that social variables were much more important to productivity. The outgrowth of the Hawthorne study was the development of the concept of human relations, or the study of human behavior for the purposes of attaining higher production levels and personal satisfaction (Kazmier, 1974, p. 12). The human relations concept has expanded into the behavioral science approach to management. A trend toward emphasizing employee satisfaction to increase production on the job can still be seen today. Employee motivation, the workplace as a social system, leadership within the organization, communication within the system, and personal and professional employee development are five major areas of concern to managers who use behavioral science methods and principles. Writings by Chris Argyris, Chester Barnard, Douglas McGregor, Kurt Lewin, Rensis Likert, Robert Tannenbaum, and others give a more in-depth perspective on the behavioral science movement.

The systems approach to management is the most recent development among management concepts (Kazmier, 1974, p. 16). With the systems approach, both the structure and the processes of an organization are analyzed. Emphasis is placed on examining how all the parts of an organization interact and interrelate to achieve the goals of the organization. Systems managers recognize that a change in one part of the organizational system affects all the other parts, just as practitioners using a systems approach recognize that a change (illness) in the family unit affects all other members of the family system.

Today, community health nurses work in complex systems. To function effectively in these modern health care systems, the community health nurse must know not only nursing theory but management theory as well. Traditionally, management concepts were not emphasized during a nurse's academic study, even though nurses were expected to fill management positions in practice. Now it is recognized that the task of organizing health care delivery can be made easier and more powerful with knowledge of management concepts. That is why principles of management are covered during a nurse's basic educational preparation.

THE ORGANIZATIONAL STRUCTURE OF HEALTH CARE DELIVERY

There are an increasing number of health care delivery systems in which the community health nurse may work. Table 2-1 in Chapter 2 delineates many of the places where community health nurses give client services.

Nurses must know the organizational structure of their employing agencies so that they can determine how to utilize agency resources and to identify appropriate ways to effect change within the organization. Organizational structure encompasses the formal and informal patterns of behavior and relationships in an organization. This includes both formal and informal position allocations, as well as the chain of command and the channels of communication.

The Informal Organizational Structure

The informal organizational structure refers to the personal and social relationships of people who work together. Informal relationships have no formal power. However, they can have a major impact on the organization and its management. The way in which a manager is viewed by the staff does influence the manner and effectiveness of her or his management.

The Formal Organizational Structure

Formal organizational structure defines what people will do which tasks so that the objectives of the organization can be accomplished. It is basically the power structure of the organization. The rules, policies, procedures, control mechanisms, and financial arrangements of the organization are all part of the formal structure (Kast and Rosenzweig, 1974, p. 208). The schematic organization is part of this formal structure and can be seen in an organizational chart.

Organizational Chart

An organizational chart diagrams the relationship between members of the organization and indicates the structure of authority, formal lines of communication, and levels of management and delegation. These all interrelate to accomplish the goals of the organization. An example of an organizational chart is presented in Figure 20-1.

An organizational manual supplements an organizational chart by supplying information about the requirements of the various job positions represented on the chart. Organiza-

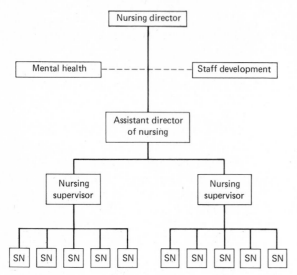

FIGURE 20-1 An organizational chart showing staff and line positions. SN = staff nurse. Line positions: nursing director, assistant director, nursing supervisor, staff nurse. Staff positions: mental health consultant, staff development director.

tional charts and manuals are useful tools which describe the formal relationships in a particular organization. They do not show the informal relationships that exist.

Usually there are two types of positions in an organization: *staff* and *line*. Figure 20-1 shows how staff and line positions are depicted on an organizational chart. The line structure is the basic framework of an organizational structure. The staff nurse is in a direct line position and is accountable to the person directly above him or her on the organizational chart. The term *staff nurse* should not be confused with *staff personnel*. The staff personnel supplement the line personnel in an advisory capacity. They are extensions of the administrator but usually have no authority to direct the actions of persons in the line position. Authority can, however, be delegated in several directions from both staff and line positions.

The line organization is characterized by a direct flow of authority from top to bottom.

Each position has general authority over the one directly below it. Authority is inherent in line positions. For example, the assistant director of nursing has authority over the nursing supervisor who in turn has authority over the staff nurse. Persons in staff positions, on the other hand, are delegated authority by top-level administrators (nursing director) to carry out specific tasks and responsibilities. Authority is not inherent in staff positions.

A manager must have a basic understanding of organizational power relationships in order to manage effectively. Four types of power relationships evolve in any organization:

1. Authority: the power to direct the actions of others

2. Responsibility: the obligation to carry out or perform tasks in an acceptable way

3. Accountability: the obligation to answer for one's actions

4. Delegation: assigning and empowering one person to act for another with the responsibility for the act remaining with the person who assigned it

Organizational structure and resulting power relationships in a health care agency assist personnel in all positions to carry out effectively the functions of management. It would be impossible to "manage" if such a structure did not exist. Effective and efficient management can occur only when personnel understand what they are responsible for and to whom they are accountable. Ignoring the power relationships in an organization can create real difficulties. Illustrative of this are the actions taken by the community health nurse in the following situation.

A community health nurse identified a need for a family planning program in two of the census tracts she served. Knowing that the county health department did not include these services, she independently arranged a group meeting in the club-house at a local park to discuss the need for these services with the people of the community. This was done without discussing the action with her supervisor.

Twenty community members attended the meeting. They quickly became emotionally involved in the issue and wanted immediate action taken by the health department to initiate such a service. The nurse became uncomfortable because she recognized that she did not have the power to make a definite commitment to establish a new program. The community members became frustrated with the nurse's lack of action.

Had proper channels within the agency power structure been utilized, this situation would probably have been handled differently.

When looking at this situation, one can quickly ask the following questions: Did the nurse have the authority to organize this meeting, and was she acting in a responsible and an accountable manner? What were her objectives for the meeting and did she clarify them for herself and the group?

When one is planning a meeting with a group such as the one above, it is crucial to seek the advice of individuals within the organization who have the authority to make decisions. When this is not done, it can result in stress and frustration for all parties involved. If the nurse had gone to her supervisor prior to the meeting, she would have been aware of the types of commitments she could make during the meeting. If, for instance, the health department did not have adequate resources to staff a family planning clinic, the group goal might be to look at alternative ways to obtain funding for family planning services in the community, rather than only to discuss how the health department could provide these services.

Organizational Policies

Another component of the formal organization structure which maximizes functioning is organizational policies. Policies define the limits of acceptable activities and provide structure and guidelines for employee decision making. They are generally developed to handle situations that occur consistently in daily practice. Policies that address how to handle referrals (see Chapter 9), when and how to conduct nursing audits (see Chapter 21), and benefits staff will have, such as travel allowance, are a few examples of policies commonly found in a community health agency that can make an impact on staff decision making.

When policies are absolute, with no flexibility, they are considered rules. Rules are usually established in order to ensure client and staff safety and quality of care. The following are examples of rules:

· "No home visits are to be made at night in census tract 3 without an escort."

· "No immunizations are to be given until an allergy history has been taken."

· "Every fifth record closed to service must be audited."

When nurses accept employment within a health setting, it is assumed that they accept responsibility for following, enforcing, and informing others about agency policies. This means that the conditions of employment should be clearly understood before the nurse accepts a position within an organization. Otherwise, the nurse may be in a situation where it is necessary to follow certain policies that are inconsistent with her or his philosophy of practice.

Nursing personnel at all levels may be involved in writing policies. Policy statements should include the following items:

1. Reason for establishing the policy (philosophy behind the policy)

2. Actual policy statement

3. Guidelines for implementing the policy

If used effectively, policies can increase the efficiency and ease with which individuals carry out their functions within an organization. Difficulties with implementing a policy will occur, however, if employees do not un-

derstand the reason for the policy, if employee input is not obtained when the policy is being formulated, if the policy is not clearly written, or if policies become numerous and prevent necessary flexibility for nursing practice.

DEFINING MANAGEMENT

Management is the planning, organizing, directing, coordinating, and controlling of activities in a system so that the objectives of that system are met. For community health nurses, that system may be represented by any number of settings in which the nurse practices, such as a public health agency, ambulatory care setting, a school, or an industrial plant.

Administration is a term that is often mistakenly used interchangeably with *management*. The principles of management and administration are the same, but the scope of functioning for managers and administrators varies. For instance, both administrators and

managers set goals, but the administrator sets goals for a department, whereas a staff nurse sets personal goals.

Administration is more comprehensive and includes such executive activities as setting goals and formulating policy, as well as managing personnel and materials. Thus, a director of nursing is an administrator who sets goals, formulates policy, and manages the nurses who provide care, or in some institutions, participates in these decision-making processes with other departmental administrators on behalf of the nursing department. (Clark and Shea, 1979, p. 6)

THE MANAGEMENT FUNCTIONS OF THE COMMUNITY HEALTH NURSE

The five management functions carried out by the community health nurse are planning, organizing, directing, coordinating, and controlling. These management functions help to link the entire organizational system together and assist the nurse in effectively managing workload responsibilities. Managing is done on many levels by nurses, depending upon their place in the organizational structure as well as their interest, skills, and educational background.

The director of nursing in an agency will probably spend more time in managing than the staff nurse, and at a level which affects all staff members. Staff nurses must, however, utilize management functions to deliver nursing services. They can also influence how a director of nurses carries out management functions.

Management is a process which has both interpersonal and technical aspects and which utilizes human, physical, and technological resources to achieve well-defined goals (Longest, 1976, p. 38). Figure 20-2 depicts all the variables that influence how the manager implements the five functions of management. It also illustrates the cyclical nature of the management process (planning, organizing, directing, coordinating, and controlling); the functions overlap and do not always follow a sequential pattern.

Planning

Planning means deciding in advance what must be done and what the organization wants to achieve. Without planning, no set goals will be accomplished.

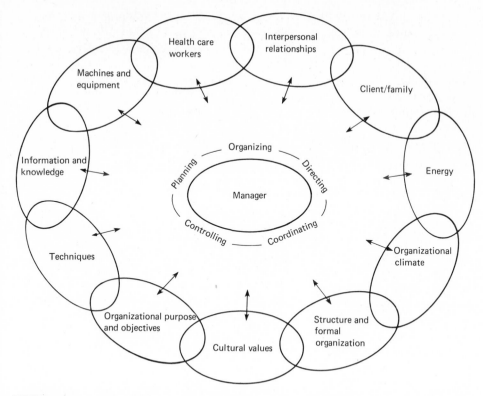

FIGURE 20-2 The manager links together subsystems of the organization. *(From C. C. Clark & C. A. Shea. Management in Nursing. A Vital Link in the Health Care System. New York: McGraw-Hill, 1979, p. 9.)*

Planning gives purpose and direction to the decision-making process. It is the management function most often neglected because of emphasis placed upon carrying out day-to-day activities, the attitude that planning takes too much time, and the tendency for an individual to resist change. Planning is an important activity because it helps the organization to remain dynamic, to identify standards, and to determine what or who requires organization or direction. It increases the likelihood that activities will be orderly, predictable, and less costly. Most important, planning improves the quality and effectiveness of nursing care. Although planning does not guarantee the quality of outcomes, the evaluation aspects of this process help a manager to identify strengths and needs within the organization.

Health care planning should include both the provider and the consumer. Emergencies may necessitate individual decision making and planning. In these situations, it is important for the decision maker to explain to others involved in the process the circumstances and reasons for the emergency decision.

Planning uses past, present, and future information projections to determine what services should be. Currently, the impact of political, social, economic, and technical forces are directly influencing the types of services provided by community health agencies and the type of personnel needed to implement these services. For instance, in health departments that provide bedside care, money allocated from taxes is increasingly scarce and third-party payments for home health care are an increasingly larger part of the health department budget. This budget change comes about because of demographic changes in the population as well as social and political policy about the appropriateness of tax money for tertiary health care. Some of the results of these changes include a greater emphasis on delivering home health care, greater use of ancillary personnel such as home health aides, and a greater focus on older people who need "hands-on" care rather than on clients who need health teaching and anticipatory guidance.

Careful planning is needed to successfully implement nursing services when the focus of these services has changed. Activities such as in-service education for staff, planning for increased time for the supervision of home health aides, and the added paperwork involved in carrying out a home health care program are a few examples of factors that should be considered when one is planning for increased home health services.

An example of when a staff nurse would put the planning process into action would be when working with the nursing supervisor to establish a well-child conference in the staff nurse's area. Together they would develop a written plan which would include the following:

1. Specific, measurable objectives related to establishment of the conference

2. Time schedule for achieving objectives

3. Process for carrying out the objectives, including necessary resources

4. Evaluation methods to measure the success of the plan in relation to completion of objectives

5. Timetable for periodic evaluation

A staff community health nurse also implements the planning function when structuring the workday and when carrying out caseload management activities. The data gathering, diagnosis, and goal-setting phases of the nursing process are used by the community health nurse to develop plans for activities such as those described above.

During planning, many needs and goals may be identified and priorities for them must be set. The following points should be considered when priorities are being set.

Economic impact. Considering the results if something is done or is not done is crucial. Although an immunization campaign against rubella may be costly, it is much less expensive socially and economically than paying for the care of children who have congenital deformities resulting from in utero rubella. The cost-benefit aspect must also be considered. In one community, for instance, the health department discontinued a screening clinic for the geriatric population because it was not cost-effective. It cost the health department $40 per client to do the screening, and 90 percent of those screened had recently received the same screening from their private physicians and planned to do so again in the future. This was duplication of services at a high cost to the health department. Methods other than a screening clinic could be utilized to reach the 10 percent of the population not receiving the screening privately.

Practicality. Is the program necessary? What is being done currently? Will enough people benefit from it to make it worthwhile? Are there sufficient resources available, such as work force and money, to accomplish the stated goals? Is there enough organizational and community support to carry out the program? Does it meet the needs of the community? All of these are questions to be answered in relation to the practicality of the program.

Feasibility. Does the program fit the organizations policies and priorities? Are the resources available to carry out the program?

Legal mandates. The organization must follow its legal mandates. The official health department, for example, has a legal mandate to control communicable disease.

Urgency of the situation. An emergency situation is usually given top priority. In one urban community, for instance, a large Mexican restaurant used home-canned chili peppers that were improperly prepared. Many of the restaurant's patrons developed botulism. This produced an emergency health situation which required urgent action to pinpoint the source of the poisoning and all patrons affected by the botulism organism. The county health department launched an immediate epidemiological investigation to pinpoint the cause. Many other health department activities were stopped or modified so that this serious problem could be given priority. Once priorities have been established, a manager must organize activities so that priority goals can be implemented.

Organizing

Organizing determines how a manager implements planning to achieve stated goals. The organizational structure, as previously discussed, facilitates decision making and assigning of tasks. There are three principal components of any organizational structure: people, work, and relationships. The interrelationship of these three variables is analyzed during the organizing phase to determine the best way to organize activities. A manager's major concerns when organizing are fourfold:

1. *Analysis of the system:* identifying strengths and needs of the present system in order to make it more effective and efficient in the future. Comparing present staff capabilities to the needs evidenced by clients being served is one example of how a system is analyzed.

2. *Analysis of functions:* defining all the tasks that are involved in a particular job and determining the relationships between various jobs. A nurse and supervisor analyzing a staff nurse's responsibilities when she or he has a caseload of 8 bedside-care clients, 40 families needing health supervision, and work in 6 schools and 2 clinics weekly is an example of this principle.

3. *Assigning job responsibilities:* grouping tasks to minimize duplication of effort and assigning responsibilities to individuals who have the knowledge and competence to carry out the job. Responsibility and authority limits should be clearly defined. Again, work with clients who need bedside care illustrates this principle. The home health aide should be assigned only basic physical care and the community health nurse should assess and supervise the care given by the home health aide.

4. *Implementation:* developing an atmosphere which allows for successful completion of the work to be done by identifying the structure of authority and support mechanisms in the system. Team meetings that provide support, case consultation, and identification of needs illustrate this concept.

Organizing requires a cooperative effort by a health care team working together to obtain the goals of the organization. This managerial function is familiar to community health nurses because they must organize the care of a family around the family's expressed needs and the resources of the health team working with them.

Directing

The purpose of directing is to convey to workers what has occurred during the planning and organizing phases of management. The activities of directing include order giving, direction, leadership, motivating, and communicating (Longest, 1976, p. 45).

Order giving involves helping an employee to identify what needs to be done in a way that fosters understanding and acceptance. A community health nurse who clearly and completely tells an aide the details of the physical care needed by a client with a cerebrovascular accident and also allows the aide to ask questions and to provide input illustrates how effective order giving can be accomplished.

Direction refers to the effort made in an organization to ensure that all the work is done. Personal and professional guidance for people is basic to the concept of direction. In the community health setting, work activities are focused on the provision of services both to families and to the community. Thus, the focus of direction should include guidance which helps staff to effectively intervene both with families and with the community. This aids staff to provide the services and helps an agency to achieve stated goals.

Employees are more likely to carry out directions if they understand the justification for them and if there is no doubt regarding what is expected to be done. If directions are clearly given, there should not be a need for constant supervision or follow-up.

Leadership is the ability to influence and inspire others to reach the objectives of the organization. Success in leadership is the result of interaction between a leader and those for whom the leader is responsible in a work situation. No single type of leadership is always successful. Rather, a successful leader chooses a method that works for her or him in a particular situation. Leadership is critical to the climate of the organization. Leaders can command people to do things, but the most effective style is to lead so that people want to reach organizational objectives. A successful leader develops a style that fits him or her and the

situation. A nursing leader, for instance, may be directive (authoritative or dictatorial) with new nursing staff members because they need more structure in an unfamiliar work environment and democratic with more experienced staff members because they need less direction. Both of these styles can be appropriate. The leader must decide what to use and when. Each person in a leadership position should analyze her or his own assumptions and develop a style that is comfortable and meets the needs of the situation.

Motivating focuses on analyzing the needs of individual workers. Maslow's hierarchy of needs can provide a theoretical framework for examining worker needs. Maslow has developed a priority schema based on a continuum of needs beginning with those that are physiological and ending with self-actualization. He believes that a worker must satisfy lower-level needs (physiological) before the higher-level ones (self-actualization) become significant (Maslow, 1954). When working with other employees or when analyzing one's own behavior in the job setting, it may be found that work is not satisfying because lower-level needs are not being met. If this is the case, an effective manager would attempt to build into the management system rewards that would help the employee to meet these basic human needs.

McGregor (1960) has done considerable research looking at the effect of management attitudes upon employee motivation. His studies have provided the X and Y theories of motivation. Theory X illustrates a negative attitude in its assumptions about human nature, and theory Y reflects positive attitudes about human nature (McGregor, 1960, pp. 33–35, 45, 49).

Theory X makes the following assumptions:

1. The average human being has an inherent dislike of work and will avoid it if at all possible.

2. Most people must be coerced, controlled,

directed, or threatened with punishment to get them to put forth adequate effort toward achievement of organizational objectives.

3. The average human being prefers to be directed, wishes to avoid responsibility, has relatively little ambition, and wants security above all.

Theory Y makes the following assumptions:

1. The expenditure of physical and mental effort is as natural as play or rest.

2. A person will exercise self-direction and self-control in the service of objectives to which that person is committed.

3. Commitment to objectives is a function of the rewards associated with their achievement.

4. The average human being learns, under proper conditions, not only to accept but to seek responsibility.

5. The capacity to exercise a relatively high degree of imagination, ingenuity, and creativity in the solution of organizational problems is widely, not narrowly, distributed in the population.

6. Under the conditions of modern industrial life, the intellectual potential of the average human being is only partially utilized.

McGregor promoted theory Y for the development of a directing style that would motivate employees. It is a more positive approach to working with people. McGregor's theories, like Maslow's framework, can be used as guidelines for managers.

When using any set of guidelines to develop a management style, it is necessary to remember that work is more satisfying when workers are able to meet their own needs in the work situation. The nurse gives care to, and cares about, clients daily, and this is emotionally taxing. The needs of the nurse must also be met in the work setting.

Communicating with workers is crucial. The manager must be able to convey what is to be done, how it is to be done, who is to do it, and why it is to be done and to provide feedback on the activity. This feedback should emphasize the strengths, as well as the weaknesses, inherent in the employee's activity. The interviewing skills that are a primary tool of community health nurses should be used in communicating with health care workers. These skills will help the manager to direct, coordinate, and control activities within the organization.

Coordination

Coordination links people on the health care team together to function in such a way that objectives are achieved. A problem arises when health care workers look at objectives in different ways. One nurse may consider nursing in the school setting as a low priority. The supervisor may think it a high priority. Thus, coordinating can mean managing conflict. Conflict can promote growth but it can also reduce productivity. Effective coordination reduces and prevents growth-restricting conflict.

Controlling

Controlling is a process that measures and corrects the activities of people and establishes standards so that objectives are reached. The controlling function has three steps: establishing standards, measuring performance criteria, and correcting deviations from normal (Longest, 1976, p. 49). The nursing audit, described in Chapter 21, is an example of a controlling function, as is a supervisory or evaluation conference between a staff nurse and a supervisor.

The following are the six characteristics of effective control:

1. *Adjustability:* a control mechanism must be flexible enough to respond to changing situations.

2. *Purposefulness:* a control measure should focus on a specific problem area, not an entire system.

3. *Practicality:* a control measure should not be instituted until it can be implemented reasonably.

4. *Meaningfulness:* a control measure must give direction to other controls and activities, not work against them.

5. *Enforceability:* a control measure should not be instituted until it is possible to put it into effect and to carry out the mandates of the control.

6. *Congruence:* the control measure should be consistent with other control measures and allow the manager to perform other responsibilities and activities.

The staff nurse who delegates care to a home health aide can utilize these characteristics of control so that quality care is given consistently. The nurse and aide must be flexible in their expectations of each other; an aide who has an ill child at home may not work as well on that day as on another. If the nurse is concerned about a particular client care problem, such as the aide's lack of understanding about maintaining skin integrity, she or he can utilize conference time to discuss that problem but should not bring all other concerns to the conference. The nurse needs the supervisor's support when working with the home health aide so that the solutions to the nurse's concerns are enforceable and not opposed by the supervisor.

The controlling function can provide direction for growth and thus should be considered a positive function. Strengths of workers as well as areas of concern are important to examine when one is implementing the controlling function of management.

APPLYING MANAGEMENT CONCEPTS IN COMMUNITY HEALTH NURSING

In the community health nursing setting, nurses have multiple responsibilities. They may have a large number of families in their caseload as well as a number of other nursing services to be performed. In addition, community health nurses need to develop collaborative relationships with other disciplines in order to coordinate family care and to establish priorities for home visits and other activities, such as school and clinic services. Community health nurses must also learn how to effectively delegate tasks to other nursing personnel.

Organizing and scheduling community health nursing activities is not an easy task for an experienced practitioner and, therefore, it is often overwhelming to a new staff member.

These activities are easier to handle, however, if a new staff member applies management concepts while carrying out daily responsibilities.

Using Planning Functions of Management as a Staff Nurse

The nurse can more readily carry out responsibilities if the following planning activites of management are utilized.

Scheduling Regular Conferences with the Nursing Supervisor

This can assist in analyzing the nurse's caseload responsibilities and in establishing priorities for service (Figure 20-3). With the supervisor's help, the nurse should do both a case analysis of each family that is being seen and a caseload analysis of all the work that is being done.

Case analysis: The nurse should learn to "diagnose" each case by answering questions such as the following:

1. What are the health problems of this family as viewed by the family and the nurse?

2. What resources does the family have for meeting these problems?

3. What movement does the family wish to make?

4. What resources are there in the community for meeting these needs?

5. What nursing activities are needed to contribute to the solution of the problems and to bring family and community resources into proper relationship with family needs?

6. Are there some parts of the problems or needs which cannot be met at present with the resources available?

7. What has the family done to work toward solving the problem?

This case analysis should be done on a periodic basis, at least every 6 months, so that families who do not wish to make progress can be closed to service until such time as they wish to again work on an area of need. In addition, case analysis helps nurses to look at their approach to families and alter it so that they can be more effective. A written summary, as well as supervisory conferences, facilitates case analyses. A written summary of work with a family, after a given number of visits in a specified time frame, aids nurses to organize their care and their work. In general, nurses find it valuable to summarize a family record after 10 visits have been made or after they have seen

the family for 6 months. The controlling function of management is in effect when case analysis is done because work with clients is being measured and corrected.

Caseload analysis. Study of the caseload will also improve the planning ability of the nurse and will reveal gaps in service. A caseload analysis differs from a case analysis in that it focuses more on examining the quantity of work the nurse is responsible for and the multiple activities assigned than on the needs of individual families. Caseload analysis is done to determine whether a nurse has sufficient time to implement all assigned responsibilities, to ascertain whether time is being used effectively and efficiently, and to identify whether the needs present in a caseload of families reflect the needs of the population being served. Analysis of the caseload may be in relation to many aspects of service—the types and numbers of cases carried, the complexity of problems in the cases visited, the age groups served, the proportion of new referrals received, and the number of emergency or crisis situations, such as individuals with positive sputums for tuberculosis. In addition, it examines all the other activities a nurse engages in, such as school visits, clinic services, group work, committee meetings, coordination with other community agencies, and recording and planning time. When the caseload is studied, it is wise to graph or tabulate the findings so that they may be readily used and compared with caseloads in other areas or with the same area over time.

Simultaneous caseload study by several nurses may be encouraged occasionally to give a general picture of the services provided by the health agency and to allow for comparisons between nurses. When this was done in one health department, it was found that 2 out of 15 census tracts had a disproportionate number of referrals. The result was that workload assignments were reallocated so that work was more evenly divided. The strength of such

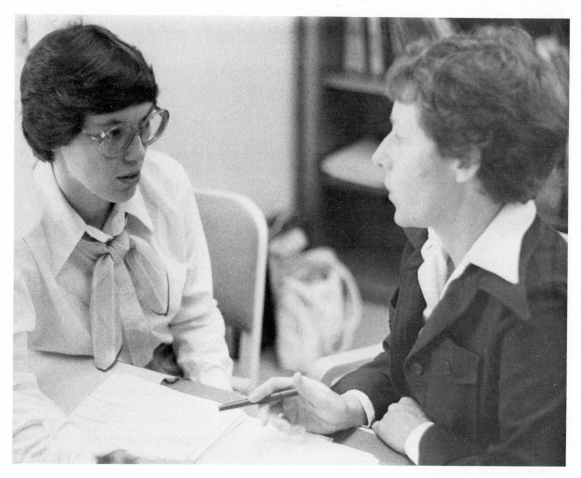

FIGURE 20-3 Staff nurse and supervisor in conference.

a procedure is its usefulness for the individual nurse to identify the uniqueness of cases in her or his own area and to examine if there is adequate time to handle the demands of the workload. Nurses should not try to develop an "average" in the caseloads they carry but to develop a caseload pattern which will provide optimum community service (Freeman, 1949, p. 358). When making comparisons, nurses must keep in mind that caseloads should reflect community needs and population characteristics (see Chapter 11 for how one deter-

mines these needs and characteristics). One nurse may have a higher geriatric clientele than another nurse because of the uniqueness of the census tract she or he serves.

Use a Tickler System

A tickler system is a card file wherein each family in the nurse's caseload has an identification card displaying data such as name, address, telephone number, and service classification. It assists in scheduling family visits and determining what families need service and when, as well as the type of service needed. When a nurse makes a home visit, the date of this visit and the month and day for the next visit are indicated on the card. The card is then placed under the appropriate month in an index file box. If a tickler system is used effectively, a new nurse can quickly identify priorities for home visiting by noting how frequently the previous nurse visited a family and when the nurse planned the next visit. When a staff nurse has a caseload of families, an organized method such as a tickler file for determining when to see whom is essential.

Set Priorities

This allows the nurse to put activities in their order of importance (caseload priority). The following should be considered when one is establishing priorities:

Nursing knowledge. The nurse has a strong theoretical background on which to base priorities for nursing service. This knowledge helps the nurse to analyze the nursing service needs of families who have particular types of problems and directs interventions as well. The developmental framework discussed in Chapters 12 through 18 of this book, along with the nurse's knowledge of crisis theory, for instance, helps a nurse to identify problems across the lifespan that present stress, and in some cases, crisis. For example, a single, pregnant adolescent may receive higher priority than a 25-year-old pregnant married person. The first client is dealing with the developmental tasks of two age periods—the adolescent and the young adult—and thus is more likely to experience a crisis than the 25-year-old, who is dealing with developmental tasks of only one age period.

Third-party payers. To be reimbursed by third-party payers for nursing services, the community health nurse must follow established guidelines. For instance, Medicare requires a home visit within a specified time of hospital discharge. If a visit is not made within the appropriate time frame, Medicare will not pay for nursing services. Nurses do need to be aware of and consider the financial input into their organization so that they meet the requirements established by funders. An organization cannot run without adequate funding.

Community needs. Statistical data, input from consumers, and reports from other professionals can often alert the community health nurse to critical community problems or lack of health services in certain areas. For example, if the herd immunity for polio is 10 percent in a certain section of a county, the community health nurse needs to spend time planning for the provision of immunization service to the total population in this section of the county. This may leave the nurse less time for home visiting. In the long run, however, an immunization campaign could reduce the time the nurse needs for home visits. It takes far more time to individually contact families who need to up-date their immunization status than to conduct a mass campaign which alerts the total community to the need for immunization protection.

Agency policies and priorities. A community health nurse is responsible for following agency policy. Some agency policies read: "Premature infants should be seen weekly for 6 weeks" or "All newborns in the community are to be visited once." If the nurse finds, after analyzing the caseload, that it is impossible to implement an agency policy, she or he should not ignore the policy, but rather take concrete action to see that it is changed. Many agencies, for instance, have recently found that it is impossible to visit all newborns in the community because of the other needs present in the community.

Unfortunately, sometimes it is found that an old policy is not changed because staff do not take the initiative to have it changed. This can create frustration, especially if staff members are trying to implement an unrealistic policy.

Nursing services should also reflect agency priorities and, hopefully, these priorities will coincide with communities' needs. If a community has a high geriatric population, a health department may place priority on delivering service, such as home health care to the elderly. If an agency places a high priority on home health services, the staff nurse will have to schedule other health supervision visits (maternal-child health, school health, mental health) around home health services. If, on the other hand, community statistics reflect high infant and maternal mortality rates, maternal-child health cases at risk may receive top priority for follow-up. Priorities may vary from one census tract to another, depending on the needs evidenced in each census tract.

Legal mandates. Communicable disease follow-up is mandated to the official health department by law and as such must receive priority when caseload needs are analyzed. Communicable disease follow-up is also a high priority because of its potential threat to the community.

Agency resources

1. *Staffing:* The availability of health personnel influences the type of services that can be provided. Where limited personnel and other resources exist, only clinic and crisis intervention services may be provided. If only limited resources are available, the community health nurse will have to examine carefully what nursing services are essential and how the most people can be reached in the time available. Some agencies have increased clinic services and group work and decreased home visits because of personnel shortages. If changes such as these do not meet the needs of the population being served, careful documentation may help the agency to obtain additional resources. Too often, however, nurses and other health professionals accept their current state and fail to document the need for increased resources.

2. *Funding:* Financing can affect the type and amount of staffing available within a health agency and also the type of services provided by a particular department. Health departments and visiting nurse associations have been able to expand nursing personnel in the past several years as a result of the increased funding for home health service (bedside nursing care) and EPDST screening through Medicaid. When the nursing division in a health agency contracts for special services, such as school health, family planning, EPDST screening, and home health services, there usually are conditions for the type of services which need to be provided, as well as a time frame designating when these services should be delivered. Health departments, for example, are sometimes paid for school health services by the board of education. Nurses in these instances may be required to visit the schools at least once a week from September through June.

Use Data from Time and Cost Studies

This is useful in determining the average time needed to accomplish certain nursing activities and costs related to these activities. Time studies help a new nurse to be more realistic about the quantity of service that can be provided and the cost of the service being delivered. Time studies are not designed to evaluate the performance of an individual staff nurse. They are done to analyze the average time it takes for all staff members to accomplish certain activities. Even though they are time-consuming and taxing, time studies are extremely valuable because they help a staff nurse and the nursing division to gain a better perspective on the cost-effectiveness of nursing service. In addition, time studies can provide the documentation needed to request additional funding for increased personnel and resources. They also provide guidelines that help a nurse to schedule nursing activities more efficiently.

Factors to Consider when Scheduling Community Health Nursing Activities

The community health nurse has a work schedule that frequently changes. As was discussed, there are guidelines that help the nurse to give priority to work. Establishing priorities helps the nurse to schedule activities more effectively. There are several other factors that need to be considered as the nurse schedules work. Ideally, at the beginning of each month, the nurse will develop a calendar that identifies her or his scheduled activities for the month and allows the nurse to see how much time is available for other requests such as new referrals. If new demands for service exceed the time available, the nurse will then have an organized calendar to share with the nursing supervisor which documents the excess demand and which helps to rearrange priorities as necessary. Figure 20-4 presents a portion of a monthly calendar to illustrate how a community health nurse uses it to schedule activities. As can be seen, the nurse's workload for this week is heavy. If too many new referrals are received, the nurse should seek assistance from the supervisor. Often it is found that staff nurses use the time set aside for office work to handle excess workload. It is not wise to do so consistently, because office time is essential for appropriate planning, adequate follow-up, and high-quality recording.

The community health nurse should consider the following parameters when scheduling community nursing activites for the coming month:

I. Schedule every case and activity requiring service during the month.

II. Schedule new visits around scheduled commitments.

III. Make daily visits at the same time each day, if possible.

IV. Establish priorities for visits according to need and timing of visits, as illustrated by the following examples:

    A. Families with new babies—around feeding or bath time, to assess how these activities are handled by the family

    B. Crisis cases as soon as possible

    C. Infectious diseases last in the day, if possible, to decrease potential for exposure to other families

V. Provide for follow-up of families with long-term and chronic diseases.

    A. Handicapped or ill individuals

    B. Chronic problems

VI. Set time aside for shared home visits, when care is delegated to:

    A. Home health aides

    B. Licensed practical nurses

VII. Plan time for:

    A. Office activities

        1. Planning of visits for the week; planning activities for next week

        2. Assignment of cases

        3. Supervisory conferences

            a. Ancillary personnel

            b. Supervisor

A.M.	Monday	Tuesday		Wednesday	Thursday	Friday
8:30	Prepare for conferences with personnel regarding assigned cases			Office Preparation Conferences with team TCs Recording		Prepare for shared home visits
9:00	TC Lerner, Mayor, and Vinant families re: time for home visit	School			Mary Jones, 16-year-old AP	Shared visit with LPN to Johnson family—diabetic
10:00	Hartsford family, cleft lip and palate, new parents	Gilbert child, recheck vision, TC to parents if indicated		Hartsford family follow-up visit		
11:00				Vinant family, premie in hospital	Spartan, first baby	Shared visit with HHA—White family
12:00 P.M.	Lunch					
1:00	Mayor family, threatened abortion	Mayor family, follow-up visit		Well-child conference set up by RN in A.M.	Endicott family, new in area, multiple sclerosis	Bond family, follow-up visit
2:00	Bond family, new TB	Lerner family, new parents		Conference		Make necessary TCs in relation to referrals or family needs
3:00				Follow-up on referrals from the well-child conference	Staff meeting	Complete recording
4:00	Recording and referrals if any; TCs to MDs or sources of referral	Ring family, rheumatic fever child		Hastings family, TB contacts encourage to go to clinic for exam		Plan for next week's work
5:00						

FIGURE 20-4 A sample weekly calendar of a staff community health nurse in a county health department.

4. Recording and reporting

5. Follow-up

   a. Referrals

   b. Phone calls to agencies, physicians, families

6. Team meetings

B. Clinic activities

1. Setting up

2. Time in clinic

3. Follow-up and evaluation

C. School activities

D. Agency or community committee activities

Organizational Staffing Patterns for Community Health Nurses

Another area of concern to nurses who are managing the care of families and groups is the staffing pattern used in a health care organization. Some agencies utilize a system of solo nursing and others use a team nursing system. The method of staffing selected by an agency will determine how the nurse schedules and implements monthly activities.

Solo nursing. If this pattern of organization is used, the community health nurse is assigned a geographical area and is responsible for all open cases, new referrals, and schools in that district. The advantages of this method of assignment are several. First, the same nurse follows all clients over time, which results in better continuity of care. Second, this method allows for independent planning and decision making, which is often less time-consuming and, therefore, less expensive than group decisions. Last, one person serves a geographic area, which requires less travel time than if the same person would have to travel in several different geographic areas.

The greatest disadvantage for solo nursing is the lack of flexibility of work assignment. If an individual nurse becomes very busy with referrals or if the nurse becomes ill, coverage for the workload is difficult.

The solo nursing organizational pattern does not, or should not, eliminate peer and supervisory guidance with case analysis. Weekly team conferences can be very important to the successful implementation of the solo nursing concept. The nurse can use weekly conferences to increase knowledge in specific areas, such as available community resources, or to analyze the needs of complex families, such as failure-to-thrive families.

Team nursing. Other agencies use team nursing. This involves assigning a personnel team consisting of one or more community health nurses, RNs, LPNs, and HHAs to serve a larger geographical area or larger caseload than that in a solo nursing assignment. Each member of the team covers the same geographic area. Team nursing offers the advantage of lending more flexibility to work assignment because there are several team members to share new referrals or care of clients. Perhaps its greatest advantage is that quality of service can improve as a result of the shared planning and problem solving which occurs in regularly planned *team conferences.* Disadvantages are that more time is needed for planning because of the number of people involved and travel expenses are often increased.

Both team and solo nursing, however, can work. Some advantages and disadvantages of each were shared so that nurses will recognize the importance of analyzing strengths and limitations of different organizational patterns. Examining both strengths and limitations helps nurses to identify mechanisms which would minimize limitations when an agency selects a particular organizational pattern.

Determining Priorities in Community Health Nursing Practice

When setting up a calendar for the month, the staff nurse may find that there is not enough time to carry out all the responsibilities that she or he would like to be able to. Community health nurses cannot meet all the health needs that are evidenced in the community setting. Money, time, and personnel are not limitless, and all three, in fact, are becoming scarcer commodities. As was indicated in Chapters 2, 10, and 11, our responsibilities to groups in need are based on their vulnerability and their degree of risk. Thus, one way of determining whom community health nurses will service is to set priorities for service. Several factors to consider when one is establishing priorities have already been discussed in the section which addresses how the community health nurse uses the planning function of management in the work setting. In addition to the variables mentioned in that section, such as funding, legal mandates, community needs, and agency priorities, determining priorities based on client needs is useful. Ruth Rives, in 1953, wrote a classic work for public health nurses on the establishment of priorities according to client needs; it was updated in 1958. Table 20-1 is another update of Rives's article which provides a basis for determining priorities for nursing services. Many priorities defined by Rives are still very appropriate. Others have been added and some have been deleted.

UTILIZATION OF VARIOUS LEVELS OF HEALTH PERSONNEL

There are a variety of staffing patterns in agencies which deliver community health nursing services. In nearly any community health setting there are staff members involved in offering nursing services who are prepared at various levels. In some agencies, RNs (BSN-, AD-, and diploma-prepared), LPNs, and home health aides (HHAs) are hired. In others, only RNs and HHAs are available. In yet others, only BSN-prepared RNs are used. Knowledge of the educational preparation of these persons and the agency job descriptions are most helpful tools when nurses need to decide how to utilize personnel appropriately and determine what type of orientation and staff development is needed.

Home health aides are prepared with non-credit courses that last from 8 weeks to 1 year. Course work usually includes classroom activities and in-hospital clinical preparation. In the community setting, HHAs can give personal care and assist with housekeeping, marketing, and preparation of meals. Home health aides can give the kinds of personal care that can be taught easily to a family member if there is someone to teach.

The licensed practical nurse is prepared to give physical care, to make observations about physical conditions, to carry out special rehabilitative measures after being instructed by the community health nurse, to continue teaching of clients begun by the registered nurse, and to contribute to the nursing care plan of a client. There is a significant difference in the level of care given by LPNs and HHAs. The licensed practical nurse has knowledge and skill that helps in making limited patient assessments and contributing to the development of nursing interventions. Home health aides have knowledge and skill to provide *unskilled* patient care. Both the LPN and HHA, however, were prepared to function under the supervision of a registered nurse.

The registered nurse prepared at the AD or diploma level has been prepared mostly in acute care institutions, where there is a patient-centered approach to care. The RN is usually very skilled in the care of home health service clients who are ill and who need expert care and observations in the home. Because the RN often has developed expertise in technical procedures, she or he can teach these techniques to other staff and family members. The RN has skill and knowledge to assist in the development of the nursing care plan, especially with clients who have disease conditions. Because the registered nurse's preparation has been primarily patient-centered, she or he should receive orientation in relation to family-centered nursing practice, concepts related to analyzing the needs of populations.

TABLE 20-1 Priorities in Community Health Nursing

PURPOSES

1. To identify target population groups requiring community health nursing service

2. To identify realistic spacing of nurse service contacts according to identified target population group

3. To utilize levels of prevention and health promotion in planning nursing service to a community

CODE

· *Classification I: intensive visiting* is defined as visits spaced every 4 to 10 days

· *Classification II: periodic visiting* is defined as visits spaced every 6 to 8 weeks

· *Classification III: widely spaced visiting* is defined as visits spaced every 6 to 12 months

	I. Intensive visiting	*II. Periodic visiting*	*III. Widely spaced visiting*
Communicable disease	To families who	To families who	To families who
A. Tuberculosis (by law a priority)	1. Have young adults and unexamined contacts living in crowded home conditions with a patient who has positive sputum 2. Have a recently diagnosed patient with positive sputum 3. Have a recently diagnosed patient without positive sputum 4. Have a diagnosed patient with positive sputum, who is recalcitrant 5. Have a patient receiving chemotherapy	1. Have the patient with positive sputum hospitalized; have no young adults in the family; have good living standards but have some unexamined contacts 2. Need preparation for the hospital admission of the patient 3. Need preparation for the discharge of the patient	1. Have an arrested patient returned to good home conditions 2. Have had all contacts examined and the patient hospitalized, under adequate medical supervision. 3. Are under adequate medical supervision, with the source of infection located
B. Acute reportable dangerous communicable diseases	To families who 1. Have been contacts to reportable dangerous communicable disease 2. Have a diagnosed patient needing home care 3. Have food handlers as a case/contact to *Salmonella*	To families who 1. Are unimmunized 2. Have a patient under medical care but complications develop 3. Need follow-up for defects after recovery from acute stage	To families who 1. Are known to have immunization against communicable disease. 2. Are receiving adequate medical care 3. Have a typhoid carrier in the home
C. Venereal disease control	To clients who 1. Need treatments and education on the prevention and spread of disease 2. Have known contacts they will name	To clients who 1. Need follow-up clinical examinations (for example, spinal taps)	

TABLE 20-1   Priorities in Community Health Nursing (*Continued*)

	I. Intensive visiting	*II. Periodic visiting*	*III. Widely spaced visiting*
	3. Need examination, advice on treatment, and education on how to arrest and prevent the transfer of infection		
	4. Need posttreatment observation		
	5. Need to be convinced of the necessity of the treatment ordered by the doctor		
	6. Need to be taught how to prevent further manifestations of the disease		
	7. Have babies born of mothers with active VD at time of delivery		
Home care of the sick			
A. Cardiovascular disease	To clients who	To clients who	To clients who
	1. Have acute rheumatic fever or chorea	1. Have a suspected heart disease, but the diagnosis is not established	1. Have inactive rheumatic heart disease regardless of history or recrudescences
	2. Have cardiac failure or have had an acute cardiac episode from any cause	2. Have a congenital heart disease: nonoperable, postoperative	2. Have a history of rheumatic fever, but no clinical heart disease
	3. Are convalescing from rheumatic fever	3. Have a murmur of undetermined origin with a history of rheumatic fever	3. Are under medical care, stablized for cardiovascular diagnoses
	4. Are suspected of having acute rheumatic fever	4. Have congenital heart disease (to be followed until a thorough medical evaluation is completed)	
	5. Have a chronic cardiac disability requiring active treatment: medical, nursing, dietetic	5. Have diagnosed hypertension	
	6. Have had a CVA and require active treatment: medical, nursing, occupational, and physical therapy		
B. Diabetes	To clients who	To clients who	To clients who
	1. Are newly diagnosed, not stabilized by diet or insulin	1. Are newly diagnosed, administering own insulin but still needing supervision	1. Are under medical care, stabilized as to diet or insulin, or both
	2. Cannot take own insulin (blind, aged, low mentality, and so forth)	2. Are suspected of having diabetes	

TABLE 20-1   Priorities in Community Health Nursing (*Continued*)

	I. Intensive visiting	*II. Periodic visiting*	*III. Widely spaced visiting*
	3. Have difficulty understanding diet or administering their own insulin		
	4. Have uncontrolled diabetes		
	5. Have diabetes with gangrene		
	6. Have diabetes complicated by an infection		
C. Kidney disease	To clients who	To clients who	To clients who
	1. Are on dialysis	1. Understand medications and diet but are not stabilized	1. Are under medical care and are stabilized
	2. Need help with medications and diet and understanding disease		
D. Cancer	To clients who	To clients who	To clients about whom
	1. Are discharged from a hospital and need active nursing care, instruction for themselves, and interpretation of their physical and emotional needs to the family	1. Have precancerous lesions and are delinquent for periodic checkups (cervical erosions, leukoplakias, keratoses, mastitis, and others)	1. Information is needed for statistical purposes (cured, deceased, or other)
	2. Have symptoms suspicious of cancer; need medical supervision, completion of all tests and examinations, and, if required, treatment on the earliest possible date	2. Have cancer apparently treated successfully but are not reporting for medical reexamination (cancer of the skin with no apparent recurrence)	
	3. Are diagnosed but who, without consulting the physician, have interrupted their treatment or discontinued having medical checkups	3. Have advanced disease and need care (some of these patients may need to be in classification I)	
	4. Are under observation for malignancy but delinquent from regular medical supervision (the urgency of a patient's problem can be determined only by the attending physician)	4. Have families that have been taught to carry out medical orders but need support in continuing medical supervision	

TABLE 20-1 Priorities in Community Health Nursing (*Continued*)

	I. Intensive visiting	*II. Periodic visiting*	*III. Widely spaced visiting*
E. Other noncommunicable diseases, acute or chronic	To clients who 1. Are acutely ill and need nursing care 2. Are helpless or bedridden and need nursing service 3. Are senile and do not receive adequate home care 4. Are acutely ill or helpless but have families who can be taught how to give the necessary care	To clients who 1. Are acutely ill or helpless but whose families can provide care under nursing supervision 2. Need encouragement to continue medical care 3. Need emotional support to carry out health instructions	To clients who 1. Are under adequate medical supervision and are given good home care (by the family, a registered nurse, or a practical nurse)

Health teaching and supervision
 	
    A. Maternity-antepartum
	To women who
	
	  1. Are primiparas
	
	  2. Are under 17 or over 40 years of age
	
	  3. Are single parents
	
	  4. Are of low socioeconomic status
	
	  5. Are hypertensive
	
	  6. Have poor nutrition
	
	  7. Are not under medical care
	
	  8. Have had six or more pregnancies
	
	  9. Have had conditions associated with pregnancy resulting in infant deaths
	
	10. Have had complications in past pregnancies or have signs of complications in the present pregnancy, including psychosomatic disturbances
	
	11. Have a chronic disease, such as tuberculosis, diabetes, syphilis, anemia, nephritis, cardiac disease, or rheumatic fever
		To women who
		
		1. Have adequate medical supervision for apparently normal pregnancies
		
		2. Are in good physical and mental condition
		
		3. Are able to follow advice
		
		4. Have questions and desire help
			(No antepartum patients in this category)

TABLE 20-1 Priorities in Community Health Nursing (*Continued*)

	I. Intensive visiting	*II. Periodic visiting*	*III. Widely spaced visiting*
	12. Have previously had premature deliveries		
B. Maternity-postpartum	To women who	To women who	To women who
	1. Delivered at home	1. Had problems but are making normal progress 7 days after delivery	1. Are receiving good care and adequate medical supervision
	2. Have nursing problems or breast complications, such as engorgement or abscess	2. Have adequate medical supervision	
	3. Are not receiving adequate medical supervision or competent nursing care		
	4. Had complications or accidents of labor: stillbirths, abortions, or other difficulties resulting in a mishap to the mother or baby		
	5. Delivered prematurely		
	6. Had multiple births		
	7. Delivered a baby with a congenital defect		
	8. Had a baby that died during the first month of life		
	9. Evidence poor maternal-infant bonding		
	10. Have no or few support systems		
	11. Are single		
	12. Are economically stressed (low socioeconomic status)		
C. Infancy (higher priority is given to infants, regardless of whether they are first-born, when they live in low economic districts where the mortality rate is highest)	To infants who	To infants who	To infants who
	1. Are premature	1. Are past the first month and are gaining slowly	1. Are receiving adequate medical supervision
	2. Are newborn, especially if firstborn	2. Are not being fed properly	2. Are receiving good home care
	3. Have difficulty in breast-feeding	3. Have questionable physical and emotional delays	
	4. Have consistently lost weight		
	5. Are being weaned		
	6. Have inadequate medical care		

TABLE 20-1   Priorities in Community Health Nursing (*Continued*)

	I. Intensive visiting	*II. Periodic visiting*	*III. Widely spaced visiting*
	7. Have a reportable dangerous communicable disease		
	8. Have a physical handicap resulting from a birth injury or a congenital defect		
	9. Need immunization		
	10. Are from substandard poorly managed homes, or homes where there are problems of inadequate parenting		
	11. Are considered "difficult" babies by parents		
D. Preschool period	To children who	To children who	To children who
	1. Have a reportable dangerous communicable disease	1. Are insecure	1. Have adequate medical supervision
	2. Have a physical defect	2. Have lost weight	2. Have good home care
	3. Need immunization	3. Lack medical supervision	
	4. Need dental care	4. Have poor health habits	
	5. Have nutritional deficiencies	5. Deviate from normal physical and emotional behavior	
	6. Are inconsistently disciplined		
	7. Are from homes where there is inadequate parenting		
	8. Are reported for suspected child abuse and neglect		
E. School health	To children who	To children who	To children who
	1. Have acute health problems	1. Need follow-up of allergies: "hives," eczema, asthma	1. Have a chronic health condition that is stabilized and under medical care
	a. Communicable diseases: immunization reactions or complications developing from acute communicable diseases	2. Have inadequate medical care	2. Have a congenital defect which does not require remedial work at the time
	b. Skin conditions: scabies, impetigo, ringworm, pediculosis	3. Have not had diagnosed defects corrected within a reasonable period of time	

TABLE 20-1 Priorities in Community Health Nursing (*Continued*)

	I. *Intensive visiting*	II. *Periodic visiting*	III. *Widely spaced visiting*
	c. Other: pregnancy, unexpected loss or gain of weight, abuse, neglect, diabetes, epilepsy	4. Are on medication for a duration of more than 3 weeks during the school year	
	2. Have had an accident in school requiring hospitalization	5. Need to be observed in relation to their growth pattern (those with structural scoliosis, those wearing braces, and so forth)	
	3. Need immediate attention for defects discovered on physical examination: vision, hearing, cardiac, kidney, scoliosis, or other serious defects	6. Need follow-up of minor defects: poor eating and health habits, poor dental and personal hygiene, foot and posture problems	
	4. Need follow-up of incidents indicating intense or serious emotional disturbance		
	5. Need follow-up as a contact of a diagnosed dangerous communicable disease		
	6. Have growth and other developmental delays		
F. Adult health	To clients who	To clients who	To clients who
	1. Are in situational or maturational crisis	1. Are in crisis but have support systems	1. Have needed nursing care, are currently coping well, but are at risk for physical, emotional, and psychosocial problems
	2. Are disorganized as a family and at risk for abuse and neglect of children or spouse	2. Recognize their disorganization and are working on ordering their lives	
	3. Have suspected dangerous communicable or chronic disease symptoms	3. Have diagnosed disease and are receiving medical treatment; need help with referral to resources	
	4. Have no medical supervision for diagnosed physical, emotional, psychosocial problems	4. Are needing help dealing with developmental tasks of parenting: sexuality and death education tasks of their children	
	5. Are needing help adapting to chronic illness: heart disease, arthritis, multiple sclerosis, depression		

TABLE 20-1   Priorities in Community Health Nursing (*Continued*)

	I. Intensive visiting	*II. Periodic visiting*	*III. Widely spaced visiting*
G. Health of aging people	To clients who	To clients who	To clients who
	1. Have no medical supervision	1. Have a diagnosed medical problem	1. Are under medical supervision
	2. Have symptoms of a dangerous communicable, nutritional, or chronic disease	2. Have a complex treatment regimen and are following it	2. Have readily available support systems
	3. Have a diagnosed disease and need help following the treatment plan	3. Are able to live independently but need referral sources and support	
	4. Have no support systems		
	5. Have evidence of situational or maturational crisis especially in relation to: loss of income, loss of spouse, loss of friends		
	6. Have evidence of intentional or unintentional alcohol or drug abuse		
	7. Are unable to maintain an environmentally safe housing situation		

SOURCE: Reproduced per permission of the Nursing Division, Oakland County Health Department, Pontiac, Michigan.

and principles relative to the coordination of care and prevention, if she or he is expected to implement all the services provided by community health nurses in a health department. This orientation is a necessity. It is unfair to expect the registered nurse, prepared at the AD or diploma level, to provide comprehensive community health nursing services. She or he has not been prepared to do so. If circumstances exist where only these registered nurses are available, an agency has the responsibility to provide them with orientation and staff development opportunities which adequately prepare them to carry out the demands of the job.

The community health nurse has been prepared at the baccalaureate level in community health, with an emphasis in the educational program on wellness and prevention as well as experience in the community health setting. She or he is expected to have a family-centered focus and to function in a comprehensive fashion. This entails identifying client strengths and needs and all variables that affect health and illness (physical, social, and emotional), facilitating identification of family health goals and assisting families to reach their goals. The community health nurse initiates, plans, and evaluates care. In addition, she or he participates in planning for the health needs of the community and works in schools, clinics, and community groups, giving service as well as functioning as a planning participant to see that needed services are provided.

The agency job description is a helpful tool for nurses who are in positions where they have to delegate care to various levels of personnel. A job description defines what tasks or functions are appropriate for each level of personnel, based on their educational preparation. Identifying tasks and functions that different levels of staff are capable of handling facilitates the utilization of all personnel and also the delegation process. The following illustrates how this is so: In the well-child, immunization, or VD clinic, many tasks need to be done, including taking histories, weighing and measuring children, teaching clients, giving immunizations or injections of medication, and drawing blood samples. Some of these are best done by the community health nurse, but others can be done effectively by the LPN or HHA. Knowledge of the educational preparation of personnel and agency job descriptions can help the nurse to decide what may be delegated or assigned. For instance, in one large health department, there were five kinds of personnel working in the well-child clinic because there were activities to be accomplished which could be handled by nurses prepared at various levels: the HHA weighed and measured children and set up the equipment needed to run the clinic; the LPNs and RNs gave immunizations; the RNs and community health nurses took immunization histories (determining with parents what their child had had and what was to be given today); the community health nurse took health and illness histories and counseled and provided education for parents. The pediatric nurse practitioner on the staff carried her own caseload of clients, doing physical examinations and teaching and counseling with parents. Assignments in this situation were based on the complexity of the tasks involved and the preparation each staff member had. Pediatric nurse practitioners, for example, usually have more in-depth preparation to handle complete physicals than does the generalized community health nurse.

Another example of how various levels of personnel can be used to implement nursing services in the community setting is the follow-up of vision and hearing failures from schools. Health departments often have hearing and vision technicians who screen school children, retest the failures, and then refer the retest failures to the community health nurse for follow-up and referral. It is then the community health nurse's responsibility to see that the follow-up is done. However, lesser-prepared personnel, such as an LPN or clerk, may be taught how to appropriately do the initial contacting of parents by phone to ascertain whether or not medical care has been obtained, and if so, what the results were. Using lesser prepared personnel to handle the above activities provides more time for the community health nurse to follow up with families who are having difficulty obtaining medical care. In addition to clinic and school activities, home health activities are commonly implemented by differing levels of personnel.

Many home health service clients need to be visited two or three times a week. After the nurse has established a plan of care, visits can often be shared with other personnel such as the LPN or HHA. Remember, though, that when care is delegated to other personnel, responsibility for care of that client or family remains with the community health nurse. The community health nurse must plan adequate time in her or his schedule to supervise the care delegated to other personnel.

Using Delegation as a Management Function in Community Health Nursing

In order to carry out the diverse responsibilities of the position, the community health nurse frequently needs to delegate tasks to other health care personnel. When planning responsibilities for others, the community health nurse should:

1. Analyze the nature of the task to be delegated, considering the complexity as well as the time involved to complete it.

2. Determine the capability of the individual staff member to handle the assigned responsibility, especially noting the staff member's educational and experience background and other workload responsibilities.

3. Identify the willingness of the staff member to accept responsibility for the assigned activity.

4. Determine how much time will be needed to supervise if tasks are delegated to others.

Delegation is the process of designating tasks and bestowing on others the authority needed to accomplish these assigned tasks. Delegation does not mean, however, that the community health nurse negates personal responsibility for providing quality care to the families she or he serves. Care given by home health aides or LPNs should never be increased so rapidly that it is impossible for the community health nurse to adequately supervise the care delegated to them. The community health nurse must have sufficient time available to apply the principles of the five management functions when carrying out the following supervisory activities with HHAs and LPNs:

1. Shared home visits with the LPN or HHA on the initial visit to a family (planning, organizing)

2. Development of nursing care plans on each family in the caseload, based on assessment data and input from the LPN or HHA (planning, organizing)

3. Regular conferences with the LPN or HHA to determine guidance and assistance needed in specific situations (directing, organizing, coordinating)

4. Periodic shared visits with the LPN or HHA for supervision and reevaluation of the status of the family (directing, coordinating, controlling)

5. Periodic review of family records to evaluate the status of the family and the level of nursing service (controlling)

6. In-service education related to the needs of the staff and the families in the nurse's caseload (directing)

In community health nursing, management functions are utilized daily by nurses at every level. The five functions of management—planning, organizing, directing, coordinating, and controlling—are useful tools to nurses as they work with peers, ancillary personnel, supervisors, and the community in providing nursing care.

SUMMARY

Community health nurses have multiple and diverse responsibilities to handle in the practice setting. They have found that by applying the principles of management they are more effective in dealing with the multiple and diverse demands in the work environment. Knowledge of the five functions of management is especially helpful. These are planning, organizing, directing, coordinating, and controlling.

The development of management thought has changed over time. Reviewing the historical evolution of management helps nurses to understand why it is useful to implement the five functions of management in the work setting. Analysis of this evolution is also beneficial because it provides a basis for defining a personal philosophy of management.

The utilization of management concepts in the community health nursing setting is essential. Management principles help the community health nurse to organize and schedule activities, to establish priorities for nursing service, to effectively and efficiently utilize time, and to appropriately delegate responsibilities. All these tasks must be accomplished if the community health nurse is going to deliver quality care to clients in the community.

REFERENCES

Clark, C. C., & Shea, C. A. *Management in nursing.* New York: McGraw-Hill, 1979.

Freeman, R. B. *Techniques of supervision in public health nursing* (2d ed.). Philadelphia: Saunders, 1949.

Kast, F. E., & Rosenzweig, J. E. *Organization and management* (2d ed.). New York: McGraw-Hill, 1974.

Kazmier, L. J. *Principles of management. A programmed-instructional approach.* New York: McGraw-Hill, 1974.

Longest, B. B. *Management practices for the health professional.* Reston, Va.: Reston Publishing Co., 1976.

Maslow, A. H. *Motivation and personality.* New York: Harper & Row, 1954.

McGregor, D. *The human side of enterprise.* New York: McGraw-Hill, 1960.

Rives, R. Priorities according to needs. In D. M. Stewart & P. A. Vincent (Eds.), *Public Health Nursing.* Dubuque, Iowa: Wm. C. Brown Company, 1968. Copyright 1958, American Journal of Nursing Company. Reproduced with permission from *Nursing Outlook,* July 1958, *6,* 404–408.

SELECTED BIBLIOGRAPHY

Cantor, M. M. Philosophy, purpose, and objectives. *Journal of Nursing Administration,* July–August 1973, *3,* 21–25.

Council of Home Health Agencies and Community Health Services. *Administrator's handbook.* New York: National League for Nurses, 1977.

Daeffler, R. J. Patient's perception of care under team and primary nursing. *Journal of Nursing Administration,* March–April 1975, *5,* 20–26.

Daniel, L., Eigsti, D. G., & McGuire, S. L. Teaching caseload management. *Nursing Outlook,* January 1977, *25,* 27–29.

Deal, J. The timing of change. *Supervisor Nurse,* September 1977, *8,* 73–79.

Heimann, C. G. Four theories of leadership. *Journal of Nursing Administration,* June 1976, *6,* 18–24.

Kissinger, C. L. Community nursing administration: Quantifying nursing utilization. *Nursing Outlook,* September–October 1973, *111,* 42–48.

Marriner, A. Organizational concepts: II. *Supervisor Nurse,* October 1977, *8,* 37–46.

———. Organizational process and bureaucratic structure. *Supervisor Nurse,* July 1977, *8,* 54–58.

Odiorne, G. S. Management by objectives: Antidote to future shock. *Journal of Nursing Administration,* February 1975, *5,* 27–30.

Passos, J. Y. Accountability: Myth or mandate? *Journal of Nursing Administration,* May–June 1973, *3,* 17–22.

Sayles, L. R. *Leadership. What effective managers really do and how they do it.* New York: McGraw-Hill, 1979.

Wobbe, R. R. Primary versus team nursing. *Supervisor Nurse,* March 1978, *9,* 36–37.

Wong, P., Doyle, M., & Strauss, D. Problem solving through process management. *Journal of Nursing Administration,* January 1975, *5,* 37–39.

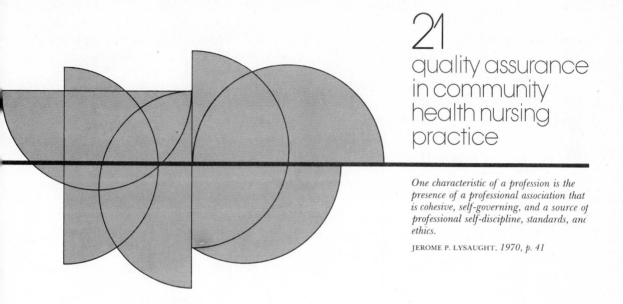

21
quality assurance in community health nursing practice

One characteristic of a profession is the presence of a professional association that is cohesive, self-governing, and a source of professional self-discipline, standards, and ethics.

JEROME P. LYSAUGHT, *1970, p. 41*

Health care professionals are entering an era of quality assurance. Increasingly they are being challenged by legislative action, third-party payers, and consumers to assume accountability for the services delivered by members of their profession. The professional standard review organizations (PSROs) established by the 1972 amendments to the Social Security Act were developed to ensure that federal monies spent for Medicaid, Medicare, and other federal health care programs would be used effectively, efficiently, and economically. The PSRO law (Public Law 92-603) mandated review of health care delivered by physicians and nonphysician health practitioners when such care was paid for by federal funds (Public Law 92-603, 1972). This has created the necessity of developing standards for practice because the review examines current practice to see how it compares with established norms for quality care.

The passage of the National Health Planning and Resources Development Act of 1974 (see Chapter 12), like the PSRO legislation,

also provided an impetus for the development of quality assurance programs. This law mandated that health care professionals promote activities that improve the quality of health care services to all segments of the population. It set forth as a national priority "equal access to quality health care at a reasonable cost" (National Health Guidelines, January 1977, p. 1). It called for the development of national health planning goals and standards.

In addition to federal influences, private nonprofit third-party payers (see Chapter 4) have encouraged professionals to monitor both the cost and quality of health services. They have established criteria for the type of care they will reimburse, and they require as well that health services be audited by professional audit committees.

Consumers are also motivating health care professionals to evaluate the care they provide. Consumers are becoming more sophisticated about the health care they desire and are demanding that current practice keep up with societal changes and needs. In addition, through legislative action, they are becoming more actively involved in reviewing services delivered by health care professionals.

Nursing shares with all health care professionals the need to examine carefully the delivery of their services in light of changing societal demands. To validate itself as a profession and to maintain the right to govern nursing practice, nursing must take the responsibility to control the activities of its members. There is no question that if nursing does not assume accountability for its actions, others will control nurses' actions for them in this era of quality assurance.

QUALITY ASSURANCE DEFINED

Quality assurance is a dynamic process through which nurses assume accountability for the quality of care they provide. It involves both the evaluation of care and the implementation of measures to improve care, based on data obtained from evaluation efforts. It is a commitment to excellence with an emphasis on ensuring that all nurses provide safe nursing care and that all clients receive quality care. Quality assurance is a guarantee to society that services provided by nurses are being regulated by members of the profession. It is a series of actions aimed at governing nursing practice so that all clients receive nursing services that are *equal to or better than* the standard of care designated appropriate for clients who have like characteristics. Quality assurance is also a systematic, ongoing evaluation of care delivered by nurses for the purpose of determining what type of care is provided and for identifying the outcome of services delivered to clients.

Selected definitions of quality assurance are presented in the accompanying chart. Schmadl (1979, p. 465) proposed an additional definition after analyzing what nurses should be assuring, for whom nurses are assuring quality, and what measures identify quality nursing care. His definition is given below because it is clearly stated, comprehensive, and provides direction for the development of a quality assurance program.

Quality assurance involves assuring the consumer of a specified degree of excellence through continuous measurement and evaluation of structural components, goal-directed nursing process, and/or consumer outcome, using pre-established criteria and standards and available norms, and followed by appropriate alteration with the purpose of improvement.

Since 1966, the American Nurses' Association has diligently pursued the development of a quality assurance program for nurses. At that time the divisions on practice, including community health nursing, geriatric nursing, maternal and child health nursing, medical-surgical nursing, and psychiatric and mental health nursing, were established with a mandate to consider the development of standards for nursing practice as their major priority. After 6 years of concentrated efforts, all divisions on practice presented standards of care for their division based on their beliefs about nursing practice at the 1972 biennial ANA convention in Detroit (American Nurses' Association, 1975, p. 1). In 1973 the community health nursing standards were made available for distribution to all members of the community health nursing division. They were delineated as follows (American Nurses' Association, 1973, unnumbered pages):

STANDARD I

The Collection of Data about the Health Status of the Consumer Is Systematic and Continuous. The Data Are Accessible, Communicated and Recorded.

STANDARD II

Nursing Diagnoses Are Derived from Health Status Data.

Selected Definitions of Quality Assurance

American Nurses' Association: Estimation of the degree of excellence in (1) the alteration of the health status of consumers attained through providers' performances of (2) diagnostic, therapeutic, prognostic, and other health care activities.[1]

Quality assurance is a relatively new term conveying the broad idea that superiority or excellence in care is made secure or certain.[2]

A program executed to make secure or certain the excellence of health care; the term is applied to programs as limited as that of an administrative unit of a health care agency or as broad as that of a community, a region, a state, or a nation. The program must have two major components:

1. The securing of measurements and ascertaining of the degree to which stated standards are met;

2. The introduction of changes based on information supplied by the measurements, with the view to improvement of the total effort and product of the unit or agency.[3]

Quality assurance is an ongoing program in the nursing profession, constructed and executed to secure and implement the excellence of health care.[4]

Brown: Quality assurance, when used in reference to

health care, refers to the accountability of health personnel for the quality of care they provide.[5]

Davidson: Quality assurance is a process for attainment of the highest degree of excellence in the delivery of patient or client care.[6]

A commitment to excellence of care; an estimation of the health status of consumers attained through nursing performance.[7]

Lang: Activities done to determine the extent to which a phenomenon fulfills certain values and activities done to assure changes in practice which will fulfill the highest levels of values.[8]

Mayers: Quality assurance has as its central goal making certain that care practices will produce good patient outcomes.[9]

Nichols: The term quality assurance is used to describe a process in which standards are set and action is taken to ensure achievement of the standards.[10] It involves the description of the level of quality desired and feasible, and a system for ensuring its achievement.[11]

Zimmer: Quality assurance is estimation of the degree of excellence in patient health outcomes and in activity and other resource cost outcomes.[12]

References

1. American Nurses' Association. *Guidelines for Review of Nursing Care at the Local Level.* (Publ. No. NP-54) Kansas City, Mo., The Association, 1976, p. A-2.
2. ———. *A Plan for Implementation of the Standards of Nursing Practice.* (Publ. No. NP-51) Kansas City, Mo., The Association, 1975, p. 5.
3. Ibid., p. 30.
4. Ibid., p. 6.
5. Brown, B. Quality Assurance (editorial) *Nurs. Admin. Q.* 1:v, Spring 1977.
6. Davidson, S. V. S. *PSRO: Utilization and Audit in Patient Care.* St. Louis, C. V. Mosby Co., 1976, p. 5.
7. ———, and others. *Nursing Care Evaluation: Concurrent and Retrospective Review Criteria.* St. Louis, C. V.

Mosby Co., 1977, p. 408.
8. Lang, N. *A Model for Quality Assurance in Nursing.* Milwaukee, Marquette University, 1974, p. 11. (unpublished doctoral dissertation)
9. Mayers, M. G. and others. *Quality Assurance for Patient Care: Nursing Perspectives.* New York: Appleton-Century-Crofts, 1977, p. 3.
10. Nichols, M. E. and V. G. Wessells, (eds.). *Nursing Standards and Nursing Process.* Wakefield, Mass.: Contemporary Publishers, 1977, p. 1–2.
11. Ibid., p. 37.
12. Zimmer, M. J. "Quality assurance in the provision of hospital care: A model for evaluating nursing care." *Hospitals,* 48:91, 131, March 1.

STANDARD III

Plans for Nursing Service Include Goals Derived from Nursing Diagnoses.

STANDARD IV

Plans for Nursing Service Include Priorities and Nursing Approaches or Measures to Achieve the Goals Derived from Nursing Diagnoses.

STANDARD V

Nursing Actions Provide for Consumer Participation in Health Promotion, Maintenance and Restoration.

STANDARD VI

Nursing Actions Assist Consumers to Maximize Health Potential.

STANDARD VII

The Consumer's Progress toward Goal Achievement Is Determined by the Consumer and the Nurse.

STANDARD VIII

Nursing Actions Involve Ongoing Reassessment, Reordering of Priorities, New Goal Setting and Revision of the Nursing Plan.[1]

Beliefs and standards for nursing practice should never be static. As societal changes, expansion of knowledge, and technological advances occur, beliefs and standards should be reevaluated to determine whether they reflect the values of the profession and society. The ANA Standards for Practice of 1973 were presented only as a working document to be continually evaluated and revised. In 1978, a Conceptual Model Task Force of the Division on Community Health Nursing Practice began working on a specific statement of beliefs about community health nursing practice (Division on Community Health Nursing Prac-

tice, March 16, 1979). These beliefs were presented to the Community Health Nursing Division of ANA at the 1980 biennial ANA convention in Texas and are delineated in the pamphlet *A Conceptual Model of Community Health Nursing* (ANA, 1980).

Model for Quality Assurance

The development of standards for practice is only one component of a quality assurance program. Quality assurance efforts should be focused on evaluating the structure, process, and outcome aspects of health care delivery, as well as on the implementation of measures to improve care when warranted (Donabedian, 1966, pp. 169–170). Actions to improve care in the community health setting include such things as securing more nursing staff, hiring better-prepared personnel, providing additional nursing supervision, increasing the frequency of home visits to given families, and planning health programs for specified high-risk population groups. All aspects of community health nursing practice, including services to individuals, families, and the community as a whole, must be evaluated when one is implementing a quality assurance program.

Like the nursing process described in Chapter 8, quality assurance involves a series of circular, dynamic actions which are client-centered. Shared responsibility between nurses and consumers is essential if clients are to be protected from incompetent practitioners. The circular nature and the shared partnership aspects of quality assurance are illustrated in the quality assurance model (Figure 21-1) developed by participants at an ANA leadership workshop (*The American Nurse*, 1976, p. 23). When graphically depicted, the monitoring of quality assurance appears simple. In reality, it is a complex process requiring time, effort, and commitment to the value of professional accountability.

[1]Reprinted with permission of ANA.

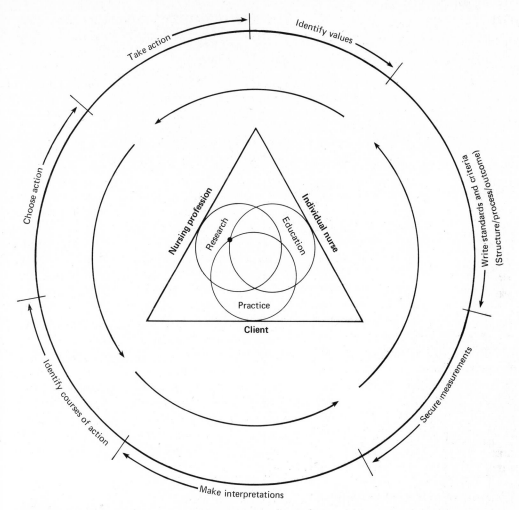

FIGURE 21-1 A quality assurance model. (*From Model shows dynamic concept of quality assurance. The American Nurse, Feb. 28, 1976, p. 23. Adapted from the ANA Quality Assurance Model, a Plan for Implementation of the Standards of Nursing Practice. Kansas City, Mo.: American Nurses' Association, 1975, 15. Reprinted with permission of ANA.*)

COMPONENTS OF A QUALITY ASSURANCE PROGRAM

The schema presented in Figure 21-1 identifies the basic components in a quality assurance program. These are listed below and will be discussed in detail later.

· Identify values

· Write standards and criteria (structure, process, and outcome)

· Secure measurements

· Make interpretations

· Identify courses of action

· Choose action

· Take action

Currently, because of external and internal pressures, quality assurance programs in many organizations and agencies are developing rapidly. Some programs are being implemented so quickly that nursing staff do not have adequate time to assimilate the changes that are occurring. Nursing personnel are frequently put in a position where they are conducting nursing audits or establishing standards and criteria for care without understanding how to do these procedures. It is crucial that careful attention be given to *how* each aspect of a quality assurance program is initiated, because many of the changes being proposed may be foreign to staff nurses. Change to the unknown produces anxiety, especially when those involved do not understand why change is necessary, how the change may affect them, or how to accomplish the specific tasks required of them.

Continuing education is often the essential first step in developing a quality assurance program. Many staff nurses have not been prepared in the academic setting to develop standards of care, because emphasis has only recently been placed on identifying standards for practice. In addition, technological advances, changes in the health care delivery system, and current views on the rights and responsibilities of clients have altered the nature of community health nursing practice. As a result of these changes, nurses have found it necessary to seek opportunities for advanced education in order to work effectively with clients in the practice setting. Keller (1978) substantiated this when she surveyed by questionnaire community health nurses and their supervisors in Michigan, to determine their continuing education needs. Her findings are presented in Table 21-1 and Table 21-2. Both

TABLE 21-1 Rank Order of Nurses' Continuing Education Needs as Perceived by Community Health Nurses in the State of Michigan

Need	Percent	N*
1. Motivation	24.2	113
2. Improving counseling techniques	23.2	110
3. Multiproblem families	17.8	83
4. Improving interviewing techniques	17.1	80
5. Changing health behavior	14.1	66
6. Drug or alcohol addictions	13.5	63
7. Effective recording	13.3	62
8. Assisting clients with problem solving	12.8	60
9. Basic processes of disease	10.7	50
10. Managing effective clinic services	10.3	48
11. Evaluating the effectiveness of your nursing care	10.1	47

N = number of times the need is identified.

SOURCE: From B. S. Keller. The continuing education needs of community health nurses in Michigan and factors influencing these needs as perceived by these nurses and their supervisors. Ann Arbor, Mich.: University of Michigan, 1978, p. 59, unpublished doctoral dissertation.

groups thought that community health nurses needed continuing education to keep current in practice. Keller's findings are not atypical. Nurses across the country recognize that they have continuing education needs and are requesting that universities offer more learning opportunities for the practitioner.

Keller's research study revealed several significant continuing education needs of community health nurses that directly relate to their ability to provide and document high-quality nursing care. First, supervisors and staff nurses alike thought that staff nurses needed assistance to better evaluate the effectiveness of their nursing care. When nurses have difficulty evaluating the results of the services they provide, it is hard for them to determine when they have reached quality standards. Second, Keller found that staff nurses needed help with documenting the care they have provided (recording). Effective documentation is essential for adequate evaluation of quality. Last, Keller identified that nurses in the study needed more knowledge to effectively utilize the family-centered nursing process. All of the needs identified in Tables 21-1 and 21-2 directly affect how well a nurse is able to implement the nursing process. For example, if a practitioner does not understand the dynamics involved in drug and alcohol addiction, it would be difficult for this practitioner to collect accurate data in relation to this problem or to formulate appropriate client goals and intervention strategies. This, in turn, would result in care that is less than the standard of quality prescribed for clients who are experiencing these types of difficulties.

When a quality assurance program is being implemented, the continuing education needs of all personnel in a community health agency should be ascertained before changes are made which personnel are not prepared to handle. All personnel need the opportunity to provide input and to have administrative support that provides time and encouragement for learning. Quality is not assured if only a small committee evaluates care.

As was previously mentioned, there are several components in a sound quality assurance program. Factors to consider when implementing each of these components will be shared in the following section of this chapter. By using the model presented in Figure 21-1 and the information presented below, the reader should be able to evaluate the progress made in implementing a quality assurance program in specific practice settings.

TABLE 21-2 Rank Order of Community Health Nurses' Continuing Education Needs in the State of Michigan as Perceived by Their Supervisors

Need	Percent	N*
1. Improving interviewing techniques	25.6	20
2. Effective recording	21.8	17
3. Motivation	20.5	16
4. Assessing family dynamics	19.2	15
5. Increasing self-awareness by nurses	17.9	14
6. Multiproblem families	16.7	13
7. Changing health behavior	16.7	13
8. Setting goals and priorities	16.7	13
9. Assisting clients with problem solving	15.4	12
10. Evaluating effectiveness of your nursing care	14.1	11
11. Improving counseling techniques	12.8	10
12. Giving family-focused service	12.8	10
13. Organizing time	12.8	10
14. Teaching and learning	10.3	8

*N = number of times the need is identified.

SOURCE: From B. S. Keller. The continuing education needs of community health nurses in Michigan and factors influencing these needs as perceived by these nurses and their supervisors. Ann Arbor, Mich.: University of Michigan, 1978, p. 60, unpublished doctoral dissertation.

Identify Values

Attitudes, beliefs, and values influence how we think, how we act, and how we evaluate. In terms of quality assurance, they affect how we define quality based upon our beliefs about health, about humanity, and about the nature of nursing practice. Identifying values in relation to quality, however, is a difficult task because many factors influence how nursing services are delivered. Available resources, consumer needs and wants, and professional philosophies all determine the scope of practice in a particular community. It is unrealistic, for instance, to assume that an agency can plan nursing services without taking into consideration the restrictions of limited resources. Providing fragmented services for all is not assuring quality.

Establishing a philosophy of nursing practice is fundamental to the identification of quality in nursing care. A philosophy provides direction for the nature and scope of services provided by both an agency and an individual practitioner. Based on available resources, it identifies clients' needs, why activities are being carried out, and the population to be served. A philosophy also describes the type of relationship the practitioner and client will have.

When a philosophy for nursing practice is being defined, there should be discussion related to key, general concepts. Often concepts are accepted as truths, but their meaning to each practitioner varies. Concepts such as the "clients' right of self-determination," "active client participation," "individualization of client care plans," and a "family-centered preventive approach" to the delivery of health care are difficult to internalize. Practitioners need time to analyze how these concepts can be applied in the practice setting. They need to understand what it means to their practice when they subscribe to a broad concept such as "the right of self-determination." When dealing with this concept, for example, nurses need time to share feelings about client situations where their value systems differ from their clients' value orientations.

It was said in Chapter 2 that a community health nurse's "dominant responsibility is to the population as a whole" (American Nurses' Association, 1973). This concept, like the above concepts, is difficult to grasp and to apply. An agency that has limited resources and subscribes to this belief must identify ways in which it can implement this concept. It is impossible for any agency to provide direct service to all individuals within a community. A community health agency can, however, identify nursing service needs it can provide and then apply the principles of health planning to see that gaps in services are met by other community agencies.

Agencies must determine what is realistic for them to accomplish in view of the resources available or potentially available to them. If this is not done, they will never be able to determine when quality has been achieved. Being "all things to all people" is an impossible goal, but defining what one can do is not impossible. For instance, in the accompanying statement of philosophy, the Visiting Nurse Association of Hartford, Inc., clearly spelled out that they would provide *skilled* nursing services, including instruction in prevention of disease and preservation of health and other therapeutic services, on a part-time basis. They are meeting the needs of the population as a whole by referring individuals to other community agencies and by participating in health planning activities when unmet needs are recognized.

It should not be assumed that all community health nurses have a clear understanding of or an appreciation for their agency's philosophy and beliefs. Even when an agency has had a written philosophy statement, discourse should occur among staff members periodically so that a common framework for practice becomes explicit to all. A philosophy document given to new employees may receive little attention. This frequently happens because new employees are naturally more interested in finding out what they have to do to achieve success in their new job situation than in the philosophy behind what they are doing. Thus agency philosophy and beliefs about nursing practice must be reinforced by supervisors as new employees become comfortable with their job responsibilities. These beliefs must also be reexamined by staff who have been employed for a length of time. When the demands of the workload become heavy it is easy to lose sight of the beliefs and goals of the agency.

Statement of Philosophy: Visiting Nurse Association of Hartford, Incorporated

In 1969 a committee composed of Board members, supervisors and administrators was formed to develop the following Statement of Philosophy of the Visiting Nurse Association of Hartford, Inc. This was approved by all staff members and the Board of Directors.

The VNA of Hartford exists to provide services to people. It draws its authority from a 1923 Constitution in which the purpose "... to furnish ... skilled services of a Visiting Nurse ... including instruction in prevention of disease and preservation of health" is stated.

More specifically, the nature of the service is:

1. To provide, with a family centered approach, skilled nursing and other therapeutic services on a part-time basis in the home or other appropriate place.

2. To promote health and prevent illness—both mental and physical.

3. To help individuals get other necessary community services appropriate to their needs.

4. To recognize and bring to the attention of appropriate people unmet needs of the community and to participate in planning to meet these needs.

We believe:

1. The agency has a responsibility to honor all requests for services and to do an assessment of the situation involving the patient and the family and other appropriate professions or agencies, e.g., doctors, social workers, etc.

2. All planning and goal setting is done with the individual being served, his family and others involved in implementing care.

3. Planning and goal setting is a continuing process between nurse, patient and family, one of the goals being maximum independence of patient and family in taking care of their health needs.

4. Plans for the termination of VNA services should be made with the individual, family and all others involved when family needs exceed the capabilities of the nursing agency and the family.

5. All planning includes the giving of consideration to the coordination of services, the appropriate use of manpower and the avoidance of duplication of effort.

6. We believe the above can be best achieved through the practice of primary nursing.

   A. The designation of the primary nurse for each patient/family will be based on geography, nurses' skill and nurses' availability.

   B. The primary nurse will interpret her role to the patient/family. The primary nurse is responsible and accountable for the nursing care delivered on a 24 hour basis until the patient is discharged. Her responsibility for directing and evaluating the care of other nurses mandates holding other nurses accountable and responsible for the care they give.

   C. The responsibilities of the primary nurse include:

      (1) Assessment of patient's/family's condition.

      (2) Identification of patient's/family's problems on the problem list.

      (3) Development of the nursing care plan to meet the identified needs.

      (4) Maintenance of the current problem list and plans, based on continuing assessment of the patient's/family's status.

      (5) Implementation of the plan of care to the extent possible.

      (6) Collaboration with nursing staff, physicians and other health workers in the care of the patient/family.

      (7) Evaluation of the effectiveness of nursing intervention.

Reproduced per permission of the Visiting Nurse Association of Hartford, Inc., 80 Coventry Street, Hartford, Connecticut.

Write Standards and Criteria: Structure, Process, and Outcome

A philosophy of practice states the values and beliefs of an agency and guides the activities of all agency staff. It does not provide measurable elements by which a practitioner can judge the quality of care given by nurses. Standards and criteria must be developed so that the measurement of quality is possible.

Standards are a "model or example established by authority, custom, or general consent" (Ramey, 1973, p. 18). They are rules that help the practitioner to establish a consistent data base in an organized manner so that consistencies and deficiencies of care are easily identified. They are specific statements that reflect the outcomes or goals toward which an agency is working. For example, in the ANA community health standards, one identified goal is to "assist consumers to maximize their health potential" (standard VI).

Criteria are predetermined measurable elements which reflect the intent of a standard (American Nurses' Association, 1975, p. 16). They identify expected levels of performance by practitioners (process criteria) or clients (outcome criteria). One process criterion for measuring ANA community health nursing standard VI might be "community health nurse provides instruction in the prevention of disease and the preservation of health when client situation warrants such activities."

The development of standards and criteria for evaluation of nursing care should occur from three perspectives: structure, process, and outcome. According to Donabedian (1966, pp. 169–170), *structure* standards appraise the environment in which health care is provided. Such things as the organizational framework, the availability of resources, the qualifications of staff, and the adherence to legal mandates are examined with structural standards. Both the American Nurses' Association and the National League for Nursing have been actively engaged in the development of structural standards. Licensure, certification, and accreditation standards provide guidelines for agencies by which to evaluate their structural characteristics. One such standard requires that agencies have adequate resources to achieve their stated goals. Criteria in relation to such things as numbers of staff and amount of funding are used to measure this standard.

Process standards and criteria describe how

care should be delivered (Donabedian, 1969, p. 1833). They focus on reviewing the activities carried out by nurses in order to help clients meet their specific health care needs. They are designed to evaluate the use of the nursing process to determine if it was appropriately applied with individual clients. Process standards and criteria help nurses to examine their behavior and skills in relation to client-nurse interactions, the formulation of nursing diagnoses and client goals, the implementation of various intervention strategies, the process of evaluation, and the coordination of care with other health professionals. Process standards and criteria are used to determine if nursing services were appropriate to the needs of the family or a specified high-risk group. They also identify where nursing intervention was needed but not implemented. The ANA community health standards listed earlier are process standards. "Community health nurse documents a biopsychosocial health history on the client service record" could be one process criterion used to determine whether the ANA standard I, in relation to recording, has been achieved.

Outcome standards and criteria focus attention on the end results of care (Donabedian, 1969, p. 1833). They measure behavioral change within the client rather than the process nurses used to effect client change. They evaluate what a client has learned, for example, not what or how a nurse has taught.

There are limitations in all three approaches—structure, process, and outcome—to the evaluation of nursing care. Structural standards and criteria define essential system characteristics necessary for successful implementation of nursing care in a particular setting. They do not ensure that system resources are used effectively or efficiently in the delivery of care. Having sufficient staff, for instance, does not guarantee that quality care will be provided. Process standards and criteria appraise only how nurses carry out their functions to effect change. They do not evaluate if change has occurred as a result of nursing activities. Outcome standards and criteria are difficult to articulate because client health outcomes are influenced by multiple, interrelated factors. The biopsychosocial characteristics of a client, the environmental conditions of the client's setting, and the contributions of various disciplines all affect the health outcome status of a client. Outcome criteria do not specify which contributing factor was most relevant (Donabedian, 1966, pp. 167–169). It takes considerable skill to isolate elements which measure client outcomes that have occurred as a result of only nursing actions.

There is a trend toward emphasizing the use of outcome standards and criteria. These types of measurements can be extremely useful, but they are not perfect. They do not eliminate the need to evaluate process and structural aspects of health care delivery.

It is apparent that all three approaches to the evaluation of care are essential if quality is to be ensured. When using any of these approaches, it is important to be realistic about what one can accomplish. The realities of an agency's situation should be analyzed carefully to determine what is possible to operationalize. Standards and criteria that are all-inclusive can seldom be reached and tend to cause frustration and anxiety among staff. In the community health setting it is often stated, for instance, that comprehensive health care services will be provided to clients in the home, school, and clinic settings. Resources, however, are frequently not sufficient to achieve this goal. What happens is that services to all clients are diluted because the available work force is not adequate to meet all the health care needs in each of these settings. It would be more realistic to identify selected services, such as consultation to teachers and follow-up on children with chronic health problems, that will be provided in any one setting.

Developing standards and criteria presents special challenges to the nurse in the community health setting. A goal of community health nursing practice is to help groups (families, populations, and communities) to obtain their maximum level of functioning. Groups in all stages of the life-span are the recipients of community health nursing services. Health supervision activities vs. curative treatment is the major orientation when community health nurses are working with these groups. Measurement of health supervision activities with groups, however, is not a well-defined art. In general, most community health agencies have not focused attention on evaluating the quality of health supervision services. Morbidity care is evaluated because third-party payers mandate that it be done.

Quantitative counts such as numbers of home, school, and clinic visits, changes in mortality and morbidity statistics, and figures obtained from cost-benefit studies have traditionally been used to determine the effectiveness of nursing services in community health. *None of these measurements evaluates quality.* These measurements do not take into consideration the types of services required based on client needs, how well services are provided, and the results of nursing interventions.

Measuring health supervision activities is not an easy task because often psychosocial variables have a greater impact on health outcomes than do biological variables. There are few absolutes when it comes to defining healthy psychosocial functioning. This is becoming increasingly true as societal values change, allowing for and accepting varying life-styles. In addition, there is little research aimed at validating the effectiveness of health supervision activities carried out by nurses. Until health supervision standards are written, it is highly unlikely that these research trends and evaluation efforts will alter.

Although it is not easy to develop health supervision standards, it is not impossible. They can and are being established. The ANA community health standards are designed to evaluate *process* with all types of nursing activities, including health promotion ones. An audit tool for evaluating the third component of a quality assurance program, "Secure Measurements," will be shared below to illustrate how one agency has used process standards, based on the nursing process framework, to evaluate health supervision visits in their agency.

Outcome standards for health supervision visits are also being developed by some agencies. These have been written in a variety of ways: according to development age categories such as infant, preschool, school, adolescent, adult, and aging; according to like conditions or health-related phenomena such as pregnancy, parenthood, mental retardation, or child abuse; or according to disease categories such as cancer, arthritis, or heart problems. There is no "right" way to develop health promotion standards. Regardless of the format selected, however, a conceptual framework should be used to provide a consistent frame of reference for all. Maslow's hierarchy of needs, the developmental task approach, Roy's adaptation model, and the systems theory approach are a few examples of frames of reference that can be used. These frameworks assist the community health nurse to examine all parameters of functioning. They are especially appropriate for use in the community health setting because they have a health rather than an illness orientation. Libey and Storfjell (1978), for example, selected Maslow's hierarchy of needs as a conceptual framework and combined this with the developmental task approach when they developed the accompanying standards of care for community health nurses who are working with aging clients (Figure 21-2). These two frameworks were selected by these authors because they provide parameters for assessing current as well as potential health needs. Hence, they help health care professionals to focus on health promotion and primary preventive activities as well as on curative services.

Libey and Storfjell's Standards of Care for the Aging

STANDARD I

Maintain optimal physical and emotional *wellness*.

STANDARD II

Adjust *living standards* to retirement income, making use of remunerative activities as a supplement when necessary.

STANDARD III

Make satisfactory *living arrangements* and establish a safe, comfortable household routine to correlate with health and economic status.

STANDARD IV

Continue a supportive, close, and warm *relationship* with spouse, or significant others, including a mutually satisfying sexual relationship.

STANDARD V

Maintain *support systems* by strengthening ties with extended family and friends.

STANDARD VI

Maintain *involvement* with society through pursuit of social, civic, and political activities as well as new and former interests in order to gain status, recognition, and a feeling of being needed.

STANDARD VII

Establish a satisfactory balance between society's role *expectations* and one's own.

STANDARD VIII

Develop a meaningful *philosophy* of life and adjust to the inevitable mortality of significant others and one's own self.

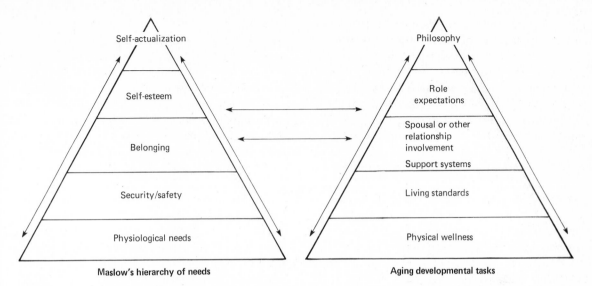

FIGURE 21-2 Standards of care for the aging, based on Maslow's hierarchy of needs and the developmental tasks of aging. Burnside (1976), Duvall (1974), and Murray and Zentner (1975) were referred to when the developmental tasks for the aging were developed. (*From Libey, Terry, & Storfjell, Judy. Standards of care for the aging, November 1978, p. 6, a course paper submitted in partial fulfillment of course requirements for N515, the Advanced Study of the Nursing Process, The University of Michigan Community Health Nursing Graduate Program, Ann Arbor, Mich.*)

Libey and Storfjell's standards for the aging are currently being used with favorable results by undergraduate baccalaureate nursing students and staff in a home care agency. Their standards help these nurses to better organize their use of the nursing process and to focus on health promotion and preventive activities, because under each standard of care, Libey and Storfjell have identified categories to assess, key considerations to note when collecting data, and optimal client-family outcomes. Under standard I, for instance, they examine family history, past health history, and general health status including hygiene, sleep, nutrition, health habits, activities of daily living, psychosocial status, and a review of functioning in relation to each body system. An example of how they have organized this material is shared in Table 21-3.

If community health nurses choose to organize standards of care according to disease categories, it is extremely important to guard against focusing attention on the disease process. How the client is *coping* with the disease

TABLE 21-3   Standard I: Maintain Optimal Physical and Emotional Wellness

Assessment	Considerations	Optimal client or family outcomes
A. Family history	A. Relatives with history of: cardiovascular or hypertensive, ocular, degenerative, lung, endocrine, or renal disease(s); cancer (breast, colorectal, prostate, lung, other); arthritis; psychosocial disorders; tuberculosis	A. Awareness of possible familial predisposition to disease and recognition of the importance of follow-up, referral, and care

condition, as well as the client's current health status, should be the major emphasis in these types of standards. The role of the community health nurse is to provide information, to help the client problem-solve, and to improve the client's self-care capabilities in a way that will facilitate adaptation to stresses being experienced. Community health nurses do not cure disease processes.

Developmental and family health supervision standards are needed in the community health setting, even when condition or disease standards are available. This is so because a major role of the community health nurse is to encourage health-promotion activities, even if disease is not present, among individuals, families, and groups across the life-span. In order to implement this role, community health nurses need a framework for assessing family structure, functions, and processes and for analyzing strengths and needs of family functioning. They also need a framework that will assist them to identify strengths and needs of individuals across the life-spectrum and that will help them to modify intervention strategies according to the individual needs of a developmental age group.

Health supervision standards must be sufficiently broad so that cultural differences are not discounted. They must be flexible enough to allow for professional judgment and client participation in the formulation of specific outcomes. They should be individualized by providers in each health care setting, based on the needs of the community and the resources of the particular organization. Use of a conceptual framework such as those previously discussed will more likely ensure that the above provisions will be included in standard formulation. Maslow's hierarchy of needs, for instance, postulates that people must meet their physical needs before they will achieve self-esteem or self-actualization. Based on this belief, a family health supervision standard which states "that the family provides for the basic needs of its members" could be developed and used with families from all cultures. Such a standard does not provide specific directives for how a family should accomplish this goal. This is important because cultures vary as to how food, shelter, and clothing are provided, as well as how health care is obtained. One criterion for evaluation of this standard could be "that family members have an adequate intake of iron, which is demonstrated by all family members having a normal hemoglobin value." This criterion does not specify that a particular type of food must be eaten and, thus, takes into consideration cultural variations in relation to eating patterns. There are several other criteria which could be used to measure whether this standard has been achieved. For any standard there will likely be many criterion measurements used to evaluate how well the standard has been met.

A strong knowledge base about specific cultural values and religious beliefs is essential in order for the community health nurse to use standards of care appropriately. Factors such as dietary patterns, traditional ways of dealing with child rearing, allocation of family roles, methods for obtaining health care and treating illness, and rituals during periods of joy or sadness must be known. Only when a community health nurse has this information can she or he make accurate professional judgments about a family's pattern of functioning. Judaism, for example, has a complex set of rituals during mourning which allows for various levels of grief and which encourages the release of emotional tension. A memorial prayer, the *Kaddish,* is recited by many Jewish families at daily services for 11 months after the death of a loved one (Kensky, 1977, p. 199). This is normal, traditional behavior. A community health nurse who is not aware of these rituals may erroneously label this behavior as "a prolonged grief reaction." The importance of an appreciation for the inherent worth of different cultural values and religious beliefs cannot be overemphasized. A community health nurse's ability to work effectively with families from different cultural groups is dependent upon the ability to understand them in terms of their background as they view it. Cultural values and religious beliefs dictate behavior and must be respected.

Secure Measurements

After standards and criteria are specified, tools and methods for evaluating and measuring quality must be selected. Nursing audits, interviews, observation of clients, peer review procedures, observation of staff performance, supervisory evaluation, and staff self-reviews are some of the most commonly used methods for evaluating the quality of nursing care. In addition, evaluative research studies are being conducted more frequently than in the past. Universities and agencies are combining their resources for the purpose of developing methodologies that assess the effectiveness and deficiencies in the delivery of nursing services.

Three evaluation tools—the Quality Patient Care Scale (Qualpacs) (Wandelt and Ager, 1974), the Slater Nursing Competencies Rating Scales (Wandelt and Stewart, 1974), and the Phaneuf Audit—are available for use by practitioners in the practice setting. The Qualpacs instrument was designed to evaluate care as it is being given. The Slater scale was developed to evaluate individual nurse performance. The Phaneuf Audit was constructed to appraise the quality of nurse care retrospectively (Phaneuf, 1976, p. 33). Of these three tools, the audit is used most often in the community health nursing setting.

Nursing Audit

Phaneuf (1976, p. 32) defines the nursing audit as "a method for evaluating quality of care through appraisal of the nursing process as it is reflected in the patient care records for dis-charged patients." How well each aspect of the nursing process was carried out is examined when a client record is audited.

The nursing audit encompasses a systematic review of a specified number of service records, in a given period of time, and the development and implementation of correction measures when deficiencies in quality are identified. It emphasizes the importance of accurately documenting nursing services because judgments about quality are made solely on the basis of what has been recorded in the client service record.

The nursing audit is a *process* evaluation method structured so that it ensures consistency of interpretation by all reviewers. This structure is obtained through the use of a nursing audit tool that has a set of care standards, criterion measurements for each care standard, and a quality rating scale. Criteria are predetermined, measurable characteristics of a variable (care standard) which are used to make judgments about the quality of care provided. One criterion used to determine how well a nurse makes assessments might read, "community health nurse collects and records data in relation to a client's family history."

The categories of care standards on a nursing audit tool should be selected so that they reflect the essential functions of nursing, not the functions of other disciplines. Phaneuf (1976, pp. 2–3) devised seven care standards from the seven nursing functions described by Lesnick and Anderson (1955, pp. 259–260). As can be seen from the listing below, Phaneuf's care standards are components of the nursing process. She selected a nursing process framework because she felt that the nursing process was a constant variable in practice not likely to change over time.

Phaneuf's seven care standards

1. Application and execution of physician's legal orders

2. Observation of symptoms and reactions

3. Supervision of the patient

4. Supervision of those participating in care

5. Reporting and recording

6. Application of nursing procedures and techniques

7. Promotion of health by direction and teaching

Phaneuf's care elements have been valuable in providing a framework for the nursing audit process. Some community health agencies, however, have found that making terminology changes in Phaneuf's list has made the nursing audit tool more usable when the agency is evaluating the delivery of health supervision services. One health department, the Oakland County Health Department, Pontiac, Michigan, redefined their categories of care standards as follows:

The Oakland County Health Department's care standards

1. Observation of situation

2. Evaluate total situation and draw up plans for nursing action

3. Implementation of nursing plans

4. Coordination of other services—intra- and inter-agency

5. Recording format

Upon examining Phaneuf's categories of care standards and the Oakland County categories of care standards, it is apparent that both use the nursing process as a framework for identifying nursing functions. The changes in terminology are due to variations in nursing approaches, roles, and responsibilities in the community setting as opposed to those in the hospital setting. A major role of the nurse in the community health setting, for instance, is to coordinate services with other community agencies. Thus, the Oakland County Health

Department believed that this responsibility should be identified as a major care standard.

The complete audit tool, including care standards, criterion measurements, and a quality rating scale, developed by the Oakland County Health Department is presented in Table 21-4. Definitions that assist their nurses in applying the criterion measurements and in using their rating scale are included in Appendix 21-1. This material is included so that the reader can gain an understanding of how one agency has chosen to look at the care delivered by community health nurses in their setting. Using these tools for several years has demonstrated to the Oakland County nursing staff that they do have consistency between reviewers.

A nursing audit tool does not eliminate the need for professional judgment. Members of the audit committee at Oakland County Health Department, for example, must use their nursing knowledge to determine if public health nurses collect sufficient data to evaluate the needs of all family members. No audit tool can list all the information needed in every family situation because needs of families vary depending on their circumstances and resources.

Donabedian (1969, p. 1835) has found that "the validity of assessments of care rests largely on agreed-upon professional judgment." He believes that "reliable judgments can be obtained through the audit of medical records." However, in order to achieve valid, reliable reviews of quality, orientation of new audit committee members is essential. They must learn how the criterion measurements are interpreted, as well as how to analyze the results of a nursing audit.

Many community health agencies find that it is necessary to change their recording format in order to achieve valid, reliable audit reviews. Traditionally, a narrative style of recording has been used in the community health setting. This type of recording is difficult to audit, especially if a nursing process framework has not been used to organize the narrative notes. Currently, use of the problem-oriented medical record (POMR) developed by Weed (1970) is increasingly popular. No one particular recording format, however, can ensure quality. Nurses must understand how to *apply the nursing process* before they can implement high-quality nursing care or before they can effectively use any recording style.

The nursing audit should not be used to evaluate individual staff performance. An agency is more likely to obtain an accurate assessment of the care provided by nurses in that agency if the audit tool is not used to identify weaknesses of individual staff. Rather, peer and supervisory conferences, observation of nursing care, staff self-evaluations, and supervisory evaluations should be used to determine the strengths and needs of individual community health nurses.

Individual Staff Evaluation

All nurses have the professional responsibility to evaluate the quality of care they are providing. Indirectly, the audit approach aids the individual nurse in examining her or his practice in relation to standards established for care. Direct mechanisms must also be used to ensure that each client serviced by the agency receives care equal to or better than established standards. Ongoing evaluation of a nurse's performance is important if the quality of care is to be safeguarded for all clients.

All nursing personnel must be evaluated on the basis of specified criteria; these criteria should reflect all aspects of nursing performance expected in a given setting. Careful attention must be given to the development of criteria that identify how well a nurse utilizes the nursing process. Often there is a greater emphasis on personal appearance, quantitative counts of visits, and adherence to time policies than to nursing care given. These factors should not be ignored when reviewing staff performance, but they should not be the only focus of the staff evaluation process.

Community health nurses at all levels, from administrators to staff, have a responsibility to become involved in the evaluation process. Nurses who actively participate in the development of tools for measurement of care and the evaluation process will be more satisfied with the results. Take the initiative to become involved. It will be a learning experience which will have long-lasting effects on the delivery of your nursing care.

Implementation of Evaluation Measurements

Developing measurement tools and procedures to facilitate use of these tools takes time and a commitment to the value of professional accountability. It took the nursing staff at the Oakland County Health Department, for example, approximately a year and a half to develop an acceptable audit tool, and then several more years to refine the audit procedures. This agency was successful in achieving its goal because adequate time was allocated for the development of a quality assurance program. Responsibilities were adjusted so that nurses could focus attention on quality assurance without feeling the pressures of caseload demands.

Administrative support during the development and implementation phases of a quality assurance program is essential. Without administrative support, it is highly unlikely that staff will be allowed sufficient time to prepare adequate measurement tools and evaluation procedures. Administrators can also help to reduce the resistance to change and to obtain funds for staff development activities. Many agencies have found that nurses feel threatened when new evaluation measurements are instituted; staff development programs can reduce this threat.

When implementing a quality assurance program, nurses should be oriented to the use of the tools as well as the *process* procedures. They should be allowed to verbalize their anxieties and lack of understanding in a suppor-

**TABLE 21-4 Oakland County Health Department:
Public Health Nurse Family Record Audit**

	Yes (8)	No (0)	Partial (4)
I. Observation of situation			
1. Physical environment			
2. Social environment			
3. Economic environment			
4. Educational environment			
5. Emotional environment			
6. Problems and needs as seen by family			
7. Problems and needs as seen by PHN			
8. Resources			
	Yes (8)	**No (0)**	**Partial (4)**
II. Evaluate total situation and draw up plans for nursing action			
1. Available information is reviewed			
2. Assessment of needs			
3. Family and patient coping abilities			
4. Acceptability of nursing service			
5. Barriers to action			
6. Nursing diagnosis			
7. Written nursing goals			
8. Written nursing plans			
	Yes (6)	**No (0)**	**Partial (3)**
III. Implementation of nursing plans			
1. Evidence of planning with family			

tive atmosphere. At times, committee members who have had the major responsibility for developing the measurement tools become frustrated when all staff members do not seem to accept the tools as readily as they have. These committee members forget how long it took them to accomplish their task and to understand the process involved. Members of evaluation committees must recognize that all personnel need time to air their concerns, just as they had time during the development phase. It should not be expected that staff will grasp the concepts of quality assurance without thought, debate, and resistance.

Make Interpretations

Data from all evaluation procedures should be examined to make interpretations about the quality of nursing care being provided in a

**TABLE 21-4   Oakland County Health Department:
Public Health Nurse Family Record Audit (*Continued*)**

2. Evidence of PHN action			
3. Evidence of follow-up			
4. Evidence of flexibility			
5. Assessment of goals			
6. Legal practice			
IV. Coordination of other services—intra- and interagency	*Yes (4)*	*No (0)*	*Partial (2)*
1. Referral to other services			
2. Follow-up of referrals made by PHN			
3. Feedback to source of referral			
4. Clarification of agency roles			
5. Conferences on behalf of the family			
V. Recording format	*Yes (2)*	*No (0)*	*Partial (1)*
1. Referral source			
2. Family record forms complete			
3. Agency dictation guide used			
4. Summaries—periodic, transfer, closing			
5. Family record in sequential order			
6. Evidence of supervisor review			
7. Evidence of PHN review			

COMMENTS: Please complete on back of this page

SOURCE: Reproduced per permission of the Nursing Division, Oakland County Health Department, Pontiac, Michigan.

particular setting. One tool alone, such as the nursing audit, cannot provide a sufficient data base to determine if quality is present or lacking. In addition, data from multiple sources are often needed to identify the real cause for inadequate care.

The purpose of evaluation is to identify discrepancies between established standards and criteria and actual nursing practice. Evaluation assessments should be specific enough to iden-

tify both strengths and needs in the current level of nursing care. In general, most agencies have found that both strengths and needs do exist. If either is found lacking when analyzing evaluation data, the measurement tools and the process for using these tools should be reevaluated. The tools may be too general and broad to discriminate between safe and unsafe care. On the other hand, the tools may be appropriate, but staff may need additional orientation to use them effectively. When they are using the nursing audit for the first time, it is not uncommon to find nurses assuming that certain care was done, even if it was not documented in the family service record. This may be an inappropriate assumption that covers up deficiencies in nursing care.

In order to make interpretations about discrepancies between standards and actual practice, measurement data must be organized and grouped so that a composite picture is clearly visualized. Summary reports should be developed so that the combined results of multiple efforts can be examined and patterns of care identified. Interpretations about overall agency quality must be based on *patterns* occurring over time, rather than on selected record reviews at a given time. Individual staff performance should be evaluated on the basis of *patterns* as well, rather than on one or two select incidents.

After individual audit committee members at the Oakland County Health Department finish their audit reviews, they complete a summary report, like the one presented in Figure 21-3. It is then shared with administration and staff. This summary report helps agency personnel to quickly identify strengths and deficiencies in nursing care. It also allows for comparisons from one audit review to another, because change is depicted numerically.

Identify Course of Action

Once strengths and weaknesses in the delivery of nursing practice have been delineated, alternative interventions should be identified to correct deficiencies in care. In addition, nurses should receive positive feedback about their strengths. Staff members who receive only negative feedback can become discouraged with nursing and may be less motivated to make necessary changes.

To identify alternative courses of action for correcting deficiencies, nurses must first ana-

lyze why certain problems are occurring. For example, perhaps the recording of the nursing staff demonstrates very little follow-up and evaluation of nursing interventions. There are several reasons why this may be happening, including lack of knowledge, insufficient time allocated for recording, inadequate caseload management skills, unshared values, limited resources, and poor staff morale. Discourse among nurses to find the reasons for the problems should occur before change actions are identified. If the problem is due to inadequate resources to meet client needs rather than to lack of knowledge, planning for continuing education programs would be inappropriate. Time allocated for continuing education in this situation would probably only increase the probability that all client needs were not being met. Administrative action to secure further resources or to reevaluate job expectations would be more appropriate.

Input from the nursing staff is essential for determining the best course of action to correct deficiencies in the delivery of nursing care. An administrative mandate which specifies that changes must occur immediately will frustrate staff members if they have not been allowed to voice their opinions about the help they need to alter their actions. Most nurses are interested in providing quality care. They will resist change, however, if they are not actively involved in selecting the appropriate course for change.

Choose Action

Two major activities should occur when choosing change actions: (1) discussion about the advantages and disadvantages of suggested remedial actions and (2) development of a plan for implementing the selected change strategy. Refer again to the situation where record audits reflect inadequate follow-up and evaluation of nursing interventions. If the major problem identified in this situation is poor doc-

Monthly summary report

Nursing audit report _____

(Month)   (Day)   (Year)

_____

/s/ Chairman, Nursing Audit Committee

Number of family folders reviewed

	Outstanding	Satisfactory	Incomplete	Unsatisfactory
Overall evaluation by number of family folders				

Category name	Outstanding	Satisfactory	Incomplete	Unsatisfactory	Total
I. Observation of situation					
II. Evaluate total situation and draw up plans for nursing plans					
III. Implementation of nursing plans					
IV. Coordination of other services—intra- and interagency					
V. Recording format					

Function	Outstanding	Satisfactory	Incomplete	Unsatisfactory
I	49–64	33–48	17–32	0–16
II	49–64	33–48	17–32	0–16
III	28–36	19–27	10–18	0–9
IV	15–20	10–14	5–9	0–4
V	12–14	8–11	4–7	0–3

Record score range

149–198 = Outstanding
100–148 = Satisfactory
51– 99 = Incomplete
0– 50 = Unsatisfactory

Summary of comments:

FIGURE 21-3 Oakland County Health Department, public health nurse family record audit: monthy summary report. (*Reproduced by permission of the Nursing Division, Oakland County Health Department, Pontiac, Mich.*)

umentation due to lack of skill, remedial actions might include conducting a continuing education program focusing on recording skills for all staff, weekly individual supervisory and staff conferences to discuss strengths and needs about recording, or self-study by individual staff members. If the majority of the nurses are having difficulty with recording, it probably would be most advantageous to ini-

tiate a staff development program. If, on the other hand, only a few nurses are having problems, a staff development program might be very costly to the agency in time and money. If it is determined that a staff continuing education activity is needed, a plan should be developed to ensure that this selected action is implemented.

When discussing the pros and cons of alternate change strategies, agency and community resources should be examined. Often, existing resources are not utilized because it is felt that an "outside expert" or a consultant can do a better job. Frequently this is not the case. Nurses are more motivated to make necessary changes when their talents and skills are recognized and supported. They also become committed to helping others during the change process when they are actively involved, because they believe they have something to contribute. The outside expert frequently does not become actively involved in the change process. This person often shares knowledge and then agency personnel are left to decide how to make changes based on newly gained information. There are times when outside resources should be used; however, such help should be used with discretion because it can be costly and may not help an agency to accomplish what it hopes to achieve.

Planning for change increases the probability that change will occur. It also increases the likelihood that activities will be orderly and predictable and less stressful to staff. Although the entire staff should be involved in developing action plans, one person must be delegated the responsibility and authority to see that changes are implemented. Group decision making spreads responsibility and often results in no one coordinating and taking responsibility for implementing alternatives.

Take Action

Improvement of nursing care is the primary objective of any quality assurance program. Action must be taken if this is to occur; merely defining problems is not enough. Decisions about various alternative approaches must be made and correction measures implemented, because merely having a discussion about change produces no results.

Taking action to alter practice is one of the most significant components of a quality assurance program. It demonstrates that nurses really do assume accountability for the care provided by members of their profession. It supports the belief that quality assurance should be the responsibility of a profession rather than the responsibility of legal authorities.

Corrective action must be carefully documented and evaluated to determine whether or not it has altered practice. Other actions may be needed if the selected one does not result in desired change. If, for instance, a staff development program does not improve the documentation on client service records, supervisors may have to increase their conference time with individual staff members to help them with their recording skills. The quality assurance cycle should continue even if change does occur. Ongoing monitoring is essential in order to maintain quality standards for practice over time.

PARTNERS IN QUALITY ASSURANCE

The quality assurance model (Figure 21-1) presented at the beginning of this chapter illustrates that individual nurses, the nursing profession, and clients all share equal responsibility for maintaining high professional standards of nursing practice (*American Nurse,* 1976, p. 23). Input from the client is essential for determining values important to recipients of care. Client feedback is also crucial for the

identification of deficiencies in practice on an ongoing basis. It is important that clients have an effect on all components of a quality assurance program because nursing is responsible for ensuring quality of care with clients.

Nursing practice, education, and research (Figure 21-1) provide knowledge and experience which aid in the development of a sound quality assurance program. Nurses involved in any of these activities must be willing to share their findings so that others can benefit from their experiences. Practitioners, educators, and researchers must be committed to quality assurance and must work toward refining tools and processes which will facilitate nurses' quality assurance efforts.

In the community health setting, research is needed to validate the effectiveness of the preventive health approach to nursing practice. Further data are also needed to determine if community health nurses are actually meeting the needs of the population as a whole. The tools discussed previously in this chapter were designed to evaluate nursing care with individual clients. Structure, process, and outcome criteria must be developed to identify discrepancies in care to the community. This is crucial if community health nurses are going to continue to subscribe to the belief that their client is the community.

SUMMARY

Members of a profession are responsible for developing and upholding standards for professional practice. They must ensure that care provided by all members is equal to or better than the standards established for quality. Monitoring of practice on an ongoing basis is essential in order to protect society from incompetent and unqualified practitioners. Changing societal demands make it even more critical that nurses evaluate the delivery of nursing care because there is a trend toward emphasizing control of professional practice. There is no question that if nursing does not assume accountability for its actions, others will govern nurses' actions for them. Professionals are in an era of quality assurance.

Quality assurance is a dynamic process involving a series of actions designed to evaluate nursing care. It also includes the implementation of measures designed to improve deficiencies found during evaluation efforts. It is a systematic, ongoing evaluation for the purpose of determining what type of nursing care is being provided, how this care is provided, and the outcome of nursing services to the client. Three partners—individual nurses, the nursing profession, and clients—all share equal responsibility for maintaining high-quality standards of professional practice. Nurses in service, education, and research must work together to refine evaluation measurements and processes that can facilitate quality assurance efforts.

APPENDIX 21-1
Oakland County Health Department Public Health Nurse Family Record Audit

Definitions

Definitions of scoring terms are as follows (except as noted in definitions):
"Yes"—clearly stated in the record.
"No"—not stated in the record.
"Partial"—stated some of the time.

   I. Observation of situation
      1. *Physical environment:* description and location of where visit occurs, and noted changes.

     2. *Social environment:* description of family constellation and living pattern, which may include religious and ethnic influences.

     3. *Economic environment:* identified source of income, which may include how it is used.

     4. *Educational environment:* description of formally and informally acquired knowledge.

     5. *Emotional environment:* description of

demonstrated feelings, verbal and/or nonverbal, such as hostility, joy, sorrow, apathy, hate, love and reverence.

6. *Problems and needs as seen by the family:* family members will have different viewpoints; therefore, we should be specific about informant.

7. *Problems and needs as seen by the PHN:* PHN evaluate need of entire family.

8. *Resources:* existing or previous individual, family or community sources of support, supply and assistance. Examples of such sources of support are occupation, and/or source of income, agency, medical or other resources such as friends, relatives, neighbors.

II. *Evaluate total situation and draw up plans for nursing action*

1. *Available information is reviewed:* information gathered from such sources as referral source, other family records, other PHN's, physicians, school records, dentists and other agencies servicing the family. The key word in definition is available.

2. *Assessment of needs:* PHN evaluates needs and assigns priorities to problems.

3. *Family and patient coping abilities:* statement of how family deals with situations or meets difficulties.

4. *Acceptability of nursing service:* statement of family response to PHN service.

5. *Barriers to action:* restraints or obstructions restricting PHN intervention or family movement. These may be as diverse as mental or physical handicaps, individual PHN limitations, social and economic factors, language barriers, or improper timing of PHN action. Absence of barriers to action is implied unless barriers are specified in dictation.

6. *Nursing diagnosis:* a labelled, concise conclusion derived from observation and evaluation and upon which nursing action is based.

7. *Written nursing goals:* goals are the desired end result. Goals must be written; i.e., appear as heading in dictation. (*See:* Guide for Recording Public Health Nursing Visits.)

8. *Written nursing plans:* written activities, designed to reach a stated nursing goal.

III. *Implementation of nursing plans*

1. *Evidence of planning with family:* PHN and family establish tasks or activities to achieve a written goal. "Evidence" is obvious data, not implied data.

2. *Evidence of PHN action:* written evidence of direct care, demonstrations, instruction, counseling, listening, supportive action, planning with family.

3. *Evidence of follow-up:* "Follow-up" is an act to carry out plans. (Example: Family might make appointment and PHN would follow-up.) Intent of follow-up can be implied, e.g., NAHFS—*moved.*

4. *Evidence of flexibility:* nursing action changes to respond to family's situation and needs. Flexibility is present unless nursing action obviously not responsive to changing family needs.

5. *Assessment of goals:* re-evaluation of written goals during service.

6. *Legal practice:* use of agency policy as mandated by law and current administrative directives.

IV. *Coordination of other services—intra- and inter-agency*

1. *Referral to other services:* family is directed toward specific services, if need indicated. May include communication with services before family is seen. If no need indicated, score as *yes.*

2. *Follow-up of referrals made by PHN:* PHN obtained information from family or services that family acted on referrals. When no referral made, score as *yes.*

3. *Feedback to source of referral:* feedback is verbal or written communication to source of referral. Verbal or written communication is necessary on all professional referrals, except birth certificates. PHN's judgement is accepted regarding feedback to non-professionals; e.g., indiscreet neighbor or hostile relative. If referral not received as written form, then feedback information should appear in dictation. Score a self-referral as *yes.*

4. *Clarification of agency roles:* PHN explained Health Department services and/or other agencies' services to family.

5. *Conferences on behalf of family:* a communication to facilitate provision of health services to individual and family as need indicated. This includes PHN's supervisor, other professionals, or non-professionals. If no need indicated, score as *yes.*

V. *Recording format*

1. *Referral source:* statement of origin and nature of referral.

2. *Family record forms complete:* admission, family data sheet, (front and back of sheet), medical data, T.B. and C.D. forms and referral forms.

3. *Agency dictation guide used:* definition: implies only that guide format, individual items (i.e., "Diagnosis," "Goals," "Plans," etc.) are audited.

4. *Summaries—periodic, transfer, closing:*

Periodic summaries are to be done every 12 direct service visits or 18 months, whichever comes first. Summaries may be done more often if evaluation of services are needed.

Transfer and closing—summary or summary statement is to be written when record is transferred or closed. Anytime service is re-initiated there must be an update of summary at the time of closure.

5. *Order of family record:* family data sheet, continuation sheets and summaries in chronological order. Reports should be grouped by department and person in reverse chronological order (current date on top). All reports, letters or miscellaneous should be taped, stapled or otherwise secured to the record.

6. *Evidence of supervisor review:* initial of supervisor at the farthest point she has reviewed and signature at the closing or transfer.

7. *Evidence of PHN review:* dictation corrected and signed in ink by PHN.

Comments
To apply only to the mechanics of the audit.

SOURCE: Reproduced per permission of the Nursing Division, Oakland County Health Department, Pontiac, Michigan.

REFERENCES

American Nurses' Association. *A conceptual model of community health nursing.* ANA Publication No. CH-10 2M, 5/80. Kansas City, Mo.: American Nurses' Association, 1980.

American Nurses' Association. *A plan for implementation of the standards of nursing practice.* Kansas City, Mo.: American Nurses' Association, 1975.

American Nurses' Association. *Standards: Community health nursing practice.* Kansas City, Mo.: American Nurses' Association, 1973, unnumbered pages.

Burnside, I. M. *Nursing and the aged.* New York: McGraw-Hill, 1976.

Division on Community Health Nursing Practice. *Conceptual model: Draft III.* Kansas City, MO.: American Nurses' Association, March 16, 1979.

Donabedian, A. Evaluating the quality of medical care. *Milbank Memorial Fund Quarterly,* July 1966, *44,* 166–206.

———. Some issues in evaluating the quality of nursing care. *American Journal of Public Health,* October 1969, *59,* 1833–1836.

Duvall, E. M. *Marriage and family development.* Philadelphia: Lippincott, 1974.

Keller, B. S. The continuing education needs of community health nurses in Michigan and factors influencing these needs as perceived by these nurses and their supervisors. Ann Arbor, Mich.: University of Michigan, 1978 (unpublished doctoral dissertation).

Kensky, Rabbi A. D. Cultural influences on the Jewish patient. In S. Clemen & M. Will, *Family and community health nursing: A workbook.* Ann Arbor, Mich.: University of Michigan, 1977.

Lesnik, M. J., & Anderson, B. E. *Nursing practice and the law.* (2d ed.). Philadelphia: Lippincott, 1955.

Libey, T., & Storfjell, J. *Standards of care for the aging.* November 1978. (A course paper submitted in partial fulfillment of course requirements for N515, the Advanced Study of the Nursing Process, the University of Michigan Community Health Nursing Graduate Program, Ann Arbor, Mich.)

Lysaught, J. P. *An abstract for action.* New York: McGraw-Hill, 1970.

——— (Ed.). Model shows dynamic concept of quality assurance. *American Nurse,* Feb. 28, 1976, p. 23.

Murray, R., & Zentner, J. *Nursing assessment and health promotion through the life span*. Englewood Cliffs, N.J.: Prentice-Hall, 1975.

Papers on the national health guidelines: Baselines for setting health goals and standards. DHEW Publication No. HRA 77-640. Washington, D.C.: Health Resource Administration, January 1977.

Phaneuf, M. C. *The nursing audit: Self-regulation in nursing practice*. New York: Appleton-Century-Crofts, 1976.

Public Law 92-603: Section 246E, Title XI, General Provisions and (B) Professional Standards Review, Social Security Amendments of 1972, Ninety-Second Congress HR1, Oct. 30, 1972.

Ramey, J. G. Setting nursing standards and evaluating care. *Journal of Nursing Administration*, May–June 1973, *3*, 17–25.

Schmadl, J. C. Quality assurance: Examination of the concept. *Nursing Outlook*, July 1979, *27*, 462–465.

Wandelt, M. A., & Ager, J. W. *Quality patient care scale*. New York: Appleton-Century-Crofts, 1974.

Wandelt, M. A., & Stewart, D. S. *Slater nursing competencies rating scale*. New York: Appleton-Century-Crofts, 1974.

Weed, L. L. *Medical records, medical education and patient care*. Chicago: Yearbook Medical Publishers, 1970.

SELECTED BIBLIOGRAPHY

American Nurses' Association. *Guidelines for peer review*. Kansas City, Mo.: American Nurses' Association, 1973.

Anderson, M. I. Development of outcome criteria for the patient with congestive heart failure. *Nursing Clinics of North America*, June 1974, *9*, 349–358.

Bailit, H., Lewis, J., Hochheiser, L., & Bush, N. Assessing the quality of care. *Nursing Outlook*, March 1975, *23*, 153–159.

Berg, H. Nursing audit and outcome criteria. *Nursing Clinics of North America*, June 1974, *9*, 331–335.

Bernal, H. Levels of practice in a community health agency. *Nursing Outlook*, June 1978, *23*, 364–369.

Bloch, D. Criteria, standards, norms: Crucial terms in quality assurance. *Journal of Nursing Administration*, September 1977, *7*, 20–30.

Burgess, A. W. *Nursing: Levels of health intervention*. Englewood Cliffs, N.J.: Prentice-Hall, 1978.

Davidson, G. Collaborating with the medical staff in developing standards of care. *Nursing Clinics of North America*, June 1973, *8*, 219–225.

Davidson, S. V. Community nursing care evaluation. *Family and Community Health*, April 1978, *1*, 37–55.

——— (Ed.). *PSRO: Utilization and audit in patient care*. St. Louis: Mosby, 1976.

De Geyndt, W. Five approaches for assessing the quality of care. *Hospital Administration*, Winter 1970, pp. 21–42.

Deuschle, J. M., Logsdon, D. N., Sollecito, W., Stahl, W., Smith, H., Sonnenshein, M., & Kreitzer, M. Implementation of a peer review system for ambulatory care. *Public Health Reports*, May–June 1978, *93*, 258–267.

Eddy, L., & Westbrook, L. Multidisciplinary retrospective patient care audit. *American Journal of Nursing*, June 1975, *75*, 961–963.

Feinstein, A. The problems of the problem-oriented medical record. *Annals of Internal Medicine*, May 1973, *78*, 751–762.

Flynn, B. C. Research framework for evaluating community health nursing practice. In M. Miller & B. Flynn (Eds.), *Current perspectives in nursing*. St. Louis: Mosby, 1977, pp. 35–45.

Froebe, D. J., & Bain, R. J. *Quality assurance programs and controls in nursing*. St. Louis: Mosby, 1976.

Gold, H., Jackson, M., Sachs, B., & Vanmeter, M. Peer review: A working experiment. *Nursing Outlook*, October 1973, *21*, 634–636.

Goldfinger, S. The problem-oriented record: A critique from a believer. *New England Journal of Medicine*, March 1973, pp. 602–608, 629–630.

Haar, L., & Hicks, J. Performance appraisal: Derivation of effective assessment tools. *Journal of Nursing Administration,* September 1976, *6,* 20–29.

Hagen, E. Appraising the quality of nursing care. *Eighth Nursing Research Conference,* March 15–17, 1972, Kansas City, Mo.: American Nurses' Association, pp. 1–8.

Hegyuary, S. T., & Dieter Haussman, R. K. Monitoring nursing care quality. *Journal of Nursing Administration,* November 1976, *6,* 3–9.

Hilger, L. Developing nursing outcome criteria. *Nursing Clinics of North America,* June 1974, *9,* 323–330.

Horn, B. J., & Swain, M. A. An approach to development of criterion measures for quality patient care. In *Issues in Evaluation Research.* Kansas City, Mo.: American Nurses' Association, 1976, pp. 74–82.

Hudak, C., Redstone, P., Hokonson, N., & Suzuki, I. *Clinical protocols: A guide for nurses and physicians.* Philadelphia: Lippincott, 1978.

Lewis, W. Health behavior and quality assurance. *Nursing Clinics of North America,* June 1974, *9,* 359–365.

Mayers, M. G., Norby, R. B., & Watson, A. B. *Quality assurance for patient care: Nursing perspective.* New York: Appleton-Century-Crofts, 1977.

Parzick, J., & Nolan, Sister M. POMR at work in a home health agency. *Family and Community Health,* April 1978, *1,* 101–108.

Passos, J. Accountability: Myth or mandate? *Journal of Nursing Administration,* May–June 1973, *3,* 17–22.

Perkins, W. Quality of care and utilization assessment: The hospital response to PSRO. *West Journal of Medicine,* October 1974, *121,* 342–348.

Pridham, K. Assessing the quality of well child care. *Nursing Clinics of North America,* June 1974, *9,* 367–379.

Ramphal, M. Peer review. *American Journal of Nursing,* January 1974, *74,* 63–67.

Rubin, C. F., Rubin, L. A., & Dietz, R. R. Nursing audit: Nurses evaluating nursing. *American Journal of Nursing,* May 1972, *72,* 916–921.

Ryan, B. Nursing care plans: A systems approach to developing criteria for planning and evaluation. *Journal of Nursing Administration,* May–June 1973, *3,* 50–58.

Taylor, J. Measuring the outcomes of nursing care. *Nursing Clinics of North America,* June 1974, *9,* 337–348.

Wandelt, M. A., & Phaneuf, M. A. Three instruments for measuring the quality of nursing care. *Hospital Topics,* August 1972, pp. 20–23, 29.

Zimmer, M. J. Quality assurance for outcomes of patient care. *Nursing Clinics of North America,* June 1974, *9,* 304–315.

———— & Associates. Guidelines for development of outcome criteria. *Nursing Clinics of North America,* June 1974, *9,* 317–321.

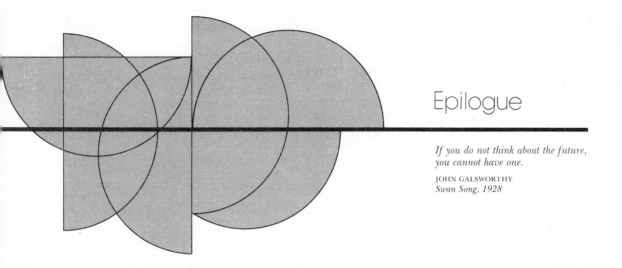

Epilogue

If you do not think about the future, you cannot have one.

JOHN GALSWORTHY
Swan Song, 1928

What is in the future for community health nursing? How can we plan for quality care and become involved in shaping tomorrow's world? As Chapter 1 demonstrated, political and social events helped to shape the development of community health nursing leaders like Nightingale and Wald, who in turn used these events to shape professional nursing. Planning for the future helps us to contribute to changes. Lack of planning forces us to be only reactive to change.

There is a certain amount of risk taking in predicting and planning the future. However, community health nursing will be viable and relevant only as we are willing to take these risks.

Leininger (1978) makes specific predictions for the year 2000 that have implications for community health nursing practice: the increased use of technology in nursing and health care services which will revolutionize nursing care services with positive and negative effects; new modes and systems of communication which will bring clients and health professionals into close and continuous contact with each other; sophistication in transcultural and nursing care practices as communication becomes more complex; and the development of aerospace and oceanic nursing as legitimate fields of practice in nursing. Leininger continues her predictions by stating that nurse leaders will be managers, economists, and political analysts. The common cold, most infectious diseases, cancer, cardiovascular diseases, and mental stress will be under control and new modes of health care delivery will be available. Health care will be conceptualized as care to the population and will be consumer based. Prevention of illness and maintenance of health will be emphasized.

What a mandate for community health nurses! We can ignore these predictions or be risk takers and build upon them! The year 2000 is 20 years away. Community health nursing by definition deals with populations and has prevention as a central focus. Let us follow Lillian Wald and lead the way.

The most powerful method that nurses can

use to shape the future is the political process. Nurses are the largest group of health care providers in the country and our number alone gives us a powerful majority. We must grow in our sophistication and use of politics.

Thelma Schorr (1976) has listed a number of political imperatives for nurses:

1. An authoritative nursing voice, at the decision-making level, in the formulation of the national health policy

2. Recognition that the umbrella service which patients need is health care, and that medical care and nursing care are two distinct, if oftentimes interdependent, entities among a number of professional services on which the nation's health depends

3. Reimbursement for nursing services as nursing services, not submerged in a bed-and-board hospital price that gets inflated by a variety of dumpings and is explained to the patients as nursing costs

4. Federal fundings for nursing research that will give us scientific underpinnings and hard data to support our legislative as well as our clinical efforts

5. Funding for nursing education that includes forgiveness mechanisms or some other kind of financial incentives to attract nurses to underserved rural and urban areas

6. Pressure for ratification of the Equal Rights Amendment to equalize opportunities and protect human rights for all people, including patients, nonpatients, families, significant others, and men and women nurses

Perhaps one of our priorities should be to get a nurse elected to Congress so that she or he can explain firsthand to fellow representatives or fellow senators what nurses could do to alleviate many of this country's serious health problems.

Let us as community health nurses think about the future so that we have the very best one possible!

REFERENCES

Leininger, M. Futurology of nursing: Goals and challenges for tomorrow. In N. L. Chaska (Ed.), *The nursing profession. Views through the mist.* New York: McGraw-Hill, 1978.

Schorr, T. Political imperatives. *American Journal of Nursing,* October 1976, *76,* 1585.